# Mineral Requirements for Military Personnel

## Levels Needed for Cognitive and Physical Performance During Garrison Training



Committee on Mineral Requirements for Cognitive and Physical Performance of Military Personnel

Committee on Military Nutrition Research

Food and Nutrition Board

INSTITUTE OF MEDICINE
*OF THE NATIONAL ACADEMIES*

THE NATIONAL ACADEMIES PRESS
Washington, D.C.
**www.nap.edu**

**THE NATIONAL ACADEMIES PRESS • 500 Fifth Street, N.W. • Washington, DC 20001**

NOTICE: The project that is the subject of this report was approved by the Governing Board of the National Research Council, whose members are drawn from the councils of the National Academy of Sciences, the National Academy of Engineering, and the Institute of Medicine. The members of the committee responsible for the report were chosen for their special competences and with regard for appropriate balance.

This study was supported by contract number DAMD17-99-1-9478 between the National Academy of Sciences and the United States Army. Any opinions, findings, conclusions, or recommendations expressed in this publication are those of the authors and do not necessarily reflect the views of the sponsoring agency that provided support for the project.

International Standard Book Number: 0-309-10126-3 (book)
International Standard Book Number: 0-309-65790-3 (PDF)

Additional copies of this report are available from the National Academies Press, 500 Fifth Street, N.W., Lockbox 285, Washington, DC 20055; (800) 624-6242 or (202) 334-3313 (in the Washington metropolitan area); Internet, http://www.nap.edu.

For more information about the Institute of Medicine, visit the IOM home page at: **www.iom.edu**.



Printed in the United States of America.

The serpent has been a symbol of long life, healing, and knowledge among almost all cultures and religions since the beginning of recorded history. The serpent adopted as a logotype by the Institute of Medicine is a relief carving from ancient Greece, now held by the Staatliche Museen in Berlin.

*"Knowing is not enough; we must apply.*
*Willing is not enough; we must do."*
—Goethe

INSTITUTE OF MEDICINE
*OF THE NATIONAL ACADEMIES*

**Advising the Nation. Improving Health.**

# THE NATIONAL ACADEMIES

***Advisers to the Nation on Science, Engineering, and Medicine***

The **National Academy of Sciences** is a private, nonprofit, self-perpetuating society of distinguished scholars engaged in scientific and engineering research, dedicated to the furtherance of science and technology and to their use for the general welfare. Upon the authority of the charter granted to it by the Congress in 1863, the Academy has a mandate that requires it to advise the federal government on scientific and technical matters. Dr. Ralph J. Cicerone is president of the National Academy of Sciences.

The **National Academy of Engineering** was established in 1964, under the charter of the National Academy of Sciences, as a parallel organization of outstanding engineers. It is autonomous in its administration and in the selection of its members, sharing with the National Academy of Sciences the responsibility for advising the federal government. The National Academy of Engineering also sponsors engineering programs aimed at meeting national needs, encourages education and research, and recognizes the superior achievements of engineers. Dr. Wm. A. Wulf is president of the National Academy of Engineering.

The **Institute of Medicine** was established in 1970 by the National Academy of Sciences to secure the services of eminent members of appropriate professions in the examination of policy matters pertaining to the health of the public. The Institute acts under the responsibility given to the National Academy of Sciences by its congressional charter to be an adviser to the federal government and, upon its own initiative, to identify issues of medical care, research, and education. Dr. Harvey V. Fineberg is president of the Institute of Medicine.

The **National Research Council** was organized by the National Academy of Sciences in 1916 to associate the broad community of science and technology with the Academy's purposes of furthering knowledge and advising the federal government. Functioning in accordance with general policies determined by the Academy, the Council has become the principal operating agency of both the National Academy of Sciences and the National Academy of Engineering in providing services to the government, the public, and the scientific and engineering communities. The Council is administered jointly by both Academies and the Institute of Medicine. Dr. Ralph J. Cicerone and Dr. Wm. A. Wulf are chair and vice chair, respectively, of the National Research Council.

**www.national-academies.org**

## COMMITTEE ON MINERAL REQUIREMENTS FOR COGNITIVE AND PHYSICAL PERFORMANCE OF MILITARY PERSONNEL

**ROBERT M. RUSSELL**, (*Chair*) Human Nutrition Research Center on Aging, Tufts University, Boston, MA
**JOHN L. BEARD**, Department of Nutrition, Pennsylvania State University, University Park
**MELINDA BECK**, School of Public Health and Medicine, University of North Carolina, Chapel Hill
**BRUCE R. BISTRIAN**, Beth Israel Deaconess Medical Center, Harvard Medical School, Boston, MA
**JOSEPH G. CANNON**, Medical College of Georgia, Augusta
**GERALD F. COMBS, JR.**, Grand Forks Human Nutrition Research Center, Grand Forks, ND
**JOHANNA T. DWYER**, Office of Dietary Supplements, National Institutes of Health, Baltimore, MD
**JOHN W. ERDMAN**, Department of Food Science and Human Nutrition, University of Illinois, Urbana-Champaign
**EMILY M. HAYMES**, Department of Nutrition, Food and Exercise Sciences, Florida State University, Tallahassee
**JANET R. HUNT**, Grand Forks Human Nutrition Research Center, Grand Forks, ND
**HELEN W. LANE**, Johnson Space Center, National Aeronautics and Space Administration, Houston, TX
**JAMES G. PENLAND**, Grand Forks Human Nutrition Research Center, Grand Forks, ND
**SUSAN S. PERCIVAL**, Department of Food Science and Human Nutrition, University of Florida, Gainesville
**CONNIE M. WEAVER**, Department of Food Science and Nutrition, Purdue University, West Lafayette, IN

*Staff*

**MARIA P. ORIA**, Study Director
**LESLIE J. SIM**, Research Associate
**JON Q. SANDERS**, Senior Program Assistant

## FOOD AND NUTRITION BOARD*



*IOM boards do not review or approve individual reports and are not asked to endorse conclusions and recommendations. The responsibility for the content of the reports rests with the authoring committee and the institution.

# Reviewers

This report has been reviewed in draft form by individuals chosen for their diverse perspectives and technical expertise, in accordance with procedures approved by the National Research Council's Report Review Committee. The purpose of this independent review is to provide candid and critical comments that will assist the institution in making its published report as sound as possible and to ensure that the report meets institutional standards for objectivity, evidence, and responsiveness to the study charge. The review comments and draft manuscript remain confidential to protect the integrity of the deliberative process. We wish to thank the following individuals for their review of this report:

**Mary R. L'Abbé**, Bureau of Nutritional Sciences Food Directorate, Health Canada, Ottawa
**Ronni Chernoff**, University of Arkansas Medical School, Little Rock
**Felicia Cosman**, Columbia-Presbyterian Medical Center, New York
**Susanna Cunningham-Rundles**, Cornell University Weill Medical College, Ithaca, NY
**Marc K. Hellerstein**, University of California, Berkeley
**Orville Levander**, USDA Human Nutrition Research Center, Beltsville, MD
**Joan Lyon**, USDA Center for Nutritional Policy and Promotion, Alexandria, VA
**Stacey L. Mobley**, Purdue University, Lafayette, IN
**Harold H. Sandstead**, The University of Texas Medical Branch, Galveston
**Richard J. Wood**, Jean Mayer USDA Human Nutrition Research Center on Aging at Tufts University, Boston, MA

Although the reviewers listed above have provided many constructive comments and suggestions, they were not asked to endorse the conclusions or recommendations nor did they see the final draft of the report before its release. The review of this report was overseen by **Michael P. Doyle**, University of Georgia. Appointed by the Institute of Medicine, he was responsible for making certain that an independent examination of this report was carried out in accordance with institutional procedures and that all review comments were carefully considered. Responsibility for the final content of this report rests entirely with the authoring committee and the institution.

# Preface

The Committee on Military Nutrition Research (CMNR) was established in October 1982 following a request by the Assistant Surgeon General of the Army that the Board on Military Supplies of the National Academy of Sciences (NAS) set up a special committee to advise the U.S. Department of Defense (DoD) on the need for and conduct of nutrition research and related issues. The CMNR, a standing committee, was eventually transferred to the Food and Nutrition Board of the Institute of Medicine, National Academies. The standing committee's primary tasks are to identify factors that may critically influence the physical and mental performance of combat military personnel under all environmental extremes, to identify knowledge gaps, to recommend research that would remedy these deficiencies, to identify approaches for studying the relationship of diet to physical and mental performance, and to review and advise on military feeding standards. It is customary that for each specific task, an ad hoc committee composed with the appropriate expertise is formed. For example, under the oversight of the CMNR, an ad hoc committee of experts provided recommendations for nutrient composition of assault rations for short-term, high intensity sustained operations in a recent report.

This report entitled, *Mineral Requirements for Military Personnel* results from the work of an ad hoc Committee on Mineral Requirements for Cognitive and Physical Performance of Military Personnel under the auspices of the CMNR. This report was produced in response to the request by the Commander, U.S. Army Medical Research and Materiel Command (USAMRMC) to the Institute of Medicine (IOM) to convene a committee to review and recommend the mineral requirements for military personnel on military garrison training, not only by considering excess losses due to physical and environmental stress, but also by considering potential enhancements of performance (e.g., mental, physical, immune). These are the personnel that, while living at military bases, engage in military training or in daily operations that entail high physical and mental demands. The specific questions posed to the committee evolved from discussions between the standing CMNR, and the Military Nutrition Division of the U.S. Army Research Institute of Environmental Medicine (USARIEM) in Natick, Massachusetts. The CMNR also provided input during the initial stages of expert selection for potential ad hoc committee members and workshop speakers.

A 14-member committee was formed with expertise on calcium, copper, iron, magnesium, selenium, and zinc, and with specific attention to areas of nutrient absorption, metabolism and functions particularly important to the military, such as immune function, physical and cognitive performance. Experts on food technology, clinical nutrition, dietetics, and psychology were also included in the committee. The committee's task was to assess the current Military Reference Dietary Intakes (MDRIs) and if needed, recommend, new mineral intakes for soldiers in garrison training. The committee was also asked to review the mineral levels of the current operational rations i.e., Meals, Ready to-Eat and First Strike Rations and determine if they are adequate. Because the committee's expertise was strong in the area of essential minerals, it was also requested that they comment on the recommendations for mineral levels in assault rations.

The committee discussed the limitations of the data, regarding minerals. First, even though there is a reasonable amount of data on mineral levels of rations, data on mineral intake by military personnel is scanty. In order to assess the adequacy of mineral levels in rations, the committee had to assume that the complete rations were consumed, which might not be the case. It is therefore a challenge to assess whether or not the intakes of military personnel are adequate. Second, there is a lack of information regarding changes in metabolism or requirements due to the unique demands arising from physical or mental stressors during military operations. The committee based its recommendations on the best available data from studies done on civilians under circumstances that paralleled the military situation as closely as possible. For example, higher mineral requirements due to sweat losses in soldiers were based on studies in exercising civilians. The committee also reviewed studies which suggested that a higher intake of minerals might improve immune function, the ability to perform physical or mental tasks, or mood states. In this case, the data were suggestive only, and no definitive conclusions were reached. Although the committee was able to recommend intakes for certain selected minerals of importance, additional data from studies performed under the circumstances encountered by soldiers in garrison training are needed, so that requirements are updated with new, more appropriate data, including data on potential improvements of functions of military importance. Undoubtedly, the committee's important recommendations relate to specific research need priorities.

The committee carried out its work over 12 months and met twice. The first meeting of the committee was held in conjunction with a two-day workshop. This workshop, designed to address this task, was hosted by The National Academies in Washington DC, June 13–15, 2004. Speakers addressed the issues brought to the committee by the USARIEM. These presentations formed the basis for the committee's deliberations and recommendations, and are included in this report as individually authored papers in Appendix B.[1]

One additional meeting of the committee was held on August 24–25, 2005. Prior to this second meeting, the committee took part in a series of conference calls to deliberate the scientific basis for the recommendations for each of the minerals. Further, additional conference calls were held to discuss and finalize recommendations. Finally, a research agenda was set forth through numerous face to face and phone interactions by committee members.

The committee wishes to express its special thanks to Andrew J. Young, Chief Nutritionist of the Nutrition Division and representative from the Department of Defense for this report, for generously giving his time and help and for being available to clarify the task of the committee. Special thanks are extended to Angus G. Scrimgeour, Research Physiologist, and James P. McClung, Nutritional Biochemist at the Nutrition Division of USARIEM. Their assistance was invaluable during the committee's work in that they helped delineate the task and provided numerous reports and other data to the committee in a timely manner. The committee wants to express its deepest appreciation to Carol J. Baker-Fulco, nutritionist at USARIEM, who offered her valuable help on numerous occasions to address the multiple questions regarding the nature of the military food and mineral intake and ration composition data. The committee wishes to extend thanks also to LTC John E. Kent, Chief, Nutrition Care Division at Darnall Army Community Hospital and LTC Sonya J.C. Corum, TRADOC Dietitian at Fort Jackson, South Carolina for their assistance in describing nutritional and environmental factors in the field. Thanks also go to COL Maria A. Worley, Nutrition Program Director and Chief Dietitian of the U.S. Army, for her frank description of practical uses of MDRIs for rations by the military. Finally, the committee wishes to thank COL Karl E. Friedl who tirelessly supports the work of the CMNR in so many different ways, from his participation in workshops to provision of appropriate contacts.

On behalf of the committee, I wish to sincerely thank the workshop participants and speakers for addressing topics critical to the completion of the committee's work. Each speaker not only provided an excellent presentation, but was available for multiple interactions during and after the workshop, and prepared a manuscript of their presentations (see Appendix B), working with IOM staff throughout the revision process. These presentations were important reference sources for the committee and, as already mentioned, were used as the scientific basis throughout the report.

The committee owes a strong debt of gratitude to the FNB staff for its professionalism and effectiveness in ensuring that our committee adhered to its task statement, for providing discipline and experience in helping to assemble

[1]The authored papers have undergone limited editorial changes, have not been reviewed by the report reviewers, and represent the views of the individual authors.

the report, for providing background research support, and for organizing our meetings. In particular, we would like to thank Senior Program Officer Maria P. Oria of the FNB, who worked tirelessly on numerous drafts and revisions. Ably assisting Maria in her efforts were Senior Program Assistant Jon Q. Sanders and Research Associate Leslie J. Sim. The committee is also grateful to the overall guidance and continuous support of Linda D. Meyers, Director of the FNB.

I also extend my deep gratitude to my fellow committee members, who participated in our discussions in this study in a professional and collegial manner, and who approached their task statement with great seriousness and intellectual curiosity.

Robert M. Russell, M.D., Chair

## Contents

# Summary

The military devotes major efforts to ensure the continuous safety, health, and performance of soldiers who are deployed to serve in combat. One such effort has focused on improving the nutrient intake levels of soldiers and, thereby, the nutrient levels of ration designs. Relevant findings from nutrition studies in the civilian population have been vital in this endeavor. However, because of the unique demands from the multiple stressors endured during many military situations, direct application of civilian-derived dietary recommendations and nutritional data is not always appropriate. For example, even though the widely applied Institute of Medicine Dietary Reference Intakes (IOM DRIs)—nutrient intake reference values for healthy U.S. and Canadian populations[1]—traditionally have been the basis of Military Dietary Reference Intakes (MDRIs), the military's nutrient standards, some values have had to be adjusted for application in military situations. In the case of essential minerals, the current military standards are the same as the IOM DRIs and are used to plan operational rations for military personnel.

Military surveys suggest that soldiers' mineral intakes might not achieve the levels recommended in the MDRIs. Mineral losses (mainly via sweat) will occur because of the physical (e.g., training or combat) and environmental (e.g., extreme temperatures) stressors. The combination of potentially low intakes and increased losses puts soldiers at greater risk of mineral deficiencies (e.g., iron, especially in women, or zinc).

---

[1]The DRIs include the Estimated Average Requirement (EAR), Recommended Dietary Allowance (RDA), Adequate Intake (AI), and Tolerable Upper Intake Level (UL).

The potential for adverse effects of marginal mineral deficiencies among soldiers engaged in training or military operations and the prospect of improving military performance through mineral intakes have spurred the military's interest in this area of nutrition. Thus, the U.S. Department of Defense (DoD) asked the IOM to study and assess mineral requirements and recommended intakes for military personnel in garrison training. The recommendations in this report also might be applicable to others who encounter situations similar to military training, such as athletes or fire fighters.

## COMMITTEE'S TASK AND APPROACH

Under the auspices of the Standing Committee on Military Nutrition Research, the Committee on Mineral Requirements for Cognitive and Physical Performance of Military Personnel was established to assess the need for setting nutrient intake reference levels specific to the military population and distinct from the IOM DRIs, and, if necessary, to recommend mineral intake levels for military personnel. Specifically, the committee was asked to select essential minerals of importance to military performance and, for those selected minerals, to recommend dietary intake levels for military personnel engaged in garrison training (i.e., training or performing operations from garrison). The basis for the recommended intake levels should be maintenance or improvement of physical and cognitive functions significant to military performance. In addition, the DoD requested an evaluation of the mineral levels in selected operational rations used in garrison training or sustained operations [i.e., meals, ready–to–eat (MREs) and first strike rations (FSRs)]. Finally, the committee also was asked to comment on the mineral recommendations for assault rations (e.g., FSRs) in the IOM 2006 report *Nutrient Composition of Rations for Short-Term, High-Intensity Combat Operations.*

To address its task, the committee convened a workshop in Washington, D.C., on June 13–15, 2005, during which speakers addressed the issues brought to the committee by the DoD. These presentations were the basis for the committee's deliberations and recommendations and are included in Appendix B of this report as individually authored papers.

The committee considered the unique circumstances that distinguish military garrison training from civilian lifestyles as well as the criteria used to establish the IOM DRIs for the general population. Next, the committee deliberated about the need to have MDRIs distinct from IOM DRIs, the risks of mineral deficiencies during garrison training as well as the potential benefits from higher mineral intakes, and the recommended mineral requirements for soldiers engaged in garrison training. Based on those new recommended intakes, the committee evaluated the mineral content of current operational rations.

## DIETARY NEEDS FOR MILITARY PERSONNEL IN GARRISON TRAINING

### Adjustment of Military Dietary Reference Intakes

Although the discussion that follows might be applicable to other nutrients, this committee has focused its deliberations on essential minerals. The current MDRIs for minerals [and the corresponding nutrient specifications for operational rations (NSORs) based on the MDRIs] are the same as the corresponding IOM DRIs. Based on discussions regarding the establishment of MDRIs, the committee reached the following recommendation:

**MDRIs should continue to reflect the IOM DRIs. Modifications should be made to specific nutrient requirements if there is sufficient scientific evidence that circumstances call for different requirements and intakes, whether to maintain nutrient or health status or to improve performance. In particular, recommended values for some minerals should take into account enhanced mineral losses caused by high-performance activity. Also, the MDRIs can be used for ration development for individual soldiers.**

The RDAs represent the nutrient intake levels that would meet the needs of nearly all of the people in a given life stage and gender group (i.e., the EAR) and are used as goals for an individual's nutrient needs. The RDA is calculated by adding two standard deviations to the EAR for the population. Often the variance of the EAR's distribution is unknown, so a standard deviation of 10 percent is used. Ideally, researchers should collect new data under the special circumstances that occur in the military (e.g., higher energy expenditures and excess sweating) to establish a new military EAR and RDA, but these data are lacking. In the absence of these data, the committee agreed that basing the current MDRIs on the IOM DRIs is appropriate and recommended that the IOM EARs for appropriate age and gender groups should be adjusted when necessary to set EARs and RDAs for military personnel. In the absence of an IOM EAR, the IOM AI (an estimated intake level that guarantees nutrient adequacy for practically everyone) could be used as a guide to ensure adequacy for an individual.

For example, sweat losses of minerals during garrison training should be measured and factored into a new garrison training EAR, and the corresponding RDA should be calculated by using the coefficient of variation of the new EAR. This new RDA will likely fulfill the needs of 97–98 percent of the military personnel in garrison training. The committee concluded that the new RDA could not appropriately be called military RDA, because the recommendations are meant to meet the unique needs only of soldiers in garrison training, not of all military personnel. For the purpose of this report, the committee refers to this new RDA as RDA for military garrison training or $RDA_{MGT}$ (and, similarly, $EAR_{MGT}$ or $AI_{MGT}$) (see Box S-1).

**BOX S-1**
**Establishment of Nutrient Military Standards**

Nutrient standards for military personnel in garrison training should be derived as follows:

1. $EAR_{MGT}$: Modify the current IOM EAR by adjusting with an adequate level of the variable of interest (e.g., sweat losses).
2. $RDA_{MGT}$: Add 2 × SD (standard deviation) of the $EAR_{MGT}$ to ensure 97–98 percent of soldiers will have adequate intake.

## Do Soldiers in Garrison Training Require Greater Mineral Intakes?

Following the recommendation to establish new reference intakes for soldiers in garrison training, the committee assessed the following research data in support of higher mineral intake requirements: (1) mineral losses with physical, psychological, or environmental stress; (2) the effects of weight loss on mineral requirements; and (3) the effects of mineral intakes on performance. In addition, the diversity in water sources as a variable for mineral intakes was evaluated (see Box S-2 for the overall finding). The committee agreed to focus the discussions and recommendations on calcium, copper, iron, magnesium, selenium, and zinc as minerals of most concern based on literature reviews about their importance to physical and cognitive performance and maintaining health status.

**BOX S-2**
**Overall Findings on Mineral Requirements for Military in Garrison Training**

The committee concluded that there is strong evidence that sweat mineral losses of copper, iron, and zinc might be significant during garrison training. There are not sufficient data on sweat losses for calcium, magnesium, and selenium to recommend an increase in dietary intake. Research demonstrating that an increase in intake of a particular mineral imparts benefits to physical or cognitive performance is still in an exploratory phase and warrants more studies. Therefore, only requirements for copper, iron, and zinc are adjusted on the basis of increased sweat losses, and revised $RDA_{MGT}$ are proposed for those minerals. The committee recommends using the current IOM AI for calcium and the current IOM RDAs for magnesium and selenium as the military requirements. All of the recommended requirements should be updated as new or confirmatory data from appropriately designed studies emerge regarding mineral losses and effects from higher intake doses of specific minerals. The derivations for the new $RDA_{MGT}$ and $AI_{MGT}$ are in Table S-1.

*Mineral Requirements Due to Stressors*

There is evidence to suggest that the mineral losses through sweat primarily, but also through feces and urine, might be significant with physical stress. However, many of the studies addressing mineral secretion with exercise either cannot be applied to the military environment or have design flaws, or both. For example, many studies were too brief and, therefore, ignored any acclimatization effects that could result in sweat losses decreasing over time. Also, it is a collection and that for more accurate determinations samples should be collected from whole-body sweat instead of from patches in specific sites, as collected in many studies. Nevertheless, because the majority of studies suggest that the losses are real, the committee has estimated the increased losses for iron, copper, and zinc, based on the best available data. It was estimated that average additional sweat losses for copper, iron, and zinc during garrison training would be respectively 0.5, 1, and 2 mg/day for men. To estimate losses for women, it was assumed that mineral losses amount to 30 percent less than in men. There is not enough evidence on other minerals' losses. These values should be revisited when studies designed as described in Chapter 4 become available.

*Mineral Requirements to Improve Performance*

There is no definitive evidence indicating that specific mineral supplementation beyond the current MDRIs will improve soldiers' physical or cognitive performance; therefore, there is no recommendation to this effect. There are, however, scientific studies that strongly suggest the potential for improved performance with higher mineral intakes. For example, a positive interaction between physical activity and calcium intake has been demonstrated in the bones of postmenopausal women; however, the same interactions have not been studied in groups that would better reflect the ages and lifestyles relevant to the military. Increased calcium intake also appears to improve mood states but needs to be demonstrated under garrison training scenarios.

Anecdotal data suggest that iron status might not be adequate for many women entering the military. The initial iron status likely will be aggravated by intense physical activity typical of garrison training. There is convincing evidence that iron supplementation improves physical performance of civilian women with low iron stores but no anemia. The data show that in women with low iron stores, iron supplementation improved endurance and the benefits of aerobic training and decreased muscle fatigability, functions that are highly relevant to military needs. There is also suggestive evidence that, in civilians, iron status is associated with improved cognitive functions and behavior. Recent studies demonstrated that civilian women who reached the highest iron status had improved measurements of attention, learning skills, and memory functions. Studies conducted to determine the effects of iron supplementation on mood states indicated that depression severity declines if iron deficiency is treated. Although there is no doubt that the data are promising, all studies linking cognition and behavior with iron status have been done in civilians. Therefore, the committee concluded that before iron requirements are increased with the objective of improving performance, more research should be conducted with the subjects and environment of interest.

A limited number of studies have examined the potential relationship between magnesium and sleep of military personnel. The association between selenium and zinc and mood states has also gained some interest, but the data for these relationships are merely suggestive and still preliminary.

### *Mineral Deficiencies During Weight Loss Diets*

Weight-loss diets are prominent among military personnel, mainly due to expectations to meet military standards for weight. If nutrient intake is not managed properly, the health and performance of individuals on weight loss diets could be compromised. For example, there is strong evidence that weight loss is associated with a loss of bone mass and a related increase in fracture risks in overweight and obese subjects as well as in postmenopausal women; calcium supplementation has been shown to minimize such bone loss. Recommending higher protein intakes and calcium intakes of at least 1,000 mg/day and as much as 1,500–1,700 mg/day is prudent to ensure minimal bone loss during weight-loss regimes. However, confirmatory research that these amounts are adequate for military personnel should be conducted. For other minerals, there is little evidence that following weight-loss diets necessitates increased requirements, especially when protein intake is high enough so that catabolism and, therefore, mineral losses are minimized. The committee emphasizes, though, that when following weight-loss diets mineral intakes should meet, at a minimum, the levels recommended in this report.

## Uses of Military Dietary Reference Intakes

DRIs are used for dietary planning and assessment for populations (IOM, 2000, 2003). In order to plan menus or rations for a large group, such as soldiers in garrison training, the EAR and the variability in intakes in a specific population are needed. In the absence of intake distribution data, the $EAR_{MGT}$ cannot be used for the actual planning of cafeteria menus for soldiers, and, for the present, managers should make sure that the food available in the cafeteria contains all the food groups so that the MDRIs are likely to be met and the menus follow nutrition guides such as the Dietary Guidelines for Americans and MyPyramid.

Conversely, although variability of nutrient intakes for military personnel eating operational rations is unknown, it can be safely assumed that it will be small if they completely consume the rations issued; therefore, planning rations for individuals (as opposed to planning rations for groups) would be appropriate and can be done by using the RDA as the reference value. In that case, rations should meet the new military RDA for minerals established in the manner described in Box S-1. In cases of a gender difference, the recommended amount in the rations should be the highest one, but lower than the UL for the age range. Accordingly, the current NSORs (based on MDRIs) are established to represent the minimal levels of minerals in operational rations and, when adjusted as described, would provide adequate levels for military personnel under specific military situations.

**The committee supports the use of NSORs as minimum levels of minerals in operational rations; NSORs should be established based on new military RDAs (e.g., $RDA_{MGT}$), developed as new scientific data become available. The NSORs might be different for specific military situations; for example, NSORs for military garrison training and those for sustained operations might differ.**

### Are the Mineral Contents of Operational Rations Adequate? Do the Mineral Levels in Water Contribute to Total Mineral Intake?

The average mineral composition of various menus for three different MREs and three different FSRs provided by the U.S. Army Research Institute of Environmental Medicine was used to assess adequacy. Although on average, most mineral content in rations meet the recommendations of this committee, some menus should be revised so that they meet the $RDA_{MGT}$ and $AI_{MGT}$ for both men and women, assuming that women will consume two MREs and men will consume three MREs.

Exceptions of minerals whose average levels do not meet the recommendations of this committee are the content of iron for women ($RDA_{MGT}$ = 24 mg versus an average of 18 mg in two MREs), zinc for men ($RDA_{MGT}$ = 15 versus an average of 14 mg in three MREs), or zinc for women ($RDA_{MGT}$ = 11 mg versus an average of 9 mg in two MREs). The mineral content of the FSRs appears to meet the recommendations of the current committee, except for calcium, whose average content in FSRs (673 mg) is slightly lower than the one recommended (750 mg, see Table S-1).

Regarding mineral levels in water, the committee concluded that, due to sanitation processes applied to fresh water for human consumption, differences in the mineral content of water are not such that will affect the total intake levels of minerals by military personnel. The committee concluded that the addition of calcium and magnesium to water consumed by military personnel is warranted only when improving the taste is the desirable outcome.

## FUTURE NEEDS

The committee stresses that the recommendations in this report regarding specific mineral requirements need confirmation based on data collected from

**TABLE S-1** Mineral Intakes: Institute of Medicine Dietary Reference Intakes, Current Military Dietary Reference Intakes, Recommended Intakes for Garrison Training ($EAR_{MGT}$, $RDA_{MGT}$, or $AI_{MGT}$), and Recommended Levels for Assault Rations

| Nutrient | IOM RDA or AI | MDRI | $RDA_{MGT}$ or $AI_{MGT}$ | Levels for Assault Rations* |
|---|---|---|---|---|
| Calcium (mg) | | | | |
| Male | 1,000 | 1,000 | 1,000 | 750–850 |
| Female | 1,000 | 1,000 | 1,000 | |
| Copper (μg) | | | | |
| Male | 900 | ND | 1,800 | 900–1,600 |
| Female | 900 | ND | 1,500 | |
| Iron (mg) | | | | |
| Male | 8 | 10 | 14 | 8–18 |
| Female | 18 | 15 | 24 | |
| Magnesium (mg) | | | | |
| Male | 420 | 420 | 420 | 400–550 |
| Female | 320 | 320 | 320 | |
| Selenium (μg) | | | | |
| Male | 55 | 55 | 55 | 55–230 |
| Female | 55 | 55 | 55 | |
| Zinc (mg) | | | | |
| Male | 11 | 15 | 15 | 11–25 |
| Female | 8 | 12 | 11 | |

NOTE: AI = Adequate Intake; EAR = Estimated Average Requirement; MDRI = Military Dietary Reference Intake; MGT = Military Garrison Training; ND = Not Determined; RDA = Recommended Dietary Allowance.
*IOM (2006).

controlled studies designed for specific military objectives and carried out under military-like environments. Conducting a comprehensive research agenda to answer all questions about mineral requirements for the military would not be feasible; therefore, the committee delineated a research agenda by prioritizing the questions on the basis of military needs and strength of the evidence, assuming that other pertinent, but less essential, information about minerals will be emerging through research at nonmilitary institutions.

First, studies to clarify concerns about soldiers' potential marginal mineral deficiencies were given the highest priority. To address those concerns, two overall, cross cutting studies that apply to more than one mineral are proposed and further explained in the following section.

Then, the most important studies to pursue have been listed and prioritized according to the strength of the available evidence, with the first study being the highest priority and so on (see specific research priorities for each mineral listed in alphabetical order at the end of this section). These are studies that would

**BOX S-3**
**Key Research Needs**

The committee recognizes that the proposed studies will be expensive to conduct; therefore, among all of the outlined research questions the following should take precedence.

*Highest Research Priorities*

- What are the effects of military garrison training conditions on mineral losses?
- What is the iron status at entry, deployment, and throughout military service? What is the total intake of calcium (i.e., from food, dietary supplements, and calcium-containing medications) at entry, deployment, and throughout military service?

*Other Research Priorities*

- Does iron supplementation prevent iron deficiency? What is the best strategy to prevent iron deficiency?
- How does physical activity during military garrison training influence calcium requirements in military personnel?
- Do iron intake amounts above the levels recommended in this report have beneficial effects on cognitive functions?
- Do magnesium intake amounts above the levels recommended in this report offer protection from sleep deprivation disturbances?
- Do zinc intake amounts above levels recommended in this report result in improved physical and cognitive performance?

confirm existing data on any potential higher requirements due to exercise or on any potential performance benefits from supplementation. The committee recognizes that the proposed studies will be expensive to conduct; therefore, a list of necessary key research questions that will assist in establishing new requirements for military personnel in garrison training has been extracted (see Box S-3).

## Priority #1: Study the Effects of Military Garrison Training on Mineral Losses and Performance

*Questions*

How do the physical, psychological, and environmental stressors encountered by military personnel (e.g., heat, physical activity, and possibly sleep restriction) effect mineral losses and what is the related impact on physical and mental performance? What are the dietary intake levels required to replenish the losses and to optimize performance?

*General Design*

These questions could be addressed through a study design conducted with a population representative of the military, including both women and men. Each subject would participate in a baseline phase (versus a stress phase with heat and heavy exercise) that includes the consumption of a controlled diet based on either the current typical MRE or rations with the NSOR mineral levels. Subsequently, each subject would receive all dietary treatments (cocktails of higher and lower mineral levels) in randomized order while being subjected to heat and physical demands similar to those experienced by military personnel. Considering possible nutrient interactions of the diet interventions is critical when designing the study and interpreting the results. Conditions could be controlled by using an environmental chamber and supervising physical activity. Because training and operational exercises may involve significant reductions in total sleep and disruptions of the normal sleep–wake cycle, both of which reliably result in severe decrements in cognitive function and mood, sleep restriction should be considered as an additional intervention.

*Measurement of Outcomes*

This experimental design evaluates a dose–response effect of minerals on ameliorating mineral losses due to heat and sweat and can be used to assess a dose–response effect of minerals on physical and mental performance. Daily, 24-hour whole-body sweat analysis and potential acclimatization over a short term (five days) and a long term (two or three weeks) can be measured.

During baseline and each treatment, cognition and behavior outcome measures could include assessments of sleep patterns; mood states; cognitive function, including attention, memory, and decision making; and psychomotor skills. The most important physical performance measurements are those for aerobic and muscular endurance, and the military should select those that have been proven to reflect the reality of military environments and physical performance demands.

## Priority #2: Mineral Status and Food and Dietary Intakes

*Questions*

What is the mineral status or dietary intake level (especially of calcium and iron) of soldiers at various times from entry to training, deployment, or combat?

*Iron Status*

The committee concluded that women's iron status is an important criterion that will determine whether a strategy to increase women's iron intake is needed;

if a strategy is needed, it is critical to identify which would be the most efficient in correcting the deficiencies. Also, surveillance programs should be established to monitor iron status (measured by serum ferritin levels) at the end of all intensive training phases as well as periodically during military service.

*Calcium Intake*

Because of calcium's potential role in preventing stress fractures during training or combat and in modulating emotional health, calcium intake from food beverages, dietary supplements, and calcium-containing medications should be surveyed periodically. There is no biomarker for calcium that can indicate calcium status; instead, an indication of status is suggested from the total dietary intake. The same studies used to analyze rations for calcium levels and to assess dietary intake could be adapted with a minimum of additional resources to analyze copper, magnesium, selenium, and zinc.

**Specific Research Priorities: Calcium**

- Quantify calcium losses due to the stressful conditions of garrison training (i.e., heat and physical exertion) (see priority #1 above).
- Assess for calcium intake the current diets of military personnel under the various environments as a practical approach to assess calcium status. This should include calcium intakes from food, beverages, dietary supplements, and calcium-containing medications (see priority #2 above).
- Conduct balance and kinetic studies to understand the role of physical activity on calcium metabolism and requirements.
- Study the potential adverse effects of weight loss and interactions with calcium supplementation in bone loss.
- Study the potential effects of dietary calcium on counteracting the negative interaction of exercise and oral contraceptives on women's bones.
- Study the association between calcium intakes above 850 mg/day and the risk of kidney stone formation.
- Study the relationship of calcium intake and mood, premenstrual syndrome, depression, and other psychological factors that affect performance.

**Specific Research Priorities: Copper**

- Quantify copper losses due to the stressful conditions of garrison training (i.e., heat and physical exertion) (see priority #1 above).
- Determine the copper concentrations of food items in operational rations, including MREs and FSRs; estimate the dietary intake levels of military personnel.

### Specific Research Priorities: Iron

- Quantify iron losses due to the stressful conditions of garrison training (i.e., heat and physical exertion) (see priority #1 above).
- Determine the prevalence of iron deficiency in women at entry to training camp and deployment; regularly survey their status to monitor the stability of their mineral nutritional status (see priority #2 above).
- Determine the relationship between iron status and cognitive and behavioral functions within the context of military garrison training.
- Determine if supplemental iron or dietary intervention approaches, or both, can alleviate the drop in iron status of female soldiers in garrison training versus iron supplementation only after screening.

### Specific Research Priorities: Magnesium

- Quantify magnesium losses due to the stressful conditions of garrison training (i.e., heat and physical exertion) (see priority #1 above).
- Determine whether increasing magnesium intake will improve sleep, protect against the effects of sleep deprivation, or regulate mood states of soldiers in garrison training.
- Determine the magnesium concentrations of food items in operational rations, including MREs and FSRs; estimate the dietary intake levels of military personnel.

### Specific Research Priorities: Selenium

- Quantify selenium losses due to the multiple stressors of garrison training (i.e., heat and physical exertion) (see priority #1 above).
- Determine whether selenium supplementation of nondeficient subjects can improve immune function.
- Determine the selenium concentrations of food items in operational rations, including MREs and FSRs; estimate the dietary intake levels of military personnel.
- Determine whether increasing selenium intake will benefit military personnel's mood states, especially depression.

### Specific Research Priorities: Zinc

- Quantify zinc losses due to the multiple stressors of garrison training (i.e., heat and physical exertion) (see priority #1 above).
- Evaluate the possible benefit of zinc supplementation on physical performance.
- Evaluate the potential benefits of zinc supplementation to enhance cognitive function.
- Determine the zinc concentrations of food items in operational rations, including MREs and FSRs; estimate the dietary intake levels of military personnel.

# 1

# Introduction

The U.S. Army Health Risk Appraisal group surveyed 400,000 active duty U.S. Army personnel in the late 1990s to determine whether or not those personnel met the dietary objectives of Healthy People 2000 (HP2000), a national agenda for health promotion and disease prevention. As reported by Yore et al. (2000), Army personnel generally did not meet the HP2000 goals for nutrition even though significant progress had been made during 1991–1998. Although the specific aspects of diet that would be relevant to this Committee on Mineral Requirements for Cognitive and Physical Performance of Military Personnel are lacking, the findings from this survey suggest that there are dietary problems in the military population. The potential for adverse effects of marginal mineral deficiencies among soldiers engaged in training or military operations and the prospect of improving military performance through mineral intakes have spurred the military's interest in this area of nutrition. This chapter discusses some background information on the current knowledge regarding soldiers' eating behaviors, mineral intakes as well as on the physical and mental stress caused by the environmental circumstances (i.e. physical and mental stress) of military garrison training.

## THE COMMITTEE'S TASK

### Study Objective

The study's objective is to review essential minerals and their potential effects—whether direct or indirect (by preventing diseases)—on military performance, including neuropsychological and physical performance. In addition, the role of minerals in preventing acute health issues, such as diarrheal diseases and infections that could affect performance, is reviewed, and possible prophylactic benefits are summarized. The role of zinc is of particular interest. In addition to zinc, the study specifically identifies the minerals of most importance for military physical and cognitive performance and evaluates if there is the potential for significant mineral deficiencies in specific military situations, which are outlined in the following section, *Specific Questions to be Addressed.* The study also assesses the adequacy of current mineral levels in operational rations and recommends new levels when appropriate. The mechanisms of action and physiological effects of interactions, including neural pathway interactions, are considered. Finally, the committee recommends delivery vehicles for adequate mineral levels and identifies research needs of military importance.

### Specific Questions to Be Addressed

The committee task addressed the following seven questions:

1. Which dietary minerals are likely to have an impact on human performance? Are these minerals provided in adequate amounts in the meals, ready-to-eat (MREs) and the current first strike rations (FSRs)?
2. Is there a potential for any significant deficiency in essential minerals when soldiers subsist on (a) MREs during garrison training (i.e., intense training and one-day missions) or (b) FSRs during combat missions (i.e., repeated cycles of three- to seven-day combat missions, with one- to three-day recovery periods that include garrison dining)?
3. During garrison training, do weight loss diets (energy or macronutrient restricted) have the potential to lead to deficiencies of specific essential minerals?
4. Do the high-performance activities of soldiers cause excessive mineral loss, thereby raising the mineral dietary requirements?
5. Is there any scientific evidence that mineral supplements (individually or in combination) improve soldiers' performance?
6. Are the Military Dietary Reference Intake (MDRIs) for dietary minerals reflective of the Institute of Medicine (IOM) Dietary Reference Intakes [Recommended Dietary Allowance (RDA) or Adequate Intake (AI)]? Should the MDRIs follow the RDAs or AIs or should differences persist because of soldiers' specific needs?
7. How do changes in the drinking water sources used during military deployment (e.g., U.S. public water supply versus bottled water versus field-purified water) affect the balance of essential dietary minerals?

## ORGANIZATION OF THE REPORT

This report is organized into an executive summary, five chapters, and seven appendixes. The chapters include an introductory chapter and subsequent chapters that answer the seven questions comprising the committee task. Appendix B is composed of the workshop speakers' written presentations; although the presentations formed the basis for the committee's answers to the military's questions, they should not be construed as representing the committee's views.

Chapter 1 provides background information on the current knowledge regarding soldiers' eating behaviors as well as on the physical and mental stress caused by military garrison training or operations. Chapter 1 also offers facts on the mineral content of rations and its intake by military personnel and addresses the potential effects of nutrient deficiencies due to inadequate intake or higher requirements during military operations. Chapter 2 provides information and recommendations on the development and uses of MDRIs and a description of strategies to increase intake of specific minerals, whether via usual foods, fortification, or supplementation. Chapter 3 features a description of the metabolism and needs for selected minerals by military personnel under garrison training, recommendations on mineral intake levels, and an assessment of mineral level adequacy in operational rations. Chapter 4 includes a prioritization of the research needed to answer information gaps and details of study designs required to gain such information. Chapter 5 presents a summary of some of the committee's findings by answering to the specific questions posed to the committee.

Appendix A presents the workshop agenda, and Appendix B features the workshop presentations organized by topic, including an introduction to information about combat rations; mineral metabolism; and the role of minerals in sustaining and improving physical and mental performance. Appendix C contains summary tables of nutrient recommendations for assault rations and of mineral levels in operational and restricted rations. The biographical sketches of the speakers and of the committee members are presented in Appendixes D and E, respectively. Appendix F lists acronyms and abbreviations, and finally, Appendix G provides a glossary.

## ENERGY EXPENDITURE AND FOOD CONSUMPTION DURING MILITARY OPERATIONS OR TRAINING

As mentioned previously, this task is concerned with soldiers mainly during garrison training. Although the unique features of high-intensity operations are not the focus of this task, they are summarized so that comments on the mineral levels in IOM (2006) are put into context. The committee has defined garrison training as situations during which soldiers spend the day performing a military mission or training exercises while living in a military base; sustained operations are defined, as in a previous IOM report (2006), as repetitive three- to seven-day high-stress missions interspersed with restorative periods of one to three days. Unfortunately, data on energy expenditure and intake and on food consumption by soldiers in the field are scarce and mostly anecdotal. The committee received no information regarding soldiers' energy expenditures performing the typical training activities addressed in this report during deployments or when the soldiers participate in one-day missions, or both. In the absence of actual data, estimated energy expenditure can be assumed from published literature that measured energy expenditures during similar military activities, albeit performed during training at home or abroad, when in noncombat situations. Fortunately, there have been a number of such studies that have been reviewed recently by Tharion et al. (2005). Because the recent report *Nutrient Composition of Rations for Short-Term, High-Intensity Combat Operations* includes a detailed description on soldiers' energy expenditure and food habits during sustained operations (IOM, 2006), this section instead will describe soldiers' expenditures during garrison training, the second scenario under consideration for this report. The reader is referred to IOM (2006), *Nutrient Composition of Rations for Short-Term, High-Intensity Combat Operations* for further description on energy expenditure and intake and on food consumption during sustained operations.

The wide range in total energy expenditures of various military groups and the factors that appear to contribute to the related differences have been described previously (Tharion et al., 2005). Field studies suggest that the typical energy intake of military personnel (soldiers, sailors, airmen, and marines) under a variety of scenarios and climatic conditions is approximately 2,400 kcal/day, even though energy expenditures of soldiers in combat units range from approximately 4,000 to 7,131 kcal/day depending on the level of physical activity and on the environment. Interestingly, these reports note that measured energy deficits for soldiers (whether in training school or in combat) were significant (Tharion et al., 2005). However, a number of these studies were conducted with soldiers in combat operations that involved an extreme level of physical exercise; the committee does not include these combat operations in its definition of garrison training. After these extremely demanding combat situations were excluded and support activities of moderate activity level were included, energy expenditures of male soldiers in garrison training varied from 3,500 (e.g., support combat soldiers involved in moderate exercise) to 4,500 kcal/day (e.g., Ranger training under intense exercise). For female soldiers, energy expenditures varied from 2,300 kcal/day while undergoing basic training to 3,000 kcal/day while running medical operations in the field. The committee assumed that the energy expenditures while in garrison training will be an average of 4,000 and 2,500 kcal/day for men and women, respectively. Conversely, for male soldiers in sustained operations (repetitive three- to seven-day missions in locations off of the military base, with rest periods of one to three days), the committee assumed an average energy expenditure of 4,500 kcal/day (IOM, 2006).

During garrison training or one-day missions in the field, soldiers typically have free access in dining facilities to cafeteria-style food for breakfast and dinner and have field rations (MREs) during the day. For these situations, and because there is access to the cafeteria-style food at least twice a day, the committee assumed that soldiers were in energy balance. In contrast, during the unique circumstances of sustained operations, soldiers' energy balance is negative, as suggested by data collected during intense combat training. Negative energy balance could be detrimental to health and performance if an adequate diet were not consumed or if the operation were too prolonged, or both. Such data indicate that with high-energy expenditures of 4,000 kcal/day or more, soldiers tend to consume an average of 3,000 kcal/day, and even less when they depend on operational rations (i.e., rations designed for a wide variety of operations and settings but consumed for a limited period of time, for example, MREs). In addition to the potential performance decrements due to a variety of stressors during short-term missions, underconsumption may result in a set of consequences ranging from body protein loss and fatigue to deficits in essential micronutrients; all of those consequences may impair physiologic functions and result in performance decrements. The adverse effects of stress combined with food underconsumption are of concern and have been the subject of a number of IOM reports. Although stress during combat operations is unavoidable, much can be done to improve soldiers' nutritional status.

## MINERAL CONTENT OF MILITARY RATIONS

The mineral content of military rations has been estimated as described by Baker-Fulco (2005; see Appendix B). The data presented are derived from a variety of sources; calculations of the estimated contents vary and are based not only on actual food analysis data but also on food composition data and on the reports by the food companies manufacturing the food items. As the author points out, multiple uncertainties translate into final estimated values that either are underestimated or overestimated depending on the calculations made. Nevertheless, the estimated values represent the best available data. Another shortcoming is that analytical data do not exist for some nutrients, for example, copper.

The mineral content of food items can be used to evaluate soldiers' mineral intake (see the following section, *Mineral Intake of Military Personnel*), and it also can be used as a benchmark for the continued improvement of rations. Tables in Appendix C show the variability in mineral content of menus to be significant and reflect the diverse nature of the individual food items included in each menu, which is necessary to ensure the menus' acceptability.

## MINERAL INTAKE OF MILITARY PERSONNEL

### Food Intake

Since the military began its continued improvement of food and rations for military personnel, there have been some studies that have examined food intake behavior and its impact on soldiers' performance and health. The military also has studied the influence of different environments (e.g., cold, high-altitude climates or hot, desert-type climates) on soldiers' nutrient requirements and eating behavior. Johnson and Sauberlich (1982) conducted a literature review on the prolonged use of operational rations and found that as early as 1966 research indicated that more nutrient-related studies were required. For example, Consolazio's (Consolazio et al., 1966) study examined energy requirements at high altitudes and concluded that for optimal military performance and energy an evaluation of nutrient requirements, including micronutrients, was necessary to improve military rations. This conclusion was reached after blood and serum tests revealed some potential nutrient inadequacies. Later, a series of laboratory metabolic studies indicated similar conclusions regarding the need for adequate levels of minerals to maintain health (Consolazio et al., 1967).

Although some studies have measured the suitability of using MREs (Edwards et al., 1991), only a few studies performed with military personnel have included mineral intake in their designs. In these cases, a comparison between the intake and the MDRIs for minerals is made (see Table 1-1 for current MDRIs for minerals). For example, the health status of 15 soldiers of average physical fitness was studied when they were eating MREs ad libitum during 12 days at 7,200 feet of altitude (Askew et al., 1986). Exercise was strenuous during 7 of the 10 of the days in the field, and a decrease in the soldiers' maximal aerobic capacity of 5 percent was reported. Caloric intake was 67 percent of energy expenditure. The mean iron intake during the study was 14 mg/day (MDRI = 10 mg/day for men [U.S. Departments of the Army, Navy, and Air Force, 2001]). Calcium and magnesium intake was 567 and 245 mg/day, respectively (MDRI = 1,000 mg/day; MDRI for magnesium = 420 mg/day for men [U.S. Departments of the Army, Navy, and Air Force, 2001]). No other essential mineral was measured. The authors concluded that the level of performance was reasonable but recommended supplementation with a carbohydrate source for energy.

A more recent study was conducted on the physiological and psychological effects of eating foods from three different menus during 12 days of military training in a tropical environment (Booth et al., 2003). Three groups of Australian Air Field Defense Guards received either freshly prepared foods or one combat ration pack (CRP) or half of a CRP. Substantial underconsumption resulted in slight weight loss, protein catabolism, and immune suppression in the groups eating rations; members of those two groups also reported greater fatigue than members of the group that ate fresh foods. Under these conditions decreased serum ferritin levels (a measure of iron status) and dehydration were observed when consuming either of the rations or the freshly prepared foods (Booth et al., 2003), possibly due to overall underconsumption. However, direct association between decreased serum ferritin and performance could not be made from this study. Other studies have attempted to investigate the effect of micronutrient supplementation on military performance; one of them showed that for healthy adults, vitamin and mineral supplement consumption for three months did not improve military physical performance (Montain and Young, 2003).

One of the military's main interests has been zinc supplementation, especially because of the potentially marginal intake of soldiers as compared to recommended requirements, difficulties in assessing zinc status, and questions regarding the body's redistribution of zinc when under stress. A lack of performance response when supplementing with zinc has been reported in two studies (Singh et al., 1994, 1999); however, in both of these studies the intake of zinc by nonsupplemented control groups was adequate. The question remains whether zinc might have beneficial effects as a supplement when dietary intake in food is compromised.

Tharion et al. (2004) evaluated the adequacy of the food-service food provided to Special Forces soldiers in garrison training. Among the data collected were the following mineral intake levels based on the food items consumed (as reported by the participants):

- Calcium, 1,065 mg (952–1,236 mg), (MDRI = 1,000 mg for men [U.S. Departments of the Army, Navy, and Air Force, 2001]);
- Copper, 1.7 mg (1.5–2.1 mg), (no set MDRI for copper, IOM RDA = 0.9 mg for men >19 years of age [IOM, 2001]);
- Iron, 19.3 mg (16.6–22.9 mg), (MDRI = 10 for men [U.S. Departments of the Army, Navy, and Air Force, 2001]);
- Magnesium, 341 mg (306–409 mg), (MDRI = 420 for men [U.S. Departments of the Army, Navy, and Air Force, 2001 ]); and
- Zinc, 16.3 mg (14.1–20.7 mg), (MDRI = 15 for men [U.S. Departments of the Army, Navy, and Air Force, 2001]).

The study also reported the amount of food and nutrients that was eaten on weekdays and weekends. The large variations were associated with more food eaten outside the cafeteria on the weekends. These results are less relevant for the current task because the soldiers were eating cafeteria food at all times and not food from rations. However, the results do show that even when having free access to food, the intake of some minerals was low. For example, only about 40 percent of the subjects achieved the dietary goal for magnesium (MDRI = 420 mg for men [U.S. Departments of the Army, Navy, and Air Force, 2001]).

A more relevant study by Thomas et al. (1995) assessed the nutritional intake of soldiers in a field environment during 30 days when the soldiers were provided either three MREs or two test rations and one MRE (standard field ration menu). The group with three MREs ate less and had mineral intake levels lower than the group eating the test ration; those intakes were also lower than the MDRI for calcium (868 versus 1,000 mg), zinc (9.3 versus 15 mg), and magnesium (306 versus 420 mg). The intake of zinc was notably low. Measurements of iron status (serum levels and ferritin) were within normal levels. Serum levels for the other minerals also were normal. Serum zinc was not measured. Performance, measured by road march times, was not altered by the two diets. General

**TABLE 1-1** Current Daily Dietary Recommended Intakes for the General Population Compared to Military Dietary Recommended Intakes for Personnel in Garrison Feeding, Operational, and Restricted Rations, Men and Women 19–30 Years of Age

| | General Population | | Military Population | | | |
|---|---|---|---|---|---|---|
| Nutrient or Energy | RDA, AI, or AMDR[a] | | MDRI[b] | | NSOR, Operational Ration, Daily Minimum Intake[b] | Restricted Ration Daily Minimum Intake[b] |
| Sex | Men | Women | Men | Women | NS | NS |
| Energy Intake (kcal) | 3,100–3,150[c] | 2,350–2,400[d] | 3,250 | 2,300 | 3,600 | 1,500 |
| Protein (g) | 56[e] | 46[e] | 63–119[f] | 50–93[f] | 91 | 50 |
| Fat (% of kcal) | 20–35%[g] | 20–35%[g] | ND | ND | ≤ 35% | ≤ 35% |
| Carbohydrate (g) | 130 | 130 | ND | ND | 494 | 200 |
| Vitamin A (μg) | 900 RAE | 700 | 1,000 RE | 800 RE | 1,000 μg RE | 500 μg RE |
| Vitamin C (mg) | 90 | 75 | 90 | 75 | 90 | 45 |
| Vitamin D (μg) | 5 | 5 | 5 | 5 | 5 | 3 |
| Vitamin E (mg) | 15 | 15 | 15 | 15 | 15 | 8 |
| Vitamin K (μg) | 120 | 90 | 80 | 65 | 80 | 40 |
| Thiamin (mg) | 1.2 | 1.1 | 1.2 | 1.1 | 1.2 | 0.6 |
| Riboflavin (mg) | 1.3 | 1.1 | 1.3 | 1.1 | 1.3 | 0.7 |
| Niacin (mg NE) | 16 | 14 | 16 | 14 | 16 | 8 |
| Vitamin $B_6$ (mg) | 1.3 | 1.3 | 1.3 | 1.3 | 1.3 | 0.7 |
| Folate (μg DFE) | 400 | 400 | 400 | 400 | 400 | 200 |
| Vitamin $B_{12}$ (μg) | 2.4 | 2.4 | 2.4 | 2.4 | 2.4 | 1.2 |
| Biotin (μg) | 30 | 30 | ND | ND | ND | ND |
| Pantothenic Acid (mg) | 5 | 5 | ND | ND | ND | ND |
| Choline (mg) | 550 | 425 | ND | ND | ND | ND |
| Calcium (mg) | 1,000 | 1,000 | 1,000 | 1,000 | 1,000 | 500 |
| Chromium (μg) | 35 | 25 | ND | ND | ND | ND |
| Copper (μg) | 900 | 900 | ND | ND | ND | ND |

| | | | | | | |
|---|---|---|---|---|---|---|
| Fluoride (mg) | 4 | 3 | 4 | 3.1 | 4 | 2 |
| Iodine (μg) | 150 | 150 | 150 | 150 | 150 | 75 |
| Iron (mg) | 8 | 18 | 10 | 15 | 15 | 8 |
| Magnesium (mg) | 400 | 310 | 420 | 320 | 420 | 210 |
| Manganese (mg) | 2.3 | 1.8 | ND | ND | ND | ND |
| Molybdenum (μg) | 45 | 45 | ND | ND | ND | ND |
| Phosphorus (mg) | 700 | 700 | 700 | 700 | 700 | 350 |
| Potassium (g) | 4.7 | 4.7 | 3.2 | 2.5 | 3.2 | 2.0 |
| Selenium (μg) | 55 | 55 | 55 | 55 | 55 | 28 |
| Sodium (g) | 1.5 (≤ 2.3) | 1.5 (≤ 2.3) | 5 (4.5–5.5) | 3.6 (3.2–3.9) | 5.0–7.0 | 2.5–3.5 |
| Zinc (mg) | 11 | 8 | 15 | 12 | 15 | 8 |

NOTE: AI = Adequate Intake, AMDR = Acceptable Macronutrient Distribution Ranges; DFE = Dietary Folate Equivalents; MDRI = Military Dietary Reference Intake; ND = Not Determined; NE = Niacin Equivalents; NS = Not Specified; NSOR = Nutritional Standards For Operational Rations; RAE = Retinol Activity equivalents; RDA = Recommended Dietary Allowance; RE = retinol equivalents.

[a]IOM (2004a) unless otherwise noted.

[b]U.S. Departments of the Army, Navy, and Air Force (2001).

[c]assuming energy intake = energy expenditure, using Institute of Medicine estimated energy requirement equation for men 19 years and older using: body reference weight = 70 kg; reference height = 1.75 m (same as military); physical activity level = active; range depicts 30 and 19 years of age respectively and rounding to the nearest 50 kcal.

[d]assuming energy inake = energy expenditure, using Institute of Medicine estimated energy requirement equation for women ages 19 years and older using: body reference weight = 57 kg; reference height =1.63 m (same as military); physical activity level = active; range depicts 30 and 19 years of age respectively and rounding to the nearest 50 kcal.

[e]using Institute of Medicine reference body weights (70 kg for men and 57 kg for women) and protein intake recommendations of. 0.8 g/kg body weight.

[f]using military reference body weights (79 kg for men and 62 kg for women) and protein intake recommendations of of 0.8 to 1.5 g/kg body weight.

[g]IOM (2002/2005).

health (constipation, diarrhea, hunger, and thirst) and mood (alertness, relaxation, confusion, and sleepiness) status were assessed by questionnaires. As with physical performance, no differences were observed with the two diets. However, the authors of this report postulated that if calcium and iron intake for male soldiers is just above the military standards, inadequate intake of these minerals by female soldiers would be likely because of their higher requirements. Thus, female soldiers could be at risk of iron and calcium deficiencies that might result in health or performance decrements.

Gender differences regarding energy and nutrient intake were examined during an 11-day field training exercise; the objective of the study was to determine if the standard MREs were adequate to meet women's nutritional needs (Baker-Fulco et al., 2002). The energy intake of the female population was lower than that of the male population among the combat-support hospital personnel studies (mean intake of 1,818 kcal/day versus 2,427 kcal/day). Likewise, a larger proportion of women did not meet the intake standards for several nutrients, including calcium, iron, magnesium, and zinc. However, when body weight was accounted for, those gender differences were mostly eliminated. More than half of the women's intake for calcium, zinc, and magnesium was inadequate if the Estimated Average Requirements (EARs) were used as reference values for group adequacy. Approximately 10 percent of the women did not meet the EAR for iron. This study also revealed an interesting observation—a significant amount of energy and nutrient sources derived from nonration foods; for example, about 7 percent of the women obtained more than 20 percent of their calories from nonration foods. The results agree with an earlier study that examined the health, performance, and nutritional status of U.S. Army women during training at Fort Jackson, South Carolina, for seven consecutive days (King et al., 1994). The meals consisted of three A-rations each day. Once again, the authors concluded that intake of calcium, magnesium, iron, and zinc was less than the MDRI.

Low mineral intake also was noted in a study that evaluated consumption, acceptability, and performance outcomes for an experimental ration (the T-ration) consumed for 60 days as compared to a B-ration (canned, dehydrated, and dried ingredients) (Tharion et al., 2000). Intake of energy, folate, magnesium, zinc, carbohydrate, and fiber was lower than recommended for the T-ration group; however, there were no notable decrements in physical performance (i.e., construction-type work) or mood.

Another study that tested the use of a supplemental carbohydrate beverage to meet the nutritional needs of soldiers (n = 63) under intense exercise in the desert, revealed significant inadequacies in calcium, magnesium, and zinc intake (Tharion et al., 1997). It is interesting that the inadequacies were more notable for those who, in addition to receiving the unitized group ration, were supplemented with carbohydrate; in this supplemented group, 59 (calcium), 34 (magnesium), 15 (iron), and 31 (zinc) percent of soldiers did not meet 70 percent of the recommended MDRI. The authors suggested that when a carbohydrate supplement is provided, changes in consumption patterns may compromise the intake of essential micronutrients.

From the few studies described, it can be inferred that the mineral intake of soldiers is compromised, even if marginally in some instances (see Table 1-1 for current MDRIs). Magnesium and zinc appear to be the minerals that are more often consumed at inadequate levels. Studies evaluating nutrient intake ideally would assess women and men separately since their needs and intake differ. In general, as Baker-Fulco concluded (Baker-Fulco, 2005; see Appendix B), the data are insufficient to have a clear picture of all the mineral intake from food. Information on nutrient intake when eating food from the dining facilities or when eating food from rations would help in designing food items with a more adequate nutrient density, especially for women; this is ultimately necessary in order to ensure that the military requirements for nutrients are met by most military personnel, both men and women. To calculate nutrient intake accurately, better data on nutrient composition of food items need to be collected.

### Supplement Intake

If data on mineral intake from foods are scarce, as the evidence in the previous section suggests, then, data on the intake of supplements by military personnel are even less abundant. Recent personal communications by U.S. Army Research Institute of Environmental Medicine (USARIEM) officials confirm that information on dietary supplement intake by soldiers is scarce (personal communication, K. Friedl, USARIEM, June 13, 2005). Nevertheless, it is a fact that soldiers have access to and readily use dietary supplements, especially weight loss supplements, protein supplements, creatine, and energy drinks. Although anecdotal data suggest that soldiers also might take calcium supplements, there are no published data either to confirm or refute that statement. The extent of dietary supplement and vitamin and mineral intake levels obtained via supplementation are unknown.

There is, however, one relatively recent study that addresses the intake of dietary supplements by U.S. Army Special Operations candidates (Arsenault and Kennedy, 1999). To collect the data, the authors administered 2,215 surveys to males entering the U.S. Army Special Forces and Ranger training schools. The results show that about 85 percent of men were using or had used dietary supplements in the past and that 35 percent were using them daily. These findings suggest that use among military personnel might be much higher than that by the general U.S. population (about 45 percent of the U.S. population reports using dietary supplements [Radimer, 2003]), possibly because of soldiers' concerns over the importance of adequate nutrition and health status for military training. For example, studies on supplement consumption by athletes, a population that might better resemble the military personnel than the general population, find that more than 50 percent use supplements (Sobal and Marquart, 1994). It is also possible that ergogenics to improve performance, such as creatine, would be favored over minerals or vitamins that could be seen as having nutritive but not performance-enhancing effects.

The study by Arsenault and Kennedy (1999) found that the majority of soldiers were taking dietary supplements for general health or performance enhancement; this finding is not surprising as soldiers perceived MREs as nutritionally poor. About 7 percent were occasional users of mineral supplements (less than once per week), 9 percent reported frequent use (one to six times per week), and 9 percent reported daily use. There was no mention, however, of the doses or forms of the supplements consumed.

The conclusion from this study and from personal communications with USARIEM officials is that the contribution of supplemental minerals to soldiers' diets is largely unknown, but it could contribute significantly to total mineral intake.

## IMPACT OF TRAINING AND MILITARY OPERATIONS ON HEALTH AND PERFORMANCE

### Physiological Consequences

As mentioned in the recent Committee on Military Nutrition Research (CMNR) report *Nutrient Composition of Rations for Short-Term, High-Intensity Combat Operations* (IOM, 2006) during combat operations (i.e., sustained operations) soldiers are often hypocaloric; as a result, the negative energy balance can affect their health and performance. Field studies that have attempted to resolve the question of the minimum energy intake that will maintain military performance were described in that report (IOM, 2006). For example, the Ranger I and II studies showed that severe hypocaloric states may result in harmful physical and cognitive effects to military personnel health (Moore et al., 1992; Shippee et al., 1994).

Protein loss is one of the main consequences of combat operations, but other consequences of stress and underconsumption during combat likely include impairments in the immune and endocrine systems, dehydration, proneness to kidney stone formation, and gastrointestinal disturbances (Montain, 2006; Montain and Young, 2003). A recent study was conducted on the physiological and psychological effects of eating foods from three different menus (two consisting of rations and one consisting of fresh foods) during 12 days of military training in a tropical environment (Booth et al., 2003). In the two groups eating the combat rations there was substantial underconsumption, which resulted in weight loss, protein catabolism, and immune suppression; members in those groups also reported greater fatigue than members of the group eating fresh foods. Despite underconsumption, all groups ate sufficient protein to meet the MDRI for protein.

In other situations, such as garrison training, underconsumption does not appear to be of concern, according to military sources. In these cases, soldiers eat mainly at dining facilities and follow a more normal eating schedule; negative energy balance and weight loss seemingly do not occur. Although during garrison training the physiological consequences are not so well described, the stress endured still could be detrimental to the immune and endocrine responses and contribute to dehydration, kidney stone formation, and gastrointestinal disturbances (Montain, 2006; Montain and Young, 2003).

## Consequences on Physical and Cognitive Performance

As described by Montain (2006), performance of simple and well-learned motor tasks (e.g., weapon handling) does not appear to be compromised by sustained operational stress (Haslam, 1982). Endurance time, however, is impaired frequently during aerobic exercise tasks (VanHelder and Radomski, 1989), and there is a higher perception among subjects of an increased effort needed to perform the same task. Nindl et al. (2002) reported a 25 percent lower level of work productivity from test group subjects, as compared to control group subjects, on a physical persistence task (building a wall for 25 minutes) after test group subjects were fed a hypocaloric diet (caloric content of diet was at least 50 percent less in kilocalories than the soldiers' energy expenditures) and allowed to sleep for only 1 h/day over a four-day period. This is consistent with the hypothesis that sustained operations compromise performance when tasks are prolonged and monotonous. Operational effectiveness also is affected if sleep is inadequate, independent of energy intake (Rognum et al., 1986).

### *Effects of Energy Balance and Nutrient Intake*

The weight loss observed during sustained operations appears to have inconsistent effects on soldiers' performance (Montain and Young, 2003); this possibly could be due to several factors—lack of the validity of the physical performance test used in the study design, severity and length of the energy deficit, or other factors related to the study design (e.g., small sample sizes). Earlier, shorter duration studies with minimal lean body mass loss generally showed little or no decrement in muscle strength, power, or fatigability (Bulbulian et al., 1996; Guezennec et al., 1994; VanHelder and Radomski, 1989). A study by Booth et al. (2003), concluded that a 3-percent weight loss after 12 days was unlikely to be detrimental to military performance. On the other hand, another study, in which male soldiers were on three different energy intake levels (1,800, 3,200, 4,200 kcal/day) while performing a sustained physical activity for one week, resulted in reduced maximal aerobic power and endurance only when consuming the lowest energy diet (1,800 kcal/day) (Guezennec et al., 1994).

Despite the seemingly contradictory results and different study designs, the data available suggest that moderate levels of weight loss (3–5 percent) have limited ill effects on the ability of soldiers to perform military tasks. The recent IOM report (2006) *Nutrient Composition of Rations for Short-Term, High-Intensity Combat Operations*, recommends that a hypocaloric ration should be used in a continuous manner during sustained operations (repetitive three- to seven-day missions with one- to three-day resting periods during which dining facilities are available) only if soldiers' weight is maintained within 10 percent of the original weight. The committee recommended that any soldier who loses more than 10 percent of his original weight not be sent to sustained operations again until he regains no less than 5 percent of his original weight.

In that same report, the committee concluded that for optimization of military performance under very short periods of time a ration with the appropriate mixture of macronutrients and micronutrients was more critical than a ration for maximizing energy intake. The available scientific data support the development of a high-protein, high-carbohydrate ration to optimize soldiers' physical and cognitive performance during short-time sustained operations. The committee recommendations, however, were limited by the scarce data available, especially in regard to specific nutrients; nevertheless, the committee recognized that preliminary data show promise for some nutrients and dietary supplements. More studies need to be conducted so that rations will continue to improve; it is particularly important that military situations in which stress and intense exercise are a daily constant be emulated in such studies.

According to the IOM report (2006), the micronutrients warranting further study are vitamins C and E; the B vitamins; and minerals, including zinc, selenium, iron, and copper. Their potential contribution to antioxidant systems, immune systems, and physical and cognitive performance is a subject of debate. There is less scientific certainty on the effects of other potential bioactive substances, such as creatine.

In addition to nutrient level and energy content, other factors—including time of meal ingestion; content of the previous meal; and psychosomatic factors that affect acceptability of the ration—might influence soldiers' eating behavior and military performance. These additional factors might explain the previously described divergent results on performance effects of eating meals with varying energy intake.

### *Effects of Mineral Status*

Minerals are essential nutrients, and researchers have observed the signs and symptoms that develop as a result of inadequate status from poor intake or from various diseases. Even when deficiencies are marginal, physical and cognitive functions that are important to military performance might be affected. Although not studied in military situations, adverse outcomes due to profound mineral deficiencies could include impairment of the immune system, decreased work productivity, increased prevalence of infections, cognitive decrements, and sleep disturbances. There is little known about the potential effects of nutritional or pharmacological interventions with dietary minerals intended either to restore normal mineral status or to enhance the status with the goal of improving a particular function (e.g., the immune responses to infection).

As explained by Friedl (2005; see Appendix B), there is no clear and direct evidence that marginal deficiencies among military personnel affect their physical or cognitive performance. The lack of evidence, however, might stem from the fact that many variables have not been taken into account or obscure other effects. For example, as stated previously, dietary intake data are limited and, moreover, data have seldom been collected by gender. Given the different requirements and activities of men and women, the absence of data by gender is an impediment when attempting to describe mineral intake and potential effects of deficiencies. Furthermore, the mineral status of "at-risk" populations (e.g., physically active women and their need for iron) has not been evaluated routinely, and therefore, the relationship between mineral status and performance of subgroups within the military cannot be established with a high level of confidence.

Many of the field-related activities and scenarios common during military life could have a measurable impact on soldiers' mineral status. For instance, higher-than-normal sweat losses or minerals redistribution among body compartments due to exercise or stress might increase the need (and therefore requirement) for certain minerals. Because numerous studies have linked certain mineral deficiencies with decreased work productivity, higher prevalences of infection, and cognitive decrements in the general population, there is interest in ensuring soldiers' optimal mineral status. Unfortunately, many of the studies on minerals and these outcomes have been conducted with children and often in developing countries where other nutrient deficiencies prevail. Even in studies that are conducted with adults, extrapolation to unique military circumstances is challenging at best. Nevertheless, the idea that mineral status could be an important factor in maintaining a soldier's performance is an interesting proposition that needs to be explored.

One of the studies performed during Ranger training provides some interesting results regarding the effect of exercise on mineral status. As indicated by Friedl (2005; see Appendix B), within the first few weeks of the exercise and training course male subjects experienced a decrease in iron status, however, their iron status was corrected by the end of the course. Likewise there were no differences in zinc or copper status between the baseline and the end of the training course. The author explains that periodic re-feeding corrected any deficiencies and that the loss of muscle mass in this study would have provided a steady supply of minerals and nutrients into the circulation.

Thus, even though the direct link between mineral deficiency and performance decrements in the military has not been established, enough scientific data derived from studies on the general population are available to suggest that a more in depth analysis of the potential link is warranted (see Appendix B). Furthermore, the limited military data available suggest that dietary intake for some minerals might not be adequate and that mineral status might be compromised by the multiple stressors of military activity.

### *Effects of Sleep Deprivation*

Anecdotal evidence indicates that during garrison training, soldiers generally do not suffer from sleep deprivation. However, as indicated in the IOM report (2006) *Nutrient Composition of Rations for Short-Term, High-Intensity Combat Operations*, surveys conducted in the field during combat missions point to frequent instances of sleep deprivation (e.g., some soldiers sleep an average of 4 h/day; most of them, however, sleep 5–6 h/day). A recent CMNR report included a review on the consequences of sleep deprivation on military personnel (IOM, 2004b). The efficiency of combatants in sustained operations can be compromised significantly by inadequate sleep (Krueger, 1991). The 2006 IOM report noted that by the end of three days without sleep, combat service members may be considered totally ineffective in the operational setting, especially if they are performing complex tasks such as operating computerized command-and-control centers. Although three days of sleep deprivation are rare in scenarios of sustained operations, decreases in cognitive function still may be expected since assault operations provide shortening of sleep time and can last up to a month. Likewise, even though it appears that a major loss of sleep during training is not usual, one can imagine that, at times, unpredictable events can happen during battle and wartime and, consequently, sleep deprivation can occur. Critical abilities such as vigilance and attention suffer, reaction time is impaired, mood declines, and some personnel begin to experience perceptual disturbances. Numerous studies have demonstrated that cognitive abilities as well as marksmanship are compromised, both of which can have irreversible, adverse consequences. Interestingly, when task durations extend beyond 15 to 20 minutes, performance deteriorations from fatigue become far more pronounced than when the task durations are shorter (Caldwell and Ramspott, 1998; Wilkinson, 1969; Wilkinson et al., 1966). Despite the fact that not all types of performance are affected to the same degree by sleep loss, fatigue from prolonged duty periods clearly jeopardizes unit readiness in the operational context. This is especially the case for tasks that are not only lengthy but also boring or devoid of performance feedback.

### *Effects of Stress*

The stress response consists of two major components—the neuroendocrine arm, or hypothalamic-pituitary-adrenal axis; and the adrenergic arm, comprising the sympathetic nervous system and adrenal medulla. Together these organs and nerves release a cascade of hormones: hypothalamic corticotropin releasing hormone (CRH), pituitary adrenocorticotropin, and adrenal glucocorticoids; and the adrenergic neurotransmitters and hormones (norepinephrine and adrenalin) that jointly constitute the physiological stress response. At the same time as the stress response is activated, the parasympathetic cholinergic mediated responses (such as digestion and gut motility) are generally inhibited (Marques-Deak et al., 2005).

Activation of the stress response and inhibition of the cholinergic nervous system set into motion a series of behavioral, physiological, and metabolic responses that prepare the organism to fight or flee. These behavioral changes include focused attention, increased vigilance, and inhibition of appetitive behaviors (including eating and drinking). At the same time, some aspects of the immune response are enhanced, and white blood cells are mobilized from immune organs and carried to injury sites (Viswanathan and Dhabhar, 2005). Although such effects are beneficial in acute stress situations, such as those that occur under assault conditions, long-term chronic stress can be detrimental to health.

During chronic stress, immune responses generally are suppressed, or shifted from a TH1 (cellular) pattern to a TH2 (humoral) pattern of immunity. Pro-inflammatory cytokine production is suppressed, and anti-inflammatory cytokine production is enhanced. At a clinical level, chronically stressed individuals show decreased antibody production to vaccination, prolonged wound-healing, and greater severity of viral infection (Cohen et al., 1997; Glaser and Kiecolt-Glaser, 2005).

Both acute and chronic stress may affect nutritional status by suppressing appetite, food intake, and digestion and by changing nutrient metabolism. In addition, nutrient metabolism and decreased food and water intake can indirectly alter immune responses and susceptibility and resistance to infection. During chronic stress, the stress response may shift from a primarily CRH-driven stress response to one that is driven by vasopressin and may be, therefore, associated with alterations in thirst, salt preference, and drinking behavior.

While the stress hormones and mediators alter appetite and feeding behavior, they also alter metabolism. Glucocorticoids increase gluconeogenesis and glucose mobilization, amino acid absorption, and protein metabolism (Barthel and Schmoll, 2003; Elnif et al., 2005; Nzang Nguema et al., 2005). Inhibition of cholinergic systems during acute stress slows gut motility and delays digestion and absorption (Chang et al., 2003).

Furthermore, activation of the stress response, and the concomitant release of stress hormones (glucocorticoids) and noradrenergic neurotransmitters and adrenalin, directly affects immune responses; glucocorticoids tend to suppress immunity (Webster et al., 2002), and adrenergic mediators tend to enhance immunity (Sanders, 2005). In addition, the cholinergic nervous system directly affects inflammation—the activation of the cholinergic pathways is generally anti-inflammatory (Pavlov and Tracey, 2005). The time-course and intensity of stress, whether acute, sub-acute, or repetitive (chronic), affect these outcome measures differently. Acute stress may enhance immunity, particularly delayed-type hypersensitivity (Dhabhar and Viswanathan, 2005). Repetitive stress without adequate recovery time between stress episodes (chronic stress) tends to suppress immunity (Glaser and Kiecolt-Glaser, 2005). Also different types of stress—whether physiological (pain, blood loss, dehydration, sleep deprivation) or psychological—may differentially activate neural pathways and different effector arms of the stress response, and thus may differentially affect appetite, thirst and drinking behavior, and immune responses (Li and Sawchenko, 1998).

Consequently, in optimizing nutrition in garrison training or combat, these physiological constraints should be taken into account. The decrease in caloric intake and change in drinking behavior and taste that personnel experience in the field may not be voluntary but might be, at least in part, related to activation of the stress response, which is in turn necessary for optimal performance. In this case, attempts to voluntarily increase intake may not be successful. Therefore, rations should be designed taking into account this acute altered physiological status and should not tax the system's coping ability. Such strategies are important in preventing further compromise, since extreme weight loss in itself may further suppress immune function (IOM, 1999).

## DEVELOPMENT AND USE OF MILITARY NUTRIENT STANDARDS

The U.S. Army's Surgeon General has the responsibility of establishing and overseeing two different types of nutrient standards for military personnel: (1) the MDRI for military feeding and (2) nutritional standards for operational rations (NSORs). The current military standards, as well as the RDAs and AIs for the general population, are shown in Table 1-1. The military standards apply to hospital and other food service programs and to the Department of Defense Combat Feeding Program.

The Surgeon General also must identify the effects of environmental factors on energy and nutrient requirements. As scientific information is gathered and new standards for the general population are updated, the Surgeon General is responsible for revising the military nutrition standards and ensuring that nutrient composition of the rations and planned menus meet the military standards. The current military nutrient standards (MDRIs and NSORs) were revised in 2001 (U.S. Departments of the Army, Navy, and Air Force, 2001). The standards were based on the recommendations for the U.S. general population as described in various IOM reports (IOM 1997, 2000b; NRC, 1989). The MRDIs are mostly identical to those used for the general population, except for cases in which the idiosyncrasies of the military environment call for different criteria to be considered. For example, working in a hot environment (as is often the case in recent years), results in larger losses of fluids, sodium, and potassium; these situations call for higher intake of those electrolytes, as described in Army Regulation 40-25 (U.S. Departments of the Army, Navy, and Air Force, 2001).

MDRIs are intended for use by nutritional specialists to develop menus and ensure adequate nutrition of military personnel. The use of MDRIs to plan menus for individuals or groups has proven to be a complex exercise; as such, it requires the involvement of nutritional experts that are versed in the development of nutrient standards, as well as in the uncertainties and limitations of IOM's nutrient standards. Failure to apply the standards appropriately could result in menus with inadequate nutrient content, and as a result, might lead to adverse consequences, including health and performance decrements. Two IOM reports (IOM, 2000a, 2003) provide advice and examples of appropriate processes to use when planning and assessing menus and rations. The advice in those reports must be applied correctly for the planning and assessment to be appropriate for and beneficial to the military.

The NSORs are specifications for the nutrient composition of rations consumed by military personnel involved in diverse off-base military activities—ranging from field training exercises to combat missions. These nutrient specifications are designed to maintain health and performance over multiple days of continuous subsistence. In practice, the rations are used in many ways. For example, during one-day training activities, soldiers might have breakfast in the cafeteria, operational rations for lunch at the training site, and dinner again in the cafeteria. However, the primary intended use of operational rations is during combat missions where there is no fixed military facility to provide meal service.

The NSOR specifications are used by both designers and manufacturers of combat rations. They represent the minimal levels of nutrients that should be in the ration. There are two types of NSORs. The first apply to standard operational rations which are intended to be nutritionally complete (if consumed as indicated) and can be used for long periods of time. The second apply to specialized rations in situations where mission requirements impose size, weight and/or water content limitations to the ration composition that significantly restrict energy and nutrient density. These restricted energy rations are inappropriate as a sole, continuous, long-term source of subsistence.

To provide some flexibility to ration designers but to avoid potential adverse effects of inadequate intakes, the average meal menu should meet one-third of the NSOR level but no single meal menu should be 20 percent above (if standard is a maximum, such as for sodium) or below (if standard is a minimum, such as for vitamin C) one-third of the NSOR limits (Baker-Fulco et al., 2001). For essential minerals, which are the nutrients of interest for the current task, the standards have been set at the highest gender-specific RDA or AI for adults. The NSORs for restricted rations are set arbitrarily by the military at 50 percent of the corresponding operational ration standard for each nutrient.

Rations developers who use these standards also consider other food-related factors—such as bioavailability and storage losses of nutrients—that may influence the actual nutrient level needed in the food items.

## REFERENCES


Arsenault J, Kennedy J. 1999. Dietary supplement use in U.S. Army Special Operations candidates. *Mil Med* 164(7):495–501.

Askew EW, Claybaugh JR, Cucinell SA, Young AJ, Szeto EG. 1986. *Nutrient Intakes and Work Performance of Soldiers During Seven Days of Exercise at 7,200 Ft Altitude Consuming the Meal, Ready-to-Eat Ration.* Technical Report T3-87. Fort Detrick, MD: U.S. Army Medical Research and Development Command.

Baker-Fulco CJ. 2005 (June 13). *Derivation of the Military Dietary Reference Intakes and the Mineral Content of Military Rations.* Paper presented at the Institute of Medicine Workshop on The Mineral Requirements for Cognitive and Physical Performance of Military Personnel, Washington, DC: Institute of Medicine Committee on Mineral Requirements for Cognitive and Physical Performance of Military Personnel.

Baker-Fulco CJ, Bathalon GP, Bovill ME, Lieberman HR. 2001. *Military Dietary Reference Intakes: Rationale for Tables Values.* Technical Report TN-00/10. Natick, MA: U.S. Army Research Insitute of Environmental Medicine.

Baker-Fulco CJ, Kramer FM, Lesher LL, Merrill E, Johnson J, DeLany J. 2002. *Dietary Intakes of Female and Male Combat Support Hosptial Personnel Subsisting on Meal-Focused or Standard Versions of the Meal, Ready-to-Eat.* Technical Report T-01/23. Natick, MA: U.S. Army Research Institute of Environmental Medicine.

Barthel A, Schmoll D. 2003. Novel concepts in insulin regulation of hepatic gluconeogenesis. *Am J Physiol Endocrinol Metab* 285(4):E685–E692.

Booth CK, Coad RA, Forbes-Ewan CH, Thomson GF, Niro PJ. 2003. The physiological and psychological effects of combat ration feeding during a 12-day training exercise in the tropics. *Mil Med* 168(1):63–70.

Bulbulian R, Heaney JH, Leake CN, Sucec AA, Sjoholm NT. 1996. The effect of sleep deprivation and exercise load on isokinetic leg strength and endurance. *Eur J Appl Physiol Occup Physiol* 73(3–4):273–277.

Caldwell JA, Ramspott S. 1998. Effects of task duration on sensitivity to sleep deprivation using the multi-attribute task battery. *Behav Res Method Instr Comp* 30(4):651–660.

Chang HY, Mashimo H, Goyal RK. 2003. Musings on the wanderer: What's new in our understanding of vago-vagal reflex? IV. Current concepts of vagal efferent projections to the gut. *Am J Physiol Gastrointest Liver Physiol* 284(3):G357–G366.

Cohen S, Line S, Manuck SB, Rabin BS, Heise ER, Kaplan JR. 1997. Chronic social stress, social status, and susceptibility to upper respiratory infections in nonhuman primates. *Psychosom Med* 59(3):213–221.

Consolazio CF, Matoush LO, Nelson RA. 1966. *The Caloric Requirements of Men Performing Moderate Physical Activities at 3475 Meters.* Technical Report 295. Denver, CO: U.S. Army Medical Research and Nutrition Laboratory.

Consolazio CF, Matoush LO, Johnson HL, Nelson RA, Krzywicki HJ. 1967. Metabolic aspects of acute starvation in normal humans (10 days). *Am J Clin Nutr* 20(7):672–683.

Dhabhar FS, Viswanathan K. 2005. Short-term stress experienced at time of immunization induces a long-lasting increase in immunologic memory. *Am J Physiol Regul Integr Comp Physiol* 289(3):R738–R744.

Edwards JSA, Askew EW, King N, Fulco CS, Hoyt RW, Delany JP. 1991. *An Assessment of the Nutritional Intake and Energy Expenditure of Unacclimatized U.S. Army Soldiers Living and Working at High Altitude.* Technical Report No. T10-91. Natick, MA: U.S. Army Medical Research and Development Command.

Elnif J, Buddington RK, Hansen NE, Sangild PT. 2005. Cortisol increases the activities of intestinal apical membrane hydrolases and nutrient transporters before weaning in mink (Mustela vison). *J Comp Physiol [B]* :1–9.

Friedl KE. 2005 (June 13). *Concerns About the Effects of Military Environments on Mineral Metabolism and Consequences of Marginal Deficiencies to Performance.* Paper presented at the Institute of Medicine Workshop on Mineral Requirements for Cognitive and Physical Performance of Military Personnel, Washington, DC: Institute of Medicine Committee on Mineral Requirements for Cognitive and Physical Performance of Military Personnel.

Glaser R, Kiecolt-Glaser JK. 2005. Stress-induced immune dysfunction: Implications for health. *Nat Rev Immunol* 5(3):243–251.

Guezennec CY, Satabin P, Legrand H, Bigard AX. 1994. Physical performance and metabolic changes induced by combined prolonged exercise and different energy intakes in humans. *Eur J Appl Physiol Occup Physiol* 68(6):525–530.

Haslam DR. 1982. Sleep loss, recovery sleep, and military performance. *Ergonomics* 25(2):163–178.

IOM (Institute of Medicine). 1997. *Dietary Reference Intakes for Calcium, Phosphorus, Magnesium, Vitamin D, and Fluoride.* Washington, DC: National Academy Press.

IOM. 1999. *Military Strategies for Sustainment of Nutrition and Immune Function in the Field.* Washington, DC: National Academy Press.

IOM. 2000a. *Dietary Reference Intakes. Applications in Dietary Assessment.* Washington, DC: National Academy Press.

IOM. 2000b. *Dietary Reference Intakes for Vitamin C, Vitamin E, Selenium, and Carotenoids.* Washington, DC: National Academy Press.

IOM. 2001. *Dietary Reference Intakes for Vitamin A, Vitamin K, Arsenic, Boron, Chromium, Copper, Iodine, Iron, Manganeses, Molybdenum, Nickel, Silicon, Vanadium, and Zinc.* Washington, DC: National Academy Press.

IOM. 2002/2005. *Dietary Reference Intakes for Energy, Carbohydrate, Fiber, Fat, Fatty Acids, Cholesterol, Protein, and Amino Acids.* Washington, DC: The National Academies Press.

IOM. 2003. *Dietary Reference Intakes. Applications in Dietary Planning.* Washington, DC: The National Academies Press.

IOM. 2004a. *Dietary Reference Intakes Tables—The Complete Set.* [Online]. Available: http://www.iom.edu/Object.File/Master/21/372/0.pdf [accessed February 24, 2005].

IOM. 2004b. *Monitoring Metabolic Status. Predicting Decrements in Physiological and Cognitive Performance.* Washington, DC: The National Academies Press.

IOM. 2006. *Nutrient Composition of Rations for Short-Term, High-Intensity Combat Operations.* Washington, DC: The National Academies Press.

Johnson HL, Sauberlich HE. 1982. *Prolonged Use of Operational Rations: A Review of the Literature.* San Francisco, CA: U.S. Department of Agriculture and Letterman Army Institute of Research.

King N, Arsenault JE, Mutter SH, Champagne C, Murphy TC, Westphal KA, Askew EW. 1994. *Nutritional Intake of Female Soldiers During the U.S. Army Basic Combat Training.* Technical Report T94-17. Natick, MA: U.S. Army Research Institute of Environmental Medicine.

Krueger GP. 1991. Sustained military performance in continuous operations: Combatant fatigue, rest and sleep needs. In: Gal R, Mangelsdorff AD, eds. *Handbook of Military Psychology.* New York: John Wiley & Sons. Pp. 255–277.

Li HY, Sawchenko PE. 1998. Hypothalamic effector neurons and extended circuitries activated in "neurogenic" stress: A comparison of footshock effects exerted acutely, chronically, and in animals with controlled glucocorticoid levels. *J Comp Neurol* 393(2):244–266.

Marques-Deak A, Cizza G, Sternberg E. 2005. Brain-imune interactions and disease susceptibility. *Mol Psychiat* e-pub February 1:1–12.

Montain SJ. 2006. Physiological demands of combat operations. In: Institute of Medicine, *Nutrient Composition of Rations for Short-Term, High-Intensity Combat Operations.* Washington, DC: The National Academies Press. Pp. 169–180.

Montain SJ, Young AJ. 2003. Diet and physical performance. *Appetite* 40(3):255–267.

Moore RJ, Friedl KE, Kramer TR, Martinez-Lopez LE, Hoyt RW, Tulley RE, DeLany JP, Askew EW, Vogel JA. 1992. *Changes in Soldier Nutritional Status & Immune Function During the Ranger Training Course*. Technical Report T13-92. Natick, MA: U.S. Army Medical Research and Development Command.

Nindl BC, Leone CD, Tharion WJ, Johnson RF, Castellani JW, Patton JF, Montain SJ. 2002. Physical performance responses during 72 h of military operational stress. *Med Sci Sports Exerc* 34(11):1814–1822.

NRC (National Research Council). 1989. *Recommended Dietary Allowances*. 10th ed. Washington, DC: National Academy Press.

Nzang Nguema G, Boghossian S, Dardevet D, Grizard J, Alliot J. 2005. Effect of treatment with dexamethasone on protein intake in adult and old Lou/c/jall rats. *Mech Ageing Dev* 126(6–7): 655–663.

Pavlov VA, Tracey KJ. 2005. The cholinergic anti-inflammatory pathway. *Brain Behav Immun* 19(6):493–499.

Radimer KL. 2003. National nutrition data: Contributions and challenges to monitoring dietary supplement use in women. *J Nutr* 133(6):2003S–2007S.

Rognum TO, Vartdal F, Rodahl K, Opstad PK, Knudsen-Baas O, Kindt E, Withey WR. 1986. Physical and mental performance of soldiers on high- and low-energy diets during prolonged heavy exercise combined with sleep deprivation. *Ergonomics* 29(7):859–867.

Sanders VM. 2005. Epigenetic regulation of Th1 and Th2 cell development. *Brain Behav Immun* October 10:E-pub ahead of print.

Shippee R, Friedl K, Kramer T, Mays M, Popp K, Askew E, Fairbrother B, Hoyt R, Vogel J, Marchitelli L, Frykman P, Martinez-Lopez L, Bernton E, Kramer M, Tulley R, Rood J, Delany J, Jezior D, Arsenault J. 1994. *Nutritional and Immunological Assessment of Ranger Students With Increased Caloric Intake*. Technical Report T95-5. Fort Detrick, MD: U.S. Army Medical Research and Materiel Command.

Singh A, Failla ML, Deuster PA. 1994. Exercise-induced changes in immune function: Effects of zinc supplementation. *J Appl Physiol* 76(6):2298–2303.

Singh A, Papanicolaou DA, Lawrence LL, Howell EA, Chrousos GP, Deuster PA. 1999. Neuroendocrine responses to running in women after zinc and vitamin E supplementation. *Med Sci Sports Exerc* 31(4):536–542.

Sobal J, Marquart LF. 1994. Vitamin/mineral supplement use among athletes: A review of the literature. *Int J Sport Nutr* 4(4):320–334.

Tharion WJ, Cline AD, Hotson N, Johnson W, Niro P, Baker-Fulco CJ, McGraw S, Shippee RL, Skibinski TM, Hoyt RW, Delany JP, Tulley RE, Rood J, Santee WR, Boquist SHM, Bordic M, Kramer M, Slade SH, Lieberman HR. 1997. *Nutritional Challenges for Field Feeding in a Desert Envrionment: Use of the Unitized Group Ration (UGR) and a Supplemental Carbohydrate Beverage*. Natick, MA: U.S. Army Medical Research and Materiel Command.

Tharion WJ, Baker-Fulco CJ, McGraw S, Johnson WK, Niro P, Warber JP, Kramer FM, Allen R, Champagne CM, Falco C, Hoyt RW, Delny JP, Lesher LL. 2000. *The Effects of 60 Days of Tray Ration Consumption in Marine Combat Engineers While Deployed on Great Inagua Island, Bahamas*. Technical Report T00-16. Natick, MA: U.S. Army Medical Research and Materiel Command.

Tharion WJ, Baker-Fulco CJ, Bovill ME, Montain SM, DeLany JP, Champagne CM, Hoyt RW, Lieberman HR. 2004. Adequacy of garrison feeding for Special Forces soldiers during training. *Mil Med* 169(6):483–490.

Tharion WJ, Lieberman HR, Montain SJ, Young AJ, Baker-Fulco CJ, Delany JP, Hoyt RW. 2005. Energy requirements of military personnel. *Appetite* 44(1):47–65.

Thomas CD, Friedl KE, Mays MZ, Mutter SH, Moore RJ, Jezior DA, Baker-Fulco CJ, Marchitelli LJ, Tulley RT, Askew EW. 1995. *Nutrient Intakes and Nutritional Status of Soldiers Consuming the Meal, Ready-to-Eat (MREXII) During a 30-Day Field Training Exercise.* Technical Report T95-6. Natick, MA: U.S. Army Research Institute of Environmental Medicine.

U.S. Departments of the Army, Navy, and Air Force. 2001. *Nutrition Standards and Education.* AR 40-25/BUMEDINST 10110.6/AFI 44-141. Washington, DC: U.S. Department of Defense Headquarters.

VanHelder T, Radomski MW. 1989. Sleep deprivation and the effect on exercise performance. *Sports Med* 7(4):235–247.

Viswanathan K, Dhabhar FS. 2005. Stress-induced enhancement of leukocyte trafficking into sites of surgery or immune activation. *Proc Natl Acad Sci* 102(16):5808–5813.

Webster JI, Tonelli L, Sternberg EM. 2002. Neuroendocrine regulation of immunity. *Ann Rev Immunol* 20:125–163.

Wilkinson R. 1969. Some factors influencing the effect of environmental stressors upon performance. *Psychol Bull* 72(4):260–272.

Wilkinson RT, Edwards RS, Haines E. 1966. Performance following a night of reduced sleep. *Psychon Sci* 5(12):471–472.

Yore MM, Bell NS, Senier L, Amoroso PJ. 2000. Progress toward attainment of the *Healthy People 2000* objectives in the U.S. Army: Measured by health risk appraisal results. *Am J Prev Med* 19(2):87–93.

# 2

# Military Dietary Reference Intakes: Process to Establish, Uses, and Delivery Methods

Nutrient standards are developed to ensure that different populations' (individuals or groups) nutrients needs are met—they serve as criteria for dietary nutrient adequacy. In the United States, the Dietary Reference Intakes (DRIs) recommended in various Institute of Medicine (IOM) reports (IOM, 1997, 1998a, 2000b, 2001, 2002/2005, 2005) are used as the nutrient standards to ensure a healthy U.S. population (see Table 1-1). The DRIs are comprised of the following four nutrient-based reference values established by gender and age group—the Estimated Average Requirement (EAR), the Recommended Dietary Allowance (RDA), the Adequate Intake (AI), and the Tolerable Upper Intake Level (UL).

The IOM EARs and RDAs are the average intake levels that meet respectively the requirements of 50 and 97–98 percent of the healthy individuals in a population in a particular life stage and gender group. An RDA is the reference value—derived mathematically from the EAR population distribution—for planning individual intakes. If an EAR cannot be determined because of a lack of experimental data (e.g., balance studies), then the AI (estimated intake by a population, based on observed or experimentally determined approximations of nutrient intakes) is used for planning individual intakes. The IOM UL is the highest intake level likely to pose no risk of an adverse health effect to almost all individuals. As mentioned previously, changes in the DRIs are the prerogative of the IOM DRI committee and will be considered and applied as new relevant information becomes available.

Military personnel engage in activities that may require higher intakes of specific nutrients to maintain health. If the objective is not only to maintain health, like with the IOM DRIs but also to optimize performance, then the nutrient needs might change even more. The establishment of standards specific to the military population requires not only expertise in nutrient metabolism but also in-depth knowledge of the military scenarios and factors that need to be considered thereof. Such standards—the Military Dietary Reference Intakes (MDRIs) and the nutritional standards for operational rations (NSORs)—were last published in 2001 Army Regulation (AR) 40-25 (U.S. Departments of the Army, Navy, and Air Force, 2001) before the publication of numerous IOM reports, including those that have provided revised IOM DRI values for some minerals (IOM, 2001). Table 1-1 in Chapter 1 shows the MDRIs, the NSORs, and the IOM RDAs (or AIs) for men and women.

MDRIs are intended to serve menu developers and other nutritional specialists with ensuring adequate nutrition of military personnel during garrison activities, that is, when the personnel are eating primarily from cafeteria-style menus in dining facilities, not from operational rations. In contrast, the NSORs have been established to represent the minimal levels of nutrients that operational rations should contain; these levels would provide adequate nutrition for most military personnel doing moderate or intense physical activity and are based on the MDRIs (see Chapter 1). AR 40-25 (U.S. Departments of the Army, Navy, and Air Force, 2001)—the 2001 regulation stating the MDRIs and NSORs—will be revised soon (Baker-Fulco, 2005; see Appendix B) to possibly reflect updated DRI values that take into account new EARs (e.g., for iron and zinc) or nutrients previously without MDRIs (e.g., copper and manganese). The 2001 MDRIs were based entirely on the DRIs but were applied to the military population, which in general tends to be a little heavier and more active than the U.S. population (Baker-Fulco, 2005; see Appendix B). Many of the MDRI values are similar to the DRIs, with the notable exception of sodium. Although the following discussion on the process of establishing mineral standards for the military might be applicable to other nutrients, the Committee on Mineral Requirements for Cognitive and Physical Performance of Military Personnel has focused its deliberations on standards for minerals, therefore, these recommendations apply mainly to the establishment of mineral standards.

There are two main types of feeding schedules in the military: garrison and operational rations. Garrison feeding refers to food consumption by military personnel who are under a variety of scenarios that range from administrative duties (e.g., office workers completing physically inactive tasks) to support tasks performed by personnel (e.g., hospital personnel involved in moderate levels of activity) to soldiers training for or performing missions while living on a military base (e.g., Rangers training at high levels of physical activity).

Operational feeding refers to the consumption of either full- or restricted-calorie rations while engaged in military operations (e.g., sustained operations as defined in Chapter 3) or training. The MDRIs are used to establish the NSORs for full-calorie, standard operational rations as well as for restricted-calorie rations. There is an expectation that operational rations will be used by men and woman who undergo much more rigorous physical activity than the average person in the same age range in the U.S. general population.

This report is concerned with soldiers in garrison who perform a moderate- to high-level of physical activity (referred to throughout the report as "garrison training" and defined in Chapter 3) and with soldiers in sustained operations while eating operational rations [i.e., first strike rations (FSRs)].

## MILITARY NUTRIENT STANDARDS

### Is There a Need for Specific Military Nutrient Standards?

Because of the different environmental and physiological circumstances often encountered by the Armed Forces, the MDRIs (traditionally variants of the IOM DRIs) have been developed to plan appropriate intakes and rations for enlisted personnel. There are several good reasons to establish the MDRIs, distinct from the IOM DRIs for the U.S. general population.

First, the reference anthropometric standards for the military are different from those for civilians. The reference military person is slightly different in height, weight, and body fat and lean mass compared to the civilian person. Second, the MDRIs are targeted to individuals who are 17–50 years old, the age range of the vast majority of enlisted men and women (for those who are 17–18 years old, AR 40-25 includes exceptions to the MDRI levels, indicated as footnotes to the MDRI tables) (U.S. Departments of the Army, Navy, and Air Force, 2001). The MDRIs are stated as a single value for men and women when they are used to establish NSOR, that is, the highest gender-specific reference value for 17–50 year olds is used. The MDRIs could be adapted for specifying different recommendations for males and females, should that be necessary. There are no ULs specifically for the military, because the UL values are judged to be the same as those for civilians.

Second, the process of developing the MDRIs involves examination and deliberation about the specific requirements of the military, not taken into account when establishing the DRI for the general population. For example, MDRIs specify appropriate nutrient intakes in especially stressful environments (e.g., those with extremes in weather) or under different levels of activity. Other groups within the military that might need special nutrient requirements are those consuming calorie-reduction diets or suffering from illnesses, such as infections or those performing tasks that demand appropriate maintenance of cognitive functions (e.g., attention or alertness). Hence, it would be possible to specify conditions for various special circumstances, such as garrison training and sustained operations, each with its own idiosyncrasies that might result in different nutrient recommendations. In fact, although the MDRIs are based generally on the IOM DRIs, there are already some exceptions to them based on unique situations; the rationale for these exceptions is stated explicitly in an accompanying document (Baker-Fulco et al., 2001), which is updated periodically by the U.S. Department of Defense. As the science addressing the unique nutrient needs of the military personnel emerges, additional exceptions will have to be made, as illustrated in the mineral level recommendations listed in Chapter 3.

The importance of establishing military-specific nutrient standards lies in the fact that the MDRIs serve as a useful basis for devising menus for the troops. The MDRIs are used as a sort of minimum standard to be supplied in developing rations for which the military provides most or all of the food. This is a critical and practical application of the MDRIs. It may be that some rations' nutrient levels would be inadequate—especially when soldiers face extreme environmental or stressful situations—if the IOM DRIs for the general population were used.

The third reason for establishing and periodically revising the MDRIs is to demonstrate that the Armed Forces have duly noted and carefully considered and updated recommendations for feeding enlisted men and women. Maintaining and promoting the health of the military who are serving public interests should be among the utmost priorities and deserve the highest consideration.

**RECOMMENDATION: The MDRIs should continue to reflect the IOM DRIs. Modifications should be made to specific nutrient requirements if there is sufficient scientific evidence that circumstances call for different requirements and intakes, whether to maintain nutrient or health status or to improve performance. In particular, some recommended values for minerals should reflect enhanced mineral losses caused by high performance activity. Also, the MDRIs can be used for rations development for the individual soldier.**

### Establishment of Nutrient Military Standards

The MDRIs have not been established using the more systematic approach followed for deriving the IOM DRIs because critical experimental studies to develop them were lacking. The foundation for setting RDAs is the EAR for a given gender and life stage within a population. As mentioned previously the EAR is the nutrient intake level for a population group that would meet the needs for 50 percent of that population and should be based on appropriate experimental data that allow an estimate of average requirements. The RDA then can be set by adding two standard deviations (SDs) of the EAR to the EAR if the requirement is normally distributed. Thus, the RDA = EAR + ($2 \times SD_{EAR}$). Often the SD of the EAR's distribution is unknown, and a coefficient of variation of 10 percent around the EAR is used. In any case, it follows that establishing an EAR is necessary for setting an RDA. Although, ideally, one should collect new data under the special circumstances that occur in the military (e.g., higher energy expenditures and excessive sweating) to establish a new military EAR, it is unlikely that such data will be collected specifically for military personnel. In the absence of these data, adjustment of the existing EAR for appropriate age and sex groups may be necessary to set an RDA for military personnel. If an IOM EAR for the U.S. population does not exist, then the U.S. population's AI (which allows estimating an intake level that will be adequate for practically everyone in a particular life stage and gender) could be used as a guide to ensure adequacy. There is less confidence, however, in using an AI as a nutrient standard than there is in using an RDA. Moreover, using an AI as a criterion for planning rations and menus as well as for assessing intake adequacy presents special challenges (IOM, 2000a, 2003).

Thus, the committee urges that research studies be designed to determine the EAR adjustments needed for those nutrients whose requirements will most likely change under the environmental conditions of higher energy expenditure and stress that accompany garrison training and other unique military situations. In addition, the standard deviation of such experimental data should be derived in order to calculate an RDA for military personnel. For example, sweat losses of minerals during garrison training should be measured and factored into a new garrison-training EAR; in other words, to calculate the military standard, the IOM EAR should be modified accordingly (see the following section, *Factors Affecting Nutrient Needs for Military Personnel*, for other considerations). Using an approach that is similar to the derivation of IOM RDAs, the new military RDA for garrison training for each nutrient could be calculated by using the new EAR's standard deviation. Such an approach will result in a new level estimated to be adequate to fulfill the needs of 97–98 percent of the military personnel in garrison training. The committee concluded that the new RDAs could not appropriately be called military RDAs, because they are meant to meet the unique needs of those in garrison training, not all military personnel. For the purpose of this report, the committee will refer to these new RDAs as RDAs for military garrison training or $RDA_{MGT}$ (also $EAR_{MGT}$ or $AI_{MGT}$). The following two-part equation—using the example of mineral losses during garrison training—demonstrates how the new standard will be calculated:

1. Current IOM EAR + additional mineral sweat losses = $EAR_{MGT}$
2. $EAR_{MGT} + 2 \times SD (EAR_{MGT}) = RDA_{MGT}$

**RECOMMENDATION: Nutrient standards for the military in garrison training should be derived as follows:**

1. **$EAR_{MGT}$ = Modify the current IOM EAR by adjusting for the variable of interest (e.g., level of sweat losses)**
2. **$RDA_{MGT}$ = Add 2 × SD of the $EAR_{MGT}$, to ensure 97–98 percent of soldiers will have adequate intake**

### Factors Affecting Nutrient Needs for Military Personnel

There are at least five different ways in which nutrients deficiencies may develop: (1) reduced intake, (2) impaired intake due to disease or trauma, (3) increased losses, (4) impaired utilization, and (5) increased requirements. One or more of these factors may be involved in increasing an individual's vulnerability toward nutrient deficiency. Except for those individuals in the military who are responsible solely for administrative tasks, military life encompasses unique circumstances that, for some nutrients, may result in nutrient requirements different from those of the general population. For example, soldiers are involved routinely in training, combat, and support operations; these activities carry with them a number of stresses that are extremely demanding, both physically and mentally, for each individual. It is important to periodically examine the nutrient needs of various groups within the military and to adjust or develop new MDRIs accordingly.

In addition to any altered nutrient requirements that emerge as a result of the unique situations in military life, it is necessary to distinguish between the nutrient requirements as defined in previous IOM reports and the nutrient requirements that will be recommended in this report, which are referred to as standards for individuals for various military situations (e.g., $RDA_{MGT}$). An underlying principle of the RDAs set by the IOM is that the desired outcome was to maintain health in already healthy people; improving performance was not relevant. Following this principle, the IOM levels are based on calculations of the amounts that must be provided to meet physiological needs under relatively normal conditions. In contrast, the task given to this committee was to determine mineral requirements that sustain but also improve military performance, including physical and cognitive performance. Accordingly, the $RDA_{MGT}$ or $AI_{MGT}$ recommended by this committee have taken into account not only requirements to meet physiological needs, but also any scientific evidence that would support potential benefits of a particular nutrient level on military performance. Outcomes that have been considered by this committee are mostly those included in the cognitive and behavioral systems, immune and endocrine systems, and musculoskeletal system.

Currently the MDRIs-based NSOR are meant for the healthy military population; they are supposed to cover the needs of military personnel under operating conditions, whether simulated or actual combat. The major feature that currently distinguishes the MDRIs from the IOM DRIs is a need for additional sodium for individuals who do hard physical work. Future reiterations of the Army Regulations should reflect other unique requirements of military personnel undergoing physical exercise under stress and extreme environmental conditions.

Variables such as nutrients' bioavailability, interactions with other nutrients, and nutrient degradation due to long-term storage should be factored in when designing rations. The rations should contain at least the level of nutrients required, plus an amount of nutrient that reflects nutrients' bioavailability or losses during food processing or storage.

**RECOMMENDATION: As more evidence becomes available, the committee recommends that military nutrient standards for unique circumstances in the military (e.g., soldiers engaging in sustained operations or in garrison training) be updated periodically by considering scientific evidence from studies on the benefits of specific nutrients (e.g., for improved cognitive function) or from studies revealing altered nutrient metabolism due to military performance (e.g., increased sweat losses).**

### Use of Nutrient Military Standards

To recommend levels for mineral nutrient standards that are scientifically-based as well as practical, it is important to consider the intended use of such standards. With this in mind, the committee asked for guidance from military personnel with experience in implementing the military nutrient standards, both the 2001 MDRIs and the previous standards, the 1985 MRDAs. In addition, the committee requested opinions from military professionals (including physicians, dietitians, and Quartermaster Corps) regarding the need for distinction between the MDRIs and the IOM DRIs. The requests revealed that the MDRIs were used as basis for the NSORs, which are used for rations planning and assessment; consequently, they affect the Combat Feeding Program for both training and combat (e.g., sustained operations) more directly than they affect the menu designs or dietary counseling activities in garrison situations. In summary, there is a place for the MDRIs as nutrient standards in the context of military operations, but they are not as useful as a basis for the garrison training situations during which cafeteria-style food is offered ad libitum.

As with other dietitians, those in the military rely on the DRIs for counseling clients or for planning garrison menus. The major goal for garrison menus is to provide variety of healthy options to military personnel who eat in the dining facilities, especially for those who are trying to lose weight. Dietitians use basic and flexible menu standards; devising menus primarily by using food-based guidelines, such as the Department of the Army Pamphlet 30-22, *Operating Procedures for the Army Food Program* (U.S. Department of the Army, 2002), rather than the nutrients standard in AR 40-25 (U.S. Departments of the Army, Navy, and Air Force, 2001). Although installation commanders are told to promote a comprehensive nutrition program for all operational dining facilities through AR 30-22, *The Army Food Program* (U.S. Department of the Army, 2005), respondents to the committee's queries indicated that implementation and oversight varied greatly by commander. Food Operations Sergeants (FOS) are asked to consider nutritional adequacy in accordance with the *Nutrition Standards and Education*, AR 40-25 (U.S Department of the Army, 2002) when they make adjustments to the dining facility menus—AR 40-25 regulations are cited in various places in Department of the Army Pamphlet 30-22.

The most practical use of the IOM DRIs is in the dietary planning and assessment for populations and individuals; these uses have been described in two reports (IOM, 2000a, 2003) that illustrate the processes with practical examples. Generally, the IOM DRIs are used for planning to ensure a low prevalence of inadequate nutrient intakes. For example, the IOM DRIs can be used by an individual to plan his or her diet and food purchases or by a food service manager to plan menus for an institution. To plan menus or rations for a large group, the EAR (the average intake for nutrients by the target population) or AI and its distribution should be known. To plan diets for individuals, however, it is appropriate and sufficient to use only the RDAs. Both the group and individual planning also use the UL as well. Similar to the IOM DRIs, the MDRIs could be used to plan and assess menus for military personnel.

The difficulty in assessing the nutritional adequacy—whether nutrient composition satisfactorily will meet nutrient needs—of menus for soldiers in garrison training is the lack of data on the intake distribution. The distribution is likely to be broad when individuals are sometimes eating cafeteria food ad libitum, as soldiers do when in garrison training. This lack of data is a limitation that partially explains the fact that the MDRIs are not typically used to plan or assess menus for soldiers with free access to cafeteria food. This committee speculates that the MDRIs could be used by cafeteria menu planners as a useful benchmark for what levels of nutrients are needed in foods on the menu. However, that task is beyond the scope of this report. The IOM report *Applications in Dietary Planning* (IOM, 2003) should serve as a guide on using MDRIs for dietary planning for populations. For the present, managers should make sure that cafeteria food is nutritionally diverse and adequate and that it contains all of the food groups so as to meet an individual's MDRIs. Food service managers should include dietitians and nutritionists who also are capable of applying nutrition guides, such as the *Dietary Guidelines for Americans* (http://www.healthierus.gov/dietaryguidelines/) and MyPyramid (http://www.mypyramid.gov/), to the design of cafeteria food choices. The committee encourages studies by the military on nutrient intake distribution data that would assist the military in using the MDRIs to plan menus.

Conversely, although the nutrient intake levels for those eating rations is not known, it can be assumed safely that such levels will not vary too much if all of the rations issued are fully consumed. Under such circumstances, group-planning methods are not needed. Instead, the goal will be that each individual eating the rations gets the recommended intake, which can be expected since each individual within the group will be provided the same level of nutrient (mineral). In particular, to plan the levels of minerals in operational rations for garrison training, rations should meet the new military RDAs (e.g., $RDA_{MGT}$) for minerals, which should be established specifically depending on the operation and environment (e.g., garrison training versus sustained operations).

In this report, the assumption is made that most soldiers in military operations will consume their complete rations. Since males and females may differ in requirements, and given that the Army cannot particularize its rations, the recommended mineral amounts in the rations for groups with gender differences should be set at the highest standards. In every case, this recommended level should be lower than the UL for the age range. Accordingly, the current NSOR are established to represent the minimal levels (or those that are maximums) of nutrients in operational rations and, when adjusted as described (where the average menu meets one-third of the NSOR and no single menu is 20 percent below set minimums or above set maximums of one-third the NSOR limits [Baker-Fulco et al., 2001]), would provide adequate levels for military personnel under specific military situations.

**RECOMMENDATION: The committee supports the use of NSORs as minimum levels of minerals in operational ration; NSORs should be established based on new military RDAs (e.g., $RDA_{MGT}$), developed as new scientific data become available. The NSORs might be different for specific military situations; for example, NSORs for military garrison training and those for sustained operations might differ.**

## THREE STRATEGIES TO INCREASE NUTRIENT INTAKE

The following three basic strategies can be used to improve intake and nutritional status of enlisted personnel: food-based approaches, fortification, supplementation (IOM, 1998b). The uses, advantages, and disadvantages of each strategy are described in the following sections.

### Typical Food-Based Approaches

The most common food-based strategies to raise nutrient intake are those that encourage dietary diversification and frequent consumption of particularly nutrient-rich food sources.

#### *Uses and Advantages*

The advantages of these strategies include greater acceptability by the target population, the ability to provide many nutrients simultaneously, and the relatively low cost. Also, concentrated doses of nutrients that may be problematic or associated with toxicities are avoided. Finally, there are potentially beneficial bioactive food components that, because they are not nutrients, are not added to foods as fortificants or supplements. Food-based strategies are relatively long-term strategies if changing diets or food habits is necessary, but they can be combined with shorter-term strategies to achieve needed results. In an ideal situation—if food access, availability, and diversity were optimal—the nutrient needs of the general population would be met solely from food sources, since there are many different food combinations in diets that sustain good health. The optimal food combinations depend on the food characteristics and the larger environments, economics, and other factors (e.g., accessibility) that may apply only to the military.

There is a general perception that nutrients from food are healthier than those that come from supplements. Although it is true that some forms of vitamins and minerals are different or more bioavailable in foods than in supplements, this is not true in all cases; bioavailability varies from nutrient to nutrient. In fact, some nutrients (e.g., various forms of calcium) are more bioavailable in fortificants and supplements than they are in food form. Many constituents that exist in a food matrix may influence not only nutrient bioavailability but also their functions in the body. In general, if the diet is complete and balanced, no supplement is needed to meet the DRI. For these reasons, most nutrition science experts favor food-based strategies and dietary patterns instead of ones that emphasize dietary supplements (Lichtenstein and Russell, 2005). Also, even though it has not been possible to show a decreased incidence of cardiovascular disease or other chronic degenerative diseases with simple single-nutrient supplementation or fortification programs, total dietary patterns do seem to make a greater difference. For example, the Dietary Approaches to Stop Hypertension (DASH) diet—which uses regular food items to provide a moderate- to low-fat diet high in calcium, potassium, and magnesium (elements that have been associated with a decreased risk of heart disease)—does seem, in fact, to have a beneficial effect on blood pressure, especially when dietary sodium is also lower (Appel et al., 1997; Harsha et al., 1999).

### *Disadvantages*

One of the disadvantages associated with food-based strategies is that it is a long-term strategy; thus, when more immediate results are necessary, they may not be achievable in a short time period. A second disadvantage is that dietary strategies involving ordinary foods are rarely helpful therapeutically. Once disease is present more radical measures, including diet therapy and supplementation, are likely to be needed. Third, educators need to be involved extensively, and, if the food is not already available, then the agricultural sector must become involved to produce it. Also, long-held food beliefs, cultures, and behaviors may need to be changed. Some advocates of supplements claim that although most Americans consume enough nutrients in their diets to prevent dietary deficiency diseases, they consume less than the amount necessary for good health. While this is an interesting hypothesis, it has yet to be tested, and at present cannot be used as a justification for supplementation. Finally, it may not be possible to obtain the necessary nutrient amounts from food sources alone, so other measures may then be taken.

### Fortification

Fortification describes adding to a food nutrient levels that are above the naturally-occurring levels; in some cases, it means adding a nutrient to a food in which it normally would not be present. Restoration is a form of fortification that involves the replacement (either partial or full) of nutrients that were lost during a stage of food production or distribution. In theory, it should be possible to add pure forms of nutrients present in minimally processed foods to highly processed foods to obtain nutritional equivalency. The original food should be an important source of one or more nutrients, especially if there is nutrient inadequacy in the population group. One standard for this is that the food that provides at least 10 percent of the Daily Value for a specific nutrient (U.S. FDA, 1999).

Nutritionally improving widely consumed foods by fortification (also called enrichment), without trying to change food habits, is a common way of ensuring and improving the food supply's nutritional adequacy. This strategy also is useful when food choices are limited or when available foods are not nutritionally complete or acceptable. Other cases exist, too, when fortification may be necessary (e.g., to meet certain nutrient standards). The term *fortification* is used to refer to the addition of nutrients not only to food but also to water and salt.

Key conditions for successful fortification include the following:

- Fortification should focus as narrowly as possible on a target population. For example, when the benefits from higher nutrient intakes extend across the population, the entire population is the target, and appropriate fortification of staple foods ensures reaching the targeted population. On the other hand, when only a subgroup of the population is deficient in a nutrient, then fortification of specific foods eaten by those at risk is more appropriate. Dietary surveys may be needed to describe the amounts and distributions of nutrient intakes in the population and to identify the most suitable food vehicle.
- Fortificants must be bioavailable.
- Fortification must be acceptable from the standpoint of final food product taste and appearance, as some fortificants, such as iron salts, change food quality.
- The food vehicle used to carry a fortificant must be easily accessible and eaten regularly in portions that are large enough to provide the appropriate dose.
- The production capacity, instructions, and monitoring of fortification must be in place.

Fortification increases costs to food manufacturers because of the cost of mixing the fortificants, quality control procedures, and the cost of acquiring particular fortificants at selected levels. Foods fortified solely for the military are more costly than foods already fortified for the civilian menu because of losses in economies of scale. In the United States, most ready-to-eat breakfast cereals have been fortified voluntarily—with a range of vitamins and iron at levels of 17 to 50 percent of the RDAs—for many years (e.g., iron levels see Johnson et al., 1998). Bread and flour have been fortified not only for iron but also, in the United Kingdom, for calcium; these fortifications appear to be acceptable even at fairly high levels. Orange juice, meal-replacement products, and sport drinks are examples of other calcium-fortified foods.

*Uses and Advantages of Fortification*

Fortification is best used as a preventive strategy or to decrease the risk of nutrient inadequacy. Its time course of effect is between that of the supplement, which is relatively rapid in achieving the change in micronutrient status (owing to the high specificity and relatively high doses), and the less rapid effects observed from eating usual diets. The fortification strategy is sustainable under most conditions, and it is often cost effective as well.

Fortification is defined by statute for certain nutrients but not for others. For example fortification is used in the United States for restoring certain nutrients to flour. Enriched products in the United States have a standard of identity that requires nutrients to be added in accordance with U.S. Food and Drug Administration (FDA) regulations, for example folic acid (U.S. FDA, 1996). The FDA also specifies enrichment and fortification levels for nutrients that are known to be essential such as minerals and it is recommended that they are fortified at levels proportional to the caloric content of the food they are added to. In the majority of cases, these specifications are FDA guidelines and are not mandated. Thus, public health measures—specified by law or regulation—that rely on fortification and enrichment have clear guidelines that must be followed. No specific fortification levels are set as regulations for other nutrients (e.g., chromium, selenium, potassium) as well as for some nutrients in other foods (e.g., for calcium in orange juice).

*Disadvantages*

One of the disadvantages of fortification is that it is rarely used for more than a few nutrients. However, some nutrients occurring in foods may function better together with or only in the presence of other nutrients. For example, the B-complex vitamins have closely interrelated metabolic functions. Failure to provide sufficient dietary amounts of one or more of those nutrients that work together may impair the functions of other B vitamins. This scenario also might be true for some combinations of minerals.

The risk of excessive intakes of specific nutrients due to voluntary, market-driven food fortification or overconsumption of the fortified food is of concern, especially when the IOM UL is relatively close to the RDA. Also, there are concerns about the potential for public confusion about nutrition education messages. For example, fortifying candies and carbonated beverages is not supported fully among nutritionists because it might be perceived as sending an inconsistent message.

Another disadvantage of providing nutrients, especially minerals, in large amounts from single sources is that bioavailability may decrease when nutrient interactions are favored by the high nutrient concentrations.

## Supplementation

The FDA defines a dietary supplement as a product (other than tobacco) that adds to the diet and contains one or more of the following dietary ingredients: a vitamin; a mineral; an herb or other botanical; an amino acid; a dietary substance that supplements the diet by increasing the total daily intake; or a concentrate, metabolite, constituent, extract; or combinations of these ingredients (U.S. FDA, 1995). Dietary supplements that provide nutrients or non-nutrients by oral means come in various forms (e.g., pills and powders) other than food and beverages.

### *Uses*

International bodies, such as the Codex Alimentarius (FAO, 2005), recently have released guidelines for the use of supplements. The guidelines state that individuals should be encouraged to select a balanced diet from which sufficient amounts of the vitamins and minerals can be obtained. Hence, supplements should be used only in cases where food does not provide sufficient vitamins and minerals. The Scientists from an International Conference on Nutrition suggests that supplementation be restricted to vulnerable groups that cannot meet their nutrient needs through food alone. Such groups include women of childbearing age, infants and young children, the elderly and the poor, those who are displaced, refugees, and those in other emergency situations (FAO and WHO, 1992).

Factors to consider when choosing supplementation as a strategy include the following:

- The intake amounts that can be obtained normally from food relative to the amounts that are needed.
- The target group or population.

- The targeted individuals' willingness to consume supplements.
- The inability to use another strategy (e.g., nutrient-rich food sources or fortified foods).

*Advantages*

Supplementation is suitable for nutrient deficiency prevention in healthy individuals, but it is especially appropriate for therapeutic purposes. However, the efficacy of using dietary supplements to provide high levels of nutrients for altering chronic disease risk is less well established (Caballero, 2003). Criteria for recommending mineral supplementation vary among expert groups.

Supplementation can generate changes in micronutrient status relatively quickly. However, when compared with fortification or dietary diversification, the approach reaches relatively small numbers of consumers and requires action on the part of many individuals to comply. For some nutrients to reach the targeted individuals in sufficient amounts supplementation is justified (Perelson and Ellenbogen, 2002).

Unlike the other strategies mentioned, dietary supplements do not require major changes in the food supply, food processing, or distribution. Moreover, in a heterogeneous population, only those who are in certain age, gender, or lifestyle groups may require dietary supplements. Within these groups, further tailoring may be possible and desirable. For example, in the past there has been a one-size-fits-all recommendation that pregnant women should use iron supplements; however, it has been suggested more recently that only pregnant women who exhibit certain hematological parameters indicative of deficits should use iron supplements (IOM, 1998b). In general, the IOM reports have endorsed supplementation with specific nutrients (including the minerals) only for situations in which there is clear evidence of potential harm due to their inadequacy.

If very high levels of mineral intakes are necessary to achieve optimal health benefits, supplementation may be the only recourse. Nonetheless, the advisability of providing such high levels of nutrients must be justified, and for many nutrients (including some of the minerals) the relationship between high-nutrient levels and associated benefits is still unclear. While there is little disagreement about the usefulness of dietary supplements in boosting nutrient intake shortfalls and thus achieving IOM RDA levels (for example, in situations of weight loss or illness), the value of consuming nutrient levels higher than the IOM RDAs continues to be debated (Lichtenstein and Russell, 2005; Perelson and Ellenbogen, 2002). There is a strong consensus that intervention studies are needed to demonstrate conclusive nutrient–health benefit links before high levels of nutrients can be recommended to the general population. The proposition that taking a multivitamin mineral supplement each day is advisable to decrease the risk of chronic degenerative disease in adults is also debatable. It presents economic as well as public health concerns if the intake is beyond the UL.

*Disadvantages*

The efficacy of most supplements in preventing chronic degenerative diseases has not been demonstrated; however, they are helpful in preventing nutrient deficiency diseases (e.g., folic acid helps fight neural tube defects) and chronic degenerative disease (e.g., vitamins A, D, C, iron). Attempts at using supplements to prevent cardiovascular disease and lung cancer have been disappointing, and the evidence to date is stronger for the association between dietary patterns and decreased chronic disease risk than it is for individual nutrients.

There are other disadvantages in using supplements. When supplementary doses of nutrients are high, nutrient interactions tend to be accelerated. There might be unknown consequences from shifting the emphasis away from food and toward nutrient supplements (Caballero, 2003; Lichtenstein and Russell, 2005), in which unusual nutrient profiles could be created and lead to alteration in absorption or metabolism of other constituents. Finally, genetic polymorphisms in the population might lead not only to increased requirements and needs for nutrients but also to lower thresholds for adverse effects from large doses of nutrients.

## Combined Strategies

The Armed Forces may find it useful to consider combined strategies that involve usual diets, fortified foods, and dietary supplements—the combination could work toward a long-term goal while rapidly remedying immediate problems. In fact, a comprehensive approach could be implemented to provide preventive measures with nutrients at normal levels for the general population of soldiers and therapeutic treatment with nutrients at pharmacological levels for those with proven deficiencies.

## Complementary Public Health Measures

Regardless of the strategy adopted, complementary public health measures are also essential. For example, to prevent anemia in regions where malaria parasites (*Plasmodium falciparum)* are present in the environment, de-worming and taking antimalarial measures are vital, as is consuming iron in adequate amounts. Sanitary water and food are indispensable since intestinal disease will cause excessive malabsorption or excretion of most nutrients.

## Choosing the Best Strategies

The best choice among these strategies for raising nutrient intakes depends on several factors and varies from one nutrient to another. Considerations include the following:

- The prevalence and severity of a population's nutritional inadequacy.
- The consequences of failing to raise intakes to RDAs or other nutrient standard levels.
- The number of nutrients that require intervention.
- The time required to affect the health outcomes linked to the nutrient in question.
- The phase, appropriateness, and feasibility of the intervention.
- Other characteristics that are unique to the particular setting (e.g., the military).
- Other characteristics of the mineral under consideration.

The recent report *Nutrient Composition of Rations for Short-Term, High-Intensity Combat Operations* (IOM, 2006) offered recommendations and suggestions that address providing the appropriate amounts of nutrients to the military personnel. The three main points made by that report's committee are the following:

- Macronutrients should be provided in whole foods, and fortification and the use of supplementation should be limited to the extent possible due to the potential for nutrient interactions. The committee acknowledges the need for fortification in some cases due to the type of foods included in some rations, for example, those rations where shelf-stability is a priority.
- Fortification with labile nutrients presents unique challenges because of potential interaction with other compounds and decreased bioavailability with storage. Shelf-life should be a factor to consider when calculating the level of fortificant in the food, and encapsulation for some nutrients may be necessary.
- Because taste is an important factor in soldiers' food preferences and operational rations should be eaten entirely, providing a variety of acceptable and palatable products becomes a primary concern. Zinc, calcium, magnesium, and other nutrients have objectionable tastes to some individuals at the levels used in fortificants. Use of appropriate chemicals with better taste or encapsulation or other means to mask objectionable tastes should be given high priority for food developers.

## WATER AS A MATRIX TO INCREASE INTAKE OF MINERALS

### Background

The military promotes consumption of water during periods of heavy exercise and elevated ambient temperatures. In addition to being a potential vehicle for nutrients and hydration, water can be a feasible vehicle for providing minerals that help meet mineral requirements as long as soldiers are consuming daily 2–10 L of water. The changes in drinking water sources that occur during military deployment could affect the balance of the essential dietary minerals that are provided. The amounts of minerals in the U.S. public water supplies, in bottled water, and in field purification water may vary.

The U.S. Environmental Protection Agency (EPA) administers the tap water (drinking water) quality standards as well as those for local and state water (U.S. EPA, 2005). The EPA standards recognize that some minerals—such as heavy metals, copper, and iron—need to be regulated for high levels. In addition to enforced levels, quality factors are considered when changing the levels of minerals in water. For instance, elevated levels of calcium make most water unpalatable and difficult to use because of associated brine qualities (WHO, 2004).

Mineral levels in U.S. tap water vary in quantity depending on the origin of the freshwater supply (See Table 2-1; NRC, 1980). For example, from the National Health and Nutrition Examination Survey III (NHANES III) data on water intake, it can be calculated that individuals consuming hard water (water with high calcium and magnesium levels) can supplement their mineral intake with tap water (median intake between 900–1,000 ml/day) (IOM, 2005). Generally, this is considered advantageous if dietary sources do not provide adequate intakes (see Combs, 2005 in Appendix B; NRC, 1980). Hard water generally contains 10–500 mg/L of calcium carbonate and traces of magnesium as compared with soft water, which contains lower levels of calcium (< 10 mg/L) (WHO, 2003). This high level of calcium can be altered with water treatments, and sodium levels may be exchanged for calcium, thus providing soft water with elevated levels of sodium (NRC, 1980; WHO, 2004).

## Water Treatment

Ground or well water is treated by various methods, including filtration and chlorination. The final mineral levels depend on the source water, for example, ground water is hard water and rain water is soft water. Combination methods like filtration, reverse osmosis, and distillation are used in some parts of the world because the local water is high in salt and debris. Desalination is used to

**TABLE 2-1** U.S. Tap Water Mineral Levels

| Mineral | Typical levels (mg/L) | Higher levels (mg/L) |
|---|---|---|
| Calcium | 26.00 | 145.00 |
| Magnesium | 6.25 | 120.00 |
| Iron | 0.24 | 2.20 |
| Copper | 0.10 | 0.45 |
| Zinc | 0.20 | 1.50 |
| Selenium | 0.00 | 0.01 |
| Sodium | 28.00 | 220.00 |

SOURCE: NRC (1980).

treat water that is high in salt content, (e.g., some lakes and the ocean). Treatments such as distillation, deionization using membranes, electrodialysis, reverse osmosis, and other technologies, significantly reduce the mineral content.

Bottled water can be obtained from tap water, treated water, and other ground water sources. In the United States, bottled water standards are under the administration of the FDA (Bullers, 2002). In general, the FDA's standards for bottled water are the same as the EPA's standards for tap water. If the bottled water is labeled *purified water*, then it is manufactured by distillation, reverse osmosis, or other suitable processes that meets the definition set by the U.S. Pharmacopeia (http://www.usp.org/). Purified water has a low mineral content unless the manufacturer adds minerals especially to improve taste. There are no known health advantages from consuming bottled water except in areas where local drinking water does not meet health standards. Table 2-2 lists an example of the mineral content from bottled water prepared for the military operations in Iraq.

### Minerals and Taste

Most sensory evaluation studies indicate that low-salt waters have poor taste for most people. The addition of calcium (at least 4 meq/L of $CaSO_4$), sodium (1.5 meq/L $NaHCO_3$), and magnesium (3 meq/L of $Mg[HCO_3]$) enhanced positive taste results (Zoeteman, 1980). On the other hand, overly high levels of calcium and sodium can decrease taste acceptability. Results vary, but in general levels of calcium that are above 100 mg/L and of sodium that are above 200 mg/L (WHO, 2004; Zoeteman, 1980) are unacceptable.

In fact, when water treatment results in low mineral content, calcium and magnesium may be added back to improve taste and to prevent the leaching of

**TABLE 2-2** Mineral Content of Bottled Water in Iraq (Danone Hayat, Product of Istanbul)

| Compound | Content (mg/L) |
|---|---|
| Calcium | 25.650 |
| Magnesium | 7.050 |
| Fluoride | 0.030 |
| Chloride | 4,900 |
| Chlorine | — |
| $NH_3$ | — |
| Sulphate | 2.560 |
| $NO_2$ | — |
| Nitrate | 1.236 |
| Silica | 1.000 |
| pH | 7.480 |

SOURCE: Personal communication, J. Kent, Darnall Army Community Hospital U.S. Army, August 25 (2005).

minerals from pipes (Cotruvo, 2005; Kozisek, 2005; Monarca et al., 2005; WHO, 2004; Zoeteman, 1980). The process results in the provision of calcium and magnesium as dietary sources. The addition of dissolved salts and calcium may be around 100 mg/L and 30 mg/L, respectively (Kozisek, 2005). Another factor that might change mineral content of water is the leaching of minerals (especially of cadmium and lead depending on nature of pipe) from pipes that occurs with desalted water (Cotruvo, 2005). Finally, water might be blended, that is, some salt water is added to increase the overall salt levels after the desalination treatment. This results in an increase primarily of sodium (Cotruvo, 2005).

## Minerals in Water and Cardiovascular Disease

Many epidemiological studies have been conducted to determine if consuming hard water decreases the risk of cardiovascular diseases (Altura and Altura, 1995; Hopps and Feder, 1986; Kousa et al., 2004; Maheswaran et al., 1999; Pocock et al., 1980; Rubenowitz et al., 2000). Studies suggest an inverse relationship between calcium and magnesium concentrations in tap water and cardiovascular mortality in the United States (Hopps and Feder, 1986), England (Pocock et al., 1980), Europe (Sonneborn et al., 1983), and Finland (Kousa et al., 2004). Recently, Monarca et al. (2005) reviewed the literature between 1979 and 2003 regarding the role of calcium and magnesium content of water on prevention of cardiovascular diseases. These studies were conducted in many geographical locations and report case-studies and correlation studies between both naturally occurring hard water and water treated to reduce hardness; this entailed replacement of calcium and magnesium with sodium, an electrolyte that at high dietary levels may be related to hypertension, which might have confounded the results. Aside from this limitation, most case-control studies show and inverse relationship between mortality (but not incidence) from cardiovascular disease and magnesium levels but not calcium levels. Most studies show an inverse correlation between water hardness and mortality from cardiovascular disease, but not all. Although many of these studies have large sample sizes and include longitudinal data to document the efficacy of hard water, government agencies (Combs, 2005; see Appendix B) do not support adding calcium and magnesium to drinking water to prevent cardiovascular diseases. There are indications that reducing hard water by the substitution of calcium and magnesium with sodium replaces valuable dietary calcium and magnesium; also, high-sodium diets may be related to hypertension for some people. Apart from the studies suggesting the benefits of consuming hard water, there are no data that show increased cardiovascular disease in communities where rain water (soft water) is the primary source of drinking water (Hopps and Feder, 1986; Maheswaran et al., 1999; Pocock et al., 1980). Also, the consumption of purified water (e.g., bottled water) showed no enhancement of health except in cases where local water cannot meet U.S. EPA standards for chemical and microbiological contaminents (Bullers, 2002).

In summary, chronic consumption of soft water has been related to cardiovascular disease in some studies but not all. Altogether, these studies were not deemed strong enough for the WHO to recommend the addition of calcium and magnesium to drinking water, but they do indicate potential importance of water as a nutrient source of calcium and magnesium.

### Bioavailability

The bioavailability of each mineral from water will vary with the salt form (Hopps and Feder, 1986; Sonneborn et al., 1983). Except for some epidemiological research (see section on *Epidemiological Cardiovascular Disease Studies*), there has been little evidence showing that adding calcium and magnesium to drinking water enhances mineral nutritional status. However, calcium and magnesium in hard water are well absorbed and can provide additional sources of these nutrients to meet dietary requirements (Kozisek, 2005). This additional source may be important when other food sources of calcium and magnesium are low.

### Water Quality During Military Operations

The military's primary concern is to provide water that meets U.S. EPA standards for chemicals and microbiological levels. During foreign deployments, drinking water may come from local water supplies and undergo additional treatments, such as chlorination for bacterial control and filtration for the removal of dissolved solids. The mineral levels with this type of treated water depend on the mineral levels of the source water, that is, hard water, which is high in minerals—primarily calcium and magnesium—would retain its minerals after treatment.

In some situations, water may be treated by reverse osmosis or distillation, both of which remove minerals. Thus, as mentioned previously, most treatment plants add minerals, especially calcium and magnesium, to prevent metal leaching and to improve the water's palatability. Bottled water generally has low concentrations of minerals.

Typical levels of minerals in tap water are similar to those in bottle water used in Iraq (Table 2-1 and 2-2). Based on these typical levels, on the known treatment processes applied to water, and on the typical consumption of 3 L of water/day the committee concluded that, differences in mineral content of water would not be such that will affect the total intake levels of minerals by military personnel. The committee also concluded that the addition of calcium and magnesium to water consumed by military personnel is warranted only when improving the taste is the desirable outcome. There is no evidence to suggest that the addition of substantial levels of calcium and magnesium would be an efficient strategy to meet nutritional standards; in addition, there is little research on bioavailability of minerals from water. Additional cost evaluation of using water as a vehicle for minerals should be conducted if it is to be considered for implementation.

## REFERENCES

Altura BM, Altura BT. 1995. Magnesium and cardiovascular biology: An important link between cardiovascular risk factors and atherogenesis. *Cell Mol Biol Res* 41(5):347–359.

Appel LJ, Moore TJ, Obarzanek E, Vollmer WM, Svetkey LP, Sacks FM, Bray GA, Vogt TM, Cutler JA, Windhauser MM, Lin PH, Karanja N. 1997. A clinical trial of the effects of dietary patterns on blood pressure. DASH Collaborative Research Group. *N Engl J Med* 336(16):1117–1124.

Baker-Fulco CJ. 2005 (June 13). *Derivation of the Military Dietary Reference Intakes and the Mineral Content of Military Rations*. Paper presented at the Institute of Medicine Workshop on The Mineral Requirements for Cognitive and Physical Performance of Military Personnel, Washington, DC: Institute of Medicine Committee on Mineral Requirements for Cognitive and Physical Performance of Military Personnel.

Baker-Fulco CJ, Bathalon GP, Bovill ME, Lieberman HR. 2001. *Military Dietary Reference Intakes: Rationale for Tables Values*. Technical Report TN-00/10. Natick, MA: U.S. Army Research Institute of Environmental Medicine.

Bullers AC. 2002. Bottled water: Better than tap? [Online]. Available: http://fda.gov/fdac/features/2002/402_h2o.html [accessed January 30, 2005].

Caballero B. 2003. Fortification, supplementation, and nutrient balance. *Eur J Clin Nutr* 57(Suppl 1):S76–S78.

Combs GF. 2005 (June 13). *Drinking Water as a Source of Mineral Nutrition*. Paper presented at the Institute of Medicine Workshop on The Mineral Requirements for Cognitive and Physical Performance of Military Personnel, Washington, DC: Institute of Medicine Committee on Mineral Requirements for Cognitive and Physical Performance of Military Personnel.

Cotruvo JA. 2005. Desalination guidelines development of drinking water: Background. In: *Nutrients in Drinking Water*. Geneva: World Health Organization.

FAO (Food and Agricultural Organization). 2005. *Guidelines for Vitamin and Mineral Food Supplements*. CAC/GL 55. Rome: FAO.

FAO and WHO (World Health Organization). 1992. *International Conference on Nutrition. World Declaration and Plan of Action for Nutrition*. Rome: FAO.

Harsha DW, Lin PH, Obarzanek E, Karanja NM, Moore TJ, Caballero B. 1999. Dietary approaches to stop hypertension: A summary of study results. DASH Collaborative Research Group. *J Am Diet Assoc* 99(8 Suppl):S35–S39.

Hopps HC, Feder GL. 1986. Chemical qualities of water that contribute to human health in a positive way. *Sci Total Environ* 54:207–216.

IOM (Institute of Medicine). 1997. *Dietary Reference Intakes for Calcium, Phosphorus, Magnesium, Vitamin D, and Fluoride*. Washington, DC: National Academy Press.

IOM. 1998a. *Dietary Reference Intakes for Thiamin, Riboflavin, Niacin, Vitamin $B_6$, Folate, Vitamin $B_{12}$, Pantothenic Acid, Biotin, and Choline*. Washington, DC: National Academy Press.

IOM. 1998b. *Prevention of Micronutrient Deficiencies*. Washington, DC: National Academy Press.

IOM. 2000a. *Dietary Reference Intakes. Applications in Dietary Assessment*. Washington, DC: National Academy Press.

IOM. 2000b. *Dietary Reference Intakes for Vitamin C, Vitamin E, Selenium, and Carotenoids*. Washington, DC: National Academy Press.

IOM. 2001. *Dietary Reference Intakes for Vitamin A, Vitamin K, Arsenic, Boron, Chromium, Copper, Iodine, Iron, Manganese, Molybdenum, Nickel, Silicon, Vanadium, and Zinc*. Washington, DC: National Academy Press.

IOM. 2002/2005. *Dietary Reference Intakes for Energy, Carbohydrate, Fiber, Fat, Fatty Acids, Cholesterol, Protein, and Amino Acids*. Washington, DC: The National Academies Press.

IOM. 2003. *Dietary Reference Intakes. Applications in Dietary Planning*. Washington, DC: The National Academies Press.

IOM. 2005. *Dietary Reference Intakes for Water, Potassium, Sodium, Chloride, and Sulfate*. Washington, DC: The National Academies Press.

IOM. 2006. *Nutrient Composition of Rations for Short-Term, High-Intensity Combat Operations*. Washington, DC: The National Academies Press.

Johnson MA, Smith MM, Edmonds JT. 1998. Copper, iron, zinc, and manganese in dietary supplements, infant formulas, and ready-to-eat breakfast cereals. *Am J Clin Nutr* 67(5 Suppl):1035S–1040S.

Kousa A, Moltchanova E, Viik-Kajander M, Rytkonen M, Tuomilehto J, Tarvainen T, Karvonen M. 2004. Geochemistry of ground water and the incidence of acute myocardial infarction in Finland. *J Epidemiol Community Health* 58(2):136–139.

Kozisek F. 2005. Health risks from drinking demineralised water. In: *Nutrients in Drinking Water*. Geneva: World Health Organization.

Lichtenstein AH, Russell RM. 2005. Essential nutrients: Food or supplements? Where should the emphasis be? *J Am Med Assoc* 294(3):351–358.

Maheswaran R, Morris S, Falconer S, Grossinho A, Perry I, Wakefield J, Elliott P. 1999. Magnesium in drinking water supplies and mortality from acute myocardial infarction in north west England. *Heart* 82(4):455–460.

Monarca S, Donato F, Zerbini M. 2005. Drinking water hardness and cardiovascular diseases: A review of the epidemiological studies 1979–2004. In: *Nutrients in Drinking Water*. Geneva: World Health Organization.

NRC (National Research Council). 1980. *Drinking Water and Health*. Volume 3. Washington, DC: National Academy Press.

Perelson AM, Ellenbogen L. 2002. Rationale for use of vitamin and mineral supplements. In: Berdanier CM, Feldman EB, Flatt WP, St. Jeor ST, eds. *Handbook of Nutrition and Food*. Boca Raton, FL: CRC Press. Pp. 1333–1361.

Pocock SJ, Shaper AG, Cook DG, Packham RF, Lacey RF, Powell P, Russell PF. 1980. British Regional Heart Study: Geographic variations in cardiovascular mortality, and the role of water quality. *Br Med J* 280(6226):1243–1249.

Sonneborn M, Mandelkow J, Schon D, Hoffmeister H. 1983. Health effects of inorganic drinking water constituents, including hardness, iodide, and fluoride. *CRC Crit Rev Environ Control* 13(1):1–22.

U.S. Department of the Army. 2002. *Operating Procedures for the Army Food Program*. DAP 30-22. Washington, DC: Department of the Army.

U.S. Department of the Army. 2005. *The Army Food Program*. AR 30-22. Washington, DC: Department of the Army.

U.S. Departments of the Army, Navy, and Air Force. 2001. *Nutrition Standards and Education*. AR 40-25/BUMEDINST 10110.6/AFI 44-141. Washington, DC: U.S. Department of Defense Headquarters.

U.S. EPA (U.S. Environmental Protection Agency). 2005. *List of Drinking Water Contaminants & MCLs*. [Online]. Available: http://www.epa.gov/OGWDW/mcl.html#mcls [accessed January 26, 2006].

U.S. FDA (Food and Drug Administration). 1995. *Dietary Supplement Health and Education Act of 1994*. [Online]. Available: http://www.cfsan.fda.gov/~dms/dietsupp.html [accessed January 26, 2006].

U.S. FDA. 1996. Food Standards: Amendment of Standards of Identity for enriched grain products to require addition of folic acid. Final Rule. *Federal Register* 61(44):8781–8797.

U.S. FDA. 1999. *The Food Label*. [Online]. Available: http://www.fda.gov/opacom/backgrounders/foodlabel/newlabel.html [accessed February 10, 2006].

WHO. 2003. *Hardness in Drinking-water*. WHO/SDE/WSH/03.04/06. Geneva: WHO.

WHO. 2004. *Guidelines for Drinking-water Quality*. 3rd ed. Vol. 1. Geneva: WHO.

Zoeteman BCJ. 1980. *Sensory Assessment of Water Quality*. In: Hutzinger O, Safe S, eds. Pergamon Series on Environmental Science Vol 2. Oxford: Pergamon Press.

# 3

# Mineral Recommendations for Military Performance

This chapter presents the available scientific evidence to support the committee's recommendations on minerals and their required intake levels for military personnel during garrison training. Garrison training is defined for the purpose of this report as situations during which military personnel living on a garrison base are either training or carrying out combat simulations or conducting one-day convoy-type operations. A specific group of known essential minerals was selected based on the minerals' importance to physical and cognitive performance and maintaining health status. The minerals group was developed after committee deliberations and was founded on results from literature reviews and from information provided by the Department of Defense. Furthermore, in-depth literature reviews on calcium, copper, iron, magnesium, selenium, and zinc were conducted. Following the approach described in this chapter, the committee makes recommendations for soldiers, both men and women, during garrison training. Also, the committee comments on the adequacy of the estimated levels of those minerals in the current meals, ready to eat (MREs) and first strike rations (FSRs), which are consumed typically during garrison training and sustained operations, respectively. Further, the committee comments on the recent Institute of Medicine (IOM) (2006) mineral level recommendations for sustained operations (i.e., FSRs). Finally, a list of priority research questions for each mineral are included. (The research questions are expanded in Chapter 4 to include descriptions of study designs.)

## THE COMMITTEE'S APPROACH

The committee's task was to review and, if necessary, to recommend new levels of dietary intakes for minerals that are of the greatest interest to the military because (1) risk factors during military operations might result in marginal deficiencies among military personnel or (2) higher intakes might be beneficial for optimizing military performance. Based on these two criteria, the committee discussed the relevance of all minerals and decided to focus its task on calcium, copper, iron, magnesium, selenium, and zinc. An in-depth literature review was conducted to gauge the relevance of studies and to evaluate using the studies' results as a basis for recommending mineral intake levels or priority research needs, or both, to answer information gaps related to the committee's task.

Subsequently, the committee was able to make recommendations for the future establishment of new military standards for the specific minerals; specifically, the committee recommended new Estimated Average Requirements (EARs) and Recommended Dietary Allowances (RDAs) or Adequate Intake (AIs) for military garrison training (MGT). The new values are referred to as $EAR_{MGT}$, $RDA_{MGT}$, and $AI_{MGT}$. Based on the outcomes of importance to the military, that is, to either maintain or improve both physical or cognitive performance under garrison training, two general types of studies were considered: (1) studies designed to examine requirement increases due to exercise, stress, or other conditions encountered during military life (e.g., sweat losses or changes in bone resorption rates) and (2) studies designed to evaluate the potential benefits of increasing mineral intakes for cognitive or performance functions.

When potential nutrient losses or low intake could put soldiers at risk for deficiencies, the recommended level for a given nutrient was increased—as long as the new level did not exceed the Tolerable Upper Intake Level (UL)—based on data from peer-reviewed scientific literature. However, when making a recommendation based on potential benefits of supplementation, the committee erred on the side of caution and only considered those effects if there was enough clear supporting evidence of the benefits to military performance. The committee cautions that most of the studies were conducted on civilians and under circumstances that might not be able to be extrapolated to military circumstances and garrison training. An effort was made to consider gender differences where the data were available. In addition to the other assumptions formulated by the committee, they considered as worst-case scenario the loss of sweat volumes of up to 10 L/day due to heat and exercise.

The committee evaluated the adequacy of the mineral content of rations. Adequacy can be evaluated for the population or for the individual. Because the committee does not know of data on mineral distribution intakes for military garrison training, the mineral content of menus for the population could not be evaluated. Instead, the calculated $RDA_{MGT}$ and $AI_{MGT}$ were used as benchmarks to evaluate mineral content adequacy of various rations for individuals. The mineral compositions of three different MREs and three different FSRs were provided by the United States Army Research Institute of Environmental Medicine and used to evaluate the rations' adequacy (see Table 3-1 and Tables C-2 through C-7 in Appendix C).

**TABLE 3-1** Summary Table of the Institute of Medicine Dietary Reference Intakes and Military Dietary Reference Intakes for Garrison Training and Combat Operations for 19–50 Year Olds and the Mineral Levels in Current Rations

| | IOM Dietary Reference Intakes (civilian population, ages 19–50 years) | | | IOM Mineral Intake Recommendations (military population, ages 19–50 years) | |
|---|---|---|---|---|---|
| Nutrient | IOM RDA or AI | IOM UL | MDRI | $RDA_{MGT}$ or $AI_{MGT}$ | FSRs |
| Calcium (mg) | | | | | |
| M | 1,000 | 2,500 | 1,000 | 1,000 | 750–850 |
| F | 1,000 | 2,500 | 1,000 | 1,000 | |
| Copper (μg) | | | | | |
| M | 900 | 10,000 | ND | 1,800 | 900–1,600 |
| F | 900 | 10,000 | ND | 1,500 | |
| Iron (mg) | | | | | |
| M | 8 | 45 | 10 | 14 | 8–18 |
| F | 18 | 45 | 15 | 22 | |
| Magnesium (mg) | | | | | |
| M | 400–420* | 350 | 420 | 420 | 400–550 |
| F | 310–320* | 350 | 320 | 320 | |
| Selenium (μg) | | | | | |
| M | 55 | 400 | 55 | 55 | 55–230 |
| F | 55 | 400 | 55 | 55 | |
| Zinc (mg) | | | | | |
| M | 11 | 40 | 15 | 15 | 11–25 |
| F | 8 | 40 | 12 | 11 | |

NOTE: AI = Adequate Intake; F = female; FSR = first strike ration; IOM = Institute of Medicine; M = male; MDRI = Military Dietary Reference Intake; MGT = military garrison training; MRE = meals, ready to eat; ND = not determined; RDA = Recommended Dietary Allowance; SUSOPS = sustained operations; UL = Tolerable Upper Intake Level.

* Lower requirement for 19–30 year olds and higher requirement for 31–50 year olds.

SOURCE: Baker-Fulco (2005); IOM (1997, 2000, 2001, 2006); U.S. Departments of the Army, Navy, and Air Force (2001).

Mineral Levels in Current Military Rations

| MRE XXII | MRE XXIV | MRE XXIII | FSR |
|---|---|---|---|
| 269–1051<br>Average: 511<br>(3 rations = 1,533) | 272–949<br>Average: 557.4<br>(3 rations = 1,672) | 269–950<br>Average: 526<br>(3 rations = 1,578) | 643–697<br>Average: 673 |
| ND | ND | ND | ND |
| 5–19<br>Average: 7.9<br>(3 rations = 24) | 6–18<br>Average: 9<br>(3 rations = 27) | 5.78–18.39<br>Average: 8.6<br>(3 rations = 26) | 15–18.4<br>Average: 17 |
| 60–195<br>Average: 114<br>(3 rations = 342) | 78–227<br>Average: 140.5<br>(3 rations= 421) | 69–299<br>Average: 177<br>(3 rations = 531) | 375–403<br>Average: 86 |
| 0.12–34<br>Average: 9.6<br>(3 rations = 30) | 0.68–38<br>Average: 12.5<br>(3 rations = 37) | 1.34–28.3<br>Average: 7.8<br>(3 rations = 23) | 63–160<br>Average: 100 |
| 1.8–8.5<br>Average: 4.2<br>(3 rations = 13) | 2–8<br>Average: 4.7<br>(3 rations = 14) | 0.96–8.14<br>Average: 4.2<br>(3 rations = 13) | 11.4–12.2<br>Average: 11 |

The committee provided comments on the recent mineral recommendations in the IOM report *Nutrient Composition of Rations for Short-Term, High-Intensity Combat Operations* (2006; see Table 3-1). The comments reflected all of the report's supportive evidence, including factors related to food technology and nutrient interactions as well as those related to the diets, consumption behaviors, and nature of the operations.

## NUTRITIONAL AND ENVIRONMENTAL FACTORS FACING SOLDIERS IN THE FIELD

The need for specific nutrients is influenced by the health status and specific scenarios and environmental conditions into which soldiers are deployed. Thus, two military scenarios were considered: (1) garrison training and (2) sustained operations. In order to delineate such scenarios, the committee made a series of assumptions regarding health, environmental conditions, and the soldiers' diets (described in the following section); the scenarios are based on the committee's deliberations, open sessions with sponsor representatives and other military personnel, information from field surveys conducted in Iraq and Afghanistan, and available literature. Specifically, the garrison training information was collected through a personal communication (Personal communication, J. Kent and S. Corum, U.S. Army, August 24, 2005).

### Garrison Training

*Environment*

Soldiers (men and women 19–50 years old) are generally in a region of operations for 12 months, although they can be there for up to 18 months, especially if serving in the National Guard or Reserves. Most military sites are large garrison bases with many facilities, however, some are small with a reduced number of facilities.

The majority of Iraqi military sites are in hot, desert climates. Soldiers are typically exposed to temperatures above 100°F for 8–10 hours per day. During 12–18-month deployments, soldiers (e.g., combat arms soldiers and soldiers performing convoy-type operations in Iraq) are typically away from base camp for 12 hours per day accomplishing a mission or training. They generally return to the camp daily, eat in a dining facility, and sleep in tents or buildings. Under high temperatures and when prescribed rest–work cycles can be followed, soldiers engage in heavy work for about 10 minutes and take long rests periods of about 50 minutes. As they become acclimated, the rest cycles often are shortened. Under combat conditions, rest cycles obviously are not possible.

*Exercise and Energy Expenditure*

There are no data on exercise schedules, and they may vary significantly. There are also no metabolic data and no data on the soldiers' energy expenditure in garrison training. However, past studies reported that male soldiers who engaged in various activities expended energy in amounts that ranged from 3,500 kcal/day for combat support and combat service support soldiers involved in moderate exercise while in garrison to 4,500 kcal/day for Ranger training under intense exercise. For female soldiers, energy expenditures may range from 2,300 kcal/day when in basic training to 3,000 kcal/day when running medical operations in the field. The committee assumes that the energy expenditures will be an average of 4,000 and 2,500 kcal/day for men and women, respectively.

*Diet*

While in base camp, soldiers have free access to dining facilities, and they typically eat three times a day. There are no recorded data on energy intake. When soldiers go on missions off the base camp they eat MREs during the day (sometimes for several days) as well as personal food items (snack foods) received through the mail or purchased at local Army and Air Force Exchange Service operations. For the purpose of evaluating the adequacy of rations' mineral content, the committee assumes that male soldiers will consume three MREs per day and that female soldiers will consume two MREs per day. If consumption differs from this assumption (e.g., if male soldiers eat two MREs per day and female soldiers eat one MRE per day, and both sets supplement the MREs with snack foods), then the conclusions regarding mineral adequacy of the rations might be different.

Soldiers have access to supplemental food and drink from the local economy, but they are highly discouraged from consuming such products. It is unknown to what extent they eat outside of the base camp. Because weight gain can be a problem, weight-loss diets are as popular as they are with the civilian population. Soldiers have access to supplements, especially weight-loss supplements, protein supplements, creatine, or energy drinks. Soldiers also might ingest calcium supplements. However, there are not enough data on supplement use in the field to make definitive conclusions.

*Water Consumption*

In Iraq, soldiers consume up to 3 L/day of mineral water that is produced at eight different sites. Since bottled water is considered a food product, members of the Veterinary Corps from Fort Dietrich, Maryland, inspect it for bacteria, contaminants, and mineral content. In order for the water to be shipped to the soldiers, the mineral content has to be as low as what is found in commercially available mineral water in the United States. Commercially purchased bottled water from the United States is used as an internal standard. Often minerals, such as calcium, are added to improve the taste.

Soldiers also have access to water that has been filtered through reverse osmosis (reverse osmosis purification unit); this water is essentially mineral free. The filtered water typically is not consumed by soldiers unless bottled water is unavailable; instead, it is used when large amounts of water are required (e.g., in hospitals, cooking, cleaning, washing).

*Health*

There is not a particular single health issue that stands out with currently deployed soldiers in garrison training. Diarrhea is fairly common, due to antimalarial drugs as well as to occasional outbreaks from consuming unapproved foods (e.g., food from the local economy). Some minor outbreaks of food-borne diseases have occurred (20–30 cases per outbreak, possibly due to consumption of local foods).

The incidence of iron deficiency among military women is unknown. Typically, they are not tested for iron status, except for when they visit the hospital with other medical problems; during these hospital visits, iron deficiencies have been observed among women in the military.

Dehydration is infrequent, and if it does occur, it happens more commonly when soldiers first arrive at base camp, mainly due to emotional issues and lack of acclimation to the heat and daily routines. Soldiers quickly learn to avoid dehydration by drinking fluids.

Anecdotal data that indicate weight gain as a problem are being studied currently. To meet military specifications weight loss diets are popular among military personnel, which might have adverse health consequences if intakes of essential nutrients are inadequate.

Sleep deprivation does not seem to be a generalized problem, although it may happen occasionally. Soldiers typically sleep for 8 h/day, but sometimes sleep time can be reduced to only 4–6 h/day.

## Sustained Operations

In the recent IOM report (2006), *Nutrient Composition of Rations for Short-Term, High-Intensity Combat Operations*, the assumptions related to the characteristics of the soldiers' diets and health, the missions, and other issues for soldiers deployed to sustained operations (assault missions) were described at length. The following list summarizes the assumptions:

- Soldiers deployed on assault missions are male, relatively fit, with an average body weight of 80 kg and approximately 16 percent body fat, and within an age range of 18–45 years (average < 25 years).

• Soldiers may be on a mission for as many as 24 out of 30 days, with each mission lasting three to seven days.

• There may be as much as 20 h/day of physical activity, with an average of 4 h/day of sleep. Total daily energy expenditure will be approximately 4,500 kcal.

• Soldiers are likely to have an average energy intake of 2,400 kcal/day.

• Soldiers are likely to have access to 4–5 L/day of chlorinated water.

• Some soldiers may experience diarrhea, constipation, or kidney stones during assault missions.

• The daily ration must fit within 0.12 cubic feet and weigh three pounds (1.4 kg) or less. It will be approximately 12–17 percent water (varying greatly from one item to the other); most items will be energy dense and intermediate in moisture.

• There will be no liquid foods in the rations, although gels and powders may be provided.

• The food available during recovery periods will provide, at a minimum, the nutritional standards for operational rations.

The recommended rations (see Table C-1 and Box C-1 in Appendix C) do not meet the MDRIs in AR 40-25 (U.S. Departments of the Army, Navy, and Air Force, 2001), nor do they meet the recommended nutrient intakes for civilians (IOM, 1997, 1998a, 2000, 2001, 2002/2005, 2004a). The assault rations (i.e., FSRs) are meant to be used only for repetitive three- to seven-day missions that last for a maximum total period of one month and that include recovery periods of 24–72 hours between missions. With the expected energy expenditures of 4,500 kcal/day during the missions and the possibility of as much as a 10-percent body weight loss, it was recommended that weight loss be measured after one month of use. If weight loss of a soldier is higher than 10 percent for a soldier, he should not be sent on assault missions until weight is regained to within 5 percent of the initial weight.

## CALCIUM RECOMMENDATIONS

Calcium is an essential mineral that plays a range of biological roles, from being a major constituent of bones and teeth to affecting nerve conduction, muscle contraction, heartbeat regulation, blood coagulation, energy production, glandular secretion, and the maintenance of immune function. Although many minerals are essential for bone health and function, the risk of calcium inadequacy in the diet is higher than risks of other deficiencies; moreover, calcium is more abundant in the bone than other minerals.

Calcium in the diet offsets obligatory calcium losses, protecting skeletal reserves and maintaining structural integrity. Bone loss might occur from inadequate caloric intake to meet energy expenditure and calcium dermal losses during exercise and will be exaggerated in females with loss of menstrual function or eating disorders. Micro-fracture repair is also dependent on calcium intake. Thus, ingested calcium prevents the net efflux of calcium from bone and by doing so may help to prevent osteoporosis and stress fractures as a result of military training and combat action (Burr, 1997; IOM, 1997). Basic training appears to first lead to increased resorption (perhaps to compensate for calcium loss due to sweat or negative energy balance), but this is followed by increased formation (stimulated by intense training) and the window between increments in these two processes may be the period of greatest risk of stress fractures. To counteract any excess in bone turnover and meet the demands of the skeleton during intense activity calcium levels higher than current AI of 1,000 mg may be needed with intense exercise. Data on the prevention of stress fractures by calcium are limited and not conclusive yet but there is ongoing research that should soon shed more light. More data are clearly needed to understand the role of nutrition in stress fracture occurrence (see Nieves and Hayes in Appendix B).

Remarkable changes in bone mineral content (BMC) have been observed in male army infantry recruits 18–21 years old who were subjected to very strenuous physical training. After 14 weeks of walking, jogging with and without weights, and calisthenics for at least 8 hours a day, 6 days a week, the average bone mineral content of the subjects increased 11 percent in the left leg and 5.2 percent in the right leg (Margulies et al., 1986). Of the 268 recruits, 110 did not complete the training, largely because of incurring stress fractures in the lower limbs. The relationship of calcium intake to bone health and fracture prevention is discussed in more detail in Appendix B (Nieves and Hayes).

### Monitoring Calcium Status, Its Metabolism, and Related Bone Health

Methods for evaluating calcium metabolism and bone health are advanced. Yet simple, inexpensive methods for assessing calcium metabolism and bone health for large numbers of people are still lacking. No biochemical measure can assess calcium status, unless calcium metabolism is grossly abnormal. Measuring calcium intake, therefore, is the only approach to evaluating current calcium status in healthy individuals. Approaches for calculating dietary calcium intakes and their limitations have been reviewed by Boushey (2006). A rapid assessment method specific for dietary calcium is given in Weaver and Heaney (2006). However, a dietary assessment tool to evaluate several key nutrients likely to be deficient in diets of military personnel would have broader utility.

A detailed description of research methods to measure all parameters of calcium metabolism is given by Weaver (2006). Isotopic calcium tracer methodology, typically in conjunction with metabolic balance studies, is the gold standard for quantifying complete calcium kinetics including calcium absorption, endogenous secretion, urinary and fecal excretion, bone formation rates, and bone resorption rates. Serum and urinary calcium and serum parathyroid hormone (PTH) levels are the best, most readily available assessment tools for evaluating disturbances in calcium metabolism [e.g., those related to premenstrual syndrome (PMS)].

Strategies for monitoring bone health are given in an IOM report (2004b), *Monitoring Metabolic Status. Predicting Decrements in Physiological and Cognitive Performance.* Total body calcium can be determined from total body BMC using bone density, because calcium is a constant fraction of BMC, and represents net cumulative calcium rather than recent dietary calcium intakes. Bone mineral density (BMD), measured by bone densitometry, quantitative computed tomography (QCT), or ultrasound, is a useful measure of bone health because of the strong inverse relationship between BMD and fracture risk (Melton et al., 1993). The large normative databases used by manufacturers of dual energy x-ray absorptiometers (DXA) allow BMD of individuals to be compared to age-matched reference values and fracture risk to be assessed as *z*-scores. Newer imaging methodologies (e.g., QCT) for assessing bone quality can provide additional useful information about bone geometry. Evaluating interventions by DXA or QCT require years to analyze small changes in bone; however, some interventions produce large changes in bone that can be observed in periods as short as six months.

Bone is a dynamic tissue that constantly turns over through a remodeling process, during which fatigued bone is resorbed and new bone is formed. In young adults, the two processes are typically coupled to achieve net bone balance. A number of commercial kits are available to estimate bone formation and bone resorption rates. They lack specificity because they do not measure calcium or bone, but rather protein fragments that are released during bone turnover. Moreover, the biochemical markers of bone turnover are typically too variable to reliably predict small changes in bone. Therefore, their use as a primary outcome measure to gauge the effect of stress on bone turnover or to evaluate the effectiveness of interventions is not recommended. However, under conditions that have a large impact on bone (e.g., microgravity associated with space flight), biochemical markers have provided useful insights to mechanisms of action (Smith et al., 1999).

## Calcium Intake Effects on Health and Performance

### *Stress Fractures*

The rate of stress fractures during basic training has varied depending on the branch of service, methods of detection, and training methods. Navy and Air Force programs consistently report a lower incidence of stress fractures than the Army and Marine Corps programs (Beck et al., 1996; Jones et al., 1989; Kelly et al., 2000; Shaffer, 2001; Shaffer et al., 1999). The fracture rates for females are consistently higher than for males (Almeida et al., 1999; Shaffer, 2001). Pre-

1989 studies of the U.S. military indicate male stress fracture rates from 0.9 percent to 3.0 percent and female rates from 2.7 to 8.2 percent (Jones et al., 1989). Since 1995, stress fracture incidence in female Marine recruits and officer cadets has ranged from 5.7 percent to 11.5 percent (Shaffer et al., 1999; Winfield et al., 1997). The female recruit stress fracture rate at the Naval Recruit Training Center Great Lakes in 1995 was reported as 3.9 percent (Shaffer et al., 1999). Stress fractures rates ascertained at the Fort Leonard Wood Army training center between October 2003 and June 2004 were 9.1 percent for males and 17.5 percent for females (Personal communication, J. Lappe and R. Ellyson, U.S. Army Training and Doctrine Command, February, 2003). Research on the benefits of calcium supplements in preventing stress fractures in females is currently being conducted and the results from these studies should be considered when developing calcium requirements for the military. See also Nieves and Hayes in Appendix B.

### *Mood and Psychological Performance*

There is evidence in the literature that inadequate dietary calcium is associated with negative emotional and mental health, which could have implications for performance. The most rigorously studied type of these conditions is PMS. Approximately 5 percent of North American women have PMS symptoms so severe that health and performance are affected (Thys-Jacobs, 2006). The symptoms—irritability, depression, anxiety, social withdrawal, headache, and abdominal cramps—can be alleviated in most women with increased dietary calcium or calcium supplementation. The supporting evidence consists of two small, single-site trials (Penland and Johnson, 1993; Thys-Jacob et al., 1989) followed by a multisite randomized, controlled trial (Thys-Jacobs et al., 1998).

The study by Penland and Johnson (1993) controlled dietary calcium at 587 or 1,336 mg/day by supplementing with calcium lactate after a 13-day equilibration diet containing calcium of 800 mg/day. Higher calcium intakes were associated with improved mood, concentration, and behavior symptoms, as well as with decreased pain. The multisite trial (Thys-Jacobs et al., 1998) randomly provided 720 women who were 18–45 years old and suffering from PMS with a placebo or with 1,200 mg/day of calcium as calcium carbonate for a duration of three menstrual cycles. A daily rating scale and diary were used to measure 17 core symptoms and 4 symptom factors (negative affect, water retention, food cravings, and pain). By the third menstrual cycle, an overall 48-percent reduction in total symptom scores was observed. All 4 symptom factors and 15 core symptoms, but not fatigue and insomnia, were reduced significantly by the calcium treatment as compared to placebo. Negative affect was reduced by 45 percent.

Results from observation studies add more evidence to the effects of calcium intake in alleviating PMS symptoms. In the Nurses' Health Study II cohort,

1,079 women with PMS and 2,154 controls 25–42 years old (on entry into the study) were followed for ten years; data showed that high intakes of calcium (median intake = 1,507 mg/day) and vitamin D (median intake = 567 International Units [IU]/day) were associated inversely with PMS. Calcium showed a relative risk (RR) of 0.76 (95 percent coefficient interval [CI], 0.56–1.04) in the highest quintile of calcium intake compared to the lowest quintile of calcium intake with P = 0.12 for trend (Bertone et al., 2005).

Thys-Jacobs (2006) attributes PMS symptoms to estrogen fluctuations during the ovulation and luteal phases of the menstrual cycle; the fluctuations and phases affect serum calcium concentrations, especially in women with inadequate dietary calcium. Estrogen inhibits bone resorption and would favor lower serum calcium concentrations. However, the menstrual cyclicity of calciotropic hormones and biochemical markers of bone turnover is controversial. Some research has demonstrated a rise in serum PTH, calcium, and 25-hydroxyvitamin D at midcycle in women with PMS (Thys-Jacobs and Alvir, 1995). Other research has shown fluctuations in biochemical markers of bone turnover during the menstrual cycle (Nielsen et al., 1990; Schlemmer et al., 1993). And yet, other research has found no appreciable fluctuations in these regulators (Lopez Moreno et al., 1992; Muse et al., 1986).

Inadequate calcium status and associated hyperparathyroidism have been associated in patients with depression (Borer and Bhanot, 1985; Cogan et al., 1978; Jimerson et al., 1979).

A discussion of general strategies for monitoring cognitive and physical performance outcome measures is given in IOM (2004b), *Monitoring Metabolic Status. Predicting Decrements in Physiological and Cognitive Performance.* PMS symptoms appear to be uniquely associated with calcium and vitamin D deficiency. An assessment of PMS symptoms can be monitored with a menstrual calendar, a daily rating scale, or a symptom diary (Alvir and Thys-Jacobs, 1991; Thys-Jacobs et al., 1995). The National Institutes of Mental Health uses a criterion of a 30-percent change in mean symptoms from the luteal phase to postmenstrual phase for diagnosis of PMS (National Institute of Mental Health, 1983). Another useful manual for diagnosis is the *Diagnostic and Statistical Manual of Mental Disorders DSM-IV* (American Psychiatric Association, 1994).

## Risk Factors for Inadequacy During Military Garrison Training

### *Inadequate Intake*

The mean calcium intake in the general population is 1,013 mg/day for 19–30-year-old males, 913 mg/day for 31–50-year-old males, 647 mg/day for 19–30-year-old females, and 637 mg/day for 31–50-year-old females (IOM, 1997). Thus, on average, men almost achieve their AI whereas only women whose intakes are at the 90th percentile or above achieve their AI (1,000 mg/day).

Calcium intakes have not been studied for many military groups. A study of 52 combat-support hospital staff consuming MREs showed that virtually all of the men and women were consuming less than their AI (Baker-Fulco, 2005; see Baker-Fulco in Appendix B). A study of 40 Special Forces male soldiers in garrison training for nine days using self-reported food records showed that calcium recommendations were met with an average intake of 1,065 mg/day (Tharion et al., 2004).

Vitamin D is important in bone health in that it maintains serum levels of calcium and phosphorus. Vitamin D deficiency might increase requirements for calcium and, therefore, it would be appropriate to assess the vitamin D status of the military population. There is, however, an on-going debate regarding the criterion for vitamin D adequacy, that is, the cutoff serum level of 25 hydroxy vitamin D (25 [OH] D) as an indicator of adequacy is currently a subject of much research. Because of its importance for bone health, this committee suggests that when the optimal cutoff is determined, the military conducts surveys to determine serum levels of 25 (OH) D of military personnel and assesses the risk of inadequacy.

*Exercise and Environmental Conditions*

**Physical activity and calcium and bone metabolism.** Researchers' understanding of the effect of physical activity on calcium metabolism and bone is incomplete. Physical activity could lead to extra losses through sweat, and thus a need for increased requirements. Alternatively, physical activity could lead to increased bone strength, which could protect against inadequate calcium intakes. But, at high-impact loading, physical activity also could result in stress fractures. In women, high-intensity physical activity also can cause amenorrhea, which can lead to bone loss.

Bone responds to changes in mechanical loading beyond habitual levels of loading. In skeletal unloading environments (i.e., environments that minimize loads on bone), such as immobilization or microgravity, bone resorption rates exceed bone formation rates, and bone is lost. Increased skeleton loading, such as the loading that can occur during military training, may lead to bone formation rates exceeding bone resorption rates, and thereby, to increased bone mass. Metaanalyses of controlled trials of exercise and bone in premenopausal women show modest positive effects, averaging about 1 percent per year, of aerobic and resistance training on BMD of the lumbar spine (Singh, 2004). Few studies have been done with male subjects. One study examined 38–68-year-old men who had no running experience but spent nine months training for a marathon and found that the men had improved BMC at the heel (Williams et al., 1984). A high-intensity free-weight exercise program resulted in a 1.9 percent gain of lumbar spine BMD after six months in 50–60-year-old men (Maddalozzo and Snow, 2000). The effects of exercise on bone are greater in prepubertal children, when bone turnover rates are higher. This also may be related to a synergy between exercise and growth hormone, which is higher during growth (Bass, 2000). Exercise training increases serum IGF-1 (insulin-like growth factor 1) levels—which may be a key regulator of bone—in both young and older adults (Vukovich and Specker, 2006).

In order to determine the effects of physical activity on dietary calcium requirements, a factorial design that varies levels of calcium intakes and exercise is required. Few studies have been designed specifically to address whether or not dietary calcium enhances the adaptive bone response to exercise. A one-year trial in which three- to five-year-old children were assigned randomly to receive either 1 g/day of calcium (calcium carbonate supplement) or a placebo and to participate in either gross-motor (weight-bearing) or fine-motor (sitting) exercise resulted in increases in BMC only in the group that both received the calcium and participated in weight-bearing exercise (Specker and Binkley, 2003). However, bone strength was improved in the exercise–placebo group; the finding was illustrated by an increase in tibia diameter, as assessed by peripheral QCT (see Figure 3-1). Small increases in the diameter of bone have a profound impact on the bone's bending strength because bone strength increases by the squared distance from the axis around which bending occurs. Another randomized trial demonstrated a significant calcium (calcium-fortified foods, 434 mg/day) and exercise interaction in bone mass in prepubertal girls at the femur, but not at the tibia or fibula (Iuliano-Burns et al., 2003). A positive interaction between dietary calcium and exercise on bone density also has been found in other age groups, including in postmenopausal women (Lau et al., 1992; Prince et al., 1991; Specker, 1996). In growing children as well as in postmenopausal women, bone turnover is higher than for the young adults of this report's target age.

Lifestyle factors are thought to influence bone conservation but to have less of an impact during the years of reduced bone turnover. Prospective studies in premenopausal women show mixed results; some show a positive interaction of

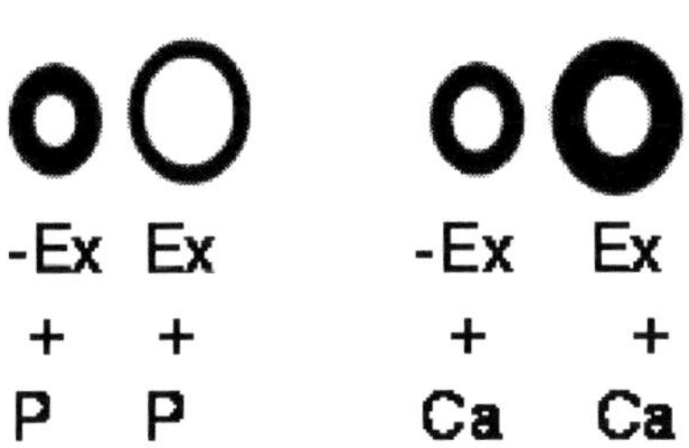


**FIGURE 3-1** Exercise increases 20 percent tibia cross-section bone strength and, when combined with calcium supplementation, increases bone mass in a 1-year randomized, controlled trial in 3–5-year-old children.
SOURCE: Specker and Binkley (2003).

dietary calcium and physical activity (Recker et al., 1992), while others do not find a significant interaction (Valimaki et al., 1994). Unfortunately, the appropriate randomized, controlled trials of calcium and exercise on calcium metabolism or on bone mass and strength have not been conducted in young and middle-aged adults, so it is unproven whether or not exercise has an impact on calcium requirements for those age groups.

If young adults' bodies react similarly to children's bodies, then exercise may provide increased bone strength and offset inadequate calcium intakes, but benefits may be greater from providing adequate calcium intakes in conjunction with training. From literature on animal models, exercise may up-regulate calcium absorption (Yeh et al., 1989) and initially increase then decrease bone resorption (Yeh et al., 1993). From studies in humans, endurance exercise lasting longer than 30 minutes can increase bone serum calcium and PTH levels (Vukovich and Specker, 2006). An increase in circulating PTH could increase calcitriol, which would increase calcium absorption, renal conservation of calcium, and bone resorption. An acute bout of moderate aerobic exercise significantly enhanced fractional strontium absorption (a surrogate of calcium absorption) in 18 male athletes, 25.2 ± 0.6 (mean ± standard error of the mean) years old and decreased a biochemical markers of bone formation but not bone resorption (Zitterman et al., 2002). Other studies have shown a single bout of exercise decreases bone resorption markers up to three days postexercise while urinary calcium increased on the day of exercise in 14 Asian males 24.5 ± 0.7 years old (Ashizawa et al., 1998). The authors explained the increase in urinary calcium excretion by an increase in renal acid excretion. The type of exercise may influence the effect on bone turnover. Anaerobic training, but not aerobic training, accelerated bone turnover in young males (Woitge et al., 1998). Ingestion of a calcium load (approximately 1,000 mg) in mineral water during endurance cycling suppressed the elevation of a biomarker of bone resorption in male athletes (Guillemant et al., 2004).

Much of what researchers know about the role of physical activity and calcium intake on bone, information that might be relevant to military personnel, is discussed by Nieves (2005; see Nieves and Hayes in Appendix B). Male military cadets in the highest-level exercise group had significantly higher tibial BMC, cortical thickness, and periosteal circumference than cadets in lower-level exercise groups. Cadets consuming more than three glasses of milk per day had greater tibial BMD, cortical thickness, and periosteal circumference. There was a significant interaction between milk intake and prior exercise on cortical thickness. In another study, training in Marine recruits resulted in significant increases in a biochemical marker of bone resorption (Sheehan et al., 2003).

Military training has been associated with an increase in stress fractures (IOM, 1998b). The role of calcium and vitamin D supplementation on preventing stress fractures in female naval recruits undergoing basic training is being investigated by Joan Lappe at Creighton University.

In summary, physical activity above habitual levels may increase bone strength and, thus, may protect against inadequate calcium intakes; bone strength may benefit further from adequate intakes. Mechanisms for the putative positive interactions of physical activity and dietary calcium may be through enhanced calcium absorption and changes in bone turnover. Suppression of bone turnover as could occur with dietary calcium and exercise has been associated with improved bone quality (Heaney and Weaver, 2005). Excess in bone turnover with high-impact exercise would increase skeletal demands for calcium.

**Calcium losses through sweat and excreta.** According to Charles et al. (1991) normal endogenous fecal calcium excretion is 3.4 mmol/day (136 mg/day), urinary calcium excretion is 5.5 mmol/day (220 mg/day), and dermal calcium loss is 1.6 mmol/day (64 mg/day). In setting the Dietary Reference Intake (DRI) for calcium for young adult males and females, the following basal losses of calcium were estimated: urinary—203 mg/day for women, 162 mg/day for men; endogenous fecal calcium—132 mg/day for women, 156 mg/day for men; sweat—63 mg/day for men and women (IOM, 1997). Whole-body integumentary calcium loss in 16 ambulatory men averaged 15.8 mg/day (8.7 mg/m$^2$/day) (Chu et al., 1979). Urinary calcium losses in the Chu study ranged from 51 to 380 mg/day depending on the calcium and protein intake. Palacios et al. (2003) found whole-body dermal calcium loss in six young women averaged 103 ± 22 mg/day. Dermal calcium measured in patches attached to the arms, legs, and back was found to overestimate the whole-body calcium more than threefold. Mitchell and Hamilton (1949) used a whole-body wash-down technique to measure sweat calcium in six men resting in a warm humid environment. Average sweat calcium concentration decreased from 52.6 mg/L during the first 30 minutes to 31.7 mg/L in the second 30 minutes to 4.0 mg/L during the third hour of exposure. Average dermal calcium loss over 7.5 hours was 20.2 mg/h in the heat compared to 6.2 mg/h while resting in a comfortable environment. Whole-body calcium loss through sweat was measured in four women resting in the heat (Johnston et al., 1950). Mean sweat calcium loss during four 1-h exposures was 8.5 mg/h (33.5 mg/L).

Several studies have examined sweat calcium losses during exercise. Consolazio et al. (1962) used arm bags to measure sweat calcium losses of eight men during 16 days of exposure to 21°C, 29.4°C, and 37.8°C environments for 7.5 hours that included 100 minutes of exercise per day. Calcium intake was 441 mg/day throughout the study. Mean calcium losses in the urine and feces were approximately the same in the three environments and ranged from 183–199 mg/day for urinary calcium and 199–226 mg/day for fecal calcium. Excretion of calcium through sweat increased from 111 mg/day at 21°C to 137 mg/day at 29.4°C and 201 mg/day at 37.8°C. These estimates were extrapolated from arm bag collections in environmental chambers for 7.5 hours plus an assumed ratio of loss outside of chambers of 3 mg/h. Sweat calcium loss measured while the men were in the environmental chamber increased gradually from 8.1 mg/h at 21°C to 11.6 mg/h at 29.4°C and 20.2 mg/h at 37.8°C.

A second experiment involved three men doing 30 minutes of moderate exercise for 16 days. In the heat (37.8°C), sweat calcium loss decreased from 36 mg/h to 17 mg/h by the second week. Mean sweat calcium loss in a neutral environment (23.9°C) was 3 mg/h. These findings suggest that sweat calcium loss decreases with acclimatization to heat. Urinary calcium loss did not change over time in the heat and was approximately the same in the hot and neutral environments.

Chu et al. (1979) measured whole-body integumentary calcium losses during 40 minutes of intense exercise. Integumentary calcium excretion ranged from 18 to 31 mg per 40 minutes of exercise but was unaffected by dietary calcium or protein intake. Urinary calcium loss increased on exercise days when dietary protein (61 to 157 mg/day) or calcium increased (116 to 150 mg/day). Shirreffs and Maughan (1997) also used a whole-body technique during moderate exercise to measure sweat calcium in a hot humid environment (34°C, 60–70 percent relative humidity). Mean sweat calcium concentration for five men and two women was 52 ± 36 mg/L. Bullen et al. (1999) examined the sweat and urinary calcium losses in 10 men who were running in a hot, humid (32°C, 58 percent relative humidity) environment. Sweat was collected in pads attached to the back. Mean sweat calcium loss was 45 mg within 45 minutes. Urinary calcium excretion was 206 mg/day on the exercise day versus 189 mg/day on the rest day.

Sweat collections with pads were used in two other studies. Verde et al. (1982) collected sweat during moderate exercise indoors and outdoors as well as while sitting in a sauna. Sweat calcium concentration was lower during exercise than while resting in the sauna. O'Toole et al. (2000) measured sweat calcium in 42 male recruits undergoing fire-fighting training. Mean sweat calcium concentration was 44 mg/L, and sweat loss averaged 2.44 liters during the 3–4-hour training session for an average sweat calcium loss of 107 mg per session. Sweat samples from male basketball players were collected from their cotton t-shirts over three days of practice by Klesges et al. (1996). Players practiced twice a day with each practice session lasting more than two hours. Average weight loss per session was 2.13 kg, and mean calcium loss during practice was 426.7 mg. Mean sweat calcium concentration decreased significantly over the three days. Urinary calcium concentration averaged 86 mg/L during the practices.

### *Bone Loss in Young Adults*

Several factors can lead to abnormal bone loss in apparently healthy adults—oral contraceptive use, weight loss, and amenorrhea.

**Oral contraceptives (OC).** The effect of OC use on bone mass is conflicting—it has been shown to be protective of spine BMD (Kleerkoper et al., 1991) as well as detrimental to spine BMD (Hartard et al., 1997). OC use also has been associated with a reduction in sex steroid hormones (Bemben et al., 1992); this reduction could result in increased bone turnover. Both exercise and OC use were detrimental to femoral neck bone mass and strength (Burr et al., 2000). A negative interaction between OC use and physical activity on spine and hip BMD was observed in 18–30-year-old-women randomized to an exercise program (Weaver et al., 2001). Three women in the exercise group who used OCs and ingested recommended calcium intakes did not lose bone, suggesting that adequate dietary calcium must be present for bone modeling to occur under the stimulus of mechanical loading. In a one year intervention of 18–30 year old women consuming < 800 mg/day of calcium, total hip and spine loss observed in OC users randomized to the control group was prevented in those randomized to a dairy supplementation to achieve > 1,000 mg/day of calcium (Teegarden et al., 2005). Use of Depro-Provera was related inversely (P = 0.007) to hip and spine BMD in U.S. military female cadets (Nieves et al., 2005). Thus, achieving calcium recommendations may be particularly important among military women who use OCs and should be investigated.

**Weight loss.** It is unclear whether weight loss results in bone loss in physically active adults who are younger than 45 years old (Shapses and Cifuentes, 2004). Women typically consume less calcium during periods of moderately low energy intake (Ricci et al., 1998). Moderate weight reduction in obese premenopausal women did not result in bone loss (Shapses et al., 2001), but rapid weight loss in leaner women might result in bone loss. Bone loss associated with weight loss in women older than 45 years old, who are more likely to be estrogen depleted, has been prevented by calcium intakes of 1,600 mg/day or more (Jensen et al., 2001; Ricci et al., 1998; Riedt et al., 2005), but not by 800 mg/day (Svendsen et al., 1993). Calcium intakes above those currently recommended may protect bone during weight loss regimens. The higher levels of physical activity typical in military personnel that protect against bone loss may offset any need for increased requirements. With the current knowledge, it is important that individuals attempting voluntary weight loss strive to consume at least the recommended levels of calcium, although higher levels might be needed. The committee recommends that individuals engaging in weight loss diets reach calcium intakes of 1,200, and maybe even 1,500–1,700, mg/day. However, this recommendation should be validated through research (see Chapter 4).

**Amenorrhea.** Amenorrhea also is associated with bone loss. Amenorrhea can result from energy-restricted diets, anorexia nervosa, or extreme exercise. Young women with exercise-induced amenorrhea are at increased risk of fractures (De Souza and Williams, 2005).

Energy restriction or weight loss, or both, are associated with reduced estrogen levels and increased glucocorticoids, which can result in decreased calcium absorption and increased serum PTH (Shapses and Cifuentes, 2004). Premenopausal women with amenorrhea are also hypoestrogenomic (De Souza and Williams, 2005).

Losses in spine and hip BMD were observed in female military cadets with subclinical eating disorders and women with fewer than six menstrual cycles per year (Nieves, 2005; see Nieves and Hayes in Appendix B).

## Requirements for the General U.S. Population

An EAR for calcium for 19–30-year-olds in the U.S. civilian population could not be calculated, because there are no studies conducted with various intakes and bone accretion and because of the uncertainties regarding calcium endogenous and obligatory losses. However, the results from balance studies that investigated the intakes needed for BMC gains made it possible to estimate an AI of 1,000 mg/day for men and women (IOM, 1997).

## Daily Intake Recommendations for Military Personnel in Garrison Training

Calcium requirements for military personnel in garrison training may be higher than those for civilians because of the stress caused by increased physical activity and potentially extreme environmental conditions and related factors like increased sweat loss or reduced bone mass and calcium loss due to oral contraceptive use or weight loss. Alternatively, the requirements might be lower because additional exercise may compensate for calcium losses by increasing calcium bone deposition and bone diameter. In addition, current research being conducted on the benefits of calcium supplements in preventing stress fractures in females naval recruits should be closely followed and the results from these studies should be considered when developing calcium requirements for the military. Further research is required before any change (especially a reduction) to the IOM AI is recommended. Therefore, until new data that answer these questions are collected, 1,000 mg/day of calcium is recommended for military personnel in garrison training.

**RECOMMENDATIONS FOR CALCIUM INTAKE:**

| | |
|---|---|
| **$AI_{MGT}$ for men** | **1,000 mg/day** |
| **$AI_{MGT}$ for women** | **1,000 mg/day** |

## Adequacy of Calcium Military Dietary Reference Intakes and Calcium Levels in Rations

The committee concluded that the current Military Dietary Reference Intake (MDRI) of 1,000 mg/day of calcium for men and women is adequate given the number of unanswered research questions.

Table 3-1 (and Tables C-2 through C-5 in Appendix C) shows the averages and ranges of calcium content for three different MREs that each include about 25 menus. Even though some of the menus appear very low in calcium (269 mg), for this interpretation it will be assumed that a mix of menus are eaten per day and that the mix is sufficient for meeting the average level of calcium in the menus. However, there is a potential for deficiencies due to not only low food consumption but also selection of MREs low in calcium. The committee recommends that the menus at the low end of the range be revised to meet the 1,000 mg/day goal for both men and women.

As an example, the average calcium content in MRE XXIII and XXIV menus is 526 and 557 mg, respectively. Assuming that women will consume two MREs and men will consume three MREs, the amount in the ration, if consumed completely, will meet the recommendation of this committee. The extra calcium that men would consume will not reach amounts that would cause any safety concerns. A seven-day study of Rangers in the field showed an average calcium intake of only 639 ± 212 mg/day (mean ± standard deviation [SD]) (Baker-Fulco, 2005; see Baker-Fulco in Appendix B). The reasons behind the discrepancy between the total amount in three rations (~1,500 mg) and the intake of calcium (639 mg) deserve further investigation; surveys regarding food intake need to be conducted (see Chapter 4).

The current FSRs contain an average of 673 mg of calcium (see Table 3-1; see Table C-6 in Appendix C). Although this amount is not grossly inadequate, a minimum amount of 750 mg was recommended in IOM (2006) report *Nutrient Composition of Rations for Short-Term, High-Intensity Combat Operations* and is endorsed by this committee.

### Adequacy of IOM Recommendations for First Strike Rations

The IOM Committee on Optimization of Nutrient Compositions of Military Rations for Short-Term, High-Stress Situations recommended 750–850 mg/day of calcium for soldiers engaged in short-term, high-stress operations (IOM, 2006; see Table C-1 in Appendix C). The lower level of the recommendation was based on needs to replace losses determined by the factorial approach, potential sweat losses during prolonged exercise, and concerns about renal stone formation. The IOM AI (1997) of 1,000 mg/day for 19–50-year-olds was determined primarily by estimating the intake for maximal calcium retention. Any extra sweat loss theoretically would increase calcium requirements unless adaptation led to decreased calcium losses by other routes. If sweat calcium losses increase from 111 mg/day at 21°C to 201 mg/day at 37.8°C, as reported by Consolazio at al. (1962), this increase in calcium loss of 90 mg/day would increase calcium requirements by about 300 mg/day, assuming 30 percent absorption efficiency. A better understanding of calcium losses through sweat and adaptive responses over time requires more research. Prolonged exercise may have the effect of strengthening bone through changes in geometry to compensate for a negative calcium balance, as explained earlier in this paper.

The upper level of the committee's recommendation (850 mg/day) was set to minimize risk of kidney stones. Hypercalciuria is associated with increasing supersaturation of the urine, an environment that increases renal stone risk, and would be aggravated by high salt intakes and reduced fluid intakes. However, dietary calcium's role in the risk of renal stone formation under conditions experienced by the military is unknown. In civilians, higher dietary calcium has been associated with decreased risk of kidney stones, unless calcium supplements were taken separately from the consumption of dietary oxalate from food (Curhan et al., 1993, 1997, 2004). The assumption is that calcium consumed with oxalate-containing foods would bind the oxalate that forms insoluble calcium oxalate, which would be excreted in the stools rather than absorbed to form kidney stones.

In the Nurses' Health Study II, 96,245 27–44-year-old women were followed for eight years and experienced 1,223 symptomatic cases of kidney stones. The age-adjusted RR of kidney stones after adjusting for body mass index, family history of kidney stones, calcium supplementation, dietary calcium, animal protein, potassium, sodium, sucrose, phytate, and fluids is shown for each quintile of calcium intake in Table 3-2 (Curhan et al., 2004). Thus, calcium intake greater than the AI for calcium was associated with reduced risk of stones compared to the lowest quintile of calcium intake. The largest reduction in risk occurred between the first and second quintiles of dietary calcium (< 626 to 627–763 mg/day). Supplemental calcium was not independently associated with risk of kidney stones. Other dietary factors showing significant associations with kidney stones between the highest and lowest intake were fluid intake (RR = 0.68, CI = 0.56–0.83), phytate (RR = 0.63, CI = 0.51–0.78), and sucrose (RR = 1.31, CI = 1.07–1.60). Dietary phytate was as protective as dietary calcium in its association with kidney stones. Dietary sodium, potassium, and magnesium were not associated independently with the risk of kidney-stone formation.

The impact of diet on the risk of kidney stones under conditions of inadequate calorie and fluid intake during periods of stress from heat, physical exertion, and combat is unknown. More research is needed to confirm whether or not calcium intake combined with low fluid intake and inadequate caloric intake will increase the risk of kidney stones in military personnel who are engaged in assault missions. The committee finds that short-term calcium intakes below the AI (e.g., 750–850 mg/day) recommended by IOM (1997) do not pose long-term risks because the skeleton's calcium reserve is large and requires prolonged periods of dietary inadequacy to disrupt. However, because of lacking evidence on the link between calcium intake and kidney-stone formation, this committee recommends 1,000 mg/day as the calcium-level upper limit for assault rations.

**TABLE 3-2** Relative Risk for Incident Kidney Stones According to Calcium Intakes in Nurses' Health Study II ($n$ = 96,245; Cases = 1,223)

| Mineral | Quintile 1 | 2 | 3 | 4 | 5 |
|---|---|---|---|---|---|
| **Calcium** | | | | | |
| Intake (mg/day) | ≤ 626 | 627–763 | 764–908 | 909–1,128 | ≥ 1,129 |
| Age-adjusted values | | | | | |
| RR | 1.00 | 0.74 | 0.72 | 0.69 | 0.54 |
| 95% CI | Ref | 0.63–0.87 | 0.61–0.84 | 0.58–0.80 | 0.45–0.63 |
| Multivariate values | | | | | |
| RR* (P = 0.007) | 1.00 | 0.85 | 0.85 | 0.87 | 0.73 |
| 95% CI | Ref | 0.72–1.01 | 0.72–1.02 | 0.73–1.05 | 0.59–0.90 |
| **Phytate** | | | | | |
| Intake (mg/day) | < 596 | 596–697 | 698–797 | 798–938 | ≥ 939 |
| Age-adjusted values | | | | | |
| RR | 1.00 | 0.92 | 0.74 | 0.64 | 0.54 |
| 95% CI | Ref | 0.78–1.08 | 0.63–0.88 | 0.54–0.76 | 0.45–0.65 |
| Multivariate values | | | | | |
| RR* (P < 0.001) | 1.00 | 0.97 | 0.85 | 0.84 | 0.84 |
| 95% CI | Ref | 0.81–1.16 | 0.70–1.02 | 0.69–1.03 | 0.68–1.04 |
| **Fluid** | | | | | |
| Intake (mL/day) | ≤ 1,431 | 1,432–1,850 | 1,851–2,252 | 2,253–2,768 | ≥ 2,769 |
| Age-adjusted values | | | | | |
| RR | 1.00 | 0.85 | 0.76 | 0.67 | 0.63 |
| 95% CI | Ref | 0.72–1.00 | 0.64–0.89 | 0.56–0.80 | 0.53–0.75 |
| Multivariate values | | | | | |
| RR* (P < 0.001) | 1.00 | 0.88 | 0.79 | 0.72 | 0.68 |
| 95% CI | Ref | | | 0.60–0.86 | |

NOTE: *Model included age, BMI, family history of kidney stones, intake of supplemental calcium, dietary calcium, animal protein, potassium, sodium, sucrose, phytate, and fluid.
Ref = Referent group, RR = Relative risk, CI = Confidence interval.
SOURCE: Adapted from Curhan et al. (2004). 

## RECOMMENDATION FOR CALCIUM IN ASSAULT RATIONS: 750–1,000 mg/day

### Strategies for Achieving Sufficient Calcium Intake

*Usual Foods*

During adulthood, calcium intakes offset daily losses and withdrawals from skeletal reserves, and thus prevent loss of bone strength and minimize the bone remodeling needed for optimal bone-structure maintenance (Heaney, 2005). The major sources of calcium in American civilian diets are dairy products, although other foods also contribute. Some vegetables—Chinese cabbage, kale, and broccoli—are relatively high in calcium, although the levels are much lower than in dairy products. The 2005 Dietary Guidelines for Americans recommend 2–3 servings of milk and milk products for most people to meet their dietary calcium needs (U.S. Department of Health and Human Services [DHHS] and United States Department of Agriculture [USDA], 2005). Following a food guide such as MyPyramid or the DASH diet ensures that most people's calcium intakes will meet IOM's AI levels. Diets that are devoid of dairy foods rarely contain more than 200–300 mg of calcium, amounts far below the current AI (Heaney, 2005), and some individuals, particularly older persons, may need to add dietary supplements or fortified foods. Only 30 percent (approximately) of calcium consumed through diet or supplements is absorbed; the remaining calcium is excreted in the feces (IOM, 1997).

*Fortified Foods*

There are many calcium-fortified food sources currently available. Fortified foods are helpful alternatives for individuals who are unable or unwilling to consume sufficient amounts of foods that are naturally high in calcium. There is little danger of excessive fortification since so few products actually contain substantial amounts of calcium, even those that are fortified.

Numerous fortificants are available, and several calcium-fortified food vehicles with stable shelf lives are successful on the market. They include fruit juices, fruit drinks, soy drinks, tofu, and highly fortified cereals, among others. For example, a six-ounce serving of calcium-fortified orange juice provides about 200–260 mg of calcium, a fortified instant breakfast drink provides about 105–250 mg, and a fortified ready-to-eat cereal provides 100–1,000 mg per serving (Office of Dietary Supplements, 2005). Caramel-like chewable candies fortified with relatively large amounts of calcium and vitamin D are also available and may be an option for certain groups with high needs.

Fortified foods help to maximize calcium absorption because the doses are relatively low (so that absorption efficiency is good), and the doses are always consumed with food, slowing release into the duodenum and increasing absorption. However, in developing fortified foods it became apparent that there were interactions between added calcium and many of the constituents in food. Thus, it was necessary to actually ascertain the bioavailability of calcium in the final products that were developed. Calcium is poorly absorbed from foods that are rich in oxalic acid (e.g., spinach, sweet potatoes, rhubarb) and that have high levels of phytic acid (e.g., bran-rich cereals). However, soybeans have calcium that is absorbed nearly as well as from milk, even though it is high in phytate (IOM, 1997).

For liquid products, it is important to ensure that the calcium is soluble in the beverage and that the suspension is stable; in many products the suspension is not stable and the calcium settles out as a sludge in the bottom of the container (Heaney et al., 2005). Therefore, whenever calcium fortification is considered, it is important to determine if the fortified food actually delivers the intended calcium dose.

*Supplementation*

Supplementation is yet another alternative for those who are unable to obtain sufficient calcium from food sources. The level of elemental calcium in supplements varies depending on their salt content. Calcium and phosphate carbonate each contain about 40 percent, calcium citrate about 21 percent, calcium lactate about 13 percent, and calcium gluconate about 9 percent (Levenson and Bockman, 1994). Supplements are absorbed best when they are given as divided doses, because absorption efficiency is inversely proportional to the logarithm of the ingested load (Heaney et al., 1990). Also, slow delivery of calcium to the absorptive sites in the upper small intestine optimizes absorption, and so it is best to take calcium supplements with meals. Variations in bioavailability, pharmaceutical formulation, the matrix, and in the amount of calcium in different supplements are substantial and can vary over a twofold range; therefore, any recommendations for supplementation should be accompanied by studies of actual absorption.

The danger of consuming excessive calcium through supplementation is low. The differences between the UL and the recommendations for calcium needs are relatively high—the recommended maximum level of calcium for adults is 1,450 mg/day, and the UL is 2,500 mg/day (IOM, 1997). The UL is based on the risk of the milk-alkali syndrome, which involves a hypercalcemia at the same time that the kidney and the skeleton are hypoperfused (insufficient blood flow) and thus effecting calcium regulation and homeostasis. However, the milk-alkali syndrome—and other adverse effects, such as nephrocalcinosis and renal insufficiency—usually occurs only at very large doses (about 5 g/day of elemental calcium or more than 12 g/day of calcium carbonate) (IOM, 1997). Milk-alkali syndrome can be managed by hydration and by maintaining blood flow to the kidneys and bones.

There is little evidence that supplementary calcium causes renal stones, although people who are at risk of kidney-stone formation should not take supplements. There is some evidence that supplemental calcium taken without food may increase the risk of kidney stones in women, and possibly in men, perhaps because doing so decreases the potential for calcium to bind oxalate in foods and subsequently to reduce oxalate kidney stones (Curhan et al., 1997, 2004). Although this risk can be avoided by taking calcium supplements with food, people who are prone to kidney stones should not take supplemental calcium at all, especially when there is a risk of dehydration.

As calcium intake increases, the efficiency of intestinal calcium falls, so that the urinary calcium levels do not rise greatly (Allen, 1998). Although there has never been a reported case of calcium overdosing from food sources, even at levels as high as 6,000 mg/day, even greater excess is possible from supplements. For that reason, intakes of more than 2,500 mg/day are not recommended (Heaney, 2005). People with low levels of stomach acid (achlorhydria) should take calcium with food. People who undergo calcitriol (active vitamin D) therapy and those who suffer from sarcoidosis (which increases calcium absorption) also should use calcium supplements with caution. There is considerable evidence that supplementation works and that people adhere to it. There are a number of calcium supplementation trials reviewed in the literature, and most have shown positive effects on bone health (Elders et al., 1994; Lloyd et al., 1993; Weisman and Matkovic, 2005; Winters-Stone and Snow, 2004).

Up to 90 percent of calcium is excreted through feces. The presence of a calcium-rich digesta might have some health-related effects. For example, high calcium intakes (over 1,000 mg/day) cause oxalic acid to be absorbed poorly from plant foods or other sources, and the formation of calcium oxalate in the gut reduces oxalate absorption and the renal oxalate load, thereby reducing the risk of kidney stones (Heaney, 2005). Calcium also complexes with free fatty acids and bile acids in the disgestate, a process that might decrease the irritant quality of the fatty acids. Finally, calcium complexes with dietary phosphorus, blocking the calcium's absorption to some extent. So, calcium salts are used to control hyperphsophatemia; every 500 mg of ingested calcium binds about 165 mg of phosphorus that is ingested at the same time (Heaney, 2005).

One of the problems with all mineral supplements is that the tablets or pills are relatively large, so many people find it difficult to swallow them. Chewable calcium products exist and are often acceptable even to those who find the tablets too difficult to swallow. Constipation problems related to calcium supplementation are poorly documented; in several clinical trials there was little evidence that constipation occurred (Clemens and Feinstein, 1977).

Many forms of calcium supplements exist, mainly as salts (carbonates, citrates, phosphates, lactates, and citrate-malate). Salts of gluconic acid, calcium acetate, and calcium chelates with amino acids are somewhat less common but are also available. The elemental calcium amounts they contain vary from about 40 percent calcium in the carbonate to 21 percent in the calcium citrate (Hendler and Rorvik, 2001). Aside from a slight advantage of calcium citrate malate and the chelates, most of the major salts of calcium are absorbed equally well (Heaney et al., 2001). Other research suggests that the citrate form of calcium is better absorbed (Kenny et al., 2004; Sakhaee et al., 1999). However, although the bioavailability may be similar, some products that are poorly formulated may not disintegrate, and thus, absorption may be decreased. This problem can be avoided by focusing on supplements that meet U.S. Pharmacopoeia Disintegration Standards or by using only products that have been tested for their bioavailability. It is also important to ensure that the supplement is stable under the expected use conditions, which in many missions in the armed forces are likely to involve extremes in temperature and humidity.

There are several interactions between calcium and other diet components or pharmaceutical drugs. Calcium supplements bind with tetracycline, and they also may interfere with thyroxin absorption. Calcium salts and foods high in calcium reduce absorption of heme and nonheme iron eaten at the same meal. With regard to drug interactions, calcium may decrease absorption of biphophonates, $H^2$ blockers, l-thyroxin, proton pump inhibitors, quinolones, and tetracyclines. Vitamin D analogues increase calcium absorption (Hendler and Rorvik, 2001).

The increased use of calcium supplements and fortified foods has raised concerns about high calcium intakes and their influence on producing relative deficiencies of several minerals. High calcium intakes have produced relative magnesium deficiencies in rats (Evans et al., 1990). However, calcium intake does not affect magnesium retention in humans (Andon et al., 1996). Similarly, except for a single report in postmenopausal women (Wood and Zheng, 1997), decreased zinc retention has not been associated with high calcium intakes (Dawson-Hughes et al., 1986; Spencer et al., 1984). The nature of this interaction is unclear and requires further study. Iron absorption from nonheme sources is decreased by 30 to 50 percent from radiolabeled test meals in the presence of calcium intakes up to 300 mg/day, after which there is no further reduction. Thus, practically speaking, it is prudent to set iron requirements assuming that individuals are going to ingest 300 mg of calcium at each meal (Gleerup et al., 1995). The inhibition of iron absorption by calcium does not appear to be a gut effect and may involve competition with the transport of iron in the intestinal mucosa (Halberg et al., 1992), possibly at the level of mobilferrin. A period of up to 12 weeks of calcium supplementation does not produce changes in iron status (Whiting, 1995). Long-term supplementation also does not reduce total body iron mass accumulation in adolescent girls (Ilich-Ernst et al., 1998). Similarly, calcium salts inhibit heme iron absorption in a single meal, but do not affect long-term iron status (Roughead et al., 2005). Single-meal iron absorption studies quite possibly exaggerate inhibitory effects that disappear in the context of the whole diet.

### Recommendations for Achieving Sufficiency

The main consideration when comparing strategies to increase calcium intake is practicality. The estimated calcium contents of rations suggest that many, but not all, MRE menus meet a calcium level for which consumption of two rations will provide the AI of 1,000 mg/day. Ideally, the calcium levels in all operational rations should be increased that the AI is achievable with two rations. The addition of dairy products would appear to be most effective since they are the main source of calcium and other nutrients; however, some situations might not lend themselves to dairy product increases and some individuals may refuse to consume dairy products or may be lactose intolerant. If these are real concerns for soldiers in garrison training, then strategies like fortification or supplementation should be tested for increasing calcium intake.

### Research Needs

*Specific Priorities*

- Quantify calcium losses due to the stressful conditions of garrison training (i.e., heat and physical exertion, psychological stressors).
- Assess the current diets and calcium intake of military personnel under the various environments as a practical approach to assess calcium status. This should include calcium intakes from food, beverages, dietary supplements, and calcium-containing mediators like antacids.
- Conduct balance and kinetic studies to understand the role of physical activity on calcium metabolism and requirements.
- Study the potential adverse effects of weight loss and the interactions with calcium supplementation in bone loss.
- Study of the potential role of dietary calcium in counteracting the negative interaction of exercise and OCs on bone in women.
- Study the relationship between calcium intakes greater than 850 mg/day and the risk of kidney-stone formation.
- Study the relationship of calcium intake and mood, PMS symptoms, depression, and other psychological factors that affect performance.

*Other Research Needs*

- Assess the effects of calcium on cognitive and psychomotor function and sleep quantity and quality.

## COPPER RECOMMENDATIONS

*Need for Copper*

Copper is an essential trace element required for the functioning of all organ systems. Because of its ubiquitous nature in many oxidation–reduction reactions, a severe deficiency of copper could have far reaching effects, in-

**TABLE 3-3** Copper Values

| Source | Amount |
|---|---|
| Total body content | 50–120 mg |
| Military Dietary Reference Intakes | Not established |
| Estimated Average Requirement (ages > 19 years) | 700 μg/day |
| Recommended Dietary Allowance | 900 μg/day |
| Urine loss (normal conditions) | 20 μg/day |
| Fecal loss | 240 μg/day |

SOURCE: Baker-Fulco et al. (2001); IOM (2001); Turnlund (1999).

cluding effects related to adenosine triphosphate (ATP) synthesis, iron transport, norepinephrine synthesis, connective tissue synthesis, and dismutation of superoxide anion. Fortunately, copper deficiency in humans has not been documented except in cases of genetic disorders (Menkes disease), in total parenteral solutions (Percival, 1995), in a prolonged jejunostomy feed (Jayakumar et al., 2005), and with high zinc consumption (Willis et al., 2005). A summary of some physiological values as well as established requirements for copper are presented in Table 3-3.

*Absorption and Metabolism*

Copper homeostasis is maintained by balancing absorption distribution, storage, and excretion. Copper is absorbed in the upper portion of the small intestine (IOM, 2001; Schumann et al., 2002), and the amount of copper absorbed is dependent on the amount consumed. Turnlund et al. (1989) estimated that copper absorption in adults has a set point rate of 0.8 to 1.0 mg in 24 hours. Adequate hydrochloric acid production facilitates copper absorption presumably by aiding protein digestion and increasing copper availability. Alkaline pH values may reduce copper bioavailability by forming copper-hydroxides. Phytates, even though they may impact zinc and iron absorption, do not impair the absorption of copper. Organic acids increase absorption of copper. For more details see Hunt in Appendix B.

Copper absorbed in the small intestine is transported to the liver, and sometimes to the kidney, predominately bound to albumin. Uptake of copper by the hepatocytes occurs with a specific copper transport proteins designated hCtr1 (Lee J et al., 2002). Once in the cytosol, copper is bound to peptides known as chaperones. Each chaperone transports copper to a specific protein. Copper is exported from the hepatocytes after incorporation into ceruloplasmin. This is accomplished with a copper binding ATP-ase located in the Golgi. Very little copper is excreted in the urine, thus the regulation of body copper is through bile and fecal excretion (Turnlund, 1999). Total body copper is regulated tightly at the level of the intestine. For more details see Hunt in Appendix B.

## Measuring Copper Status

There is no one single measure that sensitively and specifically reflects copper status. Copper status measures have been discussed extensively (IOM, 2001), and no standard has yet been agreed on (Keen, 2005; see Keen and Uriu-Adams in Appendix B). For example, serum copper and serum ceruloplasmin activity are reduced when the deficiency is overt but do not appear to be sensitive enough to detect marginal deficiency (Hopkins and Failla, 1995). Other copper dependent enzymes located in peripheral blood cells have been suggested as potential status indicators, but research has not yet progressed to an agreement on any of them. Extracellular superoxide dismutase and ceruloplasmin activity are not particularly sensitive, especially in searching for marginal copper deficiency (IOM, 2001). Cytochrome C oxidase and copper–zinc superoxide dismutase (CuZnSOD) have been measured in erythrocytes, lymphocytes, platelets, and neutrophils; although these enzymes reflect copper status in animal models, rigorous testing in humans has not established any one method as superior over another. Obviously, better balance data are needed on copper and measures of copper status for marginal deficiencies.

Newer research on copper transporters and copper chaperones suggests that these are not likely to help with status measurements either. The only chaperone that changes in copper deficiency is the one that delivers copper to CuZnSOD, and it is expressed greater when dietary copper is low (Bertinato and L'Abbe, 2004).

Although there is no consensus on biomarkers of copper status, experts agree that more than one index should be used for determining human copper status. The specific activity of ceruloplasmin (the ratio of ceruloplasmin activity to ceruloplasmin protein), copper concentration of platelets or lymphocytes, and cytochrome C oxidase activity in platelets or CuZnSOD activity in erythrocytes, or both, have been used as biomarkers of copper in various studies (Koury et al, 2004; Metin et al., 2003; Milne and Nielsen, 1996; Schumann et al., 2002; Turnlund et al., 1997).

## Copper Intake Effects on Health and Performance

### *Physical Performance*

Because copper is required for cytochrome C oxidase and takes part in electron transport, a lack of copper theoretically could result in reduced physical performance due to reduced ATP synthesis. However, even though several studies using animals show a reduction in ATP levels in severe copper deficiency

(Davies and Lawrence, 1986; Kopp et al., 1983; Reiser et al., 1983; Rusinko and Prohaska, 1985), other studies show that reduced levels cytochrome C oxidase in copper deficiency do not impair ATP production (Rusinko and Prohaska, 1985). Still other studies show impaired mitochondrial respiratory complexes with copper deficiency; increased heme oxygenase-1 expression during copper deficiency in rats results from increased mitochondrial generation of hydrogen peroxide (Johnson and DeMars, 2004). Nevertheless, it is not known how this increase of hydrogen peroxide influences performance.

Most of the research on athletes shows no changes in serum copper or ceruloplasmin (Buchman et al., 1998; Gropper et al., 2003; Koury et al., 2004; Nuviala et al., 1999), whether measured after competition or compared to a sedentary control group. A moderate increase in serum copper was found in professional sportsmen compared to that found in the controls, especially if the sportsmen were involved in anaerobic exercise (Rodriguez Tuya et al., 1996). Anderson et al. (1995) found serum copper was elevated moderately immediately following strenuous exercise in trained (15–17 μmol/L) as well as in untrained (13–15 μmol/L) individuals. Metin et al. (2003) found a slight decrease in serum copper and ceruloplasmin in football players (74.9 μg/dL) as compared with the sedentary controls (137.7 μg/dL). These values are within the normal range for plasma copper. Concentration of copper in the sweat was not reported. Physical activity or training does not appear to impact serum copper levels to a great extent, and therefore does not appear to impact copper status.

Since exercise generates free radicals, scientists have hypothesized that more copper may be required for optimal CuZnSOD activity during physical activity. Despite the fact that some studies show an increase in CuZnSOD activity (Koury et al., 2004; Lukaski et al., 1990; Metin et al., 2003), some authors suggest that since the study showed no decrease in copper status with physical training (Lukaski et al., 1990) the increase might be due to a biological adaptation to minimize oxidative damage to the tissue rather than to an increase in copper requirement.

In summary, there is not a strong body of knowledge that supports increasing copper intake for physical performance benefits.

*Immune System*

Copper, like all nutrients, is essential for optimal immune function (Percival, 2005; see Percival in Appendix B). Evidence in rats suggests that marginal copper deficiency will impair peripheral blood mononuclear cell proliferation without reducing conventional markers of copper status (Hopkins and Failla, 1995). Evidence in humans suggests that peripheral blood mononuclear cell proliferation reduction will result only after consuming diets very low copper (0.4 mg/d) for several months (Kelley et al., 1995). In general, alterations in functional immune tests due to copper deficiency are not specific to copper; other nutrient deficiencies result in similar alterations in functional immunity. Neutropenia may be the one sign of copper deficiency that is specific to copper, however, neutropenia occurs only after several months of a very copper-deficient diet and may require other factors (such as inflammation) to manifest itself (Percival, 1995).

*Cognitive Performance*

Very little data are available on the relationship between copper and cognition. Research in the elderly has examined the effect of copper on cognitive tests and on dementia. Smorgon et al. (2004) and Squitti et al. (2002) showed high serum copper in Alzheimer's dementia and suggested that copper influenced the evolution of cognitive impairment. Squitti et al. (2002) also showed that serum copper levels were higher in subjects with Alzheimer's disease. However, Pajonk et al. (2005) showed that cognitive decline correlated with a low plasma concentration of copper in mild to moderate Alzheimer's patients. This same group (Bayer et al., 2003) investigated β-amyloid precursor protein (APP), a copper binding protein, and showed that chronic overexpression of APP formation reduces CuZnSOD activity, which was restored by copper supplementation. Dietary copper also was able to reduce the amyloid plaque formation in transgenic mice. A supplement (500 mg of vitamin C, 400 IU of vitamin E, 15 mg of β-carotene, 80 mg of zinc, and 2 mg of copper) used for prevention of macular degeneration in the Age-Related Eye Disease Study did not show either harmful or beneficial effects on cognition in older adults (Yaffe et al., 2004).

Rodent models of severe prenatal copper deficiency show profound effects on brain and motor function (Penland and Prohaska, 2004). There appears to be a critical prenatal window during which copper deficiency can cause permanent damage to the central nervous system. However, postnatal copper deficiency, even if severe, does not cause neurological disorders. Two genetic diseases—Wilson's disease (copper overload and accumulation in liver, brain, and kidneys) and Menkes disease (copper deficiency)—result in neurological disorders (Schumann et al., 2002). Neurological effects of Wilson's disease take years to develop, however, with Menkes disease, the neurological consequences (severe developmental delay and loss of early development skills) already are present at birth.

There are no previous studies that have made direct correlations between soldiers' copper intake or status and their cognitive function or behavior, and only two studies, both from the same laboratory, have been conducted with civilians (Penland, 1988; Penland et al., 2000). In studies on women, restricted dietary copper has been associated with impaired verbal memory, disrupted sleep, and mood states (see Table 3-4). In a double-blind, metabolic study of 23 healthy postmenopausal women (Penland et al., 2000), short-term memory and immediate recall of words presented verbally (i.e., list recall) worsened when women

**TABLE 3-4** Aspects of Cognitive Changes in Copper Deficiency

| Source | Copper Levels | Cognitive Changes* |
|---|---|---|
| Penland, 1988 | 1 versus 3 mg | Increased sleep time<br>Increased sleep latency<br>Decreased feeling restless<br>Increased depression<br>Increased confusion |
| Penland et al., 2000 | 1 versus 3 mg | Decreased short-term memory<br>Increased distraction |

*Effect of lower, compared with higher intake.

were fed diets low in copper as compared to diets high in copper (1 versus 3 mg/day) and also zinc (53 mg/day). Low copper intakes also were associated with increased difficulty in discriminating between relevant and irrelevant responses. Plasma copper and ceruloplasmin were associated positively with improved verbal memory and long-term memory and with increased clustering of verbal material (strategy), but fewer intrusions (reduced distractions) during recall (Penland et al., 2000).

In depletion-repletion experiments (Penland, 1988), research showed the following when dietary copper was low (< 1 versus > 2 mg/day): increased sleep times, increased sleep latency and feeling less rested on awakening, and increased confusion, depression, and total mood disturbances. In an unpublished study, Penland reviewed the medical charts of adult participants in long-term, live-in metabolic studies to examine the incidence of requests for medication to relieve pain unrelated to injury or illness (Penland, 2005; see Penland in Appendix B).

The activities of two copper-dependent enzymes may explain at least partially the diverse putative effects of copper intake on memory, mood, and sleep. Dopamine-β-monooxygenase is required for the synthesis of norepinephrine from dopamine, and CuZnSOD protects catecholamines from oxidation by reactive oxygen species (Johnson, 2005). Dysregulation of the locus coeruleus-noradrenergic system, which supplies norepinephrine throughout the central nervous system, may result in cognitive and arousal dysfunction, including sleep and mood problems (Berridge and Waterhouse, 2003). Although copper impacts biological functions as a catalyst of enzyme activity—that is, it regulates iron absorption, neurotransmitter metabolism, antioxidant defense, and oxygen use—there is no clear evidence that copper status affects cognitive function and behavior.

In summary, the cognitive and psychological impairments (e.g., sleep disturbances, short-term memory loss, depression, confusion, and distraction) found in civilians with marginal copper deficits are consistent with the same problems reported in soldiers during active training and operations (Reeves et al., 2005;

Ritchie and Owens, 2004). However, the importance of copper for cognitive function and behavior has received little attention and is largely unknown. Only two studies suggest that low copper intakes may affect sleep and memory performance. The limited data on copper intake and status of soldiers in various types of training do not provide evidence of overt nutritional deficiencies, however, mild or marginal copper deficiencies in the absence of sensitive biomarkers of copper status cannot be ruled out.

*Bone Health*

Copper is essential for proper bone formation and bone health. Severe copper deficiency in humans (low-birth weight infants and children in developing countries) is associated with osteoporosis, changes in bone similar to those from scurvy, fractures of the long bones and ribs, and epiphyseal separation (Danks, 1980; IOM, 2001; Velin et al., 1989).

## Risks Factors for Inadequacy Under Military Garrison Training

*Inadequate Intake*

Results from the National Health and Nutrition Examination Survey III (NHANES III) estimate the median copper consumption for 19–30-year-old women and men to be 1.1 and 1.6 mg/day, respectively (IOM, 2001). Although copper concentration in military rations has not been calculated, the study by Tharion et al. (2004) on garrison feeding situations for Special Forces soldiers indicates that copper is consumed at an overall average daily intake of 1.7 mg. This intake, in garrison feeding, is presumed to be more than adequate to maintain copper status. In this study, however, soldiers were allowed to eat food from outside the military dining facilities, so the results are less relevant because soldiers deployed to military bases in foreign countries are discouraged from eating from the local economies. Analysis of copper levels in operational rations and data on food intake are needed in order to assess copper intake adequacy.

*Exercise and Environment*

Exercise has been associated with an increased urinary excretion of copper, but not all of the studies show substantial increases. Kikukawa and Kobayashi (2002) studied air rescue trainees during four phases of their curriculum: classroom instruction, daily exercise to build stamina, demanding physical exercise, and simulated mountain rescue. This research was performed in 11 Japanese Air Self-Defense soldiers. Urine was collected in the morning and again in the afternoon for 3–4 consecutive days in each phase. Diet was not altered during the urine collection, and no supplements were allowed. Urinary copper increased almost twofold during all physical activity phases and remained unchanged for the classroom instruction (assuming urinary copper for normal individuals is 20 μg/day or less [IOM, 2001]).

In a study that compared 78 women athletes with 65 sedentary women, urinary excretion of copper was not related to the type of physical activity performed (karate, handball, basketball, and running) (Nuviala et al., 1999). Another study in marathon runners found that copper in the urine was below the level of detection (Buchman et al., 1998). These, and other studies, do not necessarily mimic the stress and physical activity of the soldier, however, overall urinary losses due to exercise may be minimal. There is mixed and limited research on the urinary excretion of copper due to exercise and its significance requires further research.

Copper losses through sweat during exercise have been measured, although none of the studies have been conducted under conditions similar to garrison training; also, methods of sweat collection and copper quantitation varied. The best sweat loss estimates are those calculated from whole-body measurements, because collection from isolated areas (e.g., arm collection) may overestimate losses. The only study to examine copper losses from whole-body measurements was published in 1981 and reported an average copper loss of 340 μg/day (see Table 3-5; Jacob et al., 1981) in individuals at rest. Turnlund et al. (1990) estimated dermal copper loss using arm bags and found copper loss ranged from 0.5 to 5.7 μg/day; as in the study reported by Jacob et al. (1981), the individuals were not exercising. The DRI report estimated 42 μg of surface copper lost per day (IOM, 2001). Omokhodion and Howard (1994) reported an average loss of 486 μg/L in an arm sweat collection during exercise. Consolazio et al. (1964) reported sweat copper losses over three consecutive collections that lasted for 4 days, resulting in reported losses of 1.94, 1.79, and 1.04 mg/day; these values appear high compared with the other studies. Aruoma et al. (1988) estimated copper losses for four sites on the body during exercise. Although the amount of copper lost from each site varied (see Table 3-5), the average loss was 10.6 μmol/L (675 μg/L). They also reported weight loss during exercise, thus allowing for an estimate of sweat losses. During 30–40 minutes of intense exercise, the average weight loss was 0.57 kg. Therefore, assuming a 1-kg weight loss = 1 L sweat, an average of 385 μg of copper were lost during exercise.

With these limited data, it appears that at least 300 μg/day of copper may be lost in sweat during exercise. An exception to this is a study by Stauber and Florence (1988) in which sweating was induced in a small area of the forearm skin with pilocarpine iontrophoresis; the artificially stimulated sweat was collected from the forearm with filters, and the copper level was analyzed by voltammetry. Males lost 103 μg/L, females lost 29 μg/L, and females who were using OCs lost 94 μg/L. The committee, however, questions the accuracy of these data as it is not clear how the induction of sweat or the method used to

**TABLE 3-5** Copper Sweat Losses

| Subjects | Comments | Copper Analysis | Sweat Collection | Sweat Loss | Reference |
|---|---|---|---|---|---|
| Males | Sedentary | Furnace atomic absorption spectrophotometer | Whole body surface | 0.042 mg/day | IOM,2001; Milne et al., 1991; |
| 15 male | Acclimatized, cycle ergometer, room temperature | Atomic absorption spectrophotometry | Arm collection during exercising | 0.486 mg/L | Omokhodion and Howard, 1994 |
| 24 males<br>39 females | Induced sweating with pilocarpine iontrophoresis | Anodic stripping voltammetry | Forearm filters | 0.103 mg/L males<br>0.029 mg/L females<br>0.094 mg/L females taking oral contraceptives | Stauber and Florence, 1988 |
| 13 males | Healthy volunteers, controlled environment | Atomic absorption spectrophotometry | Whole body surface | 0.34 mg/day | Jacob et al., 1981 |
| 3 males | Healthy volunteers in 37°C chamber at 50% relative humidity, 7.5 h/day. | Emission spectrograph | Arm collection over three consecutive four day trials | 1.94 mg/day<br>1.79 mg/day<br>1.04 mg/day | Consolazio et al., 1964 |
| 11 males | No exercise | Furnace atomic absorption spectrophotometry | Arm bag collection | 0.5–5.7 μg/day | Turnlund et al., 1990 |
| 12 males | 30–40 minutes of hard exercise | Atomic absorption spectrophotometer | Arm<br>Back<br>Abdomen<br>Chest | 0.52 mg/L<br>0.56 mg/L<br>0.89 mg/L<br>0.73 mg/L | Aruoma et al., 1988 |

measure copper influenced the results. It is obvious that military personnel in hot climates may lose a significant amount of copper if sweat volumes as high as 7–10 L/day are secreted.

### *Stress*

When an individual is stressed, serum copper levels increase due to an increase in ceruloplasmin. This stress-induced increase would occur even if the individual was mildly or moderately copper deficient. Inflammation also results in higher ceruloplasmin copper in the serum. The consequences of elevated serum copper due to stress or inflammation is unknown (Turnlund, 1999).

### *Bioavailability and Interactions*

Copper absorption is dependent on other dietary minerals, and it is negatively impacted by zinc (25–50 mg/day and above) (IOM, 2001). Copper may be absorbed less efficiently from a vegetarian diet as compared to a nonvegetarian diet, but because plant foods are rich in copper more total copper may be absorbed (Agte et al., 2005; Hunt and Vanderpool, 2001).

Animal studies have shown that copper absorption is affected by high levels of iron, molybdenum, ascorbate, fiber, sucrose, and fructose; the impact on human copper absorption, however, is probably not significant unless the diet is very unusual or a very high level of the antagonist compound is consumed (Turnlund, 1999).

Table 3-6 shows the results from two studies focusing on copper absorption with various dietary intake levels (Turnlund et al., 1989, 1998). An increase in copper intake from 0.8 to 7.5 mg/day only doubled the amount of copper absorbed (Turnlund et al., 1989), and an increase from 0.4 to 2.5 mg/day quadrupled the amount absorbed (Turnlund et al., 1998). Although a similar method was used in both studies (i.e., quantification of stable isotope $^{65}Cu$), true copper absorption in the 1998 study includes in the amount absorbed, not only the copper not excreted in the gastrointestinal tract but also endogenous excretion of

**TABLE 3-6** Copper Absorption

| Dietary Copper (mg/day) | Absorption (mg/day) | True Absorption (mg/day) | Reference |
|---|---|---|---|
| 0.38 | 67% (0.26) | 77% (0.29) | Turnlund et al., 1998 |
| 0.66 | 54% (0.35) | 73% (0.48) | |
| 2.49 | 44% (1.08) | 66% (1.64) | |
| 0.8 | 56% (0.45) | Not available | Turnlund et al., 1989 |
| 1.7 | 36% (0.61) | | |
| 7.5 | 12% (0.90) | | |

copper eliminated over 12 days after the infusion. It is therefore a more accurate determination of copper absorption rate.

Copper's bioavailability also is dependent on the form in which it is added to foods. Cupric sulfate and cupric chloride are more bioavailable than copper oxide. According to a study that reviewed dietary supplements, infant formulas, and ready-to-eat cereal products, more than 25 percent of the 18 vitamin and mineral supplements examined contained no copper, 40 percent contained cupric oxide (a form that has low absorption), and under 30 percent contained the more bioavailable form (either cupric sulfate or cupric chloride) (Johnson et al., 1998).

### Requirements for the General U.S. Population

The IOM EAR and RDA for copper for 19–50-year-old individuals is 700 and 900 μg/day, respectively (IOM, 2001; Table 3-1). Currently, there is no MDRI because there was not an IOM RDA at the time when the MRDI was established. A few human studies on the copper intake and status assessment were used to calculate the EAR (Milne and Nielson, 1996; Milne et al., 1990; Turnlund et al., 1990, 1997). The estimated value of 700 μg/day was confirmed by calculating obligatory losses. Basal copper excretion has been estimated as follows: endogenous fecal copper (240 μg/day); urinary copper (< 20 μg/day); surface copper losses (42 μg/day); and other copper losses, such as through semen or menstruation (42 μg/day) (IOM, 2001). Therefore, total basal copper loss is estimated to be 344 μg/day. The IOM EAR correct for an absorption value of 75 percent and result in a requirement of 460 μg/day. An additional 50 μg were added to account for endogenous fecal losses. This results in 510 μg/day, which is slightly lower that the estimated by obligatory losses (700 μg/day). For copper, two standard deviations are added to the EAR to obtain the IOM RDA (IOM, 2001).

### Daily Intake Recommendations for Military Personnel in Garrison Training

Evidence for changing copper requirements is scant and weak. It is unclear on the significance of copper losses in urine and feces attributable to exercise. Copper losses in sweat have not been very well established but will be considered as the basis for increased requirements by military personnel. Unfortunately, as described previously, there are no data from studies to estimate copper losses during exercise beyond an exercise duration of 30–40 minutes (Aruoma et al., 1988). Using the mean sweat copper concentrations of 0.52 and 0.56 mg/L from the arm and back, respectively, sweat copper loss would be 300–320 μg during 30–40 minutes of heavy exercise. Higher copper losses occurred in the abdominal and chest areas, 0.73 to 0.89 mg/L, respectively; thus, estimated sweat copper loss during the 30–40 minutes of exercise was 420 to 510 μg. However, such short-time exercise does not provide information regarding potential sweat concentration decreases with time, as happens with iron and zinc.

The study by Consolazio et al. (1964), which was conducted under moderate exercise and high temperature for 16 days, shows a decrease in average sweat copper from 1.95 mg/day on days 5–8 to 1.04 mg/day on days 13–16; this decrease suggests a possible acclimatization to heat effect. However, sweat was collected by an arm bag method, which likely led to overestimation of copper losses as the data suggest. The only study to examine copper losses from whole-body measurements reported an average copper loss of 340 μg/day (see Table 3-5; Jacob et al., 1981); the study used 13 male volunteers who were sitting in the heat. This average is in contrast to the sweat losses estimated in the same study by an arm sweat collection method in which copper losses of 214 μg/L were estimated from six subjects who also were sitting in the heat. Assuming that soldiers may lose up to 10 L/day of sweat when exposed to a hot environment, the total copper loss would be 2 mg/day. Data reported by Consolazio et al. (1964) estimates copper loss on days 13–16 of 1.04 mg/day.

No study has been conducted to determine copper sweat losses with appropriate methodology and under conditions of exercise similar to those in garrison training. The studies available suggest that copper levels of at least 300 μg/day and as much as 1,000 μg/day can be secreted under conditions of physical activity in heat and humidity. The committee concluded that it would be prudent to assume sweat losses of 500 μg/day—this is a conservative value that can be used until appropriate data are collected. There is an imminent need to conduct research that will determine accurately the level of sweat copper losses under military garrison training.

Based on these potential sweat losses, requirements for military garrison feeding in hot conditions might increase by at least 500 μg/day with respect to the current requirements. Assuming a rate of absorption for copper to be approximately 75 percent (Turnlund et al., 1998), then the additional requirement would be 666 μg/day. Although there are no data that demonstrate a gender difference in copper sweat losses, studies conducted to measure zinc and iron reported that women lose 30 percent less of those minerals due to less total sweat volume not to differences in concentration of either of the minerals (DeRuisseau et al., 2002). The committee assumed 30 percent less sweat losses for women. Following the same calculation as for men, total copper losses would be 350 μg/day for women. The $EAR_{MGT}$ was calculated by applying a 75 percent rate of absorption and adding these amounts to the IOM EAR (700 μg/day); the levels were rounded to the nearest 100 μg. For males the $EAR_{MGT}$ is 1,400 μg/day [500/0.75 + 700] and for females it is 1,200 μg/day [350/0.75) + 700]. The $RDA_{MGT}$ were calculated by adding two times the coefficient of variation of the $EAR_{MGT}$.

**RECOMMENDATIONS FOR COPPER INTAKE:**

| | |
|---|---|
| **$EAR_{MGT}$ for men** | **1,400 μg/day** |
| **$EAR_{MGT}$ for women** | **1,200 μg/day** |
| **$RDA_{MGT}$ for men** | **1,800 μg/day** |
| **$RDA_{MGT}$ for women** | **1,500 μg/day** |

## Adequacy of IOM Recommendations for First Strike Rations

The assault rations report recommended a copper level range of 900–1,600 μg/day in the ration used for short-term, sustained operations (IOM, 2006; Table C-1 in Appendix C). This range is based on the current IOM RDA for adult men and on the potential for sweat losses derived by Consolazio et al. (1964). The committee considered the worst-case scenario, which in the case of this experiment meant that the subjects were not heat acclimatized, and concur that sweat loss is the one factor that needs to be considered in the case of copper; until better data on sweat losses are collected, this range is appropriate, although preliminary.

## Strategies for Achieving Sufficient Copper Intake

### *Usual Foods*

Dietary copper is usually adequate in the United States, and copper deficiency is reported rarely. Food sources do not seem to vary much in copper bioavailability. Phytates do not seem to affect copper absorption. Bioavailability of copper is about 12–75 percent, considerably higher than most of the other trace elements. Foods high in copper include legumes, mushrooms, chocolate, nuts and seeds, and liver. Although there are other foods like bread, potatoes, milk, chicken, and tomatoes that are not so high in copper, they are eaten in such high amounts that they contribute substantially to copper intakes (IOM, 2001; Turnlund, 1999). In most food composition tables, the copper content is higher than in chemically analyzed diets. In some studies of pooled intakes from various studies, the intakes were compared to analyzed diets, and again the analyzed diets clearly had a lower copper content (Gibson and Scythes, 1982; Klevay et al., 1993; Rawson and Medeiros, 1989).

### *Food Fortification*

Copper has not been used as a fortificant in major foodstuffs, but a few of the newer snacks on the market are now copper fortified. Since there is little experience in use of copper as a fortificant, the efficacy and acceptability of copper fortification is unknown. Some fortificants are available, but there is little information on appropriate vehicles or on interactions between copper and food constituents.

*Supplementation*

The danger of excess copper from supplementation cannot be overlooked. The typical supplementation doses are about 1.3 to 2.2 mg/day. The UL for adults is about 10 mg (IOM, 2001). Although this amount includes a 50- to 400-fold safety factor, copper in high amounts (above 1 gram) is extremely toxic.

Several copper supplements are available on the market; however, the only supplement listed on the U.S. Pharmacopeia convention for oral use on the market is copper gluconate and cupric sulfate (http://www.healthtouch.com/bin/EContent_HT/drugShowLfts.asp?fname=usp0477.htm&title=Cupric+Sulfate&cid=HT). Instead, some research scientists have used copper salts of amino acids. Copper oxide also is present in some vitamin-mineral supplements; it is a poorly absorbed form of the nutrient but commonly used because it has a high elemental copper content per unit weight (Baker, 1999).

Drugs and nutrients that can cause interactions with high levels of copper include penicillin and iron (nonheme iron decreases copper status). Excess zinc decreased absorption of copper and vice versa. Vitamin C in very large doses (500 mg or more) can decrease the activity of the copper transport protein ceruloplasmin (Hendler and Rorvik, 2001). Sugars, including high-fructose corn syrup, also can interfere with copper absorption (Turnlund, 1999).

### Recommendations for Achieving Sufficiency

MREs and FSRs might need to be fortified with bioavailable forms of copper (copper sulfate or copper chloride are more bioavailable than copper oxide). Copper may need to be encapsulated due to its capability to oxidize other food macromolecules.

### Research Needs

- Quantify copper losses due to stressful conditions during garrison training (i.e., heat and physical exertion, psychological stressors).
- Determine copper concentrations of food items in operational rations, including MREs and FSRs, and dietary intake levels of military personnel.

## IRON RECOMMENDATIONS

Iron functions as a component of a number of proteins, including enzymes and hemoglobin (the latter being important for the transport of oxygen to tissues throughout the body for metabolism).

Iron can exist in oxidation states ranging from –2 to +6. In biological systems, four major classes of iron-containing proteins exist: iron-containing heme proteins (e.g., hemoglobin, myoglobin, and cytochromes), iron sulfur enzymes (e.g., flavoproteins and heme-flavoproteins), proteins for iron storage and transport (e.g., transferrin, lactoferrin, ferritin, and hemosiderin), and other iron-containing or activated enzymes (e.g., non-iron sulfur, nonheme enzymes). Hemoglobin, myoglobin, and the cytochromes are key functional proteins essential for the movement of oxygen from the environment to the functioning cells. These proteins, in combination with other cellular iron proteins, function in a broad variety of roles in oxidative metabolism and gene regulation and constitute the essential iron pool (IOM, 2001).

The components of iron requirements—which increase during pregnancy and growth (IOM, 2001)—include basal iron losses and menstrual iron losses and may change significantly in environmentally extreme conditions where there are further substantial losses of iron in sweat.

### *Body Content*

A 75-kg adult man contains about 4 g of iron (50 mg/kg) (Bothwell et al., 1979). A menstruating woman has about 40 mg/kg of iron because of a smaller erythrocyte mass and iron store. Almost two-thirds of the body's iron is found in hemoglobin of circulating erythrocytes. A readily-mobile iron store contains another 25 percent in the form of lactoferrin, ferritin, and hemosiderin. Most of the remaining 15 percent is in the myoglobin of muscle tissue and in a variety of enzymes necessary for oxidative metabolism and many other functions in all cells.

### *Absorption*

The body's iron content is highly conserved and tightly regulated by a number of processes from absorption to the transportation from the enterocyte to the serum. In the absence of bleeding (including menstruation) or pregnancy, only a small quantity is lost each day (Bothwell et al., 1979). The addition of all iron losses predicts that adult men need to absorb only about 1 mg/day to maintain iron balance; although variability is high for women's losses through the menses, the average requirement for menstruating women is somewhat higher, approximately 1.5 mg/day.

The two main regulators of the amount of iron absorbed in humans are (1) the total amount and form of iron compounds ingested and (2) the iron status of the individual (Finch and Huebers, 1982). Thus, individuals with an adequate iron status will absorb proportionally less of the dietary iron than will iron-deficient individuals and vice versa. This process of selective absorption is the fundamental mechanism whereby humans regulate iron balance (Bothwell et al., 1979). Although the details of regulation still are not entirely clear, major discoveries in the last decade have revealed substantial mechanistic details. At supra-physiological levels (i.e., high-dose iron supplementation), iron apparently can move across the gut by paracellular diffusion following a concentration gradient. At physiological concentrations, (i.e., those expected from food consumption), iron uptake is mediated by a series of receptors and binding proteins, specific for heme and nonheme iron.

**Heme iron absorption.** Specific transporters exist and have been characterized for the heme molecule on the surface of enterocytes (Conrad and Umbreit, 2000; Shayeghi et al., 2005). After binding to its receptor; the heme molecule is internalized and acted on by heme oxygenase to release the iron to the soluble cytoplasmic pool (Raffin et al., 1974; Shayeghi et al., 2005). The intestine is far more efficient at heme iron absorption than it is at nonheme iron absorption (Bothwell et al., 1979). In a typical American diet, it is reasonable to expect that overall dietary nonheme iron is absorbed at a rate of approximately 5–10 percent, whereas heme iron is nearly 40 percent absorbed.

**Nonheme iron absorption.** The divalent metal transporter (DMT) 1 and serum transferrin receptor (sTfR) are transmembrane proteins that reside on the luminal membrane and have a strong preference for divalent metals (Aisen et al., 2001; Gunshin et al., 1997). The nonheme iron in the lumen of the gut has variable solubility depending on the various amounts of ferric and ferrous iron and the amount of iron-binding compounds. The rapid conversion of ferric to ferrous iron is accomplished by a membrane-bound member of the cytochrome P450 family, duodenal cytochrome B (Anderson and Frazer, 2005), which is in sufficient abundance as to not be limiting to the transport capacity of DMT1 and the internalization via vesicle endocytosis. The internalized vesicle undergoes further modification and acidification with a resulting release of iron to the cytoplasmic space. The released iron is then free to be transported to the basolateral membrane for export by an intracellular iron-binding protein(s) or to be incorporated into ferritin (Eisenstein, 2000).

**Transportation from gastrointestinal cell to plasma.** Given the regulation of absorption by iron status, it long has been predicted that a signal in the plasma may communicate to enterocytes, consequently resulting in homeostatic control (Lee P et al., 2002; Nicolas et al., 2001). The signal compound, hepcidin, has been characterized as a low molecular weight protein secreted by hepatocytes in amounts proportional to iron stores (Nicolas et al., 2002). Hepcidin appears to be released from liver in response to both iron accumulation and the cytokines released during inflammation. It appears to have two primary targets—the macrophage and the basolateral membrane of the enterocyte. In the macrophage, it regulates the release of iron from ferritin stores into the plasma pool. Hepcidin binds to another transmembrane protein, ferroportin, and results in internalization and destruction (Nemeth et al., 2006). The newly described iron exporter, ferroportin, contains an iron response element motif in its mRNA sequence of nucleotides that makes it sensitive to the iron status of the cell. Mutant forms of this protein are associated with very severe iron overload (Nemeth et al., 2006; Nicolas et al., 2002). External signals, such as hepcidin from the liver, interact with proteins like ferroportin and the hemochromatosis gene product, HFE, to regulate the release of iron from the abluminal side of the enterocyte (Nicolas et al., 2002).

## Measuring Iron Status

A number of biomarkers are accepted widely as indications of iron status in populations [World Health Organization (WHO) and U.S. Centers for Disease Control and Prevention (CDC), 2005]. Laboratory tests can be used in combination to identify the evolution of iron deficiency through iron deficiency stages; the indicators and stages are described in this section and in Table 3-7. The three iron deficiency stages are (1) depleted iron stores, with no limitation in the supply of iron to the functional compartment; (2) early functional iron deficiency (iron-deficient erythropoiesis), when the supply of iron to the functional compartment is suboptimal but not reduced sufficiently to cause measurable anemia; and (3) iron deficiency anemia, when there is a measurable deficit in the most accessible functional compartment, the erythrocyte (IOM, 2001).

Since the current knowledge about iron atatus in the military is limited because of a lack in field data, developing data collection approaches that are practical and feasible in the field would be helpful. As stated previously, iron status cannot be evaluated with one simple measurement; new approaches use blood and sera samples collected on filter paper, which makes more feasible the collection of field samples, their preservation, and their transfer to a central laboratory for analysis.

### *Storage Iron Depletion*

Storage iron depletion is normally characterized by the measurement of serum ferritin, because no other biomarkers are sensitive to variations in the storage iron pool until it is nearly empty (e.g., total iron binding capacity, see Table 3-7). The ratio of log(ferritin)/(sTfR) is a newly suggested index of body iron status and is sensitive to storage pool depletion as well as to the stages of functional iron deficiency (Cook et al., 2003). See the section below titled *Early Iron Deficiency*.

The biomarker is sensitive to changes in body iron due to acute blood loss as well as changes in body iron status with more gradual increases or decreases in iron balance (WHO and CDC, 2005). However, this biomarker is not widely used yet since an agreement on reference levels related to specific outcomes has not been reached yet.

**Serum ferritin.** The concentration of plasma and serum ferritin is propor-

**TABLE 3-7** Indicators of Iron Status and Functional Outcomes

| Indicator | Comments | Level | Outcome |
|---|---|---|---|
| Serum ferritin | Direct correlation with iron stores is altered by inflammation | ≥ 15 µg/L | Iron stores are present |
| | Median iron stores for menstruating women 36–40, for men 112–156 µg/L | < 12 µg/L | Iron stores totally depleted |
| Total iron binding capacity | Less precise than serum ferritin<br>30–40% of individuals with low iron storage do not have increased binding capacity | > 400 µg/dL | Storage iron depletion |
| Serum transferrin saturation | Responsive to change in plasma iron (e.g., inflammation) as well as fed/fasted and depleted iron delivery to plasma<br>Median transferring Saturation:<br>26–30% (men)<br>21–24% (women) | < 16% | Early functional iron deficiency |
| Free erythrocyte protoporphyrin | Indicator of sufficiency of iron delivery to bone marrow | > 70 µg/dL | Early functional iron deficiency<br>Measures severity of iron deficiency |
| Serum transferrin receptor | Specific and sensitive to tissue iron deficiency | > 8.5 mg/L | Early functional iron deficiency<br>Measures severity of iron deficiency erithropoiesis |
| Hemoglobin concentration | Not sensitive or specific<br>Only 50% positive predictive value for iron deficiency when used alone<br>Median:<br>144–154 g/L (men)<br>132–135 g/L (women | < 130 g/L (men)<br>< 120 g/L (women) | Anemia |
| Mean cell volume | Not specific | < 80 fL (femtoliters) | Anemia |
| Body iron log ([ferritin]/[sTfR]) | As specific and sensitive as components of formula | Not available | NA |

NOTE: sTfR = serum transferrin receptor. NA = Not applicable
SOURCE: Cook et al., 2003; IOM (2001); WHO and CDC (2005).

tional to the size of body iron stores in healthy individuals and those with uncomplicated iron deficiencies. In an adult, each 1 μg/L of serum ferritin indicates the presence of approximately 8 mg of storage iron (Bothwell et al., 1979). Based on NHANES III, for adults living in the United States, the median serum ferritin concentrations are 36 to 40 μg/L in menstruating women (approximately 0.36 to 0.4 g of storage iron) and 112 to 156 μg/L in men (slightly greater than 1 g of storage iron) (see Appendix Table G-3 of IOM, 2001). When the serum ferritin concentration falls below 12 μg/L, the iron stores are depleted totally (IOM, 2001).

Serum ferritin concentrations are affected by factors other than the size of iron stores: infections, inflammatory disorders, cancers (Valberg, 1980) and liver disease. High serum ferritin concentrations have also been associated with ethanol consumption (Leggett et al., 1990; Osler et al., 1998), increasing body mass index (IOM, 2001), and elevated plasma glucose concentration (Tuomainen et al., 1997). Dinneen et al. (1992) reported high serum ferritin concentration in association with newly diagnosed diabetes mellitus but in a later study reported that liver iron concentrations were not significantly different in such patients (Dinneen et al., 1994). Despite this limitation, a recent study by the CDC on 10 large intervention trial data sets confirms that serum ferritin remains the single best indicator of storage iron pool size (Mei et al., 2005).

**Serum transferrin saturation.** Transferrin saturation is defined as [serum] iron/TIBC (total iron binding capacity). Transferrin is a metalloprotein with a very high affinity for iron, and virtually all plasma iron is bound to the transporter transferrin. Transferrin is normally about 21 to 30 percent saturated with iron (IOM, 2001). Therefore, it is convenient to measure plasma transferrin concentration and saturation with iron. While the iron-bound iron is highly variable, TIBC is more stable and can be upregulated as the iron status of the individual declines (Garby et al., 1969). As the iron supply decreases, serum iron concentration falls and transferring concentration increases so that more iron is available to organs, resulting in a decrease in transferrin saturation.

*Early Iron Deficiency*

Early iron deficiency is signaled by evidence indicating that the iron supply to the bone marrow and other tissues is only marginally adequate. A measurable decrease in the hemoglobin concentration is not yet present, and therefore there is no anemia.

**Serum transferrin saturation.** Levels below 16 percent saturation indicate that the rate of iron delivery is not sufficient to maintain the normal rate of hemoglobin synthesis. Low saturation levels are not specific for iron deficiency and are encountered in other conditions such as anemia or chronic diseases, which is associated with the impaired release of iron from stores.

**Erythrocyte protoporphyrin concentration.** The heme molecule is formed in developing erythrocytes by iron's incorporation into protoporphyrin IX by ferrochetalase. If there is insufficient iron for optimal hemoglobin synthesis, then erythrocytes accumulate an excess of protoporphyrin, which remains in the cells for the duration of their life spans (Cook, 1999). An increased erythrocyte protoporphyrin concentration in the blood therefore indicates that the erythrocytes matured at a time when the iron supply was suboptimal. Erythrocyte protoporphyrin concentration is not specific for iron deficiency and is also associated with inadequate iron delivery to developing erythrocytes (e.g., due to anemia or chronic disease) or impaired heme synthesis (e.g., due to lead poisoning). In iron deficiency zinc can also incorporate into protoporphyrin. The zinc protopophyrin:heme ratio is also used as an indicator of impaired heme synthesis and is sensitive to an insufficient iron delivery to the erythrocyte (Braun, 1999).

**Soluble sTfR concentration.** All cells' surfaces express transferrin receptors in proportion to their requirement for iron. A truncated form of the receptor's extracellular domain is produced by proteolytic cleavage and released into the plasma in direct proportion to the number of receptors expressed on the surfaces of body tissues. As functional iron depletion occurs, more transferrin receptors appear on cell surfaces and the concentration of sTfR rises in parallel. The magnitude of the increase is proportional to the functional iron deficit. The sTfR concentration appears to be a specific and sensitive indicator of early iron deficiency (Akesson et al., 1998; Cook et al., 1990). Furthermore, sTfR concentration is not affected by infectious, inflammatory, and neoplastic disorders (Ferguson et al., 1992). The lack of an external standard for sTfR cross-validation has limited its universal acceptance despite the very strong evidence that it can be used in combination with serum ferritin to indicate the point at which there is depletion of the storage iron pool (WHO and CDC, 2005). Because commercial assays for sTfR have been available for 5–8 years, there is a lack of data relating iron intake to sTfR concentration as well as relating sTfR concentration to functional outcomes.

**Body iron index.** The combination of ferritin and sTfR yields a metric called body iron index (log ferritin/sTfR), which is derived from the serial phlebotomy study of Cook et al. (2003). This indicator may prove to be very useful in identifying iron deficiency as the sTfR assay becomes increasingly sensitive to decreasing iron stores at the same time that ferritin measurements become less sensitive. Thus, the iron status marker becomes a continuous variable across the distribution of a population's iron status and allows the computation of dietary intake adequacy to be based less on the proportion of individuals that are defined as "iron deficient anemic" or "iron deficient" and more on the proportion of the population that has positive body iron as defined above (Cook et al., 2003; WHO and CDC, 2005). The marker is specific and sensitive to body iron but has the same limitations with regard to interpreting the ferritin data during inflammation as to measuring ferritin by itself. There is, however, a dearth of information regarding functional outcomes related to a certain amount of body iron and, hence, the clear acceptance of this metric for characterizing body iron status remains to happen.

*Anemia*

Anemia is the most easily measurable condition to identify functional iron deficiency. Iron deficiency leads to the formation of small erythrocytes and reduced hematocrit (i.e., mean corpuscular hemoglobin, mean corpuscular volume). Mean corpuscular hemoglobin (MCH) is the amount of hemoglobin in erythrocytes. The mean corpuscular volume (MCV) is the volume of the average erythrocyte. MCH and MCV both are reduced in iron deficiency; however, decreased MCH and MCV values are not sensitive or specific for mild to moderate iron deficiency. They occur in all conditions that cause impaired hemoglobin synthesis, particularly the thalassemias (IOM, 2001). Therefore, the diagnosis of iron deficiency anemia based solely on the presence of anemia can result in misdiagnosis in many cases (Garby et al., 1967, 1969).

## Iron Intake Effects on Health and Performance

Functional abnormalities historically have been thought to occur only when iron deficiency is severe enough to cause measurable anemia (IOM, 2001). More recent observations, however, suggest that this assumption should be re-examined. Data from animal models support the concept that tissue iron depletion has significant physiological consequences that are independent of anemia's consequences (Dallman et al., 1982; Davies et al., 1984).

Important consequences of iron deficiency with implications for the military are impaired physical work performance, impaired cognitive functioning, poor immune function, and altered emotional states. Once the degree of iron deficiency is severe enough to deplete essential pools of body iron (e.g., cytochromes oxidases and oxygen transport proteins), functional disabilities become evident. It is difficult to determine whether any particular functional abnormality is a specific consequence of a particular dysfunction of an iron dependent protein or process. In many situations where people have examined consequences of poor iron status, both anemia and tissue iron depletion were present. Nevertheless, it has been shown that anemia and tissue iron deficiency exert independent effects on skeletal muscle (Davies et al., 1984; Finch et al., 1976). Anemia primarily affects maximal oxygen consumption, whereas endurance in muscle contraction is impaired more markedly by intracellular iron deficiency. From a practical point of view, the distinction may be relatively unimportant since anemia and tissue iron deficiency develop simultaneously in humans who suffer from iron deficiency.

### *Physical Performance and Anemia*

Various factors may contribute to impaired work performance as a result of iron deficiency. As mentioned above, anemia and tissue iron deficiency have been shown to exert independent effects on organ function (e.g., skeletal muscle) (Davies et al., 1984; Finch et al., 1976). Anemia primarily affects maximal oxygen consumption. Mild anemia reduces performance during brief but intense exercise (Viteri and Torun, 1974) because of the impaired capacity of skeletal muscle for oxidative metabolism. On the other hand, iron deficiency in skeletal muscle cells more markedly impairs endurance exercise (Dallman et al., 1982).

Adult men studied in the Harvard Step Test protocol, which involves brief intense exercise, showed a linear positive correlation between performance and hemoglobin concentration over the entire hemoglobin range normally seen in man (Viteri and Torun, 1974). In contrast, the data of Edgerton et al. (1981) clearly demonstrate that the duration (or time to exhaustion) of submaximal exercise has a curvilinear relationship to hemoglobin. The apparent conflict between these two data sets may be explained by results from animal experiments, which suggest that the mechanisms of iron deficiency effects on performance differ. Lower intensity, endurance exercise is correlated tightly with tissue iron deficiency, whereas a brief, intense exercise (like the Harvard Step Test) is correlated more tightly with severity of anemia, measured as hemoglobin concentration (Davies et al., 1982; Finch et al., 1979).

Arterial oxygen content, oxygen bound to hemoglobin, and cardiac output are all key determinants of the amount of work that exercising muscle can do. Research evaluated the physical work capacity and metabolic stress in iron deficient workers of a tea farm in Sri Lanka (Edgerton et al., 1981). In this study, men and women with hemoglobin levels of 40–120 g/L showed that exercise tolerance was reduced dramatically in the anemic subjects, who transported 15 percent less $O_2$ per pulse compared to treated controls. Iron treatment eventually restored cardiorespiratory and work performance variables to normal levels. There is no doubt that anemia with co-existing iron deficiency is associated with dramatic declines in endurance performance as well as maximal aerobic capacity.

### *Physical Performance and Iron Deficiency Without Anemia*

Three recent iron supplementation trials with iron deficient non-anemic women provide evidence that physical performance is altered in individuals without demonstrable anemia (Brutsaert et al., 2003; Hinton et al., 2000; Zhu and Haas, 1998). In the Zhu and Haas study (1998), the metabolic response to exercise was measured by assessing $VO_2max$ and time to complete a simulated 15-km time trial with a cycle ergometer, an indicator of endurance. The iron-supplemented group (135 mg ferrous sulfate or 50 mg of iron) completed the task at a lower percentage of their $VO_2max$ (83 versus 88 percent) and with 5.1

percent less energy expended than the placebo group. The second study examined energetic efficiency (Hinton et al., 2000). The estimated $VO_2max$ did not differ between the groups after iron supplementation, but after six weeks of supplementation the iron-supplemented women (20 mg/day of ferrous sulfate) showed a 5.7 percent lower energy cost to perform the work. A third study of 20 women tested maximal voluntary static contraction using a dynamic knee extension exercise to assess local muscle fatigue (Brutsaert et al., 2003). After six weeks of supplementation the iron-supplemented women (20 mg/day of ferrous sulfate or 7 mg/day of iron) performed the task with significantly less muscle fatigue than the placebo group. The final set of studies examined adaptation to physical training (Brownlie et al., 2002, 2004; Hinton et al., 2000). Some subjects received 16–20 mg/day of iron (ferrous sulfate) and others received a placebo. All subjects completed 20 days of significant aerobic training during the final four weeks of the supplementation trial. Both groups benefited from the training by increasing their $VO_2max$ (Brownlie et al., 2002, 2004; Hinton et al., 2000) and by reducing their times on a simulated 15-km time trial with a cycle ergometer (Brownlie et al., 2004; Hinton et al., 2000). The iron-supplemented group improved its time by more than twice as much as the nonsupplemented group, showing the additive benefit of iron supplementation. Notably, the greatest improvement in time-trial time and work efficiency was seen in the iron-supplemented women who were most depleted in tissue iron at baseline (Brownlie et al., 2004). From this study, researchers can conclude that tissue iron deficiency reduces the potential benefits of aerobic training in both endurance and $VO_2max$.

*Cognition, Behavior, and Iron Deficiency*

The existing scientific literature relating iron status to cognition and behavior applies almost exclusively to the civilian population with the exception of several recently published reports (Booth, 2003; Booth et al., 2003) and one in-house military report (Cline et al., 1998). The latter report (by Cline et al., 1998) evaluated cognitive performance and physical performance in 75 female officers going through basic training. At the start of the study, about 33 percent of the officers were iron deficient, and 7 percent were anemic. After training, 64 percent of the women had low ferritin levels despite reporting iron intakes of higher than 16 mg/day. The authors collected data on iron status and negative emotions (tension, depression, and anger) and on positive emotion scale (vigor) by using the Profile of Mood States (POMS) battery of tests.

The results demonstrated a modest positive correlation between iron status and mood states but, as a group, there were few differences between iron-deficient women and iron-sufficient women in any of the behavioral measures. Neither the cognitive task, a four-choice reaction time paradigm, nor the POMS tests show any significant difference in iron-deficient compared with iron-sufficient subjects. Other reports on the relationship of iron status to cognition or behavior in military personnel are very sparse and inconclusive (Booth, 2003; Booth et al., 2003). In two studies on Australian military personnel who consumed either a fresh-food diet or combat ration packs while training during 12 or 23 days, the soldiers had significant declines (approximately 15 percent) in serum ferritin and folate as well as a decline in antioxidant status. Poor baseline antioxidant status improved in all of the soldiers, especially in those who consumed the combat ration packs; the effect could be due to the vitamin C–fortified food items. An increase in fatigue was reported, but specific relationships to a micronutrient could not be established in either study. The available studies in military personnel do not support specific changes in iron status being related to mood, behavior, or cognitive performance, but, based on civilian data, more research in this area with both men and women should be conducted before definitive conclusions are made.

There are a number of studies performed on civilian adults and adolescents that have focused on the relationship between iron status and cognitive or behavioral functioning. Several cross-sectional designs examined General Health Questionnaire subscales showing that low ferritin and oral contraceptive use was required to observe a relationship between ferritin and depression (Fordy and Benton, 1994; Rangan et al., 1998). Other work—using the Minnesota Multiphasic Personality Inventory and fatigue, depression, and anxiety scales—showed no effect of iron status on these emotional states (Hunt and Penland, 1999). One exception is the Verdon et al. (2003) study in which women with serum ferritin concentrations ≤ 50 μg/L showed greater benefit of supplementation in terms of fatigue scores compared with women with ferritin concentrations > 50 μg/L. One difference between the two studies is that the Verdon study indicated that it was a blind study design.

Studies on iron supplementation of iron deficient individuals have shown positive effects on cognition and behavior domains (see Table 3-8). Groner et al. (1986) used a high-dose iron supplementation trial as ferrous fumarate (180 mg/

**TABLE 3-8** Effects of Iron Supplementation on Cognition and Behavioral Outcomes

| Subjects | Study Design | Outcome | Reference |
|---|---|---|---|
| Women | +90 mg/day of ferrous fumarate | ↑Attention, ↑Memory | Groner et al., 1986 |
| Women | 60 mg/day of iron during four months | ↑Learning, ↑Memory of women whose iron status improved | Beard and Murray-Kolb in Appendix B |
| Women | 5 versus 15 mg of iron | ↑Sleep duration, ↑Awakenings | Penland, 1988 |
| Men | Not reported | ↓Alertness, ↓Visual detection | Tucker et al., 1982, 1984 |

day for 30 days) to demonstrate an improvement in short-term memory and vigilance with iron treatment. Bruner et al. (1996) conducted a blinded placebo-controlled study in adolescent girls and demonstrated that iron depletion without anemia alters learning and memory tasks. The strength of the intervention trial was the use of a wide variety of functioning tasks and a conservative statistical approach to the data analysis. Verbal learning and memory improved significantly in the young women, demonstrating an improvement in ferritin with the iron intervention.

A study on iron status and cognition in women of reproductive age was completed recently, and the results have been reported (Beard and Murray-Kolb in Appendix B). The strength of association between iron status variables and cognitive variables was explored by principal component analysis of data from a 16-week iron intervention trial during which 149 women whose iron status varied from sufficient to iron-deficient anemic consumed iron supplementation of 60 mg/day. Attention, memory, and learning were related significantly to iron status. That is, the amount of time that it took to complete the memory tasks was significantly longer for the women in the lower quintile iron status than those in the upper quintile. In women whose iron status improved, whether due to iron supplementation or other unknown reasons, attention and learning improved more than five times than in the women whose iron status remained low. This improvement was seven times greater for memory in those whose iron status improved.

Ballin et al. (1992) used a double-blind placebo-controlled study to measure lassitude, the ability to concentrate in school, and mood of 16–17-year-old girls. The authors noted an improvement in affect and in concentration in the iron-deficient anemic adolescents who were treated with iron (as iron polystyrene sulfonate adsorbate syrup). A recent cross-sectional study in postpartum women revealed a strong inverse relationship between the severity of anemia and depression (Corwin et al., 2003). The stronger design of a placebo intervention trial showed iron-deficient anemic women (recent mothers) given iron for 28 weeks had significant declines in depression and anxiety compared to iron-deficient women given the placebo (Beard et al., 2005). The latter study was conducted in a high-stress, complex environment of poverty, poor health care, and other potential confounding factors. This finding suggests that even in situations of high stress, treatment of iron deficiency can result in less depression and anxiety.

Several other pertinent observations exist that may explain possible biological mechanisms whereby iron deficiency in adults can alter cognitive and behavioral functioning. One such observation is that variations in iron status, as reflected by variations in serum ferritin, are related to electroencephalogram (EEG) asymmetry (i.e., activity recorded with occipital electrodes); in this study, however, specific relationships between regional activity and cognition and brain iron were not tested (Tucker et al., 1982). The biochemical explanation for these alterations in electrical activity may very well lie in fundamental alterations in brain energy metabolism with brain iron deficiency (DeUngria et al., 2000) as well as in neurotransmission efficacy and degree of myelination (Beard and Connor, 2003). Researchers measured auditory brainstem-evoked potentials in 6-month-old iron-deficient anemic infants and found absolute and interpeak latency values to be longer in the anemic infants when compared with the nonanemic controls; this finding suggests altered myelination (Roncagliolo et al., 1998). Increased turnover of catecholamines (urine or tissues) in iron deficient individuals also have been reported (Beard, 1987; Webb et al., 1982). These levels returned to normal following iron repletion. Iron may impact cognition through its role in the synthesis and function of these compounds, since they can modulate the capacity for information processing (Izquierdo, 1989).

*Immune Function*

In a conceptual model of nutritional immunity, the host must effectively sequester iron away from pathogens to provide an iron supply that is not limiting to its immune system (Hershko, 1996). There is new evidence that unicellular organisms and larger, multicellular organisms, like humans, share a common lineage of metal transporters (Fishbane, 1999). These divalent metal transporters have been identified and cloned in both bacteria and humans and are used to internalize iron from extracellular spaces, suggesting that transport of iron is key to the survival of many pathogens as well as to the host organism. As mentioned in an earlier section, DMT1 (also called divalent cation transporter-1 [DCT-1]) is known now to be able to transport iron, copper, zinc, manganese, and other divalent metals from endosomal vesicles into the cytoplasmic space. Bacterial virulence is associated with the genes that code for iron acquisition by both *Escherichia coli* and *Vibrio* (Fishane 1999; Ike et al., 1992). Thus, one route of obtaining essential iron is from biologic fluids by siderophores secreted by bacteria. Sequestration of iron seems to be an important part of the host response to infection. Administration of a potent iron chelator, desferrioxamine, to humans was examined to explore the potential antimalaria impact (Byrd and Horwitz, 1989; Fahmy and Young, 1993; Lane et al., 1991). However, the human data on the common use of iron by bacteria and humans and its consequences are far less convincing (Damodaran et al., 1979; Murray et al., 1978) and was reviewed by others (Hamer, 2005; see Hamer in Appendix B). Experimental and clinical data suggest that there is an increased risk of infection during iron deficiency. Hershko (1996) urges caution in the interpretation of many studies as the confounding issues of poverty, generalized malnutrition, and multimicronutrient deficiencies often are present in those studies.

Nonspecific immunity of human immune systems, as assessed in vitro, is affected by iron deficiency in several ways. Macrophage phagocytosis generally is unaffected by iron deficiency, but bactericidal activity of these macrophages is attenuated (Hallquist et al., 1992). Iron deficiency of the iron-containing enzyme myeloperoxidase—which produces reactive oxygen intermediates responsible for intracellular killing of pathogens—reduces activity of neutrophils (Mackler et al., 1984). A decrease in T-lymphocyte number and T-lymphocyte blastogenesis and mitogenesis in iron deficiency in response to a number of different mitogens also has been observed. Interestingly, this alteration is reversed greatly with iron repletion (Kuvibidila et al., 1999). On the other hand, other studies have found that iron deficiency does not affect T-lymphocyte proliferative response to mitogens (Canonne-Hergaux et al., 1999). Recent studies of T-lymphocytes in iron deficiency note that protein kinase C activity and translocation of both splenic and purified T-cells are altered by iron deficiency (Kuvibidila et al., 1999).

Iron deficiency affects humoral immunity less than cellular immunity. In iron-deficient humans, antibody production in response to immunization with most antigens is preserved (Hallquist et al., 1992; Spear and Sherman, 1992).

The molecular and cellular defects responsible for immune deficiency are complex since almost every effector of the immune response is limited in number, or action, by experimental iron deficiency. Iron is essential for proper cell differentiation and cell growth. In addition, iron is a critical component of peroxide-generating enzymes and nitrous oxide–generating enzymes that are critical for the proper enzymatic functioning of immune cells. And finally, iron is probably involved in the regulation of cytokine production and mechanism of action through its influence on second messenger systems (Hershko, 1996). In one of few studies on the role of iron nutrition in the development of the immune system, authors noted a delay in the development of cell-mediated immunity (Kochanowski and Sherman, 1985).

There are several possible mechanisms that could explain the effects of iron deficiency on the immune system. DNA synthesis, initiated by the iron-containing enzyme ribonucleotide reductase, is a rate-limiting factor in cellular replication and may be limited by iron deficiency. Control of cell differentiation is influenced by the available iron and iron transport into cells via the sTfR. Galan et al. (1992) reported a reduction in interleukin-2 (IL-2) production by activated lymphocytes in iron deficient subjects. The release of IL-2 is fundamental to communication between lymphocyte subsets and natural killer cells, but it does not appear to be the only cytokine that is altered by iron status (Sussman, 1974).

Conversely, other cytokines such as tumor necrosis factor (TNF-$\alpha$), IL-1, and interferon-$\gamma$ are all effectors of iron movement. These cytokines operate in a coordinated fashion to reduce the size of the intracellular labile iron pool by a reduction in the amount of TfR on the cell surface, an increased synthesis of ferritin for iron storage, and activation of nitric-oxide systems (Fishbane, 1999; Hallquist et al., 1992; Ike et al., 1992; Kochanowski and Sherman, 1985; Murray et al., 1978). These effects might be regulated by gene transcription. Although with the acute phase response system, there is a well-known decrease in the plasma iron concentration and ferritin concentration, the role of plasma ferritin in the sequestration of plasma iron and the response to infection remain uncertain. It is less apparent, whether the iron status of the individual can modify the acute phase response system.

In conclusion, iron deficiency reduces functioning of the immune system in a generalized fashion as well as in certain cell types. Whether this is a specific effect of iron deficiency or a general effect of nutritional deprivation is not clear.

## Risk Factors for Inadequacy During Military Garrison Training

### *Iron Status and Consumption*

In the United States, the median iron intake from foods is 17.9 mg/day, and the 95th percentile is 31.1 mg/day for 19–50-year-old men (IOM, 2001). Median intakes for 19–50-year-old women are 12.1 mg/day, and the 95th percentile is 20 mg/day.

The estimates of intakes among military groups are sparse (Baker-Fulco, 2005; see Baker-Fulco in Appendix B) and mostly derived from very small surveys rather than a systematic survey of iron's nutritional status of soldiers joining the military or being deployed to the field. In one such study, it was estimated that male Rangers consuming MREs had an average iron intake of 15 mg/day, about 1.5 times the MDRI for adult males (Baker-Fulco, 2005; see Baker-Fulco in Appendix B). Consumption patterns and choice selections likely change dramatically in field settings, however, and data on food intakes in those situations are lacking. Baker-Fulco reports iron intakes for most participants of these studies that are above the IOM RDA.

There are much less data on iron status of servicemen and women. A study, focusing on women, reveals that about 33 percent of 57 subjects were low in serum ferritin while seven percent were anemic at the time of entry in the military (Cline et al., 1998). After basic training, 64 percent of the women had low ferritin levels. The average reported iron intakes were greater than 16 mg/day, and only eight subjects reported consuming less than 80 percent of the MRDIs. This finding suggests that diet composition and amounts consumed during training should have been adequate for most of the women (Cline et al., 1998). The increased prevalence of iron deficiency at the end of training, however, is suggestive evidence that high levels of physical training increased iron requirements substantially and that the MDRI level (15 mg for women; see Table 3-1) was insufficient to meet metabolic requirements in these conditions. Booth et al. (2003) reported underconsumption of rations, compared with a diet of fresh foods, during 12 days of training in hot humid environment and observed significant reductions in serum ferritin, irrespective of diet, a finding that is suggestive of stress-released cytokines.

It is difficult to assess soldiers' iron status only by collecting food intake data, since high amounts of supplement consumption have been reported. For example, when the food choices of females during Officer Training Corps were examined (Arsenault and Cline, 2000), the women often chose food items that were lower in energy density than normal food choices in an apparent attempt to meet military weight requirements. A recent report on Special Forces soldiers' garrison feeding during training (Tharion et al., 2004) reported a mean intake of iron of 19 mg/day, which is already above the MDRIs. Two studies reported that during training Rangers (Deuster et al., 2003) and Special Operations candidates (Arsenault and Kennedy, 1999) frequently used supplements. This frequent use of supplement might have included iron intakes well above the MRDIs.

All of these studies support the idea that soldiers consume large amounts of supplemental iron or other supplements during active training and, possibly, field operations. The contribution of iron supplements to the diet is unknown but could be substantial and requires surveying military personnel (see Chapter 4).

Other data regarding either habitual intakes or status are unavailable, but iron deficiency rates may be similar to those of the general population [i.e., estimated to be < 3 percent for males and approximately 11–14 percent for reproductive-age females (IOM, 2001)].

### *Iron Losses*

**Basal urine, feces, and skin loss.** Body iron generally is conserved, and in the absence of bleeding (including menstruation) or pregnancy only a small quantity of iron is lost each day (Bothwell et al., 1979). Daily iron losses from urine, the gastrointestinal tract, and skin total about 1 mg/day (i.e., approximately 0.08, 0.6, and 0.2–0.3 mg/day, respectively) but may drop to 0.5 mg/day in iron deficiency or may increase as high as 2 mg/day in iron overload (Bothwell et al., 1979).

**Menstrual loss.** Results from menstrual loss have been estimated in many studies (Beaton, 1974; Cole et al., 1971; Hefnawi et al., 1980) and are fairly consistent. A community survey conducted in Sweden (Hallberg et al., 1966) served as the basis for calculating an average blood loss per period of 30.9 ml. Based on this average blood loss, the average hemoglobin concentration (135 g/L) and the concentration of iron in hemoglobin (3.4 mg/g) (Smith and Rios, 1974), the average iron loss in the menses is calculated as 0.51 mg/day.

**Iron loss in exercise and intense endurance training.** Many scientific reviews conclude that iron status is inadequate in a large number of individuals, particularly females, who exercise regularly (Clarkson and Haymes, 1995; Raunikar and Sabio, 1992; Weaver and Rajaram, 1992). Dietary intake patterns of these individuals frequently are suboptimal and include a reduced intake of several micronutrients. Many reports focus on runners and running, but analogous changes in iron status also occur in people engaged in swimming, rowing, and other aerobic activities (Beard and Tobin, 2000). In contrast to a whole-body iron loss of approximately 1.08 mg/day in postpubescent males and of 1.4 mg/day in menstruating females (IOM, 2001), Weaver and Rajaram (1992) estimated that with prolonged training daily iron loss of male and female athletes may increase to 1.75 and 2.3 mg/day, respectively. These losses were calculated by a factorial approach analysis using data from various literature sources. In that way, and assuming the athletes were excreting 3 L/day of sweat that contained 0.21 mg/L of iron, the authors estimated 0.6 mg/day for sweat iron loss and added that amount to the estimated physically active basal requirements for men and women.

Two studies have used whole-body retention of radioactively labeled iron ($^{59}Fe$) to examine the impact of exercise training on whole-body iron turnover rates (Ehn et al., 1980; Nachtigall et al., 1996). The study by Ehn et al. (1980) demonstrated that eight highly trained long-distance runners have an estimated half-life of body iron of approximately 1,000 days. Although not statistically significant, this value was substantially shorter than the 2,100 and 1,300 days half-life of body iron in trained runners for nonexercising males and females, respectively, derived from another study using the same methodology (Heinrich, 1970). The study by Nachtigall et al. (1996) also studied eight athletes after they received an oral dose of radioactive iron. By whole-body counting, two out of the eight subjects had daily elimination rates within the normal range established by that laboratory. The other six subjects had mean elimination rates slightly increased beyond the normal range. Inclusion of fecal and urine radioactivity losses showed that heavy training was associated with significant increases in fecal iron but not in urine or sweat iron. Intestinal iron loss was approximately 2.4–3.3 mg/day compared with baseline iron loss of 0.6–0.9 mg/day. The data, determined by highly sensitivity methods, suggest a strong association between substantial fecal loss and vigorous exercise. Increased fecal loss and perhaps sporadic hematuria contribute to depressed iron stores in athletic segments of the population (Siegel et al., 1979; Stewart et al., 1984). Nonetheless, the nature of the exercise seems to be more extreme in the Nachtigall study than in military garrison training. In addition, neither of these studies directly included control subjects that were provided with radioactive iron, a fact that limits the strength of the evidence.

There is also a notable reduction in hematological parameters that could be the result of increased intravascular hemolysis of erythrocytes as many studies have found an increased rate of erythrocyte turnover and fragility in athletes (Lampe et al., 1991; Newhouse and Clement, 1995; Rowland et al., 1991). Thus, several mechanisms by which iron balance could be affected by intense physical exercise have been advanced (Fogelholm, 1995; Magnusson et al., 1984; Weight, 1993), including increased gastrointestinal blood loss after running and hemoglobinuria as a result of erythrocyte rupture within the foot during running. The committee concluded that, all together these studies suggest that fecal and urine losses may increase with heavy exercise but that the data are not decisive yet.

**Sweat loss.** Although the IOM report (2001) *Dietary Reference Intakes. Vitamin A, Vitamin K, Arsenic, Boron, Chromium, Copper, Iodine, Iron, Manganese, Molybdenum, Nickel, Silicon, Vanadium, and Zinc* did not consider sweat as a major contributor to iron requirements, military men and women may have sizeable additional requirements due to the sweat loss from exercise in a hot environment. Table 3-9 summarizes this and other studies mentioned below.

Many studies have examined the sweat's iron concentration. Green et al. (1968) estimated dermal uptake and loss of iron using $^{59}Fe$ to be 0.24 mg/day. Slightly higher dermal iron loss (0.33 ± 0.15 mg/day) was found using a whole-body dermal collection method by Jacob et al. (1981). Mean sweat iron concentration measured using an arm bag was 0.076 mg/L in the same subjects. Wheeler et al. (1973) measured dermal iron loss using a whole-body technique during habitual daily activity and with the addition of two hours of exercise with two different levels of dietary iron; estimated sweat loss was approximately 0.32–0.38 mg/day. The amount of iron lost per unit time appears to decrease over time whether sweating is due to exercise (DeRuisseau et al., 2002; Paulev et al., 1983; Waller and Haymes, 1996) or exposure to sauna (Brune et al., 1986). Paulev et al. (1983) observed sweat iron on the back decreased from 0.20 mg/L to 0.13 mg/L during 30 minutes of exercise. Waller and Haymes (1996) found arm-bag sweat iron concentrations decreased from 30 to 60 minutes of exercise in warm (from 0.21 mg/L to 0.08 mg/L) and neutral environments (from 0.31 mg/L to 0.14 mg/L). Significant decreases in sweat iron concentration also were found between 30 minutes (0.19 mg/L) and 120 minutes (0.11 mg/L) by DeRuisseau et al. (2002). As explained by Brune and et al. (1986), this result could be due to cellular debris and external contaminants in the first sweat. In this study, the iron in sweat collected during sequential sauna exposure sessions of 25–30 minutes each decreased from 0.213 to 0.119 mg/L of sweat contaminated with cells and from 0.051 to 0.023 mg/L after removal of cellular debris (Brune et al., 1986). These very low sweat iron concentrations were consistent with the minimal amounts observed in sweat losses when the radioisotopic tracer $^{59}Fe$ was employed (Nachtigall et al., 1996), but considerably less than several other reports by analytical methods that did not correct for cellular debris.

Another source of sweat concentration variation is the location of the sweat collection. Regional sweat iron concentrations vary with higher concentrations found in sweat from the chest (0.50 mg/L) and abdomen (0.49 mg/L) than from the arm (0.28 mg/L) and back (0.20 mg/L) (Aruoma et al., 1988).

Although there is wide variability in concentrations from the studies described here because of differences in methodologies and study designs, overall the studies suggest that iron loss from sweat can be substantial for military personnel under garrison training and hot climates.

## Requirements for the General U.S. Population

The 2001 IOM EAR calculation was based on the need to maintain a normal, functional iron concentration but only a minimal store (serum ferritin concentration of 15 μg/L) (IOM, 2001). Physiological requirements for absorbed iron were calculated by factorial modeling of the iron requirement components,

**TABLE 3-9** Iron Sweat Losses

| Subjects | Comments | Iron Analysis | Sweat Collection | Sweat Loss | Reference |
|---|---|---|---|---|---|
| 9 males<br>8 females | Sedentary | $^{59}Fe$ dermal uptake | Whole body by plasma iron turnover | 0.24 mg/day | Green et al., 1968; IOM, 2001 |
| 6 males | 2 hours of exercise, acclimatized | Bathophenan-throlinie method | Whole body surface | 0.32–0.34 mg/day | Wheeler et al., 1973 |
| 9 males<br>1 female | 30 minutes of strenuous exercise | Ferrozine method | Back | 0.2 decreased to 0.13 mg/L after 30 minutes | Paulev et al., 1983 |
| 12 males | 30–40 minutes of exercise | Atomic absorption | Arm<br>Back<br>Chest<br>Abdomen | 0.28 mg/L<br>0.20 mg/L<br>0.50 mg/L<br>0.49 mg/L | Aruoma et al., 1988 |
| 9 males<br>9 females | 60 minutes of exercise in the heat | Ferrozine method | Arm bag | 0.21 decreased to 0.08 mg/L; at 30 compared with 60 minutes of exercise | Waller and Haymes, 1996 |
| 9 males<br>9 females | 120 minutes of exercise | Ferrozine method | Arm bag | 0.19 decreased to 0.11 mg/L; at 30 compared with 120 minutes of exercise | DeRuisseau et al., 2002 |
| 11 males | 20–30 minutes of sauna at rest, two times separated by 15 minutes | Colorimetric iron analysis, after $^{59}Fe$-controlled evaporation of samples filtered of cellular debris | Whole body surface | 0.051 decreased to 0.022 mg/L with consecutive 30 min saunas; higher values of 0.213 and 0.119 mg/L without cellular filtration | Brune et al., 1986 |

that is, basal losses, which refer to the obligatory loss of iron in the feces, urine, sweat, and skin cell exfoliation. The basal iron losses were derived from a single study (Green et al., 1968) that reported an average calculated daily iron loss of 0.9–1.0 mg/day in three groups of men (from South Africa, the United States, and Venezuela) with normal iron storage status. Since some components are not normally distributed within the U.S. population, simple addition was inappropriate and Monte Carlo simulation was used to generate a large theoretical population with the characteristics described by the component distributions (IOM, 2001, see the Introduction). Next, iron requirement estimates were made directly from this data distribution set; the IOM EAR and the RDA were calculated as the median and the 97.5th percentile of the total requirement. The upper limit of dietary iron absorption was estimated to be 18 percent and was used to set the IOM EAR and the RDA. Basal iron losses for men were computed as 14 μg/kg/day (Green et al., 1968). The median daily iron loss for American men is (77.4 kg × 0.014 mg/kg/day) = 1.08 mg/day. The 97.5th percentile of the distribution of absorbed iron requirements is 1.53 mg/day. After applying an 18 percent absorption rate to the median and 97.5th, an IOM EAR and RDA can be estimated as 6 and 8 mg/day, respectively (see Table 3-1) (IOM, 2001).

The additional requirements estimated for the female population between ages 15–50 years are based on data from Hallberg et al. (1966). Since the distribution of menstrual blood loss in the data reported was skewed, it was modeled as a log-normal distribution fitted to the reported percentiles of the blood loss distribution. Using previously described information (see section on menstrual loss), the daily menstrual iron loss (0. 51 mg/day) can be calculated as follows: blood loss/28 days × (hemoglobin) × (iron in hemoglobin). The same rationale as the one above was used to derive a women's IOM EAR and RDA of 8.1 and 18 mg/day, respectively, for menstruating women who were not using OCs. It is important to note that these calculations ignore the fact that men have higher iron stores than women as a consequence of men's higher iron intakes and lower iron needs.

There are special considerations for women who use OCs. Approximately 17 percent of women in the United States use OCs (Abma et al., 1997), which are known to reduce menstrual blood loss; a similar or even higher use rate is assumed for military personnel. The IOM (2001) report, *Dietary Reference Intakes. Vitamin A, Vitamin K, Arsenic, Boron, Chromium, Copper, Iodine, Iron, Manganese, Molybdenum, Nickel, Silicon, Vanadium, and Zinc* suggested that a reasonable estimate of effect would be the equivalent of a 60-percent reduction from expected loss. Therefore, the IOM EAR and the RDA for reproductive-age women taking OCs are 6.4 and 10.9 mg/day, respectively.

## Daily Intake Recommendations for Military Personnel in Garrison Training

The preceding discussions regarding the IOM EAR and the RDA do not consider the effect of exercise and extensive sweating, a possibility for those military personnel in garrison training who could be spending six or more hours each day in a very hot environment and expending considerable amounts of energy in physical activities; these conditions could significantly change iron requirements.

The whole-body iron loss data collected by Ehn et al. (1980) and Nachtigall et al. (1996) suggest that the EAR for iron could be as much as 30 percent greater for those who engage in regular intense exercise, such as military garrison training. The committee members caution that this suggestion is based on data from two studies with design limitations and should not be taken as definitive until more research is conducted. For example, neither of the studies included an appropriate control group. In addition, in the study by Ehn et al. (1980) the difference in iron half-time elimination between controls and runners might be magnified if the variability in iron decay was large. The committee recommends conducting a study that mimics the military situation and includes a sensitive measurement of isotopic tracers.

Because such a study has not been conducted yet, the committee used the estimates by Weaver and Rajaram (1992) to base its recommendations on iron requirements for military personnel under garrison training. As mentioned above, Weaver and Rajaram (1992) estimated increased iron losses for men and women athletes to be 1.75 and 2.3 mg/day, respectively, if the sweat losses are assumed to be 0.6 mg/day in 3 L of volume (calculated from Brune et al., 1986 at 0.21 mg/L). Based on new iron sweat loss data, the committee concluded that a recalculation of the requirements was needed. If sweat losses are subtracted from the Weaver and Rajaram findings (1992), a basal iron requirement of 1.15 mg/day for exercising men and of 1.7 mg/day for exercising women is necessary. Although data on iron sweat concentration are somewhat variable and decrease with time, it currently seems reasonable to assume that the concentration is about 0.11 mg/L (DeRuisseau et al., 2002). Although sweat iron concentration of individuals in heavy military gear during garrison training are unavailable, it is unlikely that heat acclimatization results in any significant decrease in iron concentration (DeRuisseau et al., 2002). Assuming about 10 L of sweat volume for soldiers under garrison training and high temperatures, the additional iron requirements due to sweat losses might be as much as 1 mg/day. As previously discussed, an upper limit of 18 percent iron absorption was used; therefore, $EAR_{MGT}$ is 12 mg/day ([1.15 + 1] /0.18 mg/day).

Similarly, the EAR for women would need to be adjusted upwards if the duration and level of physical effort were close to that of the men. There is however, a difference in sweat loss rates between women and men in that women sweat 30 percent less (DeRuisseau et al., 2002); sweat losses for women will amount to 0.6 mg/day. Based on the suggestive whole-body iron loss data collected by Ehn et al. (1980), the EAR for iron will be conservatively 30 percent greater for those who engage in regular intense exercise; therefore, the $EAR_{MGT}$ for women is 12.8 mg/day ([1.7 + 0.6]/0.18 mg/day), which was rounded to 13 mg/day.

To calculate the $RDA_{MGT}$ the committee assumed that the combination of exercise training and sweat losses are additive to requirements and that the distribution of requirements does not change shape. From the distribution of basal losses, the SD for basal losses males and females is estimated to be 0.22 and 0.87 mg/day, respectively (IOM 2001; Tables I-3 and 9-13, respectively). To calculate the SD for requirements, an 18 percent bioavailability rate should be applied, resulting in an SD of 1.22 and 4.66 mg/day for males and females. Therefore, the RDAs for military garrison training ($RDA_{MGT} = EAR_{MGT} + 2SD$) were derived and rounded as 14 and 22 mg/day for men and women, respectively.

The committee cautions that even though there is enough evidence to conclude that additional iron is needed for military personnel under garrison training versus the general population, the actual additional level needs to be confirmed with appropriately design studies. Since there is no data from which to accurately estimate true iron loss in soldiers in garrison, the recommendations made by this committee are posited as best estimates of requirements. In addition to these limitations, the committee lacked information regarding the distributions of requirements due to exercise and sweat iron losses. This is an area where more research clearly is warranted.

**RECOMMENDATIONS FOR IRON INTAKE:**

| | |
|---|---|
| **$EAR_{MGT}$ for men** | **12 mg/day** |
| **$EAR_{MGT}$ for women** | **13 mg/day** |
| **$RDA_{MGT}$ for men** | **14 mg/day** |
| **$RDA_{MGT}$ for women** | **22 mg/day** |

## Adequacy of Iron MDRIs and Iron Levels in Rations

The MDRIs for iron are 10 and 15 mg/day for men and women, respectively (see Table 3-1). Even though 17–18-year-old men typically need a higher level (12 mg/day) of iron, the nutritional standards for operational rations (NSORs) generally follows the highest MDRIs (15 mg/day), and consequently the iron needs for those younger men will be met. The NSOR are based on the IOM RDAs and, therefore, are appropriate for military personnel with a lifestyle similar to the civilian population. These amounts, however, might not meet the needs of exceptionally physically active people, such as military personnel under training or combat (see recommendation section). The committee concluded that, given the higher iron needs for military personnel under garrison training, the

$RDA_{MGT}$, and therefore the corresponding NSOR for garrison training, should be higher.

Table 3-1 (and Tables C-2–C-5 in Appendix C) shows the averages and ranges of iron for three different MREs that each include approximately 25 menus. Consideration should be given to the fact that some menus seem to be very low in iron (5.78 mg); for this exercise it will be assumed that a mix of menus are eaten per day sufficient to meet the average level of iron in the menus. However, there is a potential for deficiencies due to not only low food consumption but also selection of a low-iron MRE. The committee recommends that the menus that are at the low end of the range be revised so that they would meet a minimum of 14 and 22 mg/day of iron for men and women, respectively.

As an example, the average iron content in MRE XXIII and XXIV menus is 8.6 and 9 mg, respectively. Assuming that women will consume two MREs and men will consume three MREs, the amount in the ration, if it is consumed completely (approximately 18 or 27 mg, for two or three MREs, respectively), will meet the recommendations of this committee for men ($RDA_{MGT}$ = 14 mg/day), but not for women ($RDA_{MGT}$ = 22 mg/day). Two MREs per day, however, will exceed female soldiers' median requirements for iron of 14 mg/day. The extra iron that men would consume would not amount to any safety concern, except perhaps for those with the genetic disorder of hemochromatosis and especially those with occult hemochromatosis.

Most of the food intake surveys have not distinguished the intakes by gender. One exception was a study with combat support hospital staff. The results showed that the iron intake was generally adequate for both male and female personnel (Baker-Fulco, 2005; see Baker-Fulco in Appendix B), if IOM RDAs are taken as reference standards. Another study on soldiers in garrison training reached the same conclusions (Tharion et al., 2004). However, this amount might be low for personnel who are in garrison training. The actual iron intake for both men and women needs to be determiened to assess if they meet this committee's recommendations (see Chapter 4).

The current FSRs contain an average of 17 mg of iron, an amount that might be adequate for men (see Table 3-1; Table C-6 in Appendix C). In the future, if women are allowed to participate in combat operations, then this recommended amount should be revisited because of women's higher iron needs.

### Adequacy of IOM Recommendations for First Strike Rations

The recommendations presented with regard to the $EAR_{MGT}$ for garrison troops might need re-evaluation when military personnel are conducting sustained operations. The physical expenditure of energy and stress levels are higher, and sleep deprivation is more common than in garrison training. However, limited data are available with regard to the impact on iron requirements of a high-stress environment with the exception of the substantial work on iron sweat loss associated with heavy or prolonged exercise. Both of these bodies of evidence are derived from the exercise physiology and training literature and may not be accurate when the additional stressors of combat are added.

The IOM report (2006) *Nutrient Composition of Rations for Short-Term, High-Intensity Combat Operations* recommends that the daily FSRs (i.e., assault rations) for sustained operations include 8–18 mg of iron. Assault rations are targeted for men, who have iron reserves in their livers and spleens that could be used in case dietary iron is insufficient. The report also suggests that the level of iron should be closer to 8 mg/day if there are stability or palatability problems. Giving these rations' size limitations and potential stability or palatability problems if levels of iron closer to 18 mg are attempted, this committee supports the recommendations in IOM (2006) until further experimental data (listed in Chapter 4) are collected. If higher requirements for these situations are necessary, then strategies to increase intake (e.g., supplementation) might warrant consideration. Also, in the event that women are allowed to participate in sustained combat operations, then higher levels of iron might be needed, and those recommendations should be revisited.

## Strategies for Achieving Sufficient Iron Intake

### *Usual Foods*

The first strategy to employ in trying to meet iron needs is choosing natural dietary sources of heme and nonheme iron and iron-fortified foods. Because of the differences in the type of iron in the diet (heme and nonheme iron), the bioavailability of iron varies greatly.

Heme iron is the best absorbed iron, and its bioavailability is less affected than nonheme iron by other dietary components. But, heme iron constitutes about only 10 percent of total dietary iron intake (IOM, 2001). Good sources of heme iron include beef and turkey. Many inhibitors of nonheme iron—including phytate, polyphenols, and tannins—occur in food and bind to the iron to make a complex that is unavailable for digestion. Good sources of nonheme iron are beans and lentils.

Some garrison personnel are near or complete vegetarians, though the exact proportion of individuals is unknown. The estimate of the iron IOM RDA is based on an assumption that heme iron contributes to the daily iron intake. Iron is more bioavailable from meat than from plant-derived foods, and factors in meat and fish also enhance the absorption of nonheme iron. Therefore, nonheme iron absorption is even lower for people who consume vegetarian diets than for those eating nonvegetarian diets (Hunt and Roughead, 1999). Hunt (2003b) carefully examined individuals' adaptation to low or high bioavailable diets and demonstrated different relationships between ferritin and absorption efficiency in individuals who habitually consume a low bioavailable diet compared with those consuming a higher bioavailable diet. That is, an individual accustomed to consuming a high bioavailable diet, for instance one with 6–8 oz/day of meat absorbs 25 percent of dietary iron if the ferritin is 25 μg/L. This increases to an efficiency of 35 percent if the serum ferritin is only 10–12 μg/L. In contrast, individuals consuming the low bioavailable diet would have an absorption efficiency of 3 percent at the higher ferritin (25 μg/L) and 5 percent at the low iron status level of a ferritin (10 μg/L). Serum ferritin concentrations have been observed to be markedly lower in vegetarian men, women, and children than in those consuming a nonvegetarian diet (Alexander et al.,1994; Dwyer et al., 1982; Shaw et al., 1995).

Individuals who typically consume vegetarian diets may have difficulty consuming bioavailable iron intakes that are sufficient to meet the $EAR_{MGT}$. Cook et al. (1991) compared iron bioavailability from single meals with that of a diet consumed over a two-week period. There was a 4.4-fold difference between maximally enhancing and maximally inhibiting single meals, but the difference was only twofold when measured over the two-week period. It is therefore estimated that the bioavailability of iron from a vegetarian diet is approximately 10 percent, instead of the 18 percent, for a mixed Western diet. Many military personnel likely consume diets somewhere in between these two extremes. Assuming an overall efficiency of absorption of 10 percent in semistrict vegetarian adult men and premenopausal women, the $EAR_{MGT}$ is estimated to be 21.5 and 24 mg/day for vegetarian men and women, respectively.

It is important to emphasize that even lower bioavailability diets (approaching 5 percent overall absorption) may be encountered with very strict vegetarianism, raising even higher the estimated requirements and recommended intakes.

### *Food Fortification*

Many iron salts are used as food fortificants. The salts vary in solubility and bioavailability, as well as in cost, reactivity with other food substances, and effects on color and taste (reviewed in IOM, 2006). The pH of the food and the presence of other compounds also influences the potential use of an iron fortificant.

Fortification has an advantage over supplementation—the risk of toxicity is reduced substantially since the iron comes in a food vehicle. In addition, iron fortification does not seem to affect zinc absorption. On the negative side, individuals with hereditary hemochromatosis (1 in 200–400 white adults) who develop iron overload should be cautious unless their iron intakes are restricted. Early identification of this problem is essential so that measures can be taken to help individuals avoid problems. Contraindications for iron fortification and supplementation therefore include exclusively to anyone with hemosiderosis, hemochromatosis, sensitivity to iron-containing products, and elevated serum ferritin levels. The most common adverse effects of iron excess are gastrointestinal (IOM, 2001).

Common drug interactions that may suppress some or all forms of iron from being absorbed are acid pump inhibitors, antacids, bisphosphonates, $H_2$ (histamine 2 receptor) blockers, penicillamine, and tetracycline (Hendler and Rorvik, 2001). Nutritional supplements that decrease iron absorption include calcium, copper, inositol, cysteine, magnesium, vanadium, and zinc (Hendler and Rorvik, 2001). Vitamin C increase iron absorption as might foods rich in proteins containing cysteine (Hendler and Rorvik, 2001). Absorption is decreased when iron is eaten with teas or with foods rich in oxalic or phytic acids.

The hedonics of iron fortification are problematic, and taste may be compromised if levels are too high. Care must be taken to avoid reactions between the fortificant and other substances in the foods, such as fats, that may form objectionable reaction products. Iron salts also may have an undesirable metallic taste (reviewed in IOM, 2006).

Among the most popular iron-fortified foods are breakfast cereals, which are highly fortified in nonheme iron and often contain up to 100 percent of the nutrient's Daily Value (DV). Fortified instant oatmeal is also a relatively high source of nonheme iron at about 60 percent of the DV per serving (Office of Dietary Supplements, 2006). The iron-fortified foods contain reduced iron, a finely powdered metallic iron that in general is assimilated poorly since it must be oxidized to ferric iron and then reduced to ferrous iron in the stomach and small intestine before it can be absorbed. There are other forms of iron that are absorbed more easily, but they are more expensive.

*Supplementation*

The IOM EAR is based on the need to maintain a normal, functional iron concentration but only a minimal store (serum ferritin concentration of 15 μg/L) (IOM, 2001). Iron supplementation is an option when iron needs cannot be met from food alone or for those with especially high needs. Iron deficiency is uncommon among adult men but somewhat more common among women. Candidates for iron supplementation are those who have serum ferritin levels less than 15 μg/L. A sign that ferritin may be low is a low hemoglobin level, which often triggers a serum ferritin measurement.

There are two forms of supplemental iron—ferrous and ferric. Ferrous iron salts include the fumarate (33 percent elemental iron), the sulfate (32 percent elemental iron), and the ascorbate (14 percent elemental iron); their rate of absorption is the greatest among iron supplements. Chewable tablets, extended-release tablets, enteric-coated tablets, and a variety of liquids are available (Hendler and Rorvik, 2001).

The efficiency of iron absorption decreases as dosage increases, and therefore, iron supplements should be consumed in two or three equally spaced doses. The intermittent iron doses, as compared to daily iron doses, appear to have preventive potential; however, adherence may be poor for multiple pills per day.

There is considerable evidence of supplementation efficacy in those who are deficient and adhere to supplements. For example, iron supplements are used extensively in pregnant women, and there is good evidence that efficacy is high for treating iron deficiency anemia. Supplementation also might be a good approach among adults who engage in regular, intense exercise (e.g., soldiers' engaging in combat or simulated combat situations), since it is estimated that they need much higher iron intake levels. It is important to determine if supplements will be a useful approach for those who—because of low initial iron status, consumption of reduced-calorie diets, or high rates or extended periods of exercise—show low iron status. Because at least 95 percent of adult males exceed these levels of serum ferritin (IOM, 2001), routine iron supplementation is not recommended for male soldiers, and excess dietary iron may increase the risk of iron storage disorders such as hemochromatosis. Further evaluation is needed to assess the possible advantage for all female soldiers of routine iron supplementation versus iron supplementation only after screening reveals a low serum ferritin. Such research should also assess whether the criterion adequate for iron status should be elevated above 15 μg/L of serum ferritin to meet any extra iron needs associated with intense exercise and stress.

As with fortification, interactions exist with various drugs and nutrients. For example, anti-ulcer drugs reduce stomach acid but also reduce iron absorption. Likewise, many antibiotics reduce iron absorption because they chelate the iron (Hendler and Rorvik, 2001).

There is a danger of excess from supplementation because iron is a mineral that could accumulate in the body. The window between excess and the recommended levels is relatively narrow; the UL for iron is 45 mg/day (IOM, 2001), based on gastroenterological side effects versus the $EAR_{MGT}$ of 12 mg/day for males and 14 mg/day for nonpregnant, nonlactating females. Some adverse effects at high doses include nausea; vomiting; constipation; diarrhea; black, tarry stools; and abdominal distress. Small, divided doses and the use of enteric-coated or delayed-release preparations may be helpful although will not be as well absorbed. The fatal amount of elemental iron is estimated to be between 180 and 300 mg per kg of body weight (Proudfoot, 1993) although at doses of 20–60 mg/kg, iron toxicity occurs (IOM 2001). Very high amounts of iron also reduce zinc absorption, but the molar ratios at which the effects are present are very high (about 25 to 1) and decrease if other foods are present (IOM, 2001). Still, it is important to guard against overzealous use of supplements.

### Recommendations for Achieving Sufficiency

Supplementation or fortification programs targeted specifically for women appear to be the only realistic approach for meeting women's iron requirements during training periods, and especially in hot environments. Educational approaches used during garrison training should aim to increased meat intake so that heme iron in the diet is maximized. However, it is unlikely that food-choice alternatives can increase iron intakes to the > 20 mg/day range. Supplementation during pregnancy and fortification have been used effectively for decades. Research should be conducted to elucidate which approach will best meet women's iron needs during military training (see Chapter 4, Research Needs).

## Research Needs

### *Specific Priorities*

- Quantify iron losses due to the stressful conditions of garrison training (i.e., heat, physical exertion, and psychological stressors).
- Determine the prevalence of iron deficiency in women at entry, during training, and during deployment to base; perform regular surveys that monitor women's iron status stability.
- Determine the relationship between iron status and cognitive and behavioral functions within the context of military garrison training.
- Determine if supplemental iron or dietary intervention approaches, or both, can alleviate the drop in female soldiers' iron status during garrison training versus iron supplementation only after screening.

### *Other Research Needs*

- Perform field testing of current filter paper technology to evaluate the feasibility of iron status biomarkers (i.e., ferritin and sTfR) as indicators of iron nutrition during long deployments.
- Develop methods to test field-friendly cognitive tasks (e.g., finger tapping, memory tasks, etc.) that can assess cognitive functioning as it relates to iron status.

## MAGNESIUM RECOMMENDATIONS

Magnesium is a cofactor in almost all phosphorylation reactions involving ATP. The nutrient can affect neurotransmitters' binding to receptors, stabilize membranes via binding to phospholipids, and modulate $Ca^{2+}$ and $K^{+}$ ionic currents through membranes (Berdanier, 1998; Shils, 1999).

Total-body magnesium in the average adult (20–28 grams) is distributed in the bone (53 percent), skeletal muscle (27 percent), and soft tissue (19 percent). Less than one percent circulates in the bloodstream. The serum concentration is 0.7–1.0 mmol/L, of which ~65 percent is free ions, 27 percent is bound to albumin, and eight percent is complexed to anions, primarily citrate or phosphate (Shils, 1999).

*Absorption and Metabolism*

Magnesium is absorbed primarily from the jejunum and ileum by passive diffusion and active transport, with a typical efficiency of 30–40 percent (Berdanier, 1998; Shils, 1999). At a daily ingestion rate of 300 mg/day, 200 mg/day are excreted in the feces, and 100 mg/day are eliminated through urine. Increasing dietary magnesium content reduces the percentage that is absorbed (Berdanier, 1998). Approximately 70 percent of serum magnesium is filtered at the glomerulus, and usually 95 percent of the filtered load is reabsorbed. Urinary output decreases during dietary restriction, and increases during dietary excess. Hormones affecting calcium deposition and mobilization have similar effects on magnesium (Shils, 1999).

As deficiency and excess both might have dire consequences, tightly regulated magnesium absorption and excretion processes have evolved. Seven men who were consuming 657 mg/day of magnesium during a 21-day adaptation period and 719 mg/day during a 28-day experimental period lost 504 ± 70 mg/day in feces during the adaptation period and 514 ± 88 mg/day during the experimental period (Schwartz et al., 1986). Their urinary magnesium losses were 178 ± 34 and 181 ± 39 mg/day in the adaptation and experimental periods, respectively. Conversely, ten men who were fed low magnesium diets, 229 and 258 mg/day, averaged urinary magnesium losses of 106 ± 21 and 119 ± 25 mg/day, and fecal magnesium losses of 111 ± 14 and 121 ± 32 mg/day (Mahalko et al., 1983). In a study of 21 young women who consumed nonvegetarian (367 mg/day magnesium) and lacto-ovo-vegetarian (260 mg/day) diets for eight weeks each (Hunt et al., 1998), fecal magnesium loss was significantly higher in the nonvegetarian diet (278 versus 169 mg/day), however, urinary magnesium loss was not significantly different (98 versus 89 mg/day) between diets. The results of these and other studies (Beisel et al., 1968; Feillet-Coudray et al., 2002; Lakshmanan et al., 1984) are summarized in Figure 3-2 and show that dietary magnesium supplementation had no influence on serum, blood cell, or skeletal muscle magnesium concentrations (Terblanche et al., 1992; Wary et al., 1999; Weller et al., 1998). The data suggest that increased dietary intake (> 250–300 mg/day) is counterbalanced by greater urinary and fecal losses. Conversely, decreased dietary intake is compensated by higher gastrointestinal absorption efficiency and renal reabsorption.

Osmotically-induced diarrhea (through the administration of polyethylene glycol, lactulose, sorbitol, or sodium sulfate) did not affect daily output of magnesium. In other words, as daily fecal weight increased, magnesium concentration decreased. In contrast, magnesium hydroxide-induced diarrhea resulted in magnesium losses that were directly proportional to fecal weight (Fine et al., 1991). Thus, excessive dietary magnesium intake can actually cause a diarrhea that can deplete fluids and nutrients, including magnesium.

Inadequate dietary magnesium availability is uncommon, but deficiencies can occur as a result of malabsorption syndromes, renal dysfunction, alcoholism,

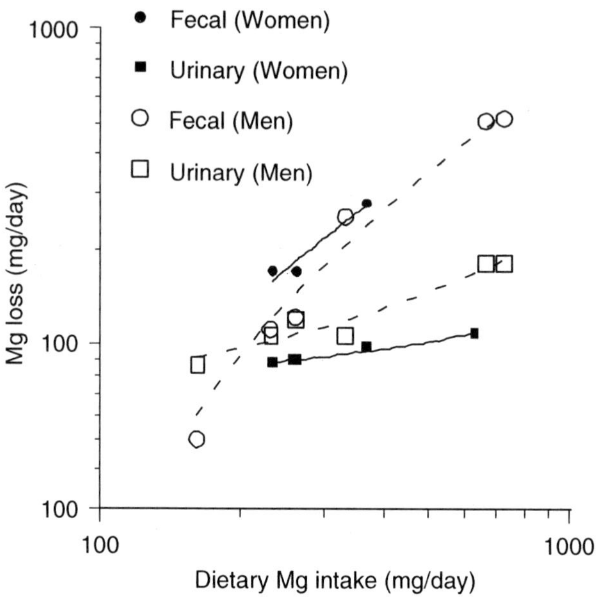


**FIGURE 3-2** Magnesium losses with increased dietary intake (> 250–300 mg/day).
SOURCE: Beisel et al. (1968); Feillet-Coudray et al. (2002); Lakshmanan et al. (1984).

or endocrine disorders. Among the endocrine disorders, diabetes mellitus often is accompanied by hypomagnesemia due to the diuresis that accompanies the disorder (Shils, 1999). The data are not clear, but researchers believe that appropriate magnesium status (i.e., meeting the IOM RDA) improves diabetes control (Hendler and Rorvik, 2001). Magnesium deficiency can lead to reduced parathyroid hormone secretion, hypokalemia, sodium retention, muscle spasms, and loss of parathyroid hormone receptor responsiveness on osteoclasts.

### *Functions*

There is some evidence that magnesium is involved in bone metabolism and in bone formation, directly and indirectly, by its interactions with hormones that regulate bone metabolism. In postmenopausal women with osteoporosis, magnesium intake is reduced along with calcium and phosphorus, compared to non-osteoporotic controls (Tranquilli et al., 1994). One study suggested that magnesium supplementation increased bone density in postmenopausal osteoporosis (Stendig-Lindberg et al., 1993).

Magnesium is suggested sometimes as an adjunctive therapy for patients with acute myocardial infarctions, although the clinical trials do not support this. Likewise, the suggested role of magnesium deficiency in causing diabetes or other chronic diseases is not proven. Epidemiological studies have associated low serum magnesium with increased risk for atherosclerosis (Liao et al., 1998) and type 2 diabetes (Kao et al., 1999).

More speculative claims involve using relatively large doses of magnesium supplements (much higher than the IOM RDA) for various purposes. There is some inconsistent evidence that magnesium supplements at levels of 350–500 mg/day lower blood pressure (Patki et al., 1990; Sacks et al., 1998), especially among those taking diuretics (Dyckner and Wester, 1983). One study suggested that magnesium (as magnesium hydroxide) had a vasodilating effect and that at doses of 250 mg supplementation increased the walking distance of individuals suffering from intermittent claudication (Neglen et al., 1985). However, these are older studies, and many of them are observational rather than experimental in nature.

Some studies claim that PMS is characterized by a magnesium deficiency (Abraham and Lubran, 1981; Sherwood et al., 1986). Some researchers argue that magnesium has the potential for reducing PMS symptoms (Bendich, 2000), and supplementation has been advocated for reducing symptoms (Facchinetti et al., 1991). However, more recent studies have not been so positive; in one such study, magnesium (200 mg of magnesium oxide) seemed to alleviate PMS-related fluid retention only in the second menstrual cycle in which it was given (Walker et al., 1998).

Magnesium excess, which can cause serum concentrations to approach 3 mmol/L, causes a drop in blood pressure, nausea, flushing, vomiting, electrocardiogram irregularities, and mental status changes. As serum concentrations increase further, depressed reflexes and respiration, coma, and cardiac arrest can develop (Mordes and Wacker, 1978).

### Measuring Magnesium Status

Plasma or serum concentrations of magnesium are used commonly to assess magnesium nutrition due to the widespread availability of such tests. However, the relative merits of measuring total-body magnesium versus free ionized magnesium (which may be more bioavailable) is a point of controversy. In addition, since less than 1 percent of total-body magnesium circulates in the blood, any measures in this compartment may not accurately reflect overall magnesium status. The more reliable methods being sought may include intracellular measurements (requiring sophisticated nuclear magnetic resonance techniques) or magnesium loading and retention tests (which are somewhat invasive and time intensive). The advantages and pitfalls of these approaches are reviewed by Keen and Uriu-Adams included in Appendix B.

## Magnesium Intake Effects on Health and Performance

### *Physical Performance*

Two studies have reported data indicating that magnesium may have a significant influence on physical performance. In the first, maximal aerobic capacity correlated significantly ($R = 0.46$, $P < 0.002$) with plasma magnesium concentration (but not red cell magnesium) in 44 male collegiate athletes (Lukaski et al., 1983). No significant correlations were observed in untrained control subjects. In the second study, 12 subjects (their gender was not reported) were supplemented with magnesium oxide to bring their total dietary magnesium intake to 8 mg/kg/day (an average of 507 mg/day per individual) (Brilla and Haley, 1992). After seven weeks of magnesium supplementation coupled with quadriceps strength training, peak torque in the trained muscles increased by 26 percent. This was significantly greater than the 11-percent strength gain in the 14 subjects who took a placebo during training.

Most other studies appearing in peer-reviewed journals report no significant influence of magnesium on physical performance:

In a double-blind, placebo-controlled study, 32 young women were supplemented with 212 mg/day magnesium oxide or a placebo and then were tested for exercise performance. After a six-week washout and treatment crossover, the women were retested. The magnesium supplementation resulted in a significant eight-percent increase in the ionic magnesium concentration of whole blood, but $VO_2$max, work load, heart rate, and blood pressure during treadmill exercise were unaffected (there was a < 2-percent difference between treatments) (Finstad et al., 2001).

Sixteen men and four women were paired according to running velocity and then assigned to magnesium-L-aspartate supplementation (365 mg/day elemental magnesium) or a placebo for four weeks before and six weeks after participation in a marathon (Terblanche et al., 1992). Magnesium supplementation had no significant effect on serum magnesium, muscle magnesium concentrations measured in biopsies, or marathon-running performance. Magnesium supplementation had no effect on creatine kinase release from muscle following the race, and in contrast to the study by Brilla and Haley (1992), had no influence on quadriceps strength before the marathon or in the rate of strength recovery after the marathon.

Athletes (16 men, four women) who had serum magnesium concentrations below 0.8 mmol/L and who reported occasional muscle cramps during exercise were assigned randomly to either a placebo or 500 mg/day of magnesium oxide in a double-blind treatment protocol for three weeks; physiological testing was performed before as well as after the treatment (Weller et al., 1998). Heart rates and oxygen consumption during submaximal and maximal exercise were unchanged in both groups. The magnesium treatment also had no effect on electromyography activity following an ischemia–hyperventilation challenge or on the number of muscle cramps reported during the treatment period.

Baseline serum magnesium concentrations were not different between runners (their genders was not reported) who did or did not experience muscle cramps during or immediately after a 56-km race (Schwellnus et al., 2004). Those who did experience cramps ($n$ = 21) exhibited a 10-percent reduction in serum magnesium by the end of the race, whereas those who did not experience cramps ($n$ = 22) actually exhibited a significantly greater reduction (19 percent) in serum magnesium.

A study of 20 female and 12 male physically-active college students sought to determine if fours weeks of dietary supplementation with magnesium oxide that brought total magnesium intake up to eight mg/kg/day (on average, 541 mg/day) had an influence on perceived exertion, heart rate, or time to exhaustion during treadmill running at 90 percent of $VO_2max$ (Brilla and Gunter, 1995). The exercise intensities apparently were different during the placebo testing versus during the magnesium-supplemented conditions because oxygen consumption was significantly lower during the latter condition. Nevertheless, no differences in perceived exertion, heart rate, or time to exhaustion were observed.

Other studies have suggested a positive effect of magnesium supplementation on exercise performance. As described below, methodological issues—such as nonrandomized supplementation schedules, lack of assessment or control of concurrent physical activity, and unsuccessful standardization of exercise testing conditions between control and magnesium-supplemented trials—make it difficult to determine if any observed performance differences can be ascribed to differences in magnesium status.

Nine male subjects performed one hour of rigorously identical exercise on cycle ergometers before and after 14 days of supplementation with 15 mmol/day of magnesium aspartate (Golf et al., 1984). At a similar work intensity, the subjects' heart rates were nonsignificantly lower and cortisol was 28 percent lower. However, these parameters were lower even before exercise, raising the question of whether familiarization with the procedure may have reduced the stress level in these subjects independent of any influence by magnesium supplementation.

Fifteen subjects (their genders were not reported) were supplemented with 20 mmol/day of magnesium aspartate, and 15 subjects were supplemented with 18 mmol/day of magnesium oxide combined with 1,500 IU $\alpha$-tocopherol for 21 days before a marathon (Bertschat et al., 1986). Fifteen additional subjects served as unsupplemented controls. Blood was taken before and immediately after the race and assayed for concentrations of intramuscular proteins that are released into the blood as a result of myocellular stress or damage. After the marathon, myoglobin, creatine kinase, and aspartate aminotransferase concentrations increased > 13-fold, > 3-fold, and > 35 percent, respectively, in the control group. The magnesium oxide supplementation had no significant effect on these increases, and the magnesium aspartate supplementation attenuated only the increase in creatine kinase (by ~20 percent). The authors also reported that magnesium concentrations were higher in the subjects' urine collected on the day of the marathon, compared to their urine that was collected on previous day. However, it is not possible to determine if magnesium excretion rates or total urinary losses actually changed, because neither creatinine concentrations nor total urine volumes were reported.

Fourteen male competitive rowers took a placebo for four weeks and then performed two six-minute trials on a rowing ergometer (Golf et al., 1989). The subjects then took magnesium aspartate (20 mmol/day) for four weeks and were retested on the rowing ergometer. It was not stated if the ergometer trials were intended to be maximal or submaximal, but the work intensity was virtually identical in the supplemented versus unsupplemented trials. The authors reported that maximal oxygen uptake decreased 14.6 percent ($p = 0.003$) after taking the magnesium supplement. It seems likely that the authors did not mean to report that maximal oxygen uptake was reduced by magnesium supplementation but instead that an equivalent amount of work was performed with less oxygen consumption after supplementation. However, because the placebo and supplementation phases were not randomized and no information was provided on any training activities during each four-week phase, it is impossible to determine if the magnesium supplementation was the actual cause of any physiological changes.

Several cardiorespiratory parameters during 30-minute cycle ergometry exercise at a work load corresponding to 70 percent of maximal heart rate (based on a preliminary maximal effort test) were assessed at baseline and at 7, 14, and 21 days into double-blind dietary supplementation trial of eight male subjects with placebo and of eight male subjects with 4.5 grams of magnesium pidolate (containing 387 mg of magnesium) (Ripari et al., 1989). The authors reported no changes in the placebo group, but significant reductions in minute ventilation, oxygen uptake, and $CO_2$ elimination at seven days compared to baseline in the supplemented group. By 14 days, heart rate and systolic pressure reportedly were decreased in the supplemented group. Although probability values were listed, no actual baseline or postsupplement data, nor the magnitude of the changes, were reported. The maximal effort test did not appear to be standardized, in that it was ended by any of three different criteria—dyspnea, muscular exhaustion, or expected heart rate maximum calculated as 220 beats per minute minus the subject's age.

Additional factors confounding many of the studies on magnesium supplementation have been described in detail in a recent review (Newhouse and Finstad, 2000).

### *Cognition and Behavior*

As described earlier, magnesium can influence cell membrane stability and ion currents and, thus, have an important influence on neuronal excitability. In the central nervous system, magnesium plays an important role in glutaminergic neurotransmission, inhibiting excitatory N-methyl-D aspartate (NMDA) (Cooper et al., 2003), and affecting monoaminergic and serotonergic systems (Singewald et al., 2004). Magnesium also is involved in regulating the hypothalamus-pituitary-adrenocortical (HPA) system (Murck, 2002). The role of magnesium as an NMDA antagonist and a gamma-aminobutyric acid agonist is a likely mechanism responsible for magnesium's effects on sleep (Held et al., 2002). The relationship between magnesium and mood is linked to increased HPA activity, which is frequently observed in depression and anxiety (Holsboer, 2000).

There are no previous studies that have directly correlated magnesium intake or status to soldiers' cognitive function or behavior, and only a few data exist from studies on civilians.

Severe magnesium deficiency has been associated with numerous neurological and psychological problems, including convulsions, dizziness, neuromuscular hyperexcitability (Chvostek and Trousseau signs), hyperemotionality (irritability and marked agitation), anxiety, confusion, depression, apathy, loss of appetite, and insomnia (Dubray and Rayssiguier, 1997; Durlach, 1980). Brain function assessed by EEGs has shown increased cortical excitability, characterized as diffuse, slow-wave activity of the type commonly found in metabolic disorders, and "diffuse irritative tracings" in the absence of focal effects, marked by spiked alpha and increased theta activity (Durlach, 1985). Authors also have reported disrupted normal sleep architecture in magnesium-deficient subjects, including greatly reduced deep, slow-wave sleep and decreased rapid eye movement sleep (Popoviciu et al., 1987).

Magnesium deficiency leads to reduced offensive and increased defensive behavior in rats (Kantak, 1988) and impaired learning and memory in mice (Bardgett et al., 2005). Magnesium deficiency in rats also leads to increased pain sensitivity (Begon et al., 2001). None of these effects have been investigated in humans. There are few data on neuropsychological effects of marginal magnesium restriction. In an early study that successfully induced magnesium deficiency by dietary restriction in seven subjects (Shils, 1969), visual evaluation revealed no changes in EEGs of subjects fed < 10 mg/day of magnesium for as long as 105 days. However, Shils' study was limited to seven subjects, and EEG analysis was visual rather than quantitative.

A study that contrasted quantitative EEGs of athletes (44 male and female kayakers) with low versus normal erythrocyte magnesium, found significantly less relative alpha (7.25–12.5 Hz) activity in the low magnesium group, particularly in the right occipital region (Delorme et al., 1992). However, magnesium intakes and status were not controlled experimentally in that study. Thirteen healthy postmenopausal women living on a metabolic research unit were fed 115 and 315 mg/day of magnesium for 42 days and had increased EEG activity (i.e., hyperexcitability) following experimentally induced marginal magnesium deficiency; the results indicated that relatively short periods of marginal magnesium deprivation can affect brain function (Penland, 1995). Compared with high dietary magnesium, the low magnesium intake increased total EEG activity in the frontal, right temporal, and parietal regions and resulted in frequency-specific increases in left occipital delta activity (1–3 Hz), theta activity (4–7 Hz) in all but the left temporal region, alpha activity (8–12 Hz) in the right frontal and right temporal regions, and beta activity (13–18 Hz) in the frontal regions. The proportion of theta activity compared with total activity in the parietal regions also increased with low magnesium intake.

Magnesium may play an important role in regulating sleep. Animal studies have shown that magnesium deficiency increases wakefulness and decreases slow-wave sleep (Depoortere et al., 1993) and total sleep time (Poenaru et al., 1984). Intravenous magnesium administration in healthy young men increased EEG activity power in sigma frequencies (11–29 Hz) during nonrapid eye movement sleep (Murck and Steiger, 1998). Magnesium supplementation (10–30 mmol/day) of older subjects (60–80 years) increased EEG power in the delta (0.8–4.5 Hz) and sigma (11.8–15.2 Hz) frequencies (Held et al., 2002). A recent study found that sleep restriction over a four-week period resulted in a seven-percent reduction of intracellular magnesium in college males (Takase et al., 2004).

Magnesium also may be involved in regulating mood states. Many correlational studies have shown a positive association between blood magnesium concentrations and mood, although a few have found either no association or a negative relationship (Imada et al., 2002). However, supplemental and intravenous magnesium have been effective in treating symptoms of mania, bipolar disorder, chronic fatigue syndrome, and PMS (Murck, 2002).

In summary, the importance of magnesium for cognitive function and behavior has received little attention and is largely unknown. Available data suggest that magnesium is involved in regulating brain electrical activity and that increasing intake may benefit sleep and mood.

*Immunity*

In animals, magnesium deficiency has been associated with thymic hyperplasia and leukocytosis. In early stages of magnesium deficiency in rats, mast cells degranulate, resulting in high blood levels of histamine and increased urinary excretion (McCoy and Kenney, 1984). Magnesium-deficient hamsters exhibited three times higher plasma concentrations of IL-1, IL-6, and TNF-α than the magnesium-sufficient control hamsters, whereas magnesium-deficient rats had 15 times higher concentrations of cytokines than the control rats (Weglicki et al., 1992).

In humans, magnesium deficiency seems to have little influence on immune function (Beisel, 1982; Wood and Watson, 1984). Only a few isolated studies have linked increased Candida infection susceptibility (Galland, 1985) and diminished cell-mediated immune responses to influenza (Henrotte et al., 1985) to a genetically-defined subpopulation (carrying the human leukocyte antigen Bw35+) with low erythrocyte magnesium concentrations.

A role for magnesium therapy in asthma has been suggested. Magnesium ions promote bronchodilation and inhibit mast cell degranulation (Chang and Gershwin, 2000). Several randomized, controlled trials have shown that administration of magnesium sulfate in aerosols along with β-2 agonists appears to improve pulmonary function during acute asthma attacks (Blitz et al., 2005). An epidemiological study of 2,633 adults found a significant, positive relationship between dietary magnesium intake and 1-sec forced expiratory volume ($FEV_1$) (Britton et al., 1994). However, a 100 mg/day difference in magnesium intake was associated with < 1 percent difference in $FEV_1$. A randomized, double-blind trial in which 99 asthma patients took magnesium supplements (as 450 mg/day of magnesium amino chelate) and 106 patients took a placebo for 16 weeks, found that magnesium had no beneficial influence on a battery of pulmonary function tests, including $FEV_1$ (Fogarty et al., 2003). Although supplementation increased urinary magnesium excretion by 34 percent, serum magnesium concentrations increased (nonsignificantly) by only 2.5 percent.

## Risk Factors for Inadequacy During Military Garrison Training

### *Dietary Intake in the U.S. Military and Special Groups*

A seven-day field study of Army Rangers who consumed MREs estimated a magnesium intake of 265 ± 61 mg/day. A three-day sample of food records on Rangers in garrison training who consumed food primarily from outside sources indicated that approximately 40 percent of the Rangers were consuming less than the IOM EAR for magnesium and approximately 30 percent were achieving or surpassing the IOM RDA. A similar study on Special Forces personnel in garrison training who ate only in military facilities found a similar distribution in magnesium consumption (Baker-Fulco, 2005; see Baker-Fulco in Appendix B).

Military personnel may fail to consume adequate amounts of magnesium, but the limited data on magnesium status of soldiers in various types of training do not provide evidence of overt nutritional deficiencies. Given the intakes reported in a few studies and the cognitive and psychological impairments, marginal magnesium deficiencies may exist in soldiers during active training and operations.

### *Bioavailability*

Magnesium bioavailability in the diet or a dietary supplement likely will affect the efficacy of treatment. Magnesium complexed with chloride, citrate, and aspartate has relatively good bioavailability. Sulfates have variable, limited bioavailability, whereas carbonates and oxides have extremely low bioavailability (Ranade and Somberg, 2001).

*Exercise and Environment*

A comprehensive evidentiary review concluded that the dietary intake and magnesium status of athletes is generally adequate, with the exception of individuals (such as wrestlers and ballerinas) who strive to maintain low body weights (Clarkson and Haymes, 1995). Nevertheless, the potential risk of excessive magnesium losses through sweat or urine in situations that military personnel may experience will be discussed in detail in the following sections.

*Sweat Loss*

Reported magnesium concentrations in sweat vary widely, from 0.2 to 1.4 mmol/L (4.8 to 34 mg/L) (Brouns, 1991). Some of the variability may be attributed to collection techniques. For example, six women demonstrated a mean magnesium loss of 35 ± 13 mg/day when the loss was measured by a whole-body collection technique. In contrast, magnesium loss determined with patches (attached to eight body sites on the arms, legs, and back) overestimated whole-body magnesium loss by 3.6-fold when the measurements were extrapolated to total body surface area (Palacios et al., 2003). Acute, short-term sweat collection also can be confounded by transiently elevated magnesium concentrations that exist early after the onset of sweating. Two studies using regional collection methods on six and eight young men found initial sweat magnesium concentrations of > 25 mg/L that subsided to < 15 mg/ml as the thermal stress progressed (Mitchell and Hamilton, 1949; Verde et al., 1982). This temporal response was observed for both passive and exercise-induced hyperthermia.

Magnesium losses from three men exposed to a hot environment (37.8°C) for 7.5 hours, including 30 minutes spent in moderate exercise, were measured using arm bags over a 16-day period (Consolazio et al., 1963). The magnesium intake was maintained at 343 mg/day throughout the study. Fecal magnesium loss declined from 110 mg/day during the first week to 76 mg/day during the last four days. Urinary magnesium loss remained relatively constant ranging from 25.7 to 21.9 mg/day. Sweat magnesium loss during the heat exposures also remained constant throughout the 16 days with a mean loss of 17.0 mg per 7.5-hour exposure. Average total sweat magnesium loss was 46.7 mg/day.

When eight men exercised on cycle ergometers in a hot (39.5°C) environment, whole-body sweat magnesium loss gradually declined from 54 mg to 50 mg to 47 mg for each collection period, resulting in a total sweat magnesium loss of 151 mg (Costill et al., 1976).

In another study, sweat magnesium was measured from the arms of five men during 90 minutes of exercise in a hot (49°C) environment (Beller et al., 1975). Mean sweat magnesium concentration was 3.4 mg/L, and sweat volume averaged 2 L for a total magnesium loss of 6.8 mg from arm collection. Mean sweat magnesium measured by a whole-body wash-down technique during moderate exercise by five men and two women in a warm, humid (34°C, 60–70 percent relative humidity) environment was 12.1 mg/L (Shirreffs and Maughan, 1997).

*Urinary Loss*

A study by Buchman et al. (1998) compared pre- and postmarathon magnesium concentration levels in 24 men and two women; magnesium concentrations (normalized to creatinine) collected after the marathon during three six-hour collection period showed a reduction of 36 percent. The runners' serum magnesium concentrations dropped 15 percent. A second study of postmarathon urinary magnesium excretion rate reported an 83-percent reduction in urinary magnesium (serum concentration dropped by eight percent, and red cell magnesium levels dropped by five percent) (Lijnen et al., 1988). In the study of progressive two-, four-, and six-percent weight loss cited previously (Costill et al., 1976), urinary magnesium loss decreased substantially from 7.1 mg to 3.5 mg to 2.5 mg in each collection period, for a total urinary magnesium loss of 13.1 mg. Although these data suggest that increased urinary reabsorption mechanisms might compensate for magnesium loss via sweat, full 24-hour urine analyses are necessary to determine if balance is maintained.

Other studies show an increase in urinary magnesium with exercise. Twenty-four hour urinary magnesium excretion actually increased by 21 percent in 13 men on the day of intermittent, high-intensity exercise (90 percent $VO_2max$) to exhaustion (Deuster et al., 1987b). This change in excretion correlated significantly with blood lactate concentration and was consistent with evidence that acidosis decreases renal magnesium reabsorption (Quamme, 1997). Excretion on the day following exercise returned to baseline but did not exhibit any compensatory decrease (Deuster et al., 1987b). Measuring passive hyperthermia in eight 22–25-year-old men for a full day showed 30 mg/day increases in urinary magnesium on the day of and on the day following heat stress (Beisel et al., 1968). Compensatory reductions in magnesium excretion (which were insufficient to restore balance) were not observed until three days after heat exposure. It should be noted that the dietary intakes of these subjects—160 mg/day—were somewhat low.

In summary, results from urinary loss associated with heat or exercise are inconsistent and might reflect different controlled mechanisms or different dietary magnesium intakes or study designs.

*Weight Loss*

Dieting and weight loss may affect magnesium status if caloric restriction is so severe that it results in ketoacidosis. In such a case, the acidosis can cause increased renal excretion of magnesium (Quamme, 1997). On reduced calorie diets, consuming at least the IOM RDA of magnesium (or of other minerals) (see Table 3-1) would be prudent.

*Infection and Trauma*

Experimental infections were introduced to 61 healthy 19–26-year-old male soldiers (Beisel et al., 1967). Bacterial (*Pasteurella tularensis*), rickettsial (*Coxiella burnetii*), and viral (sandfly fever) infections all caused negative magnesium balance, which was attributed almost entirely to a reduced dietary intake, with only slight increases in urinary magnesium excretion. Decreases in muscle magnesium also have been reported in one study of severe physical trauma (Bergstrom et al., 1987).

*Menstrual Cycle and Oral Contraceptives*

The literature is divided regarding menstrual cycle-related variations in magnesium. The magnesium content of plasma, red blood cells, and peripheral blood mononuclear cells was measured 3–5 day/week through three menstrual cycles in each of five healthy women. Plasma concentrations were highest during menses and significantly lower during the follicular phase (–8 percent) and at ovulation (–12 percent), the concentrations then rose during the luteal phase (Deuster et al., 1987a). These variations were independent of any changes in plasma albumin concentrations. No significant differences in red cell or mononuclear cell magnesium content were observed. Several other studies also reported maximal concentrations of serum ionized magnesium at menses and significantly lower concentrations at ovulation (Das and Chowdhury, 1997; Muneyyirci-Delale et al., 1998). In contrast, four studies have reported no menstrual cycle variations in serum magnesium (Goldsmith and Goldsmith, 1966; M'Buyamba-Kabangu et al., 1985; Pitkin et al., 1978). Free intracellular magnesium in skeletal muscle, measured by nuclear magnetic resonance spectroscopy, was reported to be stable across the menstrual cycles of 16 women (Rosenstein et al., 1995). Using the same analysis technique, two studies have reported that free intramuscular magnesium is significantly higher in women than men (Ryschon et al., 1996; Ward et al., 1996).

The influence of OCs on magnesium status is also equivocal, perhaps because sampling times were not standardized with any particular phase of the menstrual (or pill) cycles. Goldsmith and Goldsmith (1966) reported that serum magnesium was 15 percent lower, and the rate of urinary magnesium excretion (collected in periods ranging from 0.5 to 5 hours) was 43 percent lower in four women using OCs, compared to five normally cycling women.

Lower urinary magnesium concentrations (19 percent, after normalization to creatinine) were reported for 117 OC users, compared to 251 normally cycling controls (Goulding and McChesney, 1977), but the total 24-hour excretion rates were not significantly different between the groups (about eight percent lower for OC users). Likewise, no differences in 24-hour excretion of magnesium were observed in 13 OC users compared with 12 nonusers (Klein et al., 1995). Fifteen OC users and 15 nonusers were tested once during the baseline period and once during caffeine-induced diuresis (which was separated from the baseline by at least seven days) (Ribeiro-Alves et al., 2003). Although habitual dietary intake of magnesium (assessed by questionnaire) was 26 percent higher among the OC users, plasma magnesium and baseline urinary magnesium excretion were identical between the two groups. Urinary magnesium loss doubled in nonusers following caffeine loading but only increased by 50 percent in the OC users.

## Requirements for the General U.S. Population

The Third Report on Nutrition Monitoring in the United States concluded that magnesium presented a potential public health issue and required further study because median intakes from food were lower than recommendations for the population (IOM, 1997). More recent surveys also indicate that mean intakes are lower than current IOM RDA levels (see Table 3-1). However, the implications on human health are unclear.

The IOM RDA for magnesium is 400 mg/day for 19–30-year-old males and 420 mg/day for males older than 30 years; for 19–30-year-old females the IOM RDA for magnesium is 310 mg/day and 320 mg/day for women older than 30 years (IOM, 1997).

There are no readily mobilized stores of magnesium (other than the skeleton). The organism activates conservation mechanisms early on in any restrictions; the deficiency in young organisms (e.g., infants and children) brings about cessation of growth so that demand for the nutrient is reduced. For these reasons, assaying the magnesium content in a body fluid or tissue may not ascertain status of the nutrient. It is not known at what level magnesium deficiency poses a problem, and there are no readily available laboratory tests of biological function that clinicians can use for diagnostic purposes. The true prevalence of hypomagnesemia is unknown because most hospitals and clinics do not include this ion in routine electrolyte testing.

## Daily Intake Recommendations for Military Personnel in Garrison Training

No changes from the current recommendations are proposed. Magnesium's current MDRI for men is 420 mg/day and for women is 320 mg/day (Baker-

Fulco et al., 2001). These levels are the same as the IOM RDAs for adults over 30 years of age (IOM, 1997). Although the intakes of military personnel appear to be lower than these recommendations (the same is true for the civilian population), there appear to be no apparent related adverse health or other effects.

Military personnel may be at risk of increased magnesium losses via sweat and possibly urine during both passive and exertional heat stress. However, there is no clear evidence that such losses have an adverse effect on physical performance. Furthermore, magnesium supplementation has not consistently produced changes in magnesium status, let alone caused significant changes in performance. The risk of magnesium-induced diarrhea mandates that careful study of the true risks and benefits of increased dietary magnesium intake be conducted under carefully controlled conditions before any changes in the current MDRIs are considered.

**RECOMMENDATIONS FOR MAGNESIUM INTAKE:**

| | |
|---|---|
| **$EAR_{MGT}$ for men** | **350 mg/day** |
| **$EAR_{MGT}$ for women** | **265 mg/day** |
| **$RDA_{MGT}$ for men** | **420 mg/day** |
| **$RDA_{MGT}$ for women** | **320 mg/day** |

### Adequacy of Magnesium MDRIs and Magnesium Levels in Rations

The committee concluded that until further data are collected the current magnesium MDRIs of 420 and 320 mg/day for men and women, respectively, are adequate.

Table 3-1 (see also Tables C-2 through C-5 in Appendix C) shows the averages and ranges of magnesium for three different MREs that each include approximately 25 menus. The average magnesium content in MRE XXII, XXIII, and XXIV menus and is 114, 177, and 140 mg, respectively. Even though some of the menus seem very low in magnesium (69 mg), for this interpretation it will be assumed that a mix of menus are eaten per day and that the mix is sufficient for meeting the average level of magnesium in the menus. However, there is a potential for deficiencies due to not only low food consumption but also selection of an MRE that is low in magnesium. The committee recommends that the menus at the low end of the range be revised so that they would meet the MDRI of 420 and 320 mg/day for men and women, respectively.

An intake of magnesium above the MDRI will not be of concern if it comes from food items. Although magnesium supplementation could be used to supplement the low-magnesium menus, to redesign the rations with higher levels of magnesium is a better option. If magnesium supplementation is needed it should not approach the UL of 350 mg/day due to safety concerns (IOM, 1997).

Two studies with Rangers and Special Forces engaging in garrison training showed that about 40 percent of individuals were not meeting the IOM EAR for magnesium and that about 60 percent of individuals were not meeting the RDA for magnesium (Baker-Fulco, 2005; see Baker-Fulco in Appendix B). Because magnesium deficiency could affect cognitive functions, the reasons for the low intakes deserve further investigation. The first issue to address would be whether this low intake relates to menus with low-magnesium density or to the selective discarding of food items.

The current FSRs contain an average of 386 mg of magnesium (see Table 3-1; Table C-6 in Appendix C). Although this amount is not overtly inadequate, a minimum amount of 400 mg was recommended in IOM (2006) *Nutrient Composition of Rations for Short-Term, High-Intensity Combat Operations* and is endorsed by this committee.

### Adequacy of IOM Recommendations for First Strike Rations

The first strike rations (i.e., assault rations) report recommends a 400–550 mg magnesium-level range based on the current IOM RDA for adult men and the 95th percentile of intake for adult men. The evidence of potential effects of magnesium on performance was not strong enough to recommend a level higher than the IOM RDA; however, it was recognized that intakes higher than the IOM RDA might be beneficial to prevent kidney stones. Researchers caution against fortificant intakes of more than 350 mg, since gastrointestinal problems might occur. The committee concurs with the recommendations until stronger evidence for different requirements is available (IOM, 2006).

### Strategies for Achieving Sufficient Magnesium Intake

#### *Usual Foods*

The usual strategy for achieving dietary magnesium adequacy is to urge that individuals follow dietary guidelines (DHHS and USDA, 2005) and food guides such as MyPyramid or the DASH diet, both of which are adequate in magnesium, and eat plenty of green leafy vegetables, which are especially high in magnesium.

#### *Food Fortification*

Fortifying foods with magnesium is uncommon; however, there are some highly fortified cereals that provide, according to the nutritional label, approximately 10 percent or more of the nutrient. The difference between excess magnesium and recommendations for its intake level is relatively large. Even with fortificants, few people obtain very high levels of magnesium from food. The adult IOM RDA is 320 mg for women and 420 mg for men. The IOM UL (350 mg) is only for supplemental magnesium and not from magnesium-providing food sources because excessive intakes from food alone have not been reported. However, if magnesium salts are added as the fortificant, then magnesium levels should be limited to no more than 350 mg/day because of concerns about osmotic diarrhea (IOM, 1997).

The availability of an appropriate cereal fortification as the delivery vehicle has been successful, and the shelf life has been satisfactory. Although interactions between supplementary magnesium and various drugs and nutrients have been reported, they have not been for magnesium-fortified products.

*Supplementation*

Magnesium supplements are on the market in various forms, including oxides, hydroxides, citrates, chlorides, gluconate, lactates, aspartates, and aspartate hydrochloride as well as the glycinate. Citrates are better absorbed than oxides, but other forms seem to be equally well absorbed (Ranade and Somberg, 2001). The fractional absorption depends not only on the solubility of the compound but also on the amount ingested. Enteric-coated supplements of magnesium chloride are less well absorbed than the magnesium acetate found in ordinary gel capsules (Shils, 1999).

A number of other dietary components can inhibit or promote the absorption of magnesium, including high levels of phosohate and zinc (IOM, 1997; Shils, 1999). Nondigestible oligosaccharides, sodium alginate, and inositol hexaphosphate also may impair magnesium absorption (Hendler and Rorvik, 2001). High levels of calcium (unless they are extremely high) do not seem to affect magnesium absorption. High doses of magnesium can lead to decreased absorption of various nutrients, for example, manganese and iron (IOM, 2001). Magnesium can also cause interactions that lead to the decreased absorption of a number of drugs, including biphosphonates, quinolones, and tetracyclines.

Drinking fluid-replacement beverages that contain magnesium had no significant effect on acute plasma magnesium concentrations during two hours of running at 60–65 percent of $VO_2$max (Deuster and Singh, 1993). Likewise, ingestion of such beverages during long-duration exercise repeated daily for weeks at a time had no significant effect on magnesium balance (Johnson et al., 1988).

## Recommendations for Achieving Sufficiency

Magnesium rarely is recommended as a fortificant or supplement for individuals in good health who are living under normal conditions, similar to military personnel in garrison training. Nutrition education efforts should stress food plans such as MyPyramid or other food-based dietary guidelines that provide information on achieving sufficient mineral intake. If rations for combat or field, noncombat are insufficient for magnesium, then using highly fortified cereals is worth consideration. Actual ration levels need to be ascertained since published values may not accurately reflect analytical values. If satisfactory intakes cannot be obtained with usual food sources alone, then a stand-alone supplement or a combination mineral product containing magnesium and calcium should be considered. The amounts of magnesium supplementation should fall substantially below 350 mg (the IOM UL for magnesium), to avoid gastrointestinal distress that may occur with excessive intakes from magnesium in dietary supplements.

### Research Needs

- Quantify magnesium losses due to the stressful conditions of garrison training (i.e., heat, physical exertion, and psychological stressors).
- Determine whether increasing magnesium intake will improve sleep, protect against the effects of sleep deprivation, or regulate mood states of soldiers; conduct cognitive tests to assess visual vigilance, reaction time, pattern recognition, and logical reasoning under simulated combat conditions.
- Determine the magnesium concentrations of food items in operational rations, including MREs and FSRs, and the dietary intake levels of military personnel.

## SELENIUM RECOMMENDATIONS

Nearly 50 years of research have established that selenium, once known only as a sulfur-like element with toxic potential, is in fact an essential nutrient. In the late 1950s, selenium was found to correct pathologies in vitamin E-deficient rats and chicks. Over the following two decades studies on selenium reported benefits for a range of animal species. In the early 1970s, selenium was found to be an essential cofactor of the antioxidant enzyme glutathione peroxidase, answering the question of how the mineral functions in concert with a fat-soluble vitamin to effect cellular antioxidant protection. In the 1980s, reports of selenium's efficacy in preventing a juvenile cardiomyopathy—Keshan Disease—in parts of rural China where people suffered from severe endemic selenium deficiency drew attention to selenium as a factor in human health. The nutritional essentiality of selenium is now unquestioned, as the element has been recognized as a vital constituent of at least a dozen enzymes, each of which contains the element in the form of selenocysteine (Burk and Levander, 1999).

The potential anticarcinogenic properties of selenium were suggested in the 1960s and were based on an inverse relationship of cancer mortality rates and forage crop selenium contents in the United States. Subsequent research indeed has shown that selenium can prevent or delay tumorigenesis in animal models, and that selenium can inhibit growth and stimulate programmed cell death in a variety of cell culture systems. The results of a randomized clinical trial with American subjects showed selenium supplementation (as brewer's yeast tablets with high selenium content) to be effective in reducing the subjects' incidence of

**TABLE 3-10** Biologically Important Selenium Compounds

| Oxidation State | Compound | Biological Relevance |
|---|---|---|
| $Se^{-2}$ | Hydrogen selenide, $H_2Se$ | Obligate metabolic precursor to selenoproteins |
| | Methyl selenol, $CH_3SeH$ | Excretory form (lung) shown to be anticarcinogenic |
| | Dimethyl selenide, $(CH_3)_2Se$ | Excretory form (lung) |
| | Trimethylselenonium, $(CH_3)_3Se^+$ | Excretory form (kidney) |
| | Methylseleno-*N*-acetyl-D-galactosamine | Excretory form (kidney) |
| | Selenomethionine (SeMet) | Common food form; in nonspecific Se-containing proteins (e.g., albumin); metabolized to SeCys |
| | Selenocysteine (SeCys) | Common food form; in selenoproteins; metabolized to $H_2Se$ |
| | Se-methylselenomethionine | Form found in some foods; metabolized to $CH_3SeH$ |
| | Se-methylselenocysteine | Form found in some foods; metabolized to $CH_3SeH$ |
| | Selenobetaine | Metabolic precursor of $CH_3SeH$ |
| | Selenotaurine | Form found in some foods |
| $Se^0$ | Selenodiglutathione | Reductive metabolite of selenite and selenate with anti-carcinogenic activity |
| $Se^{+4}$ | $Na_2SeO_3$ | Commonly used feed supplemental form |
| $Se^{+6}$ | $Na_2SeO_4$ | Potential food and feed supplement form |

major cancers (Clark et al., 1996) and consequently stimulated enormous current interest in this area of research.

### *Chemical Forms of Selenium*

The chemical properties of selenium are similar to those of sulphur; however, unlike sulphur, which tends to be oxidized in biological systems, selenium tends to undergo reduction in the tissues of microbes, plants, and animals. Elemental selenium can be reduced to the $^-2$ (selenide, $Se^{-2}$) oxidation state or oxidized to the $^+4$ (selenite, $Se^{+4}$) or $^+6$ (selenate, $Se^{+6}$) oxidation states (NRC, 1983). Organic selenides are electron donors and, thus, can be converted to higher oxidation states. The selenium compounds of greatest relevance in biology are listed in Table 3-10.

### *Absorption and Metabolism*

Despite the fact that some dietary supplements and fortificants of foods and livestock feeds include selenium compounds of higher oxidation states (e.g.,

$Se^{+4}$, $Se^{+6}$), the major metabolites are in the fully reduced ($Se^{-2}$) state (NRC, 1983). Selenium is present in foods at very low concentrations and almost exclusively bound to proteins, mostly as analogues of the sulphur-containing amino acids selenomethionine (SeMet) and selenocysteine (SeCys). Because each form is absorbed via an active transport mechanism, their bioavailabilities tend to be high (50–100 percent) depending on the digestibility of the proteins in which they are contained (Burk and Levander, 1999; IOM, 2000).

The principal dietary forms of selenium, SeMet and SeCys, share a common pathway for incorporation into selenoproteins—through the intermediate, hydrogen selenide ($H_2Se$) (see Figure 3-3). Because SeCys does not carry a transfer-RNA (tRNA), it is not incorporated directly into proteins but instead is catabolized by lyases to yield $H_2Se$. In contrast, SeMet has two metabolic options: it can be incorporated into general proteins as methionine mimic because it can carry $tRNA^{Met}$, and it can also be transselenated to SeCys and then be converted to $H_2Se$. The metabolite $H_2Se$ occupies a central role in selenium metabolism; it is the obligate selenium-donor in the biosynthesis of SeCys-proteins.

Those proteins currently identified include the following: four glutathione peroxidase (GPX) isoforms, two isoforms of thioredoxine reductase (TR), one or more isoforms of the iodothyronine 5′-deiodinases (DI), and selenophosphate synthatase (Allan et al., 1999). In addition, at least four other proteins are recog-

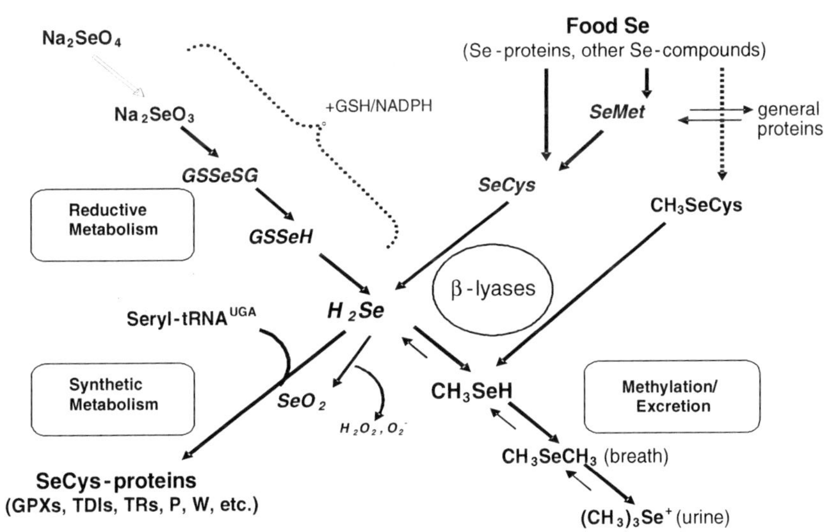


**FIGURE 3-3** Metabolism of inorganic selenium and selenoamino acids.
NOTE: selenomethionine = SeMet; selenocysteine = SeCys; selenodiglutathione = GSSeSG; glutathioneselenol = GSSeH; hydrogen selenide = $H_2Se$; selenium dioxide = $SeO_2$; methylselenol = $CH_3SeH$; dimethylselenide = $CH_3SeCH_3$; trimethylslenonium = $(CH_3)_3Se+$.
SOURCE: Material adapted from Raiche et al. (2001).

nized for specifically incorporating selenium even though their metabolic functions remain unclear. The four proteins are plasma selenoprotein P (SeP) (Allan et al., 1999; Hill et al., 1991, 1996), muscle selenoprotein W (Allan et al., 1999; Vendeland et al., 1995), and selenoproteins in the prostate and placenta (Behne et al., 1996; Gladyshev et al., 1998). Genomic analyses have indicated 25 selenoprotein genes, suggesting more, still uncharacterized selenium enzymes (Kryukov et al., 2003). In each of these proteins, selenium (from $H_2Se$) is incorporated into the amino acid SeCys by the co-translational modification of tRNA-bound serinyl residues (see Figure 3-3) at certain loci encoded by UGA codons containing SeCys-insertion sequences in their 3′-untranslated regions (Berry et al., 1993; Stadtman, 1996). The nutritional essentiality of selenium, therefore, appears to be due to the functions of SeCys-proteins—antioxidant protection by the GPXs, energy metabolism affected by the DIs, and redox regulation of transcriptional factors and gene expression by the TRs.

H2Se also can be methylated to a series of excretory metabolites, including methylselenol, which appears to have anticarcinogenic activity (Ip, 1998).

Neve (1995) reviewed several human studies and concluded that the minimum concentration of selenium that might be expected in plasma under conditions of maximal expression of plasma GPX is at least 70 μg/L. This level corresponds roughly to the amount of selenium contained in maximally expressed plasma selenoproteins (Hill et al., 1996). Plasma selenium concentrations at this level appear to be supported by dietary selenium intakes of as little as 40 μg/day (Yang et al., 1989b).

## Measuring Selenium Status

There is no parameter of selenium status that reflects both medium-term (days to weeks) selenium intake and metabolic function. Therefore, the clinical assessment of selenium status has relied on measurements of blood selenium concentration to indicate selenium intake and of blood GPX-3 activity to indicate selenium function (IOM, 2000). Each parameter has significant limitations. The selenium contents of blood cells, serum, or plasma are affected not only by the amount but also by the chemical species of dietary selenium. For example, because SeMet (e.g., found in plant foods) can replace methionine in protein synthesis as well as be converted to SeCys, sources of SeMet enter nonspecifically into blood proteins as well as specifically into SeCys-proteins, thus supporting greater blood selenium values than sources of SeCys (e.g., found in animal products) could at equivalent selenium intakes. Although almost all of serum and plasma selenium is protein-bound, most is present in two SeCys-proteins, GPX-3 of renal origin and SeP of hepatic origin, plus in more variable amounts (in Se-adequate individuals) of nonspecific SeMet-containing proteins such as albumin of hepatic origin.

Hill et al. (1996) calculated that maximal expression of these proteins contributed about 80 μg/L to plasma selenium, indicating that those parameters are useful only in populations with relatively low selenium intakes, a condition typical of few, if any, healthy Americans. Neve (1995) reviewed the results of several clinical trials and noted that subjects with plasma and serum selenium levels above 70 μg/L showed no further GPX responses to selenium supplementation. On the basis of these observations, the plasma and serum level of 80 μg/L would appear to be a useful criterion of nutritional adequacy.

## Selenium Intake Effects on Health and Performance

### *Selenium Deficiency Diseases in Humans*

Two diseases have been associated with severe endemic selenium deficiency in humans—a juvenile cardiomyopathy (Keshan disease) and a chondrodystrophy (Kaschin-Beck disease). Each disease occurs in rural areas of China and Russia (eastern Siberia) in food systems with exceedingly low selenium supplies (IOM, 2000).

Keshan disease is a multifocal myocarditis occurring primarily in children and, to a lesser extent, in women of child-bearing age (Keshan Disease Research Group, 1979; Xu et al., 1997). It is manifested as acute or chronic insufficiency of cardiac function, cardiac enlargement, arrhythmias, and electrocardiographic and radiographic abnormalities. Low selenium status is not a general feature of cardiomyopathy patients in most countries. Kashin-Beck disease is an osteoarthropathy affecting the epiphyseal and articular cartilage and the epiphyseal growth plates of growing bones. The disease is manifested as enlarged joints (especially of the fingers, toes, and knees); shortened fingers, toes, and extremities; and, in severe cases, dwarfism. The few studies on the effects of selenium supplementation in the prevention and therapy of Kashin-Beck disease have yielded encouraging results (Burk and Levander, 1999; IOM, 2000).

### *Infection and Immunity*

Several studies have demonstrated increased immune function in selenium-supplemented individuals or animals with marginal selenium status prior to the supplementation (Ferencik and Ebringer, 2003). This has been shown for asthmatics (Gazdik et al., 2002), cancer patients (Kiremidjian-Schumacher and Roy, 2001), and elderly patients (Lesourd, 1997). Animal models of selenium deficiency generally have shown a decrease in T-cell functioning, including a reduction in cytokine and chemokine production and a decrease in T-cell proliferation against mitogen and specific antigens. Humoral immune function does not appear to be impaired by a deficiency in selenium (Ferencik and Ebringer, 2003).

Patients with HIV and AIDS generally have lower circulating levels of selenium than healthy people. Taylor et al. (1997, 2000) proposed that this may reflect the extremely high turnover of CD4+ cells (billions of new cells are lost and replaced daily) that leads to progressive selenium depletion. Study findings that demonstrate decreased plasma or serum levels as a sensitive marker of disease progression indicate that selenium status may have a direct association to the HIV disease (Baum and Shor-Posner, 1998; Baum et al., 2000). In fact, the studies by Baum et al. (1997) and Campa et al. (1999) indicate that low plasma selenium level increases the relative risk of HIV-related mortality by nearly 20-fold and 6-fold respectively. Burbano et al. (2002) conducted a randomized, double-blind, placebo-controlled study of selenium therapy (200 μg/day) with 186 HIV-positive drug users. They found the selenium treatment group showed a marked decrease in hospital admission rates, particularly admissions due to infection. A nested study within that trial (Shor-Posner et al., 2003) found that selenium-treated subjects reported more vigor and less anxiety than the subjects in the placebo group.

Recent research in animal models has found that selenium deficiency results in increased viral mutation rates. A normally benign Coxsackievirus B3 infection of selenium-deficient mice (four weeks on a selenium-deficient diet resulting in a fivefold decrease in GPX levels) results in the development a severe cardiac disease. This change in viral virulence was due to mutations occurring in the genome of the virus, changing an avirulent virus into a virulent virus (Beck, 1997). Similarly, a mild strain of influenza virus becomes highly pathogenic in selenium-deficient mice due to changes in the influenza virus genome. Once these viral mutations occur, even mice with normal selenium status become susceptible to the newly virulent virus (Beck et al., 2003). In England, marginal selenium status in adults was associated with increased mutations in a poliovirus vaccine strain and decreased immune function, whereas supplementation with selenium resulted in improved immune functions (increased gamma interferon production, increased numbers of helper T-cells) and increased viral clearance (Broome et al., 2004; Jackson et al., 2004). Hence, a deficiency in selenium may lead to viral mutations in a number of viruses and provide a driving force for the emergence of new viral strains or old strains with new pathogenic potential. See also Sheridan and colleagues in Appendix B.

Studies on immune function with selenium supplementation generally have been confounded by the addition of other antioxidants to the supplement. In general, selenium supplementation of selenium-adequate animals has not resulted in enhanced immune function (Albers et al., 2003).

### *Cognitive Performance and Behavior*

It has been suggested that very low selenium intakes (< 40 μg/day) may impair mood states by causing subclinical thyroid hormone deficiency (Beckett et al., 1993, Sait Gonen et al., 2004), but this hypothesis has not been tested in low-selenium subjects. A recent supplementation trial evaluated the efficacy of a combined antioxidant supplement (vitamins E and C, β-carotene, selenium, and zinc) on parameters of oxidative stress in young men exposed to hyperbaric hypoxia and found no significant effects (Subudhi et al., 2004).

The role of selenium in cognitive function and behavior has received little attention, but available data suggest that increasing the selenium intakes of non-deficient individuals may benefit mood. It has been proposed that selenium-adequate individuals may respond to supplemental selenium through effects on dopamine turnover (Castano et al., 1997) or on brain levels of n-6/n-3 fatty acids (Clausen, 1991), or both; women with relatively low GPX-3 activities but apparently adequate selenium intakes have been found to have elevated fasting glucose and glucose intolerance (Hawkes et al., 2004), which has been associated with depression.

Several studies have shown effects of selenium supplementation on mood states in apparently selenium-adequate subjects. Benton and Cook (1991) randomized 50 men and women to 100 μg/day of selenium or to a placebo for five weeks, in a double-blind crossover design with a six-month washout period between treatments. Use of the supplement was associated with less anxiety, less depression, and more energy as reported on POMS-BI. One laboratory (Finley and Penland, 1998; Penland and Finley, 1995) randomized 30 healthy men consuming for 15 weeks mixed diets that contained either 30 or 230 μg/day of selenium. Men fed the high-selenium diet reported less confusion and depression on the POMS-BI over the course of the study. Although dietary effects were apparent for all mood states, high variability made this apparent difference highly questionable. Within the group fed low selenium, platelet GPX-1 activity was significantly correlated with all six mood states; higher activity was associated with more positive mood states.

Hawkes and Hornbostel (1996) fed 11 healthy men living in a metabolic research unit either 13 or 356 μg/day of selenium for 99 days. They found selenium intakes to be unrelated to mood states as assessed by the POMS-BI; however, they noted a significant positive relationship between erythrocyte selenium concentration and elated (versus depressed) and agreeable (versus hostile) mood states in the low-selenium group.

More recently, Penland et al. (in press) studied 51 male and female New Zealanders with the low selenium intakes typical of their native country. The subjects were randomized to supplements of 0, 10, 20, 30, or 40 μg/day of for a six-month period. As the study progressed, the 33 females showed increased agreeableness, confidence, and energy and fewer total mood disturbances as assessed by the POMS-BI. In contrast, the males showed no dietary effects on mood states, but the sample size (18) was insufficient to yield acceptable statistical power.

*Physical Performance*

There have been no studies of the effects of selenium deprivation on physical performance; however, it is expected that vigorous physical activity may enhance selenium needs, particularly in individuals with low protein intakes. Because much of the body's selenium is present as SeMet nonspecifically incorporated into various proteins, it can be expected that factors affecting protein turnover will enhance the mobilization of selenium from these stores and that the turnover of SeMet through the general protein pool will be affected by the level of methionine intake. Thus, it can be expected that periods of methionine-undernourishment may serve to increase SeMet uptake into proteins, reducing its availability for incorporation into the functional selenoproteins, and that diets providing ample amounts of methionine may serve to enhance the losses of methylated selenium metabolites under conditions of protein catabolism. This prospect has not been investigated.

There have been no studies addressing the effects of supranutritional selenium supplementation on human physical performance; however, the known biology of selenium offers no reason to expect such an effect.

## Risk Factors for Inadequacy During Military Garrison Training

### *Dietary Intakes*

The median dietary intake of selenium was 154 μg/day for 19–30-year-old males, and the 95th percentile of dietary intake was 231 μg/day. The median intake of selenium of 19–30-year-old females was 99 μg/day, and the 95th percentile of dietary intake was 159 μg/day (NHANES III, IOM, 2000). These intakes meet the required levels for the U.S. population. There are no data on selenium intakes of military personnel. These data should be collected to ensure that intake levels are appropriate. As with other minerals, meeting adequate selenium levels in rations does not always ensure that the actual intake meets the nutrient requirements.

### *Selenium Loss*

Selenium is excreted from the body after conversion to a number of methylated metabolites (see Figure 3-3). These include methylselenol, dimethylselenide (which is excreted across the lung), selenium sugars (1β-methylseleno-N-acetyl-D-galactosamine] and its deacylated analogue comprising as much as 80 percent of human urinary selenium [Kobayashi et al., 2002; Kuehnelt et al., 2005]), and trimethylselenonium (which is excreted across the kidney). Selenium also is excreted through feces, hair, and nails.

Changes in dietary intake affect the amount of selenium excreted, with high-selenium diets increasing excretion and low-selenium diets decreasing excretion (Hawkes et al., 2003; Srikumar et al., 1992). A Swedish cohort of nine men and women consuming 36 μg/10 MJ of selenium was shifted from a mixed diet to a lacto-vegetarian one that provided only 60 percent as much selenium (20–23 μg/

10 MJ of selenium) (Srikumar et al., 1992). This dietary shift resulted in an 19-percent decrease in plasma selenium concentration (from 73 to 59 μg/L) over 12 months. Within three months, comparable decreases were observed in urinary selenium (21 percent, from 19 to 15 μg/day), fecal selenium (35 percent, from 26 to 17 μg/day), and hair selenium (22 percent, from 5.3 to 4.1 μg/g).

Hawkes et al. (2003) studied the effects of changing dietary selenium intakes on the excretion of selenium by 12 subjects whose baseline selenium status (plasma selenium = 113 μg/L) reflected the higher dietary selenium intake typical of the U.S. population. Subjects randomized to a low-selenium diet (14 μg/day) for 99 days showed decreases in plasma selenium (–34 percent, from 118 to 78 μg/L) accompanied by marked reductions in selenium losses in the urine (–55 percent, from 33.0 to 14.9 μg/day), and feces (–49 percent, from 17.5 to 8.9 μg/day). In contrast, subjects randomized to a high-selenium diet (297 μg/day) for the same time period showed increases in plasma selenium (+91 percent, from 107 to 204 μg/L) accompanied by high increases in the selenium contents of the urine (+307 percent, from 28 to 114 μg/day) and feces (+290 percent, from 18.7 to 73 μg/day). Hair selenium proved less responsive to these dietary changes, showing a marked reduction (–43 percent, from 0.56 to 0.32 μg/g) in response to the low-selenium diet but only a modest increase (+14 percent, from 0.79 to 0.90 μg/g) in response to the high-selenium diet. Although it did not cause an apparent problem in either of these studies, some shampoos contain selenium sulfide as an antidandruff agent. Therefore, depending on shampoo selection, hair selenium content may not always reflect integumentary selenium content. An earlier study by Levander et al. (1981) measured urinary, plasma, and sweat selenium levels in 6 subjects after 45 days on a low-selenium diet (about 20 μg/day) and then after another 25 days on a high-selenium diet (approximately 200 μg/day). Results from this study are in agreement with the dietary effects seen in urine and plasma in the 2003 study above. It appeared that increasing selenium intake had no effect on sweat losses; however, conclusions on effects selenium dietary levels on sweat losses are not conclusive since sweat rates were not reported and, moreover, there were no details on the method of sweat collection.

Only two studies have reported selenium excretion measurements during periods of exercise and prolonged physical stress. The only report of sweat selenium concentrations is that by Consolazio et al. (1964), who measured sweat selenium loss in three men during 7.5-hour exposures in a hot environment (37.8°C) that included 30 minutes of moderate exercise for 16 days. The reported sweat selenium losses averaged 0.37 mg/day during days 5–8, 0.34 mg/day during days 9–12, and 0.30 mg/day during days 13–16. These results, which would suggest sweat losses equivalent to more than five times the DRI, must be considered highly questionable as the analyses were done by a method that was not standard for the time (emission spectroscopy) and no quality control data were presented.

*Stress and Physical Performance*

Plasma selenium concentrations seem to decrease, at least transiently, in response to stress. Singh et al. (1991) studied 66 Navy SEALS before and immediately after five days of Hell Week, which included substantial physical and psychological stress. Although dietary selenium intake increased by 50 percent during Hell Week (from 61.5 ± 5.9 μg/day to 92.5 ± 26.7 μg/day, reflecting an increased protein intake during that time), plasma selenium decreased 12 percent (from 129 ± 4 μg/L to 113 ± 5 μg/L) immediately after Hell Week but returned to pre-Hell Week levels within seven days. Urinary selenium loss did not change (before: 106 ± 23 μg/day versus after: 111 ± 14 μg/day). Singh et al. (1991) suggested that the change in plasma selenium was an acute phase response to tissue damage and the inflammatory effect of prolonged physical exertion.

It is reasonable to suggest that low selenium status may compromise physiological function under conditions of oxidative stress, as several SeCys-containing enzymes are involved directly in the antioxidant–antinitrosant defense systems. The GPXs catalyze the reduction of $H_2O_2$ and organic hydroperoxides (Arthur, 2000), and the TRs maintain a favorable redox balance of two important redox factors—ascorbate (May et al., 1997) and thioredoxin (Powis et al., 1997). The GPXs as well as the TRs also participate in the reduction of peroxynitrate ($ONOO^-$) and prevent a number of oxidation and nitration reactions (Arteel et al., 1999; Briviba et al., 1998; Sies et al., 1997). In addition to its role in the direct elimination of reactive oxygen species (ROS) and reactive nitrogen species (RNS), selenium also can regulate oxidative stress-mediated cell signaling. Treatment of cultured cells with selenium has been shown to inhibit nuclear factor (NF)-κB (a eukaryotic transcription factor) activation and NF-κB-dependent gene expression induced by oxidants or pro-inflammatory cytokines (Makropoulos et al., 1996; Tolando et al., 2000). Selenium deprivation sufficient to decrease GPX and TR expression, therefore, can impair the protective capacity of the antioxidant defense systems resulting in increased sensitivity to ROS and RNS. The consequences of this hypothesis on physical performance are unknown.

## Requirements for the General U.S. Population

The current IOM RDA for selenium, 55 μg/day for both males and female adults (IOM, 2000), is based on two studies, one conducted on young Chinese men (Yang et al., 1987) and one on New Zealand adult men and women (Duffield et al., 1999). Yang et al. (1987) found that providing a selenium supplement of 30 μg/day to subjects with a dietary selenium intake of 11 μg/day seemed to support maximal activities of GPX-3 in plasma. Duffield et al. (1999) found that providing a selenium supplement averaging 15 μg/day to subjects with a dietary selenium intake of 28 μg/day seemed to support maximal activities of GPX activities. In a more recent study that evaluated GPX-3 and SeP in a low-selenium diet that provided 10 μg/day, a Chinese cohort found that a selenium supplement of 37 μg/day as SeMet supported optimal GPX-3 activities; however, within the 20 weeks of observation SeP was not optimized even at a supplemental level of 61 μg of selenium as SeMet (Xia et al., 2005). While 6–9 months are required for the establishment of a new equilibrium of plasma selenium level after the commencement of selenium supplementation (Combs et al., 2005), these results suggest that more selenium may be required to support the maximal expression of other selenoproteins, for which SeP may be a proxy.

### Daily Intake Recommendations for Military Personnel in Garrison Training

The committee does not recommend any change to the current MDRIs of 55 μg/day for females and males (see Table 3-1). There is no strong evidence of substantial losses or that an increase intake of selenium will impart any benefit to military personnel in garrison training. However, as there appears to be no data on selenium intake in the field or in garrison training, it is necessary to collect food intake data (intake under garrison training conditions) to assess if these intake levels are reached.

**RECOMMENDATIONS FOR SELENIUM INTAKE:**

| | |
|---|---|
| **$EAR_{MGT}$ for men** | **45 μg/day** |
| **$EAR_{MGT}$ for women** | **45 μg/day** |
| **$RDA_{MGT}$ for men** | **55 μg/day** |
| **$RDA_{MGT}$ for women** | **55 μg/day** |

### Adequacy of Selenium MDRIs and Selenium Levels in Rations

As mentioned above, the recent finding that daily selenium intakes of 61 μg (as SeMet) were insufficient to support maximal SeP levels (Xia et al., 2005), raises questions about the adequacy of the MRDI level to support overall selenoprotein expression. That question would take on greater relevance under environmental or physical performance conditions that might substantially increase excretory losses. Unfortunately, available data are insufficient to address the question, making the current MDRI a reasonable working value.

Estimates of the selenium content in MREs have been made from the U.S. Department of Agriculture National Nutrient Database for Standard Reference and mineral content summaries of the MRE menus (See http://www.nal.usda.gov/fnic/foodcomp/search/). Because of the known variation in the selenium contents of many core foods, particularly grain products, such estimates must be viewed with some reservation. With that caveat, the MREs would appear to average only 7.8-12.5 μg of selenium per meal (see Table 3-1; Tables C-2 through C-5 in

Appendix C), which is at most only 66 percent of the NSOR (see Table 3-1). The variability (range of estimates = 0.12–38 μg of selenium or approximately 1–169 percent of NSOR) suggests that a number of menus do not meet the NSOR. Determining whether this is truly the case will require actual analysis of those rations for selenium.

Although apparently low in selenium, there is no evidence to suggest that the use of such rations is likely to have physiological impact, particularly in the context of personnel having periodic access to higher selenium meals or dietary supplements of selenium, or both, and presuming that the personnel are not of marginal selenium status. The latter may not always be the case. Nicklas et al. (1993) found that less than 20 percent of military wives consumed selenium at the IOM RDA, suggesting that the self-selected diets of at least some military personnel may be low in selenium.

As with MREs, the selenium contents of FSRs have been estimated from data in the U.S. Department of Agriculture National Nutrient Database for Standard Reference; due to the variability of as much as an order of magnitude according to the selenium content and availability of the soils in which those foods were grown, these values should be considered gross estimates. With that caveat, estimated selenium contents of three FSRs averaging 100 μg per meal (see Table C-6 in Appendix C; range: 63–160 μg of selenium per meal) are well above the recommended 55–230 μg of selenium for FSRs (See Table C-1 in Appendix C). On the basis of this limited evidence, it would appear that FSRs are likely to provide ample selenium.

### Adequacy of IOM Recommendations for First Strike Rations

IOM's report on FSRs (i.e., assault rations) (IOM, 2006) recommended including 55–230 μg/day of selenium in the rations based on the IOM RDA and on the 95th percentile intake (see Table 3-1). Based on a lack of evidence to increase the intake for soldiers engaging in combat, this committee agrees with the recommended selenium range for FSRs until more information becomes available.

### Strategies for Achieving Sufficient Selenium Intake

*Usual Foods*

In most diets, the primary sources of selenium are cereals, meats, and fish; 22 foods provide 80 percent of the total selenium in the American diet, with five (beef, white bread, pork, chicken, and eggs) providing 50 percent of the total selenium in the diet (Schubert et al., 1987). However, the selenium content of foods varies (NRC, 1983). Plant foods vary according to the location of their production, as the selenium contents of their tissues are related directly to the selenium content of the soil in which they were produced. For this reason, the selenium content of American wheat can vary from 0.1 to 3 ppm. Few other foods naturally contain high amounts of selenium, although one example is Brazilian nuts, which can contain selenium in amounts as much as 16.5 ppm (Schubert et al., 1987). Therefore, strategies to increase selenium intakes would address wheat grown in the Northern Plains and meats from selenium-fed livestock (poultry, pork, and beef).

There is a paucity of information concerning the chemical forms of selenium in plant and animal tissues. Because plants cannot synthesize SeCys, it is generally believed that SeMet is the predominant form of the element in plant tissues, where it acts as a methionine mimic in general protein metabolism. This is not the case for animals, which can produce SeCys from $H_2Se$ in the synthesis of selenoenzymes (NRC, 1983). Therefore, the tissues of selenium-fed animals and humans typically contain SeCys from selenoproteins as well as SeMet derived from the diet and used nonspecifically in general protein synthesis. Plant tissues also can contain smaller amounts of certain other selenium metabolites, including selenium-methylselenomethionine, selenium-methylselenocysteine, and low amounts of a number of unidentified selenium metabolites.

### *Food Fortification*

In Finland, selenium is added to agricultural fertilizers as a strategy to increase the selenium contents of foods and, ultimately, of Finnish consumers. This program, which was implemented 20 years ago, has been effective in doubling mean plasma selenium levels of the Finnish population (Aro et al., 1995).

Selenium has not been used widely as a food or water fortificant, although some selenium-fortified products have been developed in China. It is possible to fortify foods with selenium in several ways—by adding inorganic selenium salts (selenate, selenite) to foods and bottled water, by adding selenium-enriched yeasts to foods, and by using food ingredients (e.g., wheat, oats, beans, buckwheat, and mustard) produced in and distributed from high-selenium production areas.

### *Supplementation*

Nutritional supplements containing selenium are currently available on the U.S. market. These include products made using high-selenium bakers' yeast (*Saccharomyces cerevisiae*)—a cultured product typically containing 1,200 ppm selenium mostly in the form of L-selenomethionine—marketed under proprietary labels and containing 50–200 μg of elemental selenium per dose (Hendler and Rorvik, 2001). There is no standard of product identity for high-selenium yeasts, however, such products have been found to be effective in increasing selenium status as measured by plasma selenium concentration in both humans and animals. It is possible to use specific selenium compounds in supplementation. L-selenomethionine is currently in use in clinical intervention trials, and selenite and selenate have been used in multivitamin–mineral supplements. Such supplements should be relatively well (50–90 percent) utilized as sources of selenium.

Selenium can be toxic in high doses, but since the difference between the IOM RDA and the UL is large, toxicity is not likely to originate from supplementation. When blood selenium concentrations exceed 12.3 μmol/L (IOM, 2000), humans show signs that include the following: gastrointestinal upset, hair loss, blotched nails, garlicky breath odor, fatigue, and irritability. Only a few cases of selenosis due to oral exposure have been reported in the United States; each one has involved misuse (accidental or intentional) of a selenium-rich product (e.g., gun bluing and antidandruff shampoo) or purified selenium compound. Chronic selenosis of dietary origin was identified in the 1960s among residents of Enshi County, Hubei Province, China, and apparently resulted from exceedingly high concentrations of selenium in the local food supplies and, in fact, throughout the local environment (Yang et al., 1989a, b). The IOM (2000), WHO (1996), and Yang et al. (1989a) set the upper safety limit of selenium intake at 400 μg/day for an adult. A review by the U.S. Environmental Protection Agency (Poirier, 1994) set a no-adverse-effect selenium level for adults of 853 μg/day.

## Recommendations for Achieving Sufficiency

In the absence of data describing the selenium status of military personnel, the use of selenium-containing supplements, and the actual selenium contents of field and garrison meals, it is impossible to determine the benefits and risks of available strategies for increasing selenium intakes. Nevertheless, the estimated selenium contents of MREs suggest that MRDI levels may not be met consistently. Thus, it may be prudent to increase the selenium contents of many of these rations, particularly if actual analyses confirm the current estimates and if the personnel for whom they are intended include appreciable numbers of low or marginal (< 80 μg /L of plasma) selenium status.

## Research Needs

### *Specific Priorities*

- Quantify selenium losses due to the stressful conditions of garrison training (i.e., heat, physical exertion, and psychological stressors).
- Determine whether selenium supplementation (of 200 μg/day) of non-deficient subjects improves immune function.
- Determine the actual selenium contents of MREs and FSRs as well as the selenium intake, including the frequency of use of supplements containing appreciable amounts (> 50 μg/day) by military personnel.

- Determine whether increasing selenium intake with a supplementation of 200 μg/day will benefit military personnel's mood states, especially depression.

*Other Research Needs*

- Screen major water sources for selenium content.

## ZINC RECOMMENDATIONS

Zinc is an essential nutrient ubiquitously distributed in the body; it serves a variety of catalytic, structural, and regulatory functions. More than 100 enzymes depend on zinc, an electron acceptor, for activity. Severe zinc deficiency results in depressed growth, immune dysfunction, diarrhea, altered cognition, and reduced appetite. Evaluating the possible effects of marginal deficiencies is difficult since sensitive biochemical criteria for detecting marginal zinc status have not been established. Changes in serum zinc are insensitive and may reflect a temporary redistribution of body pools.

*Absorption and Metabolism*

Both zinc absorption and excretion adapt to control total body zinc in animals with zinc intakes from marginal to luxuriant (Hunt et al., 1987; IOM, 2001; Weigand and Kirchgessner, 1976a, b). The vast majority of zinc is absorbed by the small intestine through a transcellular process with the jejunum probably being the site with the greatest transport rate (Cousins, 1989; Lee et al., 1989; Lonnerdal, 1989). Zinc transporters (ZnT) regulate the membrane transfer of zinc to maintain cellular function. ZnT-1 and ZnT-2 are two such transporters expressed in the small intestine that are regulated by zinc intake. Humans absorb zinc more efficiently when dietary zinc is low (Lee et al., 1993; Taylor et al., 1991; Wada et al., 1985), but this at least partly reflects the immediate effect of the amount ingested, rather than a long-term adaptation to changed zinc intake (Sandstrom and Cederblad, 1980; Sandstrom et al., 1980), and suggests saturation kinetics. As more zinc is ingested, absorptive efficiency decreases considerably, but the absolute amount absorbed increases.

Homeostatic regulation of zinc metabolism occurs through control of excretion as well as of absorption. Endogenous zinc is excreted primarily in the feces, derived from both pancreatic and intestinal cell secretions. Isotopic tracers can be used to measure endogenous zinc excretion and correct for it to measure true absorption (Taylor et al., 1991).

More than 85 percent of total body zinc is found in skeletal muscle and bone (King and Keen, 1999). Plasma zinc represents only 0.1 percent of total body zinc, and its concentration is tightly maintained at about 10–15 μmol/L without notable change when zinc intake is restricted or increased, unless the changes in intake are severe and prolonged. Plasma zinc consequently provides only an insensitive index of zinc status.

Although knowledge of the numerous biochemical and molecular roles of zinc has been developed extensively, mechanistic explanations for the nutritional functions revealed by severe zinc deficiency—evidenced by depressed growth, immune dysfunction, diarrhea, or altered cognition—have not been established conclusively. A factorial calculation that quantifies normal zinc losses and applies knowledge of the efficiency of zinc absorption from common Western diets is used as the basis to estimate zinc requirements because established functional or biochemical markers for the nutritional adequacy of zinc do not exist.

## Zinc Intake Effects on Health and Performance

### *Physical Performance*

Two reports describe impaired physical performance of research subjects who were fed zinc-depleted diets for several weeks. Men who consumed controlled diets containing 3.7 versus 18.7 mg/day of zinc (supplemented with zinc sulfate) for nine weeks had decreased oxygen consumption and respiratory exchange ratios under peak and submaximal exercise conditions (Lukaski, 2005). Total muscular work capacity, but not peak muscular force, was impaired in men who consumed controlled diets containing 0.3 versus 12 mg/day of zinc (supplemented with zinc sulfate) for 33–41 days (Van Loan et al., 1999). Although these studies suggest the need for adequate zinc intake to support physical performance, the extended low-zinc diets of these depletion studies may not apply to military personnel for extended time periods outside of a research setting.

A limited number of studies have evaluated the effects of zinc supplementation, alone or in combination with other nutrients, on physical performance. Zinc supplements in doses substantially greater than the IOM RDA or UL (135 mg/day for 14 days; the supplement form was not specified) improved dynamic isokinetic strength in a randomized, placebo-controlled, cross-over trial with adult women (Krotkiewski et al., 1982). More moderate supplemental doses, 5–25 mg/day of zinc provided as part of vitamin and mineral supplements, did not affect the blood zinc concentrations (Singh et al., 1992; Telford et al., 1992b; Weight et al., 1988b) or the performance (Telford et al., 1992a; Weight et al., 1988a) of active males or of male and female athletes. Results from a double-blinded, placebo-controlled that examined supplementation with 25 mg of zinc (as zinc picolinate) and 1.5 mg of copper (as copper sulfate) taken twice daily for six days before testing treadmill run time to exhaustion did not show an enhancement of the exercise performance of five male runners (Singh et al., 1994). Similar negative results were obtained with 10 trained female runners given the same supplement for four days (Singh et al., 1999).

Two studies of zinc supplementation and the oxidative stress associated with physical exertion have yielded mixed results. In the previous Singh et al. study of five male runners (1994), supplementation with 25 mg of zinc (as zinc picolinate) and 1.5 mg of copper (as copper sulfate) blocked an exercise-induced increase in neutrophil production of superoxide anion (when exposed to opsonized zymosan) in vitro, a possible indicator of respiratory burst activity. In contrast, Subudhi et al. (2004) found no effect of antioxidant supplementation on measures of oxidative stress with exercise under conditions of high altitude and negative energy balance in 18 physically-fit, healthy men. In that placebo-controlled trial, supplemental zinc (30 mg/day, in addition to the 11 mg/day from the diet at high altitude)—in addition to β-carotene, α-tocopherol, ascorbic acid, and selenium—was consumed for three weeks before, as well as throughout, a 14-day, high-altitude (4,300 meters) intervention characterized by increased energy expenditure (~40 percent), decreased energy intake (3,357 versus 4,270 kcal/day at sea level), and negative energy balance (~1,400 kcal/day). Testing conditions included standardized, prolonged, submaximal exercise as well as peak aerobic power. Supplementation did not significantly reduce oxidative stress under these conditions, as measured with markers of lipid peroxidation and DNA damage.

In conclusion, there is no clear evidence that moderate increases in zinc intake (5–30 mg/day), in addition to amounts commonly consumed, will improve physical performance or reduce the oxidative stress associated with exercise (See also Montain and Young, 2003).

### *Cognition and Behavior*

No studies have investigated directly the relationship between zinc intake or status and cognitive function or behavior in soldiers. Most studies relating zinc intake or status to cognitive function and behavior have been conducted in infants and children. Penland (2005; see Penland in Appendix B) has summarized the research related to this topic. There are no peer-reviewed, controlled-intervention trials providing evidence that soldiers in garrison conditions have zinc requirements different than those already established for healthy adults.

### *Immunity and Infection*

The importance of zinc nutrition for immune function has been emphasized in studies of diarrhea and respiratory morbidity in children in developing countries. In a three-month prospective study of New Delhi children who recently recovered from nondysenteric diarrhea, those with low plasma zinc (≤ 8.4 μmol/L) had a greater risk of diarrhea (Bahl et al., 1998). Zinc supplementation (in many forms, including acetate, gluconate, and sulfate) protects at-risk children in developing countries against diarrheal disease, acute lower respiratory infection, and possibly malaria (Black, 1998; Hamer, 2005; see Hamer in Appendix B). There are no data to suggest that increasing the zinc intake of adults from Western countries would be protective or therapeutic for diarrheal, respiratory, or malarial conditions.

Zinc supplements have been evaluated extensively for treatment of the common cold. In a double-blind, placebo-controlled trial, treatment of the common cold with lozenges containing 12.8 mg of zinc acetate, taken every 2–3 hours that subjects were awake, reduced the duration of cold symptoms from 8.1 to 4.5 days (Prasad et al., 2000). A meta-analysis of eight studies found no consistent effect of zinc supplements (zinc gluconate) on cold signs or symptoms at seven days, and concluded that there is not clear evidence that zinc lozenges reduce the duration of the common cold (Jackson et al., 2000).

Studies of zinc supplementation and immune function in elderly subjects have produced a mix of negative, beneficial, and adverse effects (Bogden et al., 1988, 1990). For example, in elderly subjects receiving additional nutrient supplements, 15 or 100 mg/day of zinc (as zinc acetate) suppressed an improvement in delayed skin hypersensitivity that was observed in the elderly subjects who took the placebo (Bogden et al., 1990). Those subjects who took a zinc supplement of 100 mg had a transient improvement in natural killer cell activity. Supplementation with 150 mg of zinc (as zinc sulfate), taken twice daily, adversely affected several measures of immune function in healthy adults (Chandra, 1984). These studies suggest that excessive zinc intake may impair the immune response.

Zinc-restricted controlled diets (4.6 mg/day for 10 weeks compared with 9.1 mg/day during a five-week baseline or a five-week repletion) had a minimal effect on several indices of immune function in eight healthy men (Pinna et al., 2002). There is no current evidence that altering the dietary zinc intake of military troops would benefit immune function.

### *Recovery from Bone or Muscle Injury*

Zinc deficiency in experimental animals and in humans who rely on total parenteral nutrition has shown that zinc has a role in wound healing. The mechanisms for this role have not been elucidated clearly and may include biochemical functions of zinc such as metallothionein induction, superoxide dysmutatase activity, or influence on cytokines and growth factors (Cannon, 2005; see Cannon in Appendix B). A review of several small studies on the benefits of zinc supplementation for the healing of arterial or venous leg ulcers concluded that there is no evidence that oral zinc supplementation is generally useful for healing these ulcers and that there is weak evidence of benefit for people with venous leg ulcers and low serum zinc (Wilkinson and Hawke, 1998a, b).

## Risk Factors for Inadequacy During Military Garrison Training

*Dietary Intakes*

The median intake and the 95th percentile intake in healthy 19–30-year-old American men are 14.8 and 23.9 mg/day, respectively. For women, the median intake and the 95th percentile intake are 9.2 and 14.9 mg/day, respectively (IOM, 2001). It appears, therefore, that the majority of the population meets the required zinc levels (11 mg and 8 mg/day for men and women, respectively) (IOM, 2001). Broad surveys of military personnel's intake levels are not available except for a few studies.

A study by Thomas et al. (1995) assessed the nutritional intake of soldiers in a field environment during 30 days when they were provided with either three MREs or two ration-A meals and one MRE. The MRE group ate less, with mineral intakes lower than the MDRI for various minerals, including the 9.3 mg/day intake for zinc. Zinc serum was not measured.

Gender differences regarding energy and nutrient intake where examined during an 11-day field-training exercise (Baker-Fulco et al., 2002). A larger proportion of women did not meet the intake standards for several nutrients, among them zinc. However, when body weight was accounted for, those gender differences were mostly eliminated.

From the few studies described, it can be inferred that the zinc intake of soldiers might be marginally compromised, especially if needs are higher due to sweat losses. More studies (ideally ones that would assess men and women separately) are needed to evaluate nutrient intakes.

*Bioavailability*

Several dietary factors may influence humans' zinc absorption (Hunt, 2005; Lonnerdal, 2000; see Hunt in Appendix B; see also the following section on *Strategies for Achieving Sufficient Zinc Intake*); some of the most important factors are the amount of zinc consumed and the phytate-to-zinc molar ratio. Other factors that affect bioavailability are proteins and amino acids (enhancing effect), and calcium, iron, and copper (inhibiting effects). Absorption rates decrease with higher intake levels of zinc. People who consume vegetarian diets, especially diets with phytate:zinc molar ratios exceeding 15, may require 20–50 percent more zinc than people who consume nonvegetarian diets (Hunt, 2003a; IOM, 2001).

*Sweat Losses*

The IOM DRI factorial derivation of the EAR for zinc estimates zinc losses from skin, including integumental and sweat losses, as 0.54 mg/day for men and

0.46 mg/day for women (IOM, 2001; Johnson et al., 1993). Under controlled diet conditions, sweat and integumental losses of zinc were reduced with a low-zinc intake (< 4 mg/day) but changed little with intakes of 8 mg/day versus 34 mg/day (Milne et al., 1983). Skin-sweat losses of zinc were regarded as constant over a broad range of zinc intakes in deriving the IOM EAR (IOM, 2001; Johnson et al., 1993).

It is difficult to measure accurately whole-body sweat losses during exercise since the measurement conditions (e.g., use of full-body absorbent suits) can influence the results. Sweat losses during exercise are usually based on measurement of sweat mineral concentrations at regional sites, but this use of regional sweat measurements overestimates whole-body losses (Jacob et al., 1981; Palacios et al., 2003; see Haymes in Appendix B).

Exercise results in a greater loss of zinc through the sweat. Consolazio et al. (1964) found very high sweat zinc losses in men during the first four days of heat exposure (37.8°C) for 7.5 hours per day, which included a daily 30-minute period of moderate exercise. Mean sweat zinc loss was 13.7 mg/day or 1.83 mg/hour. Sweat zinc losses were much lower during days 5–12, ranging from 2.16 to 2.41 mg/day (0.29–0.32 mg/hour), which suggests that heat acclimatization may reduce sweat zinc losses. Tipton et al. (1993) measured sweat zinc loss in men and women during one hour of exercise in neutral (25°C) and hot (35°C) temperatures. The rate of sweat zinc loss for men was 0.65 mg/hour and for women was 0.39 mg/hour. Another study required men and women to exercise for two hours at 23°C; estimated whole-body sweat zinc loss for men was 0.50 mg/hour and for women was 0.33 mg/hour (DeRuisseau et al., 2002). Sweat zinc concentration was significantly lower during the second hour of exercise. The rate of zinc loss in the second hour for the men was 0.46 mg/hour and for the women was 0.29 mg/hour (DeRuisseau et al., 2002). Using the mean zinc loss for the second hour, estimated daily zinc loss through sweating for eight hours would be 3.68 mg/day for men and 2.34 mg/day for women.

Research is needed to determine if sweat zinc loss decreases over time during exercise lasting more than two hours. There are no data on possible adaptive reductions in such losses beyond 16 days (Consolazio et al., 1964), or on possible adaptive increases in zinc absorptive efficiency and decreases in endogenous fecal excretion in response to such losses. Table 3-11 summarizes these studies.

### *Other Losses*

Average urinary zinc excretion is estimated at 0.63 mg/day for men and 0.44 mg/day for women (IOM, 2001). Although urinary zinc increases with zinc intake (Johnson et al., 1993), urine is a minor route for zinc excretion, and requirement estimates are based on the conclusion that urinary zinc is not substantially affected by a broad range of zinc intakes (4 to 25 mg/day) (IOM, 2001).

**TABLE 3-11** Zinc Sweat Losses

| Subjects | Comments | Zinc Analysis | Sweat Collection | Sweat Loss | Reference |
|---|---|---|---|---|---|
| 11 males | Healthy volunteers; 48 hours; sedentary | Inductively coupled argon plasma spectroscopy | Whole body surface | 0.54 mg/day | IOM, 2001; Johnson et al., 1993; |
| 13 males | Healthy volunteers | Atomic absorption spectrophotometer | Whole body surface | 0.50 mg/day | Jacob et al., 1981 |
| 3 males | Exercise in the heat for 7.5 hours/day | Emission spectrograph | Arm bag over three, 4-day trials | 13.7 mg/day first 4 days decreased to 2 mg/day on days 5–12 | Consolazio et al., 1964 |
| 12 males | 30–40 minutes of exercise | Atomic absorption spectrophotometer | Arm<br>Back<br>Chest<br>Abdomen | 0.44 mg/L<br>0.48 mg/L<br>0.42 mg/L<br>0.83 mg/L | Aruoma et al., 1988 |
| 9 males<br>9 females | 120 minutes of exercise | Atomic absorption spectrophotometer | Arm bag | 0.46 mg/hour for men; 0.29 for women for second hour | DeRuisseau et al., 2002 |
| 9 males<br>9 females | 60 minutes of exercise in 30°C | Atomic absorption spectrophotometer | Arm bag | Male: 0.65 mg/hour<br>Female: 0.39 mg/hour | Tipton et al., 1993 |

Data on urinary zinc excretion with exercise are inconsistent. Urinary zinc increased (from 0.4 to 0.7 mg/day) as serum zinc decreased within a normal range (from 114 to 100 μg/dL) during a 34-day training exercise, however the baseline urinary samples were obtained before the training exercise, when zinc intake was likely lower (Miyamura et al., 1987). Urinary zinc excretion of trained distance runners elevated during the 24 hours after a six-mile run, from 0.5 mg/day compared with 0.7 mg/day on a nonrun day (Anderson et al., 1984). However, the same authors later published that, under controlled-diet conditions, urinary zinc did not change significantly with acute strenuous exercise of short duration (30 seconds) independent of training status for moderately trained and untrained men (Anderson et al., 1995). Van Rij et al. (1986) found increased urinary zinc excretion two hours following a 10-mile road race (0.061 mg/hour) as compared with the excretion before the race (0.036 mg/hour), however, total urinary zinc excretion postrace (0.95 mg/day) was not significantly different from the prerace excretion (0.86 mg/day). Men's urinary zinc losses during 16 days of heat exposure and exercise ranged between 0.57 and 0.75 mg/day (Consolazio et al., 1964). Together, these data do not indicate clearly that there is a relationship between exercise and an increase in urinary zinc. Any such increase appears to be limited to 0–0.3 mg/day.

Fecal zinc excretion is correlated positively with the amount of zinc absorbed (IOM, 2001). Body zinc retention is controlled through regulation of absorption and of intestinal excretion. Intestinal zinc losses are increased in young children with diarrhea (Castillo-Duran et al., 1988; Ruz and Solomons, 1990) and in adult patients with gastrointestinal disorders (Wolman et al., 1979), but chronic diarrhea is not likely to influence zinc requirements of healthy troops.

### *Impact of Weight Loss on Zinc Requirements*

As with the nonmilitary population, people on low-energy diets for weight loss may need to meet their micronutrient requirements by using supplements. There is little evidence that weight loss changes zinc requirements.

## Daily Intake Recommendations for Military Personnel in Garrison Training

The IOM EAR for zinc—9.4 mg/day for men and 6.8 mg/day for women, both reflecting the 19 and older age range—was based on a factorial calculation of the dietary zinc needed to replace measured endogenous losses (IOM, 2001). Using an assumed coefficient of variation (CV) of 10 percent (based on variation in basal metabolic rates), the IOM RDA to meet the requirement of 97.5 percent of the population has been set at 11 mg/day for men and 8 mg/day for women (see Table 3-1). The IOM UL was established at 40 mg/day for men as well as for women and was based on the possible adverse effects of supplemental zinc on copper status.

With limited available data, and with conservative judgment in favor of substantial rather than marginal zinc intake, the estimated requirement for garrison training ($EAR_{MGT}$) is increased based on increased zinc losses through sweat. Because there are no data on possible adaptation in such losses beyond 16 days (Consolazio et al., 1964) or on adaptive absorption or intestinal excretion changes in response to such losses, this estimate is highly uncertain. The 2001 IOM EAR was based on endogenous zinc losses of 0.54 mg/day (for men) from combined integumental and sweat losses (IOM, 2001). For garrison training, the recommendation is increased based on replacement of additional sweat losses of 2.0 mg/day of for men and 1.3 mg/day of for women (due to lower sweat loss). This is based on the data of Consolazio et al. (1964) at days 5–12 of testing and on the relative differences observed by DeRuisseau et al. (2002) between men and women during the second hour of exercise. Under these conditions of an increased requirement, it is estimated that zinc may be absorbed more efficiently or retained, or both (King et al., 2000; Taylor et al., 1991; Wada et al., 1985), and an absorptive efficiency of 60 percent is estimated to replace these increased zinc losses. Accordingly, the recommendations for garrison training conditions are based on the existing EARs for men and women, plus 2.0/0.60, or 3.3 mg for men and 1.3/0.60, or 2.2 mg for women. Studies indicate no effect of zinc supplementation on physical performance and therefore, no additional zinc supplementation to improve physical performance was recommended. The RDA for garrison training ($RDA_{MGT}$) is set by using a CV of 10 percent (IOM, 2001) to cover the needs of 97–98 percent of the individuals in the groups.

**RECOMMENDATIONS FOR ZINC INTAKE:**

| | |
|---|---|
| **$EAR_{MGT}$ for men** | **13 mg/day** |
| **$EAR_{MGT}$ for women** | **9.0 mg/day** |
| **$RDA_{MGT}$ for men** | **15 mg/day** |
| **$RDA_{MGT}$ for women** | **11 mg/day** |

### Adequacy of Zinc MDRIs and Zinc Levels in Rations

The MDRIs for zinc are 15 and 12 mg/day for men and women, respectively. These are based on the IOM RDAs from 1989 (NRC, 1989) and are higher than the current IOM RDAs (IOM, 2001); for military personnel with a life style similar to that of the civilian population, the current RDAs of 11 and 8 mg/day should be considered. These amounts, however, might not meet the needs of very physically active people, such as military personnel engaged in training or combat (See recommendation section). The committee concluded that, given the higher needs for military personnel under garrison training, the $RDA_{MGT,}$ should be higher as described previously.

Table 3-1 (see also Tables C-2 through C-5 in Appendix C) show the averages and ranges of zinc for three different MREs that each include about 25 menus. The average zinc content in MRE XXIII and XXIV menus and is 4.2 and 4.7 mg, respectively; some menus seem to be very low in zinc (0.96 mg), so it will be assumed that a mix of menus are eaten a day and are sufficient to meet the average menu level of zinc. However, there is a potential for deficiencies due to not only low food consumption but also selection of an MRE low in zinc. The committee recommends that the menus at the low end of the range be revised so that they would meet 15 and 11 mg/day for men and women, respectively. Assuming that women will consume two MREs and that men will consume three MREs, the amount in the rations, if consumed completely (approximately 9 or 14 mg, for two or three MREs, respectively), will not meet the recommendations of this committee for men ($RDA_{MGT}$ = 15 mg/day) or women ($RDA_{MGT}$ = 11 mg/day). The zinc density in MREs should be increased; also, the actual zinc intakes for men and women need to be evaluated to see if the recommendations made by this committee are met.

The current FSRs contains an average of 11.9 mg of zinc, which is adequate based on the IOM recommendation of 11–25 mg/day (IOM, 2006) (see Table 3-1; see also Table C-6 in Appendix C).

### Adequacy of IOM Recommendations for First Strike Rations

For short-term, high-intensity combat operations, a range of 11–25 mg/day of zinc in FSRs has been recommended (IOM, 2006; see Table 3-1). This recommendation, constructed under the assumption that only men conduct combat operations, was based conservatively on uncertainties in variable sweat losses, difficulties in assessing zinc status, and a possible marginal zinc status of male soldiers and is appropriate for these short-term conditions of underconsumption. Palatability considerations and size limitations were considered and should dictate the final level included in the FSRs.

### Strategies for Achieving Sufficient Zinc Intake

*Usual Foods*

As more zinc is ingested, absorptive efficiency decreases, and the absolute amount absorbed increases. Several dietary factors may influence human zinc absorption (Hunt, 2005, Lonnerdal, 2000; see Hunt in Appendix B). The zinc content and phytate content, or phytate-to-zinc molar ratio are primary factors, and the impact of these factors on fractional zinc absorption from adult diets can be estimated by using a dietary algorithm (IZiNCG, 2004). Other dietary factors that may influence bioavailability include the enhancing effect of proteins and amino acids and the inhibiting effects of calcium, iron, and copper, although these do not have as strong an effect on zinc absorption from practical whole diets as do phytic acid and the amount of zinc consumed. Most of the zinc in Western diets is derived from animal foods—including shellfish, red meat, liver, poultry, and dairy products—from which zinc is highly bioavailable. Beef supplies almost 25 percent of dietary zinc (Subar et al., 1998). Plant sources such as legumes, whole grains, nuts, and seeds also are rich in zinc, which is less bioavailable because these sources are high in phytic acid, a zinc chelator (Harland and Oberleas, 1987). Refined cereals contain less zinc, because zinc is in the outer layers of the kernel and the germ. Although phytic acid in unrefined foods reduces fractional zinc absorption, the higher zinc content may make these foods preferable to more refined products (Sandstrom et al., 1980). Because of lower zinc absorption, people who consume vegetarian diets, especially diets with phytate:zinc molar ratios exceeding 15, may require 20 to 50 percent more zinc than people who consume nonvegetarian diets (Hunt, 2003; IOM, 2001). It is possible as well as desirable to meet the zinc recommendations adjusted for garrison training conditions by using natural food sources.

*Fortified Foods*

Zinc sulfate and zinc oxide are the forms used most commonly for food fortification (Hunt, 2005; see Hunt in Appendix B). Food fortification with zinc has been limited but has been successful for the few products that are on the market. The bioavailability of appropriate fortificants is high, although absorptive efficiency decreases as the amount of added zinc increases. There is little information about taste or texture concerns relating to fortified foods. Highly fortified breakfast cereal is one appropriate vehicle for fortification, and the stability of the cereal is apparently good. Plans to routinely fortify or supplement military rations with zinc should test for changes in the palatability of the rations. Fortified foods appear to be efficacious and may be helpful in meeting recommended zinc intakes.

*Supplementation*

Zinc supplements come in several forms, including zinc gluconate, oxide, aspartate, citrate, methionine, and histidine. The efficiency of absorption (fractional absorption) of low doses of zinc salts on an empty stomach is from 40 to 90 percent (Hendler and Rorvik, 2001). Zinc histidine, zinc methionine, and zinc cysteine complexes appear to be absorbed more efficiently than other forms of supplements. The supplements usually come in doses of about 15 mg (as elemental zinc), either alone or in combination products (Hendler and Rorvik, 2001). All strengths are expressed as total zinc content. Most commonly, supplements add about 10 mg to the diet in those who take supplements in addition to consuming zinc through food. Zinc supplements are available in tablets, liquid, lozenges, and capsules.

The danger of excess from zinc supplementation appears to be slight, and there are very few reports of overdoses. However, with a combination of diets rich in zinc, zinc-fortified foods, and zinc supplements, it is possible to exceed the UL for zinc of 40 mg/day. The difference between excess and the recommendations for needs is great. Evidence of zinc supplementation safety is good, at least up to 30 mg/day. The most common adverse effects at higher doses are nausea, vomiting, gastrointestinal discomfort, metallic taste, headache, and drowsiness (Hendler and Rorvik, 2001). Long-term zinc intakes between 140 and 450 mg/day are associated with decreased copper status, altered iron function, reduced immune function, and reduced levels of high-density lipoproteins. At even higher levels (e.g., 4 g of zinc taken acutely) nausea and vomiting occur; however, there are no reports of lethal overdosing with zinc.

Zinc can interact with the following drugs and decrease their bioavailability: biphophonates, quinolones, penicillamine, and tetracyclines. Supplementation or fortification should result in an appropriate dietary balance of trace elements so that the proportion of consumed copper, iron, and zinc is roughly similar to the proportions found in natural food diets or in the current nutrient recommendations.

### Recommendations for Achieving Sufficiency

Studies have shown no beneficial effect of zinc supplementation on physical performance or measures of oxidative stress for military personnel engaged in garrison training. Researchers urge caution in fortifying foods with chemical forms of zinc, so the palatability of the rations is not adversely affected. Zinc sulfate and zinc oxide are the forms most commonly used for food fortification (Hunt, 2005; see Hunt in Appendix B). Fortification or supplementation with zinc should not be implemented without consideration of possible adverse effects on the balance of trace elements such as iron and copper. It is possible as well as desirable to meet the above RDAs adjusted for garrison training conditions by using natural food sources.

### Research Needs

- Quantify zinc losses due to the stressful conditions experienced during garrison training (e.g., heat, physical exertion, and psychological stressors).
- Evaluate the possible benefits of zinc supplementation on physical performance.
- Evaluate the potential benefits of zinc supplementation for enhancing mental function.
- Determine zinc concentrations of food items in operational rations, including MREs and FSRs, and the dietary intake levels of military personnel.

## REFERENCES

Abma JC, Chandra A, Mosher WD, Peterson LS, Piccinino LJ. 1997. Fertility, family planning, and women's health: New data from the 1995 National Survey of Family Growth. *Vital Health Stat* 23(19).

Abraham GE, Lubran MM. 1981. Serum and red cell magnesium levels in patients with premenstrual tension. *Am J Clin Nutr* 34(11):2364–2366.

Agte V, Jahagirdar M, Chiplonkar S. 2005. Apparent absorption of eight micronutrients and phytic acid from vegetarian meals in ileostomized human volunteers. *Nutrition* 21(6):678–685.

Aisen P, Enns C, Wessling-Resnick M. 2001. Chemistry and biology of eukaryotic iron metabolism. *Int J Biochem Cell Biol* 33(10):940–959.

Akesson A, Bjellerup P, Berglund M, Bremme K, Vahter M. 1998. Serum transferrin receptor: A specific marker of iron deficiency in pregnancy. *Am J Clin Nutr* 68(6):1241–1246.

Albers R, Bol M, Bleumink R, Willems AA, Pieters RH. 2003. Effects of supplementation with vitamins A, C, and E, selenium, and zinc on immune function in a murine sensitization model. *Nutrition* 19(11–12):940–946.

Alexander D, Ball MJ, Mann J. 1994. Nutrient intake and haematological status of vegetarians and age-sex matched omnivores. *Eur J Clin Nutr* 48(8):538–546.

Allan CB, Lacourciere GM, Stadtman TC. 1999. Responsiveness of selenoproteins to dietary selenium. *Annu Rev Nutr* 19:1–16.

Allen L. 1998. Calcium. Physiology. In: Sadler MJ, Strain JJ, Caballero B, eds. *Encyclopedia of Human Nutrition*. San Diego, CA: Academic Press. Pp. 214–218.

Almeida SA, Williams KM, Shaffer RA, Brodine SK. 1999. Epidemiological patterns of musculoskeletal injuries and physical training. *Med Sci Sports Exerc* 31(8):1176–1182.

Alvir JM, Thys-Jacobs S. 1991. Premenstrual and menstrual symptom clusters and response to calcium treatment. *Psychopharmacol Bull* 27(2):145–148.

American Psychiatric Association. 1994. *Diagnostic and Statistical Manual of Mental Disorders: DSM-IV*. 4th ed. Washington, DC: American Psychiatric Association.

Anderson GJ, Frazer DM. 2005. Recent advances in intestinal iron transport. *Curr Gastroenterol Rep* 7(5):365–372.

Anderson RA, Plansky MM, Bryden NA. 1984. Acute effects on chromium, copper, zinc, and selected clinical variables in urine and serum of male runners. *Biol Trace Elem Res* 6:327–336.

Anderson RA, Bryden NA, Polansky MM, Deuster PA. 1995. Acute exercise effects on urinary losses and serum concentrations of copper and zinc of moderately trained and untrained men consuming a controlled diet. *Analyst* 120(3):867–870.

Andon MB, Ilich JZ, Tzagournis MA, Matkovic V. 1996. Magnesium balance in adolescent females consuming a low- or high-calcium diet. *Am J Clin Nutr* 63(6):950–953.

Aro A, Alfthan G, Varo P. 1995. Effects of supplementation of fertilizers on human selenium status in Finland. *Analyst*. 120(3):841–843.

Arsenault JE, Cline AD. 2000. Nutrient intakes and characteristics of normal weight, female military personnel consuming foods reduced in fat or energy content. *Appetite* 34(3):227–233.

Arsenault J, Kennedy J. 1999. Dietary supplement use in U.S. Army Special Operations candidates. *Mil Med* 164(7):495–501.

Arteel GE, Mostert V, Oubrahim H, Briviba K, Abel J, Sies H. 1998. Protection by selenoprotein P in human plasma against peroxynitrite-mediated oxidation and nitration. *Biol Chem* 379 (8–9):1201–1205.

Arthur JR. 2000. The glutathione peroxidases. *Cell Mol Life Sci* 57(13–14):1825–1835.

Aruoma OI, Reilly T, MacLaren D, Halliwell B. 1988. Iron, copper and zinc concentrations in human sweat and plasma; the effect of exercise. *Clin Chim Acta* 177(1):81–87.

Ashizawa N, Ouchi G, Fujimura R, Yoshida Y, Tokuyama K, Suzuki M. 1998. Effects of a single bout of resistance exercise on calcium and bone metabolism in untrained young males. *Calcif Tissue Int* 62(2):104–108.

Bahl R, Bhandari N, Hambidge KM, Bhan MK. 1998. Plasma zinc as a predictor of diarrheal and respiratory morbidity in children in an urban slum setting. *Am J Clin Nutr* 68(2 Suppl):414S–417S.

Baker DH. 1999. Cupric oxide should not be used as a copper supplement for either animals or humans. *J Nutr* 129(12): 2278–2279.

Baker-Fulco CJ. 2005 (June 13). *Derivation of the Military Dietary Reference Intakesand the Mineral Content of Military Rations*. Paper presented at the Institue of Medicine Workshop on The Mineral Requirements for Cognitive and Physical Performance of Military Personnel, Washington, DC: Institute of Medicine Committee on Mineral Requirements for Cognitive and Physical Performance of Military Personnel.

Baker-Fulco CJ, Bathalon GP, Bovill ME, Lieberman HR. 2001. *Military Dietary Reference Intakes: Rationale for Tables Values*. TN-00/10. Natick, MA: U.S. Army Research Insitute of Environmental Medicine.

Baker-Fulco CJ, Kramer FM, Lesher LL, Merrill E, Johnson J, DeLany J. 2002. *Dietary Intakes of Female and Male Combat Support Hospital Personnel Subsisting on Meal-Focused or Standard Versions of the Meal, Ready-to-Eat*. Frederick, MD: U.S. Army Medical Research and Materiel Command.

Ballin A, Berar M, Rubinstein U, Kleter Y, Hershkovitz A, Meytes D. 1992. Iron state in female adolescents. *Am J Dis Child* 146(7):803–805.

Bardgett ME, Schultheis PJ, McGill DL, Richmond RE, Wagge JR. 2005. Magnesium deficiency impairs fear conditioning in mice. *Brain Res* 1038(1):100–106.

Bass SL. 2000. The prepubertal years: A uniquely opportune stage of growth when the skeleton is most responsive to exercise? *Sports Med* 30(2):73–78.

Baum MK, Shor-Posner G. 1998. Micronutrient status in relationship to mortality in HIV-1 disease. *Nutr Rev* 56(1 Pt 2):S135–S139.

Baum MK, Shor-Posner G, Lai S, Zhang G, Lai H, Fletcher MA, Sauberlich H, Page JB. 1997. High risk of HIV-related mortality is associated with selenium deficiency. *J Acquir Immune Defic Syndr Hum Retrovirol* 15(5):370–374.

Baum MK, Miguez-Burbano MJ, Campa A, Shor-Posner G. 2000. Selenium and interleukins in persons infected with human immunodeficiency virus type 1. *J Infect Dis* (182 Suppl 1): S69–S73.

Bayer TA, Schafer S, Simons A, Kemmling A, Kamer T, Tepest R, Eckert A, Schussel K, Eikenberg O, Sturchler-Pierrat C, Abramowski D, Staufenbiel M, Multhaup G. 2003. Dietary Cu stabilizes brain superoxide dismutase 1 activity and reduces amyloid A β production in APP23 transgenic mice. *Proc Natl Acad Sci* 100(24):14187–14192.

Beard J. 1987. Feed efficiency and norepinephrine turnover in iron deficiency. *Proc Soc Exp Biol Med* 184(3):337–344.

Beard JL, Connor JR. 2003. Iron status and neural functioning. *Annu Rev Nutr* 23:41–58.

Beard J, Tobin B. 2000. Iron status and exercise. *Am J Clin Nutr* 72(2 Suppl):594S–597S.

Beard JL, Hendricks MK, Perez EM, Murray-Kolb LE, Berg A, Vernon-Feagans L, Irlam J, Isaacs W, Sive A, Tomlinson M. 2005. Maternal iron deficiency anemia affects postpartum emotions and cognition. *J Nutr* 135(2):267–272.

Beaton GH. 1974. Epidemiology of iron deficiency. Jacobs A, Worwood M, eds. *Iron in Biochemistry and Medicine*. New York: Academic Press. Pp. 477–528.

Beck MA. 1997. Rapid genomic evolution of a non-virulent coxsackievirus B3 in selenium-deficient mice. *Biomed Environ Sci* 10(2–3):307–315.

Beck MA, Levander OA, Handy J. 2003. Selenium deficiency and viral infection. *J Nutr* 133(5 Suppl 1):1463S–1467S.

Beck TJ, Ruff CB, Mourtada FA, Shaffer RA, Maxwell-Williams K, Kao GL, Sartoris DJ, Brodine S. 1996. Dual-energy X-ray absorptiometry derived structural geometry for stress fracture prediction in male U.S. Marine Corps recruits. *J Bone Miner Res* 11(5):645–653.

Beckett GJ, Nicol F, Rae PW, Beech S, Guo Y, Arthur JR. 1993. Effects of combined iodine and selenium deficiency on thyroid hormone metabolism in rats. *Am J Clin Nutr* 57(2 Suppl): 240S–243S.

Begon S, Pickering G, Eschalier A, Mazur A, Rayssiguier Y, Dubray C. 2001. Role of spinal NMDA receptors, protein kinase C and nitric oxide synthase in the hyperalgesia induced by magnesium deficiency in rats. *Br J Pharmacol* 134(6):1227–1236.

Behne D, Kyriakopoeulos A, Weiss-Nowak C, Kalckloesch M, Westphal C, Gessner H. 1996. Newly found selenium-containing proteins in the tissues of the rat. *Biol Trace Elem Res* 55(1–2): 99–110.

Beisel WR. 1982. Single nutrients and immunity. *Am J Clin Nutr* 35(2 Suppl):417–468.

Beisel WR, Sawyer WD, Ryll ED, Crozier D. 1967. Metabolic effects of intracellular infections in man. *Ann Intern Med* 67(4):744–779.

Beisel WR, Goldman RF, Joy RJ. 1968. Metabolic balance studies during induced hyperthermia in man. *J Appl Physiol* 24(1):1–10.

Beller GA, Maher JT, Hartley LH, Bass DE, Wacker WE. 1975. Changes in serum and sweat magnesium levels during work in the heat. *Aviat Space Environ Med* 46(5):709–712.

Bemben DA, Boileau RA, Bahr JM, Nelson RA, Misner JE. 1992. Effects of oral contraceptives on hormonal and metabolic responses during exercise. *Med Sci Sports Exerc* 24(4):434–441.

Bendich A. 2000. The potential for dietary supplements to reduce premenstrual syndrome (PMS) symptoms. *J Am Coll Nutr* 19(1):3–12.

Benton D, Cook R. 1991. The impact of selenium supplementation on mood. *Biol Psychiatry* 29(11): 1092–1098.

Berdanier CD. 1998. *Advanced Nutrition. Micronutrients*. Boca Raton, FL: CRC Press.

Bergstrom JP, Larsson J, Nordstrom H, Vinnars E, Askanazi J, Elwyn DH, Kinney JM, Furst PJ. 1987. Influence of injury and nutrition on muscle water and electrolytes: Effect of severe injury, burns and sepsis. *Acta Chir Scand* 153(4):261–266.

Berridge CW, Waterhouse BD. 2003. The locus coeruleus-noradrenergic system: Modulation of behavioral state and state-dependent cognitive processes. *Brain Res Brain Res Rev* 42(1):33–84.

Berry MJ, Banu L, Harney JW, Larsen PR. 1993. Functional characterization of the eukaryotic SECIS elements which direct selenocysteine insertion at UGA codons. *EMBO J* 12(8):3315–3322.

Bertinato J, L'Abbe MR. 2004. Maintaining copper homeostasis: Regulation of copper-trafficking proteins in response to copper deficiency or overload. *J Nutr Biochem* 15(6):316–322.

Bertone ER, Hankinson SE, Bendich A, Manson JE. 2005. Intake of calcium and vitamin D and risk of premenstrual syndrome (abstract). *J Womens Health* 12:425.

Bertschat F, Golf SW, Riediger H, Graef V, Ising H. 1986. Protective effects of magnesium on release of proteins from muscle cells during a marathon run. *Magnesium Bull* 8:310–313.

Black RE. 1998. Therapeutic and preventive effects of zinc on serious childhood infectious diseases in developing countries. *Am J Clin Nutr* 68(2 Suppl):476S–479S.

Blitz M, Blitz S, Beasely R, Diner BM, Hughes R, Knopp JA, Rowe BH. 2005. Inhaled magnesium sulfate in the treatment of acute asthma. *Cochrane Database System Rev* (4):CD003898.

Bogden JD, Oleske JM, Lavenhar MA, Munves EM, Kemp FW, Bruening KS, Holding KJ, Denny TN, Guarino MA, Krieger LM. 1988. Zinc and immunocompetence in elderly people: Effects of zinc supplementation for 3 months. *Am J Clin Nutr* 48(3):655–663.

Bogden JD, Oleske JM, Lavenhar MA, Munves EM, Kemp FW, Bruening KS, Holding KJ, Denny TN, Guarino MA, Holland BK. 1990. Effects of one year of supplementation with zinc and other micronutrients on cellular immunity in the elderly. *J Am Coll Nutr* 9(3):214–225.

Booth CK. 2003. Combat rations and military performance—Do soldiers on active service eat enough? *Asia Pac J Clin Nutr* 12(Suppl):S2.

Booth CK, Coad RA, Forbes-Ewan CH, Thomson GF, Niro PJ. 2003. The physiological and psychological effects of combat ration feeding during a 12-day training exercise in the tropics. *Mil Med* 168(1):63–70.

Borer MS, Bhanot VK. 1985. Hyperparathyroidism: Neuropsychiatric manifestations. *Psychosomatics* 26(7):597–601.

Bothwell TH, Charlton RW, Cook JD, Finch CA. 1979. *Iron Metabolism in Man*. Oxford: Blackwell Scientific Publications.

Boushey CJ. 2006. Nutritional epidemiology: Dietary assessment methods. In: Weaver CM, Heaney RP, eds. *Calcium in Human Health*. Totowa, NJ: Humana Press. 2006. Pp. 39–63.

Braun J. 1999. Erythrocyte zinc protoporphyrin. *Kidney Int Suppl* 69:S57–S60.

Brilla LR, Gunter KB. 1995. Effect of magnesium supplementation on exercise time to exhaustion. *Med Exerc Nutr Health* 4:230–233.

Brilla LR, Haley TF. 1992. Effect of magnesium supplementation on strength training in humans. *J Am Coll Nutr* 11(3):326–329.

Britton J, Pavord I, Richards K, Wisniewski A, Knox A, Lewis S, Tattersfield A, Weiss S. 1994. Dietary magnesium, lung function, wheezing, and airway hyperreactivity in a random adult population sample. *Lancet* 344(8919):357–362.

Briviba K, Kissner R, Koppenol WH, Sies H. 1998. Kinetic study of the reaction of glutathione peroxidase with peroxynitrite. *Chem Res Toxicol* 11(12):1398–1401.

Broome CS, McArdle F, Kyle JA, Andrews F, Lowe NM, Hart CA, Arthur JR, Jackson MJ. 2004. An increase in selenium intake improves immune function and poliovirus handling in adults with marginal selenium status. *Am J Clin Nutr* 80(1):154–162.

Brouns F. 1991. Heat—sweat—dehydration—rehydration: A praxis oriented approach. *J Sports Sci* 9 Spec No:143–152.

Brownlie T 4th, Utermohlen V, Hinton PS, Giordano C, Haas JD. 2002. Marginal iron deficiency without anemia impairs aerobic adaptation among previously untrained women. *Am J Clin Nutr* 75(4):734–742.

Brownlie T 4th, Utermohlen V, Hinton PS, Haas JD. 2004. Tissue iron deficiency without anemia impairs adaptation in endurance capacity after aerobic training in previously untrained women. *Am J Clin Nutr* 79(3):437–443.

Brune M, Magnusson B, Persson H, Hallberg L. 1986. Iron losses in sweat. *Am J Clin Nutr* 43(3): 438–443.

Bruner AB, Joffe A, Duggan AK, Casella JF, Brandt J. 1996. Randomised study of cognitive effects of iron supplementation in non-anaemic iron-deficient adolescent girls. *Lancet* 348(9033): 992–996.

Brutsaert TD, Hernandez-Cordero S, Rivera J, Viola T, Hughes G, Haas JD. 2003. Iron supplementation improves progressive fatigue resistance during dynamic knee extensor exercise in iron-depleted, nonanemic women. *Am J Clin Nutr* 77(2):441–448.

Buchman AL, Keen C, Commisso J, Killip D, Ou CN, Rognerud CL, Dennis K, Dunn JK. 1998. The effect of a marathon run on plasma and urine mineral and metal concentrations. *J Am Coll Nutr* 17(2):124–127.

Bullen DB, O'Toole ML, Johnson KC. 1999. Calcium losses resulting from an acute bout of moderate-intensity exercise. *Int J Sport Nutr* 9(3):275–284.

Burbano X, Miguez-Burbano MJ, McCollister K, Zhang G, Rodriguez A, Ruiz P, Lecusay R, Shor-Posner G. 2002. Impact of a selenium chemoprevention clinical trial on hospital admissions of HIV-infected participants. *HIV Clin Trials* 3(6):483–491.

Burk RF, Hill KE. 2005. Selenoprotein P: An extracellular protein with unique physical characteristics and a role in selenium homeostasis. *Annu Rev Nutr* 25:215–235.

Burk RF, Levander OA. 1999. Selenium. In: Shils ME, Olson JA, Shike M, Ross AC, eds. *Modern Nutrition in Health and Disease*. 9th ed. Baltimore, MD: Williams & Wilkins. Pp. 265–276.

Burr DB. 1997. Bone, exercise, and stress fractures. *Exerc Sport Sci Rev* 25:171–194.

Burr DB, Yoshikawa T, Teegarden D, Lyle R, McCabe G, McCabe LD, Weaver CM. 2000. Exercise and oral contraceptive use suppress the normal age-related increase in bone mass and strength of the femoral neck in women 18-31 years of age. *Bone* 27(6):855–863.

Byrd TF, Horwitz MA. 1989. Interferon gamma-activated human monocytes downregulate transferrin receptors and inhibit the intracellular multiplication of Legionella pneumophila by limiting the availability of iron. *J Clin Invest* 83(5):1457–1465.

Campa A, Shor-Posner G, Indacochea F, Zhang G, Lai H, Asthana D, Scott GB, Baum MK. 1999. Mortality risk in selenium-deficient HIV-positive children. *J Acquir Immune Defic Syndr Hum Retrovirol* 20(5):508–513.

Cannon JG. 2005 (June 14). *The Influence of Minerals on Muscle Injury and Recovery.* Paper presented at the Institue of Medicine Workshop on The Mineral Requirements for Cognitive and Physical Performance of Military Personnel, Washington, DC: Institute of Medicine Committee on Mineral Requirements for Cognitive and Physical Performance of Military Personnel.

Canonne-Hergaux F, Gruenheid S, Ponka P, Gros P. 1999. Cellular and subcellular localization of the Nramp2 iron transporter in the intestinal brush border and regulation by dietary iron. *Blood* 93(12):4406–4417.

Castano A, Ayala A, Rodriguez-Gomez JA, Herrera AJ, Cano J, Machado A. 1997. Low selenium diet increases the dopamine turnover in prefrontal cortex of the rat. *Neurochem Int* 30(6): 549–555.

Castillo-Duran C, Vial P, Uauy R. 1988. Trace mineral balance during acute diarrhea in infants. *J Pediatr* 113(3):452–457.

Chandra RK. 1984. Excessive intake of zinc impairs immune responses. *J Am Med Assoc* 252(11): 1443–1446.

Chang C, Gershwin ME. 2000. Nutrition and allergy. In: Gershwin ME, German JB, Keen CL, eds. *Nutrition and Immunology. Principles and Practice.* Totowa, NJ: Humana Press. Pp. 221–231.

Charles P, Eriksen EF, Hasling C, Sondergard K, Mosekilde L. 1991. Dermal, intestinal, and renal obligatory losses of calcium: Relation to skeletal calcium loss. *Am J Clin Nutr* 54(1 Suppl): 266S–273S.

Chu JY, Margen S, Calloway DH, Costa FM. 1979. Integumentary loss of calcium. *Am J Clin Nutr* 32(8):1699–1702.

Clark LC, Combs GF Jr, Turnbull BW, Slate EH, Chalker DK, Chow J, Davis LS, Glover RA, Graham GF, Gross EG, Krongrad A, Lesher JL Jr, Park HK, Sanders BB Jr, Smith CL, Taylor JR. 1996. Effects of selenium supplementation for cancer prevention in patients with carcinoma of the skin. A randomized controlled trial. Nutritional Prevention of Cancer Study Group. *J Am Med Assoc* 276(24):1957–1963.

Clarkson PM, Haymes EM. 1995. Exercise and mineral status of athletes: Calcium, magnesium, phosphorus, and iron. *Med Sci Sports Exerc* 27(6):831–843.

Clausen. 1991. Uptake and distribution in rat brain of organic and inorganic selenium. *Biol Trace Elem Res* 28(1):39–45.

Clemens JD, Feinstein AR. 1977. Calcium carbonate and constipation: A historical review of medical mythopoeia. *Gastroenterology* 72(5 Pt 1):957–961.

Cline AD, Patton FJ, Tharion WJ, Strowman SR, Champagne CM, Arsenault J, Reynolds KL, Warber JP, Baker-Fulco C, Rood J, Tulley RT, Lieberman HR. 1998. *Assessment of the Relationship Between Iron Status, Dietary Intake, Performance, and Mood State of Female Army Officers in a Basic Training Population.* Report No. T-98. Natick, MA: U.S. Army Research Institute of Environmental Medicine.

Cogan MG, Covey CM, Arieff AI, Wisniewski A, Clark OH, Lazarowitz V, Leach W. 1978. Central nervous system manifestations of hyperparathyroidism. *Am J Med* 65(6):963–970.

Cole SK, Billewicz WZ, Thomson AM. 1971. Sources of variation in menstrual blood loss. *J Obstet Gynaecol Br Commonw* 78(10):933–939.

Combs G, Patterson B, Brindak M, Midthune D, Taylor P, Patterson K, Levander O. 2005. Thyroid hormone levels in subjects supplemented with oral selenomethionine. *FASEB J* 19(5):a1016.

Conrad ME, Umbreit JN. 2000. Iron absorption and transport-an update. *Am J Hematol* 64(4): 287–298.

Consolazio CF, Matoush LO, Nelson RA, Hackler LR, Preseon EE. 1962. Relationship between calcium in sweat, calcium balance, and calcium requirements. *J Nutr* 78:78–88.

Consolazio CF, Matoush LO, Nelson RA, Harding RS, Canham JE. 1963. Excretion of sodium, potassium, magnesium and iron in human sweat and the relation of each to balance and requirements. *J Nutr* 79:407–415.

Consolazio CF, Nelson RA, Matoush LO, Hughes RC, Urone P. 1964. *The Trace Mineral Losses in Sweat.* 284. Denver, CO: U.S. Army Medical Research and Nutrition Laboratory.

Cook J. 1999. The nutritional assessment of iron status. *Arch Latinoam Nutr* 49(3 Suppl 2):11S–14S.

Cook JD, Dassenko S, Skikne BS. 1990. Serum transferrin receptor as an index of iron absorption. *Br J Haematol* 75(4):603–609.

Cook JD, Dassenko SA, Lynch SR. 1991. Assessment of the role of nonheme-iron availability in iron balance. *Am J Clin Nutr* 54(4):717–722.

Cook JD, Flowers CH, Skikne BS. 2003. The quantitative assessment of body iron. *Blood* 101(9): 3359–3364.

Cooper JR, Bloom FE, Roth RH. 2003. *The Biochemical Basis of Neuropharmacology.* 8th ed. Oxford: Oxford University Press.

Corwin EJ, Murray-Kolb LE, Beard JL. 2003. Low hemoglobin level is a risk factor for postpartum depression. *J Nutr* 133(12):4139–4142.

Costill DL, Cote R, Fink W. 1976. Muscle water and electrolytes following varied levels of dehydration in man. *J Appl Physiol* 40(1):6–11.

Cousins RJ. 1989. Theoretical and practical aspects of zinc uptake and absorption. *Adv Exp Med Biol* 249:3–12.

Curhan GC, Willett WC, Rimm EB, Stampfer MJ. 1993. A prospective study of dietary calcium and other nutrients and the risk of symptomatic kidney stones. *N Engl J Med* 328(12):833–838.

Curhan GC, Willett WC, Speizer FE, Spiegelman D, Stampfer MJ. 1997. Comparison of dietary calcium with supplemental calcium and other nutrients as factors affecting the risk for kidney stones in women. *Ann Intern Med* 126(7):497–504.

Curhan GC, Willett WC, Knight EL, Stampfer MJ. 2004. Dietary factors and the risk of incident kidney stones in younger women: Nurses' Health Study II. *Arch Intern Med* 164(8):885–891.

Dallman PR, Refino C, Yland MJ. 1982. Sequence of development of iron deficiency in the rat. *Am J Clin Nutr* 35(4):671–677.

Damodaran M, Naidu AN, Sarma KV. 1979. Anaemia and morbidity in rural preschool children. *Indian J Med Res* 69:448–556.

Danks DM. 1980. copper deficiency in humans. *Ciba Found Symp* 79:209–225.

Das K, Chowdhury AR. 1997. Metallic ion concentration during menstrual cycle in normally menstruating women. *Indian J Med Sci* 51(2):52–54.

Davies KJ, Maguire JJ, Brooks GA, Dallman PR, Packer L. 1982. Muscle mitochondrial bioenergetics, oxygen supply, and work capacity during dietary iron deficiency and repletion. *Am J Physiol* 242(6):E418–E427.

Davies KJ, Donovan CM, Refino CJ, Brooks GA, Packer L, Dallman PR. 1984. Distinguishing effects of anemia and muscle iron deficiency on exercise bioenergetics in the rat. *Am J Physiol* 246(6 Pt 1):E535–E543.

Davies NT, Lawrence CB. 1986. Studies on the effect of copper deficiency on rat liver mitochondria. III. Effects on adenine nucleotide translocase. *Biochim Biophys Acta* 848(3):294–304.

Dawson-Hughes B, Seligson FH, Hughes VA. 1986. Effects of calcium carbonate and hydroxyapatite on zinc absorption and iron retention in postmenopausal women. *Am J Clin Nutr* 44(1):83–88.

De Souza MI, Williams NI. 2005. Beyond hypoestrogenism in amenorrheic athletes: Energy deficiency as a contributing factor for bone loss. *Curr Sports Med Rep* 4(1):38–44.

Delorme O, Bourdin H, Viel JF, Rigaud ML, Kantelip JP. 1992. Spectral analysis of electroencephalography data in athletes with low erythrocyte magnesium. *Magnes Res* 5(4):261–264.

Depoortere H, Francon D, Llopis J. 1993. Effects of a magnesium-deficient diet on sleep organization in rats. *Neuropsychobiology* 27(4):237–245.

DeRuisseau KC, Cheuvront SN, Haymes EM, Sharp RG. 2002. Sweat iron and zinc losses during prolonged exercise. *Int J Sport Nutr Exerc Metab* 12(4):428–437.

deUngria M, Rao R, Wobken JD, Luciana M, Nelson CA, Georgieff MK. 2000. Perinatal iron deficiency decreases cytochrome c oxidase (CytOx) activity in selected regions of neonatal rat brain. *Pediatr Res* 48(2):169–176.

Deuster PA, Singh A. 1993. Responses of plasma magnesium and other cations to fluid replacement during exercise. *J Am Coll Nutr* 12(3):286–293.

Deuster PA, Dolev E, Bernier LL, Trostmann UH. 1987a. Magnesium and zinc status during the menstrual cycle. *Am J Obstet Gynecol* 157(4 Pt 1):964–968.

Deuster PA, Dolev E, Kyle SB, Anderson RA, Schoomaker EB. 1987b. Magnesium homeostasis during high-intensity anaerobic exercise in men. *J Appl Physiol* 62(2):545–550.

Deuster PA, Sridhar A, Becker WJ, Coll R, O'Brien KK, Bathalon G. 2003. Health assessment of U.S. Army Rangers. *Mil Med* 168(1):57–62.

DHHS and USDA (U.S. Department of Health and Human Services and U.S. Department of Agriculture). 2005. *Dietary Guidelines for Americans, 2005*. 6th ed. Washington, DC: U.S. Government Printing Office.

Dinneen SF, O'Mahony MS, O'Brien T, Cronin CC, Murray DM, O'Sullivan DJ. 1992. Serum ferritin in newly diagnosed and poorly controlled diabetes mellitus. *Ir J Med Sci* 161(11): 636–638.

Dinneen SF, Silverberg JD, Batts KP, O'Brien PC, Ballard DJ, Rizza RA. 1994. Liver iron stores in patients with non-insulin-dependent diabetes mellitus. *Mayo Clin Proc* 69(1):13–15.

Dubray C, Rayssiguier Y. 1997. Magnesium, inflammation, and pain. In: Theophanides T, Anastassopoulou J, eds. *Magnesium: Current Staus and New Developments. Theoretical, Biological, and Medical Aspects*. Boston, MA: Kluwer Academic. Pp. 303–311.

Duffield AJ, Thomson CD, Hill KE, Williams S. 1999. An estimation of selenium requirements for New Zealanders. *Am J Clin Nutr* 70(5):896–903.

Durlach J. 1980. Clinical aspects of chronic magnesium deficiency. In: Cantin M, Seelig MS, eds. *Magnesium in Health and Disease. Proceedings of the 2nd International Symposium on Magnesium. Montreal, Quebec, May 30–June 1, 1976*. New York: SP Medical and Scientific Books. Pp. 883–909.

Durlach J. 1985. Neurological disturbances due to magnesium imbalance. In: Gabay S, Harris J, Ho BT, eds. *Metal Ions in Neurology and Psychiatry*. New York: Alan R. Liss. Pp. 121–128.

Dwyer JT, Dietz WH Jr, Andrews EM, Suskind RM. 1982. Nutritional status of vegetarian children. *Am J Clin Nutr* 35(2):204–216.

Dyckner T, Wester PO. 1983. Effect of magnesium on blood pressure. *Br Med j* 286:1847–1849.

Edgerton VR, Ohira Y, Hettiarachchi J, Senewiratne B, Gardner GW, Barnard RJ. 1981. Elevation of hemoglobin and work tolerance in iron-deficient subjects. *J Nutr Sci Vitaminol (Tokyo)* 27(2): 77–86.

Ehn L, Carlmark B, Hoglund S. 1980. Iron status in athletes involved in intense physical activity. *Med Sci Sports Exerc* 12(1):61–64.

Eisenstein RS. 2000. Iron regulatory proteins and the molecular control of mammalian iron metabolism. *Annu Rev Nutr* 20:627–662.

Elders PJ, Lips P, Netelenbos JC, van Ginkel FC, Khoe E, van der Vijgh WJ, van der Stelt PF. 1994. Long-term effect of calcium supplementation on bone loss in perimenopausal women. *J Bone Miner Res* 9(7):963–970.

Evans GH, Weaver CM, Harrington DD, Babbs CF Jr. 1990. Association of magnesium deficiency with the blood pressure-lowering effects of calcium. *J Hypertens* 8(4):327–337.

Facchinetti F, Borella P, Sances G, Fioroni L, Nappi RE, Genazzani AR. 1991. Oral magnesium successfully relieves premenstrual mood changes. *Obstet Gynecol* 78(2):177–181.

Fahmy M, Young SP. 1993. Modulation of iron metabolism in monocyte cell line U937 by inflammatory cytokines: Changes in transferrin uptake, iron handling and ferritin mRNA. *Biochem J* 296 (Pt 1):175–181.

Feillet-Coudray C, Coudray C, Tressol JC, Pepin D, Mazur A, Abrams SA, Rayssiguier Y. 2002. Exchangeable magnesium pool masses in healthy women: Effects of magnesium supplementation. *Am J Clin Nutr* 75(1):72–78.

Ferencik M, Ebringer L. 2003. Modulatory effects of selenium and zinc on the immune system. *Folia Microbiol (Praha)* 48(3):417–426.

Ferguson BJ, Skikne BS, Simpson KM, Baynes RD, Cook JD. 1992. Serum transferrin receptor distinguishes the anemia of chronic disease from iron deficiency anemia. *J Lab Clin Med* 119(4):385–390.

Finch CA, Huebers H. 1982. Perspectives in iron metabolism. *N Engl J Med* 306(25):1520–1528.

Finch CA, Miller LR, Inamdar AR, Person R, Seiler K, Mackler B. 1976. Iron deficiency in the rat. Physiological and biochemical studies of muscle dysfunction. *J Clin Invest* 58(2):447–453.

Finch CA, Gollnick PD, Hlastala MP, Miller LR, Dillmann E, Mackler B. 1979. Lactic acidosis as a result of iron deficiency. *J Clin Invest* 64(1):129–137.

Fine KD, Santa Ana CA, Fordtran JS. 1991. Diagnosis of magnesium-induced diarrhea. *N Engl J Med* 324(15):1012–1017.

Finley JW, Penland JG. 1998. Adequacy or deprivation of dietary selenium in healthy men: Clinical and psychological findings. *J Trace Elem Exp Med* 11(1):11–27.

Finstad EW, Newhouse IJ, Lukaski HC, Mcauliffe JE, Stewart CR. 2001. The effects of magnesium supplementation on exercise performance. *Med Sci Sports Exerc* 33(3):493–498.

Fishbane S. 1999. Review of issues relating to iron and infection. *Am J Kidney Dis* 34(4 Suppl 2):S47–S52.

Fogarty A, Lewis SA, Scrivener SL, Antoniak M, Pacey S, Pringle M, Britton J. 2003. Oral magnesium and vitamin C supplements in asthma: A parallel group randomized placebo-controlled trial. *Clin Exp Allergy* 33(10):1355–1359.

Fogelholm M. 1995. Inadequate iron status in athletes: An exaggerated problem? In: Kies CV, Driskell JA, eds. *Sports Nutrition. Mineralsand Electrolytes*. Boca Raton, FL: CRC Press. Pp. 81–95.

Fordy J, Benton D. 1994. Does low iron status influence psychological functioning? *J Hum Nutr Diet* 7:127–133.

Galan P, Thibault H, Preziosi P, Hercberg S. 1992. Interleukin 2 production in iron-deficient children. *Biol Trace Elem Res* 32:421–426.

Galland L. 1985. Normocalcemic tetany and candidiasis. *Magnesium* 4(5–6):339–344.

Garby L, Irnell L, Werner I. 1967. Iron deficiency in women of fertile age in a Swedish community. I. Distribution of packed cell volume and the effect of iron supplementation. *Acta Soc Med Ups* 72(1):91–101.

Garby L, Irnell L, Werner I. 1969. Iron deficiency in women of fertile age in a Swedish community. II. Efficiency of several laboratory tests to predict the response to iron supplementation. *Acta Med Scand* 185(1–2):107–111.

Gazdik F, Horvathova M, Gazdikova K, Jahnova E. 2002. The influence of selenium supplementation on the immunity of corticoid-dependent asthmatics. *Bratisl Lek Listy* 103(1):17–21.

Gibson RS, Scythes CA. 1982. Trace element intakes of women. *Br J Nutr* 48(2):241–248.

Gladyshev VN, Jeang KT, Wootton JC, Hatfield DL. 1998. A new human selenium-containing protein. Purification, characterization, and cDNA sequence. *J Biol Chem* 273(15):8910–8915.

Gleerup A, Rossander-Hulthen L, Gramatkovski E, Hallberg L. 1995. Iron absorption from the whole diet: Comparison of the effect of two different distributions of daily calcium intake. *Am J Clin Nutr* 61(1):97–104.

Goldsmith NF, Goldsmith JR. 1966. Epidemiological aspects of magnesium and calcium metabolism. Implications of altered magnesium metabolism in women taking drugs for the suppression of ovulation. *Arch Environ Health* 12(5):607–619.

Golf SW, Happel O, Graef V, Seim KE. 1984. Plasma aldosterone, cortisol and electrolyte concentrations in physical exercise after magnesium supplementation. *J Clin Chem Clin Biochem* 22(11):717–721.

Golf S Munch J, Graef V, Temme H, Brustle A, Roka L Beuther G, Heinz N, Buhl C, Nowacki PE. 1989. Effect of a 4-week magnesium supplementation on lactate elimination in competitive rowers during exhaustive simulated rowing. *Magnesium Res* 2:71.

Goulding A, McChesney R. 1977. Oestrogen-progestogen oral contraceptives and urinary calcium excretion. *Clin Endocrinol (Oxf)* 6(6):449–454.

Green R, Charlton R, Seftel H, Bothwell T, Mayet F, Adams B, Finch C, Layrisse M. 1968. Body iron excretion in man. A collaborative study. *Am J Med* 45:336–353.

Groner JA, Holtzman NA, Charney E, Mellits ED. 1986. A randomized trial of oral iron on tests of short-term memory and attention span in young pregnant women. *J Adolesc Health Care* 7(1):44–48.

Gropper SS, Sorrels LM, Blessing D. 2003. Copper status of collegiate female athletes involved in different sports. *Int J Sport Nutr Exerc Metab* 13(3):343–357.

Guillemant J, Accarie C, Peres G, Guillemant S. 2004. Acute effects of an oral calcium load on markers of bone metabolism during endurance cycling exercise in male athletes. *Calcif Tissue Int* 74(5):407–414.

Gunshin H, Mackenzie B, Berger UV, Gunshin Y, Romero MF, Boron WF, Nussberger S, Gollan JL, Hediger MA. 1997. Cloning and characterization of a mammalian proton-coupled metal-ion transporter. *Nature* 388(6641):482–488.

Hallberg L, Hogdahl AM, Nilsson L, Rybo G. 1966. Menstrual blood loss and iron deficiency. *Acta Med Scand* 180(5):639–650.

Hallberg L, Rossander-Hulten L, Brune M, Gleerup A. 1992. Calcium and iron absorption: Mechanism of action and nutritional importance. *Eur J Clin Nutr* 46(5):317–327.

Hallquist NA, McNeil LK, Lockwood JF, Sherman AR. 1992. Maternal-iron-deficiency effects on peritoneal macrophage and peritoneal natural-killer-cell cytotoxicity in rat pups. *Am J Clin Nutr* 55(3):741–746.

Hamer DH. 2005 (June 14). *Mineral Intake Needs and Infection Diseases.* Paper presented at the Institue of Medicine Workshop on The Mineral Requirements for Cognitive and Physical Performance of Military Personnel, Washington, DC: Institute of Medicine Committee on Mineral Requirements for Cognitive and Physical Performance of Military Personnel.

Harland BF, Oberleas D. 1987. Phytate in foods. *World Rev Nutr Diet* 52:235–259.

Hartard M, Bottermann P, Bartenstein P, Jeschke D, Schwaiger M. 1997. Effects on bone mineral density of low-dosed oral contraceptives compared to and combined with physical activity. *Contraception* 55(2):87–90.

Hawkes WC, Hornbostel L. 1996. Effects of dietary selenium on mood in healthy men living in a metabolic research unit. *Biol Psychiatry* 39(2):121–128.

Hawkes WC, Alkan FZ, Oehler L. 2003. Absorption, distribution and excretion of selenium from beef and rice in healthy North American men. *J Nutr* 133(11):3434–3442.

Hawkes WC, Alkan Z, Lang K, King JC. 2004. Plasma selenium decrease during pregnancy is associated with glucose intolerance. *Biol Trace Elem Res* 100(1):19–29.

Heaney RP. 2005. Calcium. In: Coates PM, Blackman MR, Cragg GM, Levine M, Moss J, White JD, eds. *Encyclopedia of Dietary Supplements.* New York: Marcel Dekker. Pp. 65–71.

Heaney RP, Weaver CM. 2005. Newer perspectives on calcium nutrition and bone quality. *J Am Coll Nutr* 24(6 Suppl):574S–581S.

Heaney RP, Weaver CM, Fitzsimmons ML. 1990. Influence of calcium load on absorption fraction. *J Bone Miner Res* 5(11):1135–1138.

Heaney RP, Dowell MS, Bierman J, Hale CA, Bendich A. 2001. Absorbability and cost effectiveness in calcium supplementation. *J Am Coll Nutr* 20(3):239–246.

Heaney RP, Rafferty K, Bierman J. 2005. Not all calcium-fortified beverages are equal. *Nutr Today* 40(1):39–44.

Hefnawi F, el-Zayat AF, Yacout MM. 1980. Physiologic studies of menstrual blood loss. II. Physiologic variables affecting the magnitude of menstrual blood loss. *Int J Gynaecol Obstet* 17(4): 348–352.

Heinrich HC. 1970. Intestinal iron absorption in man—methods of measurement, dose relationship, diagnostic, and therapeutic applications. In: Hallberg L, Harwerth HG, Vannotti A, eds. *Iron Deficiency. Pathogenesis, Clnical Aspects, Therapy*. New York: Academic Press. Pp. 213–296.

Held K, Antonijevic IA, Kunzel H, Uhr M, Wetter TC, Golly IC, Steiger A, Murck H. 2002. Oral Mg(2+) supplementation reverses age-related neuroendocrine and sleep EEG changes in humans. *Pharmacopsychiatry* 35(4):135–143.

Hendler SS, Rorvik D, eds. 2001. *Physicians Desk Reference for Nutritional Supplements*. Montvale, NJ: Medical Economics Company.

Henrotte JG, Hannoun C, Benech A, Dausset J. 1985. Relationship between postvaccinal anti-influenza antibodies, blood magnesium levels, and HLA antigens. *Hum Immunol* 12(1):1–8.

Hershko C. 1996. Iron and infection. In: Hallberg L, Asp NG, eds. *Iron Nutrition in Health and Disease*. London, UK: John Libbey and Company. Pp. 231–238.

Hill KE, Lloyd RS, Yang JG, Read R, Burk RF. 1991. The cDNA for rat selenoprotein P contains 10 TGA codons in the open reading frame. *J Biol Chem* 266(16):10050–10053.

Hill KE, Xia Y, Akesson B, Boeglin ME, Burk RF. 1996. Selenoprotein P concentration in plasma is an index of selenium status in selenium-deficient and selenium-supplemented Chinese subjects. *J Nutr* 126(1):138–145.

Hinton PS, Giordano C, Brownlie T, Haas JD. 2000. Iron supplementation improves endurance after training in iron-depleted, nonanemic women. *J Appl Physiol* 88(3):1103–1111.

Holsboer F. 2000. The corticosteroid receptor hypothesis of depression. *Neuropsychopharmacology* 23(5):477–501.

Hopkins RG, Failla ML. 1995. Chronic intake of a marginally low copper diet impairs in vitro activities of lymphocytes and neutrophils from male rats despite minimal impact on conventional indicators of copper status. *J Nutr* 125(10):2658–2668.

Hunt JR. 2003a. Bioavailability of iron, zinc, and other trace minerals from vegetarian diets. *Am J Clin Nutr* 78(3 Suppl):633S–639S.

Hunt JR. 2003b. High-, but not low-bioavailability diets enable substantial control of women's iron absorption in relation to body iron stores, with minimal adaptation within several weeks. *Am J Clin Nutr* 78(6):1168–1177.

Hunt JR. 2005 (June 13). *Bioavailability of Iron, Zinc, and Copper as Influenced by Host and Dietary Factors*. Paper presented at the Institue of Medicine Workshop on The Mineral Requirements for Cognitive and Physical Performance of Military Personnel, Washington, DC: Institute of Medicine Committee on Mineral Requirements for Cognitive and Physical Performance of Military Personnel.

Hunt JR, Penland JG. 1999. Iron status and depression in premenopausal women: An MMPI study. Minnesota Multiphasic Personality Inventory. *Behav Med* 25(2):62–68.

Hunt JR, Roughead ZK. 1999. Nonheme-iron absorption, fecal ferritin excretion, and blood indexes of iron status in women consuming controlled lactoovovegetarian diets for 8 wk. *Am J Clin Nutr* 69(5):944–952.

Hunt JR, Vanderpool RA. 2001. Apparent copper absorption from a vegetarian diet. *Am J Clin Nutr* 74(6):803–807.

Hunt JR, Johnson PE, Swan PB. 1987. Influence of usual zinc intake and zinc in a meal on $^{65}Zn$ retention and turnover in the rat. *J Nutr* 117(8):1427–1433.

Hunt JR, Matthys LA, Johnson LK. 1998. Zinc absorption, mineral balance, and blood lipids in women consuming controlled lactoovovegetarian and omnivorous diets for 8 wk. *Am J Clin Nutr* 67(3):421–430.

Ike K, Kawahara K, Danbara H, Kume K. 1992. Serum resistance and aerobactin iron uptake in avian Escherichia coli mediated by conjugative 100-megadalton plasmid. *J Vet Med Sci* 54(6): 1091–1088.

Ilich-Ernst JZ, McKenna AA, Badenhop NE, Clairmont AC, Andon MB, Nahhas RW, Goel P, Matkovic V. 1998. Iron status, menarche, and calcium supplementation in adolescent girls. *Am J Clin Nutr* 68(4):880–887.

Imada Y, Yoshioka S, Ueda T, Katayama S, Kuno Y, Kawahara R. 2002. Relationships between serum magnesium levels and clinical background factors in patients with mood disorders. *Psychiatry Clin Neurosci* 56(5):509–514.

IOM (Institute of Medicine). 1997. *Dietary Reference Intakes for Calcium, Phosphorus, Magnesium, Vitamin D, and Fluoride*. Washington, DC: National Academy Press.

IOM. 1998a. *Dietary Reference Intakes. Thiamin, Riboflavin, Niacin, Vitamin $B_6$, Folate, Vitamin $B_{12}$, Pantothenic Acid, Biotin, and Choline*. Washington, DC: National Academy Press.

IOM. 1998b. *Reducing Stress Fracture in Physically Active Military Women*. Washington, DC: National Academy Press.

IOM. 2000. *Dietary Reference Intakes for Vitamin C, Vitamin E, Selenium, and Carotenoids*. Washington, DC: National Academy Press.

IOM. 2001. *Dietary Reference Intakes. Vitamin A, Vitamin K, Arsenic, Boron, Chromium, Copper, Iodine, Iron, Manganese, Molybdenum, Nickel, Silicon, Vanadium, and Zinc*. Washington, DC: National Academy Press.

IOM. 2002/2005. *Dietary Reference Intakes. Energy, Carbohydrate, Fiber, Fat, Fatty Acids, Cholesterol, Protein, and Amino Acids*. Washington, DC: The National Academies Press.

IOM. 2004a. *Dietary Reference Intakes. Water, Potassium, Sodium, Chloride, and Sulfate*. Washington, DC: The National Academies Press.

IOM. 2004b. *Monitoring Metabolic Status: Predicting Decrements in Physiological and Physical Performance*. Washington, DC: The National Academies Press.

IOM. 2006. *Nutrient Composition of Rations for Short-Term, High-Intensity Combat Operations*. Washington, DC: The National Academies Press.

Ip C. 1998. Lessons from basic research in selenium and cancer prevention. *J Nutr* 128(11):1845–1854.

Iuliano-Burns S, Saxon L, Naughton G, Gibbons K, Bass SL. 2003. Regional specificity of exercise and calcium during skeletal growth in girls: A randomized controlled trial. *J Bone Miner Res* 18(1):156–162.

IZiNCG (International Zinc Nutrition Consultative Group). 2004. Overview of Zinc Nutrition In: Assessment of the Risk of Zinc Deficiency in Populations and Options for its Control. *Food Nutr Bull* 25(1 Suppl 2):S99–S129.

Izquierdo I. 1989. Different forms of post-training memory processing. *Behav Neural Biol* 51(2):171–202.

Jackson JL, Lesho E, Peterson C. 2000. Zinc and the common cold: A meta-analysis revisited. *J Nutr* 130(5S Suppl):1512S–1515S.

Jackson MJ, Dillon SA, Broome CS, McArdle A, Hart CA, McArdle F. 2004. Are there functional consequences of a reduction in selenium intake in UK subjects? *Proc Nutr Soc* 63(4): 513–517.

Jacob RA, Sandstead HH, Munoz JM, Klevay LM, Milne DB. 1981. Whole body surface loss of trace metals in normal males. *Am J Clin Nutr* 34(7):1379–1383.

Jayakumar S, Micallef-Eynaud PD, Lyon TD, Cramb R, Jilaihawi AN, Prakash D. 2005. Acquired copper deficiency following prolonged jejunostomy feeds. *Ann Clin Biochem* 42(Pt 3):227 231.

Jensen LB, Kollerup G, Quaade F, Sorensen OH. 2001. Bone minerals changes in obese women during a moderate weight loss with and without calcium supplementation. *J Bone Miner Res* 16(1):141–147.

Jimerson DC, Post RM, Carman JS, van Kammen DP, Wood JH, Goodwin FK, Bunney WE Jr. 1979. CSF calcium: Clinical correlates in affective illness and schizophrenia. *Biol Psychiatry* 14(1):37–51.

Johnson HL, Nelson RA, Consolazio CF. 1988. Effects of electrolyte and nutrient solutions on performance and metabolic balance. *Med Sci Sports Exerc* 20(1):26–33.

Johnson MA, Smith MM, Edmonds JT. 1998. Copper, iron, zinc, and manganese in dietary supplements, infant formulas, and ready-to-eat breakfast cereals. *Am J Clin Nutr* 67(5 Suppl):1035S–1040S.

Johnson PE, Hunt CD, Milne DB, Mullen LK. 1993. Homeostatic control of zinc metabolism in men: Zinc excretion and balance in men fed diets low in zinc. *Am J Clin Nutr* 57(4):557–565.

Johnson WT. 2005. Copper and brain function. In: Lieberman HR, Kanarek RB, Prasad C, eds. *Nutritional Neuroscience*. Boca Raton, FL: Taylor and Francis. Pp. 289–305.

Johnson WT, DeMars LC. 2004. Increased heme oxygenase-1 expression during copper deficiency in rats results from increased mitochondrial generation of hydrogen peroxide. *J Nutr* 134(6): 1328–1333.

Johnston FA , McMillan T, Evans ER. 1950. Perspiration as a factor influencing the requirement for calcium and iron. *J Nutr* 42(2):285–296.

Jones BH, Harris JM, Vinh TN, Rubin C. 1989. Exercise-induced stress fractures and stress reactions of bone: Epidemiology, etiology, and classification. *Exerc Sport Sci Rev* 17:379–422.

Kantak KM. 1988. Magnesium deficiency alters aggressive behavior and catecholamine function. *Behav Neurosci* 102(2):304–311.

Kao WH, Folsom AR, Nieto FJ, Mo JP, Watson RL, Brancati FL. 1999. Serum and dietary magnesium and the risk for type 2 diabetes mellitus: The Atherosclerosis Risk in Communities Study. *Arch Intern Med* 159(18):2151–2159.

Keen CL. 2005 (June 14). *Assessment of Zinc, Copper and Magnesium Status: Current Approaches and Promising New Directions*. Paper presented at the Institue of Medicine Workshop on The Mineral Requirements for Cognitive and Physical Performance of Military Personnel, Washington, DC: Institute of Medicine Committee on Mineral Requirements for Cognitive and Physical Performance of Military Personnel.

Kelley DS, Daudu PA, Taylor PC, Mackey BE, Turnlund JR. 1995. Effects of low-copper diets on human immune response. *Am J Clin Nutr* 62(2):412–416.

Kelly EW, Jonson SR, Cohen ME, Shaffer R. 2000. Stress fractures of the pelvis in female navy recruits: An analysis of possible mechanisms of injury. *Mil Med* 165(2):142–146.

Kenny AM, Prestwood KM, Biskup B, Robbins B, Zayas E, Kleppinger A, Burleson JA, Raisz LG. 2004. Comparison of the effects of calcium loading with calcium citrate or calcium carbonate on bone turnover in postmenopausal women. *Osteoporos Int* 15(4):290–294.

Keshan Disease Research Group. 1979. Observations on effect of sodium selenite in prevention of Keshan Disease. *Chinese Med J* 92(7):471–476.

Kikukawa A, Kobayashi A. 2002. Changes in urinary zinc and copper with strenuous physical exercise. *Aviat Space Environ Med* 73(10):991–995.

King JC, Keen CL. 1999. Zinc. In: Shils ME, Olson JA, Shike M, Ross AC, eds. *Modern Nutrition in Health and Disease*. 9th ed. Baltimore, MD: Williams & Wilkins. Pp. 223–239.

King JC, Shames DM, Woodhouse LR. 2000. Zinc homeostasis in humans. *J Nutr* 130(5S Suppl): 1360S–1366S.

Kiremidjian-Schumacher L, Roy M. 2001. Effect of selenium on the immunocompetence of patients with head and neck cancer and on adoptive immunotherapy of early and established lesions. *Biofactors* 14(1–4):161–168.

Kleerekoper M, Brienza RS, Schultz LR, Johnson CC. 1991. Oral contraceptive use may protect against low bone mass. Henry Ford Hospital Osteoporosis Cooperative Research Group. *Arch Intern Med* 151(10):1971–1976

Klein CJ, Moser-Veillon PB, Douglass LW, Ruben KA, Trocki O. 1995. A longitudinal study of urinary calcium, magnesium, and zinc excretion in lactating and nonlactating postpartum women. *Am J Clin Nutr* 61(4):779–786.

Klesges RC, Ward KD, Shelton ML, Applegate WB, Cantler ED, Palmieri GM, Harmon K, Davis J. 1996. Changes in bone mineral content in male athletes. Mechanisms of action and intervention effects. *J Am Med Assoc* 276(3):226–230.

Klevay LM, Buchet JP, Bunker VW, Clayton BE, Gibson RS, Medeiros DM, Moser-Veillon PB, Patterson KY, Taper LJ, Wolf WR. 1993. Copper in the western diet (Belgium Canada, U.K., and USA). In: Anke M, Meissner D, Mills CF, eds. *Trace Elements in Man and Animals—TEMA-8. Proceedings of the Eigth International Symposium on Trace Elements in Man and Animals.*Gersdorf, Germany: Verlag Media Touristik. Pp. 207–210.

Kobayashi Y, Ogra Y, Ishiwata K, Takayama H, Aimi N, Suzuki KT. 2002. Selenosugars are key and urinary metabolites for selenium excretion within the required to low-toxic range. *Proc Natl Acad Sci* 99(25):15932–15936.

Kochanowski BA, Sherman AR. 1985. Decreased antibody formation in iron-deficient rat pups—effect of iron repletion. *Am J Clin Nutr* 41(2):278–284.

Kopp SJ, Klevay LM, Feliksik JM. 1983. Physiological and metabolic characterization of a cardiomyopathy induced by chronic copper deficiency. *Am J Physiol* 245(5 Pt 1):H855–H866.

Koury JC, de Olilveria AV Jr, Portella ES, de Olilveria CF, Lopes GC, Donangelo CM. 2004. Zinc and copper biochemical indices of antioxidant status in elite athletes of different modalities. *Int J Sport Nutr Exerc Metab* 14(3):358–372.

Krotkiewski M, Gudmundsson M, Backstrom P, Mandroukas K. 1982. Zinc and muscle strength and endurance. *Acta Physiol Scand* 116(3):309–311.

Kryukov GV, Castellano S, Novoselov SV, Lobanov AV, Zehtab O, Guigo R, Gladyshev VN. 2003. Characterization of mammalian selenoproteomes. *Science* 300(5624):1439–1443.

Kuehnelt D, Kienzl N, Traar P, Le NH, Francesconi KA, Ochi T. 2005. Selenium metabolites in human urine after ingestion of selenite, L-selenomethionine, or DL-selenomethionine: A quantitative case study by HPLC/ICPMS. *Anal Bioanal Chem* 383(2):235–246.

Kuvibidila SR, Kitchens D, Baliga BS. 1999. In vivo and in vitro iron deficiency reduces protein kinase C activity and translocation in murine splenic and purified T cells. *J Cell Biochem* 74(3):468–478.

Lakshmanan FL, Rao RB, Kim WW, Kelsay JL. 1984. Magnesium intakes, balances, and blood levels of adults consuming self-selected diets. *Am J Clin Nutr* 40(6 Suppl):1380–1389.

Lampe JW, Slavin JL, Apple FS. 1991. Iron status of active women and the effect of running a marathon on bowel function and gastrointestinal blood loss. *Int J Sports Med* 12(2):173–179.

Lane TE, Wu-Hsieh BA, Howard DH. 1991. Iron limitation and the gamma interferon-mediated antihistoplasma state of murine macrophages. *Infect Immun* 59(7):2274–2278.

Lau EM, Woo J, Leung PC, Swaminathan R, Leung D. 1992. The effects of calcium supplementation and exercise on bone density in elderly Chinese women. *Osteoporos Int* 2(4):168–173.

Lee DY, Prasad AS, Hydrick-Adair C, Brewer G, Johnson PE. 1993. Homeostasis of zinc in marginal human zinc deficiency: Role of absorption and endogenous excretion of zinc. *J Lab Clin Med* 122(5):549–556.

Lee HH, Prasad AS, Brewer GJ, Owyang C. 1989. Zinc absorption in human small intestine. *Am J Physiol* 256(1 Pt 1):G87–G91.

Lee J, Pena MM, Nose Y, Thiele DJ. 2002. Biochemical characterization of the human copper transporter Ctr1. *J Biol Chem* 277(6):4380–4387.

Lee P, Gelbart T, West C, Halloran C, Beutler E. 2002. Seeking candidate mutations that affect iron homeostasis. *Blood Cells Mol Dis* 29(3):471–487.

Leggett BA, Brown NN, Bryant SJ, Duplock L, Powell LW, Halliday JW. 1990. Factors affecting the concentrations of ferritin in serum in a healthy Australian population. *Clin Chem* 36(7): 1350–1355.

Lesourd BM. 1997. Nutrition and immunity in the elderly: Modification of immune responses with nutritional treatments. *Am J Clin Nutr* 66(2):478S–484S.

Levander OA, Sutherland B, Morris VC, King JC. 1981. Selenium metabolism in human nutrition. In: Spallholz JE, Martin JL, Ganther HE, eds. *Selenium in Biology and Medicine.* Westport, CT: AVI. Pp. 256–268.

Levenson DI, Bockman RS. 1994. A review of calcium preparations. *Nutr Rev* 52(7):221–232.

Liao F, Folsom AR, Brancati FL. 1998. Is low magnesium concentration a risk factor for coronary heart disease? The Atherosclerosis Risk in Communities (ARIC) Study. *Am Heart J* 136(3): 480–490.

Lijnen P, Hespel P, Fagard R, Lysens R, Vanden Eynde E, Goris M, Goossens W, Amery A. 1988. Erythrocyte 2,3-diphosphoglycerate concentration before and after a marathon in men. *Eur J Appl Physiol Occup Physiol* 57(4):452–455.

Lloyd T, Andon MB, Rollings N, Martel JK, Landis JR, Demers LM, Eggli DF, Kieselhorst K, Kulin HE. 1993. Calcium supplementation and bone mineral density in adolescent girls. *J Am Med Assoc* 270(7):841–844.

Lonnerdal B. 1989. Intestinal absorption of zinc. In: Mills CF, eds. *Zinc in Human Biology.* London, Springer-Verlag. Pp. 33–55.

Lonnerdal B. 2000. Dietary factors influencing zinc absorption. *J Nutr* 130(5S Suppl):1378S–1383S.

Lopez Moreno JM, Gonzalez G, Campino C, Salvatierra AM, Croxatto HB. 1992. Serum osteocalcin in normal menstrual cycle. *Medicina (B Aires)* 52(1):37–40.

Lukaski HC. 2005. Low dietary zinc decreases erythrocyte carbonic anhydrase activities and impairs cardiorespiratory function in men during exercise. *Am J Clin Nutr* 81(5):1045–1051.

Lukaski HC, Bolonchuk WW, Klevay LM, Milne DB, Sandstead HH. 1983. Maximal oxygen consumption as related to magnesium, copper, and zinc nutriture. *Am J Clin Nutr* 37(3):407–415.

Lukaski HC, Hoverson BS, Gallagher SK, Bolonchuk WW. 1990. Physical training and copper, iron, and zinc status of swimmers. *Am J Clin Nutr* 51(6):1093–1099.

Mackler B, Person R, Ochs H, Finch CA. 1984. Iron deficiency in the rat: Effects on neutrophil activiation and metabolism. *Pediatr Res* 18(6):549–551.

Maddalozzo GF, Snow CM. 2000. High intensity resistance training: Effects on bone in older men and women. *Calcif Tissue Int* 66(6):399–404.

Magnusson B, Hallberg L, Rossander L, Swolin B. 1984. Iron metabolism and "sports anemia." I. A study of several iron parameters in elite runners with differences in iron status. *Acta Med Scand* 216(2):149–155.

Mahalko JR, Sandstead HH, Johnson LK, Milne DB. 1983. Effect of a moderate increase in dietary protein on the retention and excretion of Ca, Cu, Fe, Mg, P, and Zn by adult males. *Am J Clin Nutr* 37(1):8–14.

Makropoulos V, Bruning T, Schulze-Osthoff K. 1996. Selenium-mediated inhibition of transcription factor NF-kappa B and HIV-1 LTR promoter activity. *Arch Toxicol* 70(5):277–283.

Margulies JY, Simkin A, Leichter I, Bivas A, Steinberg R, Giladi M, Stein M, Kashtan H, Milgrom C. 1986. Effect of intense physical activity on the bone-mineral content in the lower limbs of young adults. *J Bone Joint Surg Am* 68(7):1090–1093.

May JM, Mendiratta S, Hill KE, Burk RF. 1997. Reduction of dehydroascorbate to ascorbate by the selenoenzyme thioredoxin reductase. *J Biol Chem* 272(36):22607–22610.

M'Buyamba-Kabangu JR, Lijnen P, Fagard R, Groeseneken D, Koninckx P, Lissens W, Van Assche F, Amery A. 1985. Erythrocyte concentrations and transmembrane fluxes of sodium and potassium and biochemical measurements during the menstrual cycle in normal women. *Am J Obstet Gynecol* 151(5):687–693.

McCoy JH, Kenney MA. 1984. Magnesium and immunocompetence. In: Watson RR, eds. *Nutrition, Disease Resistance, and Immune Function.* New York: Marcel Dekker. Pp. 223–247.

Mei Z, Cogswell ME, Parvanta I, Lynch S, Beard JL, Stoltzfus RJ, Grummer-Strawn LM. 2005. Hemoglobin and ferritin are currently the most efficient indicators of population response to iron interventions: An analysis of nine randomized controlled trials. *J Nutr* 135(8):1974–1980.

Melton LJ 3rd, Atkinson EJ, O'Fallon WM, Wahner HW, Riggs BL. 1993. Long-term fracture prediction by bone mineral assessed at different skeletal sites. *J Bone Miner Res* 8(10):1227–1233.

Metin G, Atukeren P, Alturfan AA, Gulyasar T, Kaya M, Gumustas MK. 2003. Lipid peroxidation, erythrocyte superoxide-dismutase activity and trace metals in young male footballers. *Yonsei Med J* 44(6):979–986.

Milne DB, Nielsen FH. 1996. Effects of a diet low in copper on copper-status indicators in postmenopausal women. *Am J Clin Nutr* 63(3):358–364.

Milne DB, Canfield WK, Mahalko JR, Sandstead HH. 1983. Effect of dietary zinc on whole body surface loss of zinc: Impact on estimation of zinc retention by balance method. *Am J Clin Nutr* 38(2):181–186.

Milne DB, Johnson PE, Klevay LM, Sandstead HH. 1990. Effect of copper intake on balance, absorption, and status indices of copper in men. *Nutr Res* 10:975–986.

Milne DB, Nielsen FH, Lykken GI. 1991. Effects of dietary copper and sulfur amino acids on copper homeostasis and selected indices of copper status in men.. In: Momcilovic B, ed. *Trace Elem Man Animals.* TEMA-7 Zagreb, Yugoslavia: IMI, 1990. New York: Springer. Pp. 5-12–5-13.

Mitchell HH, Hamilton TS. 1949. The dermal excretion under controlled environmental conditions of nitrogen and mineral sin human subjects with particular reference to calcium and iron. *J Biol Chem* 178:345–361.

Miyamura JB, McNutt SW, Wenkam NS. 1987. Altered zinc status of soldiers under field conditions. *J Am Diet Assoc* 87(5):595–597.

Montain SJ, Young AJ. 2003. Diet and physical performance. *Appetite* 40(3):255–267.

Mordes JP, Wacker WEC. 1978. Excess magnesium. *Pharmacol Rev* 29(4):273–300.

Muneyyirci-Delale O, Nacharaju VL, Altura BM, Altura BT. 1998. Sex steroid hormones modulate serum ionized magnesium an dcalcium levels throughout the menstrual cycle in women. *Fertility Sterility* 69(5):958–962.

Murck H. 2002. Magnesium and affective disorders. *Nutr Neurosci* 5(6):375–389.

Murck H, Steiger A. 1998. Mg2+ reduces ACTH secretion and enhances spindle power without changing delta power during sleep in men—possible therapeutic implications. *Psychopharmacology (Berl)* 137(3):247–252.

Murray MJ, Murray AB, Murray MB, Murray CJ. 1978. The adverse effect of iron repletion on the course of certain infections. *Br Med J* 2(6145):1113–1115.

Muse KN, Manolagas SC, Deftos LJ, Alexander N, Yen SS. 1986. Calcium-regulating hormones across the menstrual cycle. *J Clin Endocrinol Metab* 62(6):1313–1316.

Nachtigall D, Nielsen P, Fischer R, Engelhardt R, Gabbe EE. 1996. Iron deficiency in distance runners. A reinvestigation using Fe-labelling and non-invasive liver iron quantification. *Int J Sports Med* 17(7):473–479.

National Institute of Mental Health. 1983. *National Institute of Mental Health Premenstrual Syndrome Workshop Guidelines.* Rockville, MD: National Institute of Mental Health. Pp. 14–15.

Neglen P, Qvarfordt P, Eklof B. 1985. Peroral magnesium hydroxide therapy and intermittent claudication—a preliminary report. *Vasa* 14(3):285–288.

Nemeth E, Preza GC, Jung CL, Kaplan J, Waring AJ, Ganz T. 2006. The N-terminus of hepcidin is essential for its interaction with ferroportin: Structure-function study. *Blood* 107(1):328–333.

Neve J. 1995. Human selenium supplementation as assessed by changes in blood selenium concentration and glutathione peroxidase activity. *J Trace Elem Med Biol* 9(2):65–73.

Newhouse IJ, Clement DB. 1995. The efficacy of iron supplementation in iron depleted women. In: Kies CV, Driskell JA, eds. *Sports Nutrition. Minerals and Electrolytes.* Boca Raton, FL: CRC Press. Pp. 48–57.

Newhouse IJ, Finstad EW. 2000. The effects of magnesium supplementation on exercise performance. *Clin J Sport Med* 10(3):195–200.

Nicklas TA, Webber LS, Kern SL, Powers CR, Harsha DW, Berenson GS. 1993. Fort Polk Heart Smart Program. Part III: Assessment of dietary intake of military wives. *Mil Med* 158(5): 312–316.

Nicolas G, Bennoun M, Devaux I, Beaumont C, Grandchamp B, Kahn A, Vaulont S. 2001. Lack of hepcidin gene expression and severe tissue iron overload in upstream stimulatory factor 2 (USF2) knockout mice. *Proc Natl Acad Sci* 98(15):8780–8785.

Nicolas G, Bennoun M, Porteu A, Mativet S, Beaumont C, Grandchamp B, Sirito M, Sawadogo M, Kahn A, Vaulont S. 2002. Severe iron deficiency anemia in transgenic mice expressing liver hepcidin. *Proc Natl Acad Sci* 99(7):4596–4601.

Nielsen HK, Brixen K, Bouillon R, Mosekilde L. 1990. Changes in biochemical markers of osteoblastic activity during the menstrual cycle. *J Clin Endocrinol Metab* 70(5):1431–1437.

Nieves JW. 2005 (June 14). *Physical Activity and Nutrition: Effects on Bone Turnover, Bone Mass, and Stress Fractures.* Paper presented at the Institue of Medicine Workshop on The Mineral Requirements for Cognitive and Physical Performance of Military Personnel, Washington, DC: Institute of Medicine Committee on Mineral Requirements for Cognitive and Physical Performance of Military Personnel.

Nieves J, Zion M, Ruffing J, Garrett P, Lindsay R, Cosman F. 2005. Eating disorders and amenorrhea are strong predictors of change in bone mass in physically active young females. Abstract presented at the 27th Annual Meeting of the American Society for Bone and Mineral Research Nashville TN. M013.

NRC (National Research Council). 1983. *Selenium in Nutrition.* Washington, DC: National Academy Press.

NRC. 1989. *Recommended Dietary Allowances.* 10th ed. Washington, DC: National Academy Press.

Nuviala RJ, Lapieza MG, Bernal E. 1999. Magnesium, zinc, and copper status in women involved in different sports. *Int J Sport Nutr* 9(3):295–309.

Office of Dietary Supplements. 2005. *Dietary Supplement Fact Sheet: Calcium.* [Online]. Office of Dietary Supplements, National Institutes of Health. Available: http://ods.od.nih.gov/factsheets/calcium.asp [accessed December 12, 2005].

Office of Dietary Supplements. 2006. *Dietary Supplement Fact Sheet: Iron.* [Online]. Office of Dietary Supplements, National Institutes of Health. Available: http://dietary-supplements.info.nih.gov/factsheets/iron.asp [accessed February 14, 2006].

Omokhodion FO, Howard JM. 1994. Trace elements in the sweat of acclimatized persons. *Clin Chim Acta* 231(1):23–28.

Osler M, Milman N, Heitmann BL. 1998. Dietary and non-dietary factors associated with iron status in a cohort of Danish adults followed for six years. *Eur J Clin Nutr* 52(6):459–463.

O'Toole ML, Johnson KC, Satterfield S, Bush AJ, Koo WW, Klesges RC, Applegate WB. 2000. Do sweat calcium losses affect bone mass during firefighter training? *J Occup Environ Med* 42(11):1054–1059.

Pajonk FG, Kessler H, Supprian T, Hamzei P, Bach D, Schweickhardt J, Herrmann W, Obeid R, Simons A, Falkai P, Multhaup G, Bayer TA. 2005. Cognitive decline correlates with low plasma concentrations of copper in patients with mild to moderate Alzheimer's disease. *J Alzheimers Dis* 8(1):23–27.

Palacios C, Wigertz K, Weaver CM. 2003. Comparison of 24 hour whole body versus patch tests for estimating body surface electrolyte losses. *Int J Sport Nutr Exerc Metab* 13(4):479–488.

Patki PS, Singh J, Gokhale SV, Bulakh PM, Shrotri DS, Patwardhan B. 1990. Efficacy of potassium and magnesium in essential hypertension: A double-blind, placebo controlled, crossover study. *Br Med J* 301(6751):521–523.

Paulev PE, Jordal R, Pedersen NS. 1983. Dermal excretion of iron in intensely training athletes. *Clin Chim Acta* 127(1):19–27.

Penland JG. 1988. Effects of trace element nutrition on sleep patterns in adult women. 2(4):A434.

Penland JG. 1995. Quantitative analysis of EEG effects following experimental marginal magnesium and boron deprivation. *Magnes Res* 8(4):341–358.

Penland JG. 2005 (June 15). *Zinc and Other Mineral Nutrients Required for Cognitive Function and Behavior in Military Personnel.* Paper presented at the Institue of Medicine Workshop on The Mineral Requirements for Cognitive and Physical Performance of Military Personnel, Washington, DC: Institute of Medicine Committee on Mineral Requirements for Cognitive and Physical Performance of Military Personnel.

Penland JG, Finley JW. 1995. Dietary selenium and mood states in healthy young men. *N Dak Acad Sci Proc* 49:26.

Penland JG, Johnson PE. 1993. Dietary calcium and manganese effects on menstrual cycle symptoms. *Am J Obstet Gynecol* 168(5):1417–1423.

Penland JG, Prohaska JR. 2004. Abnormal motor function persists following recovery from perinatal copper deficiency in rats. *J Nutr* 134(8):1984–1988.

Penland JG, Milne DB, Davis CW. 2000. Moderately high zinc intake impairs verbal memory of healthy postmenopausal women on a low copper diet. In: Roussel AM, Anderson RA, Favrier AE, eds. *Trace Elements in Man and Animals 10*. New York: Kluwer Academic/Plenum Publishers. Pp. 1025–1030.

Penland JG, Duffield-Lillico AJ, Tompson CD. in press. Selenium supplementation and mood states of adults with low-selenium status. *Br J Nutr.*

Percival SS. 1995. Neutropenia caused by copper deficiency: Possible mechanisms of action. *Nutr Rev* 53(3):59–66.

Percival S. 2005 (June 14). *Copper, Zinc, and Immunity*. Paper presented at the Institue of Medicine Workshop on The Mineral Requirements for Cognitive and Physical Performance of Military Personnel, Washington, DC: Institute of Medicine Committee on Mineral Requirements for Cognitive and Physical Performance of Military Personnel.

Pinna K, Kelley DS, Taylor PC, King JC. 2002. Immune functions are maintained in healthy men with low zinc intake. *J Nutr* 132(7):2033–2036.

Pitkin RM, Reynolds WA, Williams GA, Hargis GK. 1978. Calcium-regulating hormones during the menstrual cycle. *J Clin Endocrinol Metab* 47(3):626–632.

Poenaru S, Rouhani S, Durlach J, Aymard N, Belkahla F, Rayssiguier Y, Iovino M. 1984. Vigilance states and cerebral monoamine metabolism in experimental magnesium deficiency. *Magnesium* 3(3):145–151.

Poirier KA. 1994. Summary of the derivation of the reference dose for selenium. In: Mertz W, Abernaty CO, Olin SS, eds. *Risk Assessment of Essential Elements*. Washington, DC: ILSI Press. Pp. 157–166.

Popoviciu L, Corfariu O, Fagaraseanu M, Kollo K, Bagathai I. 1987. Polysomnographic research in sleep disorders associated with magnesium deficiency. *Neurol Psychiatr (Bucur)* 25(2): 83–90.

Powis G, Gasdaska JR, Gasdaska PY, Berggren M, Kirkpatrick DL, Engman L, Cotgreave IA, Angulo M, Baker A. 1997. Selenium and the thioredoxin redox system: Effects on cell growth and death. *Oncol Res* 9(6–7):303–312.

Prasad AS, Fitzgerald JT, Bao B, Beck FW, Chandrasekar PH. 2000. Duration of symptoms and plasma cytokine levels in patients with the common cold treated with zinc acetate. A randomized, double-blind, placebo-controlled trial. *Ann Intern Med* 133(4):245–252.

Prince RL, Smith M, Dick IM, Price RI, Webb PG, Henderson NK, Harris MM. 1991. Prevention of postmenopausal osteoporosis. A comparative study of exercise, calcium supplementation, and hormone-replacement therapy. *N Engl J Med* 325(17):1189–1195.

Proudfoot AT. 1993. *Acute Poisoning: Diagnosis and Management*. 2nd ed. Oxford: Butterworth-Heinemann. Pp. 133–137.

Quamme GA. 1997. Renal magnesium handling: New insights in understanding old problems. *Kidney Int* 52(5):1180–1195.

Raffin SB, Woo CH, Roost KT, Price DC, Schmid R. 1974. Intestinal absorption of hemoglobin iron-heme cleavage by mucosal heme oxygenase. *J Clin Invest* 54(6):1344–1352.

Raich PC, Lu J, Thompson HJ, Combs GF Jr. 2001. Selenium in cancer prevention: Clinical issues and implications. *Cancer Invest* 19(5):540–553.

Ranade VV, Somberg JC. 2001. Bioavailability and pharmacokinetics of magnesium after administration of magnesium salts to humans. *Am J Ther* 8(5):345–357.

Rangan AM, Blight GD, Binns CW. 1998. Iron status and non-specific symptoms of female students. *J Am Coll Nutr* 17(4):351–355.

Raunikar RA, Sabio H. 1992. Anemia in the adolescent athlete. *Am J Dis Child* 146(10):1201–1205.

Rawson JR, Medeiros DM. 1989. Macronutrient, copper, and zinc intakes of young adult males as determined by duplicate food samples and diet records. *Nutr Rept Int* 39(6):1149–1159.

Recker RR, Davies KM, Hinders SM, Heaney RP, Stegman MR, Kimmel DB. 1992. Bone gain in young adult women. *J Am Med Assoc* 268(17):2403–2408.

Reeves RR, Parker JD, Konkle-Parker DJ. 2005. War-related mental health of today's veterans. *J Psychosoc Nurs Ment Health Serv* 43(7):18–28.

Reiser S, Ferretti RJ, Fields M, Smith JC Jr. 1983. Role of dietary fructose in the enhancement of mortality and bioch emical changes associated with copper deficiency in rats. *Am J Clin Nutr* 38(2):214–222.

Ribeiro-Alves MA, Trugo LC, Donangelo CM. 2003. Use of oral contraceptives blunts the calciuric effect of caffeine in young adult women. *J Nutr* 133(2):393–398.

Ricci TA, Chowdhury HA, Heymsfield SB, Stahl T, Pierson RN Jr, Shapses SA. 1998. Calcium supplementation suppresses bone turnover during weight reduction in postmenopausal women. *J Bone Miner Res* 13(6):1045–1050.

Riedt CS, Cifuentes M, Stahl T, Chowdhury HA, Schlussel Y, Shapses SA. 2005. Overweight post-menopausal women lose bone with moderate weight reduction and 1 g/day calcium intake. *J Bone Miner Res* 20(3):455–463.

Ripari P, Pieralisi G, Giamberardino MA, Resina A, Vecchiet L. 1989. Effects of magnesium pidolate on some cardiorespiratory submaximal effort parameters. *Magnesium Res* 2:70.

Ritchie EC, Owens M. 2004. Military issues. *Psychiatr Clin North Am* 27(3):459–471.

Rodriguez Tuya I, Pinilla Gil E, Maynar Marino M, Garcia-Monco Carra RM, Sanchez Misiego A. 1996. Evaluation of the influence of physical activity on the plasma concentrations of several trace metals. *Eur J Appl Physiol Occup Physiol* 73(3–4):299–303.

Roncagliolo M, Garrido M, Walter T, Peirano P, Lozoff B. 1998. Evidence of altered central nervous system development in infants with iron deficiency anemia at 6 mo: Delayed maturation of auditory brainstem responses. *Am J Clin Nutr* 68(3):683–690.

Rosenstein DL, Ryschon TW, Niemela JE, Elin RJ, Balaban RS, Rubinow DR. 1995. Skeletal muscle intracellular ionized magnesium measured by 31P-NMR spectroscopy across the menstrual cycle. *J Am Coll Nutr* 14(5):486–490.

Roughead ZK, Zito CA, Hunt JR. 2005. Inhibitory effects of dietary calcium on the initial uptake and subsequent retention of heme and nonheme iron in humans: comparisons using an intestinal lavage method. *Am J Clin Nutr* 82(3):589–597.

Rowland TW, Stagg L, Kelleher JF. 1991. Iron deficiency in adolescent girls. Are athletes at increased risk? *J Adolesc Health* 12(1):22–25.

Rusinko N, Prohaska JR. 1985. Adenine nucleotide and lactate levels in organs from copper-deficient mice and brindled mice. *J Nutr* 115(7):936–943.

Ruz M, Solomons NW. 1990. Mineral excretion during acute, dehydrating diarrhea treated with oral rehydration therapy. *Pediatr Res* 27(2):170–175.

Ryschon TW, Rosenstein DL, Rubinow DR, Niemela JE, Elin RJ, Balaban RS. 1996. Relationship between skeletal muscle intracellular ionized magnesium and measurements of blood magnesium. *J Lab Clin Med* 127(2):207–213.

Sacks FM, Willett WC, Smith A, Brown LE, Rosner B, Moore TJ. 1998. Effect on blood pressure of potassium, calcium, and magnesium in women with low habitual intake. *Hypertension* 31(1):131–138.

Sait Gonen M, Kisakol G, Savas Cilli A, Dikbas O, Gungor K, Inal A, Kaya A. 2004. Assessment of anxiety in subclinical thyroid disorders. *Endocr J* 51(3):311–315.

Sandstrom B, Cederblad A. 1980. Zinc absorption from composite meals. II. Influence of the main protein source. *Am J Clin Nutr* 33(8):1778–1783.

Sandstrom B, Arvidsson B, Cederblad A, Bjorn-Rasmussen E. 1980. Zinc absorption from composite meals. I. The significance of whest extraction rate, zinc, calcium, and protein content in meals based on bread. *Am J Clin Nutr* 33(4):739–745.

Sakhaee K, Bhuket T, Adams-Huet B, Rao DS. 1999. Meta-analysis of calcium bioavailability: A comparison of calcium citrate with calcium carbonate. *Am J Ther* 6(6):313–321.

Schlemmer A, Hassager C, Risteli J, Risteli L, Jensen SB, Christiansen C. 1993. Possible variation in bone resorption during the normal menstrual cycle. *Acta Endocrinol (Copenh)* 129(5):388–392.

Schubert A, Holden JM, Wolf WR. 1987. Selenium content of a core group of foods based on a critical evaluation of published analytical data. *J Am Diet Assoc* 87(3):285–299.

Schumann K, Classen HG, Dieter HH, Konig J, Multhaup G, Rukgauer M, Summer KH, Bernhardt J, Biesalski HK. 2002. Hohenheim consensus workshop: Copper. *Eur J Clin Nutr* 56(6):469–483.

Schwartz R, Apgar BJ, Wien EM. 1986. Apparent absorption and retention of Ca, Cu, Mg, Mn, and Zn from a diet containing bran. *Am J Clin Nutr* 43(3):444–455.

Schwellnus MP, Nicol J, Laubscher R, Noakes TD. 2004. Serum electrolyte concentrations and hydration status are not associated with exercise associated muscle cramping (EAMC) in distance runners. *Br J Sports Med* 38(4):488–492.

Shaffer RA. 2001. Incidence and prevalence of stress fractures in military and athletic populations. In: Burr D, Milgrom C, eds. *Muscoloskeletal Fatigue and Stress Fractures*. New York: CRC Press. Pp. 1–14.

Shaffer RA, Brodine SK, Ito SI, Le AT. 1999. Epidemiology of illness and injury among U.S. Navy and Marine Corps female training populations. *Mil Med* 164(1):17–21.

Shapses SA, Cifuentes M. 2004. Body weight/composition and weight change. Effects on bone health. In: Holick MF, Dawson-Hughes B, eds. *Nutrition and Bone Health*. Totowa, NJ: Humana Press. Pp. 549–573.

Shapses SA, Von Thun NL, Heymsfield SB, Ricci TA, Ospina M, Pierson RN Jr, Stahl T. 2001. Bone turnover and density in obese premenopausal women during moderate weight loss and calcium supplementation. *J Bone Miner Res* 16(7):1329–1336.

Shaw NS, Chin CJ, Pan WH. 1995. A vegetarian diet rich in soybean products compromises iron status in young students. *J Nutr* 125(2):212–219.

Shayeghi M, Latunde-Dada GO, Oakhill JS, Laftah AH, Takeuchi K, Halliday N, Khan Y, Warley A, McCann FE, Hider RC, Frazer DM, Anderson GJ, Vulpe CD, Simpson RJ, McKie AT. 2005. Identification of an intestinal heme transporter. *Cell* 122(5):789–801.

Sheehan KM, Murphy MM, Reynolds K, Creedon JF, White J, Kazel M. 2003. The response of a bone resorption marker to marine recruit training. *Mil Med* 168(10):797–801.

Sherwood RA, Rocks BF, Stewart A, Saxton RS. 1986. Magnesium and the premenstrual syndrome. *Ann Clin Biochem* 23(Pt 6):667–670.

Shils ME. 1969. Experimental human magnesium depletion. *Medicine (Baltimore)* 48(1):61–85.

Shils ME. 1999. Magnesium. In: Shils ME, Olson JA, Shike M, Ross AC. *Modern Nutrition in Health and Disease*. Baltimore, MD: Williams and Wilkins. Pp. 169–192.

Shirreffs SM, Maughan RJ. 1997. Whole body sweat collection in humans: An improved method with preliminary data on electrolyte content. *J Appl Physiol* 82(1):336–341.

Shor-Posner G, Lecusay R, Miguez MJ, Moreno-Black G, Zhang G, Rodriguez N, Burbano X, Baum M, Wilkie F. 2003. Psychological burden in the era of HAART: Impact of selenium therapy. *Int J Psychiatry Med* 33(1):55–69.

Siegel AJ, Hennekens CH, Solomon HS, Van Boeckel B. 1979. Exercise-related hematuria. Findings in a group of marathon runners. *J Am Med Assoc* 241(4):391–392.

Sies H, Sharov VS, Klotz LO, Briviba K. 1997. Glutathione peroxidase protects against peroxynitrite-mediated oxidations. A new function for selenoproteins as peroxynitrite reductase. *J Biol Chem* 272(44):27812–27817.

Singewald N, Sinner C, Hetzenauer A, Sartori SB, Murck H. 2004. Magnesium-deficient diet alters depression- and anxiety-related behavior in mice—influence of desipramine and Hypericum perforatum extract. *Neuropharmacology* 47(8):1189–1197.

Singh A, Smoak BL, Patterson KY, LeMay LG, Veillon C, Deuster PA. 1991. Biochemical indices of selected trace minerals in men: Effect of stress. *Am J Clin Nutr* 53(1):126–131.

Singh A, Moses FM, Deuster PA. 1992. Vitamin and mineral status in physically active men: Effects of a high-potency supplement. *Am J Clin Nutr* 55(1):1–7.

Singh A, Failla ML, Deuster PA. 1994. Exercise-induced changes in immune function: Effects of zinc supplementation. *J Appl Physiol* 76(6):2298–2303.

Singh A, Papanicolaou DA, Lawrence LL, Howell EA, Chrousos GP, Deuster PA. 1999. Neuroendocrine responses to running in women after zinc and vitamin E supplementation. *Med Sci Sports Exerc* 31(4):536–542.

Singh MAF. 2004. Exercise and bone health. In: Holick MF, Dawson-Hughes B, eds. *Nutrition and Bone Health.*Totowa, NJ: Humana Press. Pp. 515–548.

Smith NJ, Rios E. 1974. Iron metabolism and iron deficiency in infancy and childhood. *Adv Pediatr* 21:239–280.

Smith SM, Wastney ME, Morukov BV, Larina IM, Nyquist LE, Abrams SA, Taran EN, Shih CY, Nillen JL, Davis-Street JE, Rice BL, Lane HW. 1999. Calcium metabolism before, during, and after a 3-mo spaceflight: Kinetic and biochemical changes. *Am J Physiol* 277(1 Pt 2): R1–R10.

Smorgon C, Mari E, Atti AR, Dalla Nora E, Zamboni PF, Calzoni F, Passaro A, Fellin R. 2004. Trace elements and cognitive impairment: An elderly cohort study. *Arch Gerontol Geriatr Suppl* (9):393–402.

Spear AT, Sherman AR. 1992. Iron deficiency alters DMBA-induced tumor burden and natural killer cell cytotoxicity in rats. *J Nutr* 122(1):46–55.

Specker BL. 1996. Evidence for an interaction between calcium intake and physical activity on changes in bone mineral density. *J Bone Miner Res* 11(10):1539–1544.

Specker B, Binkley T. 2003. Randomized trial of physical activity and calcium supplementation on bone mineral content in 3- to 5-year-old children. *J Bone Miner Res* 18(5):885–892.

Spencer H, Kramer L, Norris C, Osis D. 1984. Effect of calcium and phosphorus on zinc metabolism in man. *Am J Clin Nutr* 40(6):1213–1218.

Squitti R, Lupoi D, Pasqualetti P, Dal Forno G, Vernieri F, Chiovenda P, Rossi L, Cortesi M, Cassetta E, Rossini PM. 2002. Elevation of serum copper levels in Alzheimer's disease. *Neurology* 59(8):1153–1161.

Srikumar TS, Johansson GK, Ockerman PA, Gustafsson JA, Akesson B. 1992. Trace element status in healthy subjects switching from a mixed to a lactovegetarian diet for 12 mo. *Am J Clin Nutr* 55(4):885–890.

Stadtman TC. 1996. Selenocysteine. *Annu Rev Biochem* 65:83–100.

Stauber JL, Florence TM. 1988. A comparative study of copper, lead, cadmium and zinc in human sweat and blood. *Sci Total Environ* 74:235–247.

Stendig-Lindberg G, Tepper R, Leichter I. 1993. Trabecular bone density in a two year controlled trial of peroral magnesium in osteoporosis. *Magnes Res* 6(2):155–163.

Stewart JG, Ahlquist DA, McGill DB, Ilstrup DM, Schwartz S, Owen RA. 1984. Gastrointestinal blood loss and anemia in runners. *Ann Intern Med* 100(6):843–845.

Subar AF, Krebs-Smith SM, Cook A, Kahle LL. 1998. Dietary sources of nutrients among U.S. adults, 1989 to 1991. *J Am Diet Assoc* 98(5):537–547.

Subudhi AW, Jacobs KA, Hagobian TA, Fattor JA, Fulco CS, Muza SR, Rock PB, Hoffman AR, Cymerman A, Friedlander AL. 2004. Antioxidant supplementation does not attenuate oxidative stress at high altitude. *Aviat Space Environ Med* 75(10):881–888.

Sussman M. 1974. Iron and infection. In: Jacobs A, Worwood M, eds. *Iron in Biochemistry and Medicine.* New York: Academic Press. Pp. 649–679.

Svendsen OL, Hassager C, Christiansen C. 1993. Effect of an energy-restrictive diet, with or without exercise, on lean tissue mass, resting metabolic rate, cardiovascular risk factors, and bone in overweight postmenopausal women. *Am J Med* 95(2):131–140.

Takase B, Akima T, Satomura K, Ohsuzu F, Mastui T, Ishihara M, Kurita A. 2004. Effects of chronic sleep deprivation on autonomic activity by examining heart rate variability, plasma catecholamine, and intracellular magnesium levels. *Biomed Pharmacother* 58 (Suppl 1):S35–S39

Taylor CM, Bacon JR, Aggett PJ, Bremner I. 1991. Homeostatic regulation of zinc absorption and endogenous losses in zinc-deprived men. *Am J Clin Nutr* 53(3):755–763.

Taylor EW, Nadimpalli RG, Ramanathan CS. 1997. Genomic structures of viral agents in relation to the biosynthesis of selenoproteins. *Biol Trace Elem Res* 56(1):63–91.

Taylor EW, Cox AG, Zhao L, Ruzicka JA, Bhat AA, Zhang W, Nadimpalli RG, Dean RG. 2000. Nutrition, HIV, and drug abuse: The molecular basis of a unique role for selenium. *J Acquir Immune Defic Syndr* 25 (Suppl 1):S53–S61.

Teegarden D, Legowski P, Gunther CW, McCabe GP, Peacock M, Lyle RM. 2005. Dietary calcium intake protects women consuming oral contraceptives from spine and hip bone loss. *J Clin Endocrinol Metab* 90(9):5127–5133.

Telford RD, Catchpole EA, Deakin V, Hahn AG, Plank AW. 1992a. The effect of 7 to 8 months of vitamin/mineral supplementation on athletic performance. *Int J Sport Nutr* 2(2):135–153.

Telford RD, Catchpole EA, Deakin V, McLeay AC, Plank AW. 1992b. The effect of 7 to 8 months of vitamin/mineral supplementation on the vitamin and mineral status of athletes. *Int J Sport Nutr* 2(2):123–134.

Terblanche S, Noakes TD, Dennis SC, Marais D, Eckert M. 1992. Failure of magnesium supplementation to influence marathon running performance or recovery in magnesium-replete subjects. *Int J Sport Nutr* 2(2):154–164.

Tharion WJ, Baker-Fulco CJ, Bovill ME, Montain SM, DeLany JP, Champagne CM, Hoyt RW, Lieberman HR. 2004. Adequacy of garrison feeding for Special Forces soldiers during training. *Mil Med* 169(6):483–490.

Thomas CD, Friedl KE, Mays MZ, Mutter SH, Moore RJ, Jezior DA, Baker-Fulco CJ, Marchitelli LJ, Tulley RT, Askew EW. 1995. *Nutrient Intakes and Nutritional Status of Soldiers Consuming the Meal, Ready-to-Eat (MRE XII) During a 30-Day Field Training Exercise*. Report No. T-95-6. Natick, MA: U.S. Army Research Institute of Environmental Medicine.

Thys-Jacobs S. 2006. Premenstrual syndrome. In: Weaver CM, Heaney RP, eds. *Calcium in Human Health*. Totowa, NJ: Humana Press. Pp. 357–369.

Thys-Jacobs S, Alvir MJ. 1995. Calcium-regulating hormones across the menstrual cycle: Evidence of a secondary hyperparathyroidism in women with PMS. *J Clin Endocrinol Metab* 80(7):2227–2232.

Thys-Jacobs S, Ceccarelli S, Bierman A, Weisman H, Cohen MA, Alvir J. 1989. Calcium supplementation in premenstrual syndrome: A randomized crossover trial. *J Gen Intern Med* 4(3): 183–189.

Thys-Jacobs S, Alvir JM, Fratarcangelo P. 1995. Comparative analysis of three PMS assessment instruments—the identification of premenstrual syndrome with core symptoms. *Psychopharmacol Bull* 31(2):389–396.

Thys-Jacobs S, Starkey P, Bernstein D, Tian J. 1998. Calcium carbonate and the premenstrual syndrome: Effects on premenstrual and menstrual symptoms. Premenstrual Syndrome Study Group. *Am J Obstet Gynecol* 179(2):444–452.

Tipton K, Green NR, Haymes EM, Waller M. 1993. Zinc loss in sweat of athletes exercising in hot and neutral temperatures. *Int J Sport Nutr* 3(3):261–271.

Tolando R, Jovanovic A, Brigelius-Flohe R, Ursini F, Maiorino M. 2000. Reactive oxygen species and proinflammatory cytokine signaling in endothelial cells: Effect of selenium supplementation. *Free Radic Biol Med* 28(6):979–986.

Tranquilli AL, Lucino E, Garzetti GG, Romanini C. 1994. Calcium, phosphorus and magnesium intakes correlate with bone mineral content in postmenopausal women. *Gynecol Endocrinol* 8(1):55–58.

Tucker DM, Sandstead HH, Swenson RA, Sawler BG, Penland JG. 1982. Longitudinal study of brain function and depletion of iron stores in individual subjects. *Physiol Behav* 29(4):737–740.

Tucker DM, Sandstead HH, Penland JG, Dawson SL, Milne DB. 1984. Iron status and brain function: Serum ferritin levels associated with asymmetries of cortical electrophysiology and cognitive performance. *Am J Clin Nutr* 39(1):105–113.

Tuomainen TP, Nyyssonen K, Salonen R, Tervahauta A, Korpela H, Lakka T, Kaplan GA, Salonen JT. 1997. Body iron stores are associated with serum insulin and blood glucose concentrations. Population study in 1,013 eastern Finnish men. *Diabetes Care* 20(3):426–428.

Turnlund JR. 1999. Copper. In: Shils ME, Olson JA, Shike M, Ross AC. *Modern Nutrition in Health and Disease*. Baltimore, MD: Williams and Wilkins. Pp. 241–252.

Turnlund JR, Keyes WR, Anderson HL, Acord LL. 1989. Copper absorption and retention in young men at three levels of dietary copper by use of the stable isotope $^{65}$Cu. *Am J Clin Nutr* 49(5):870–878.

Turnlund JR, Keen CL, Smith RG. 1990. Copper status and urinary and salivary copper in young men at three levels of dietary copper. *Am J Clin Nutr* 51(4):658–664.

Turnlund JR, Scott KC, Peiffer GL, Jang AM, Keyes WR, Keen CL, Sakanashi TM. 1997. Copper status of young men consuming a low-copper diet. *Am J Clin Nutr* 65(1):72–78.

Turnlund JR, Keyes WR, Peiffer GL, Scott KC. 1998. Copper absorption, excretion, and retention by young men consuming low dietary copper determined by using the stable isotope $^{65}$Cu. *Am J Clin Nutr* 67(6):1219–1225.

U.S. Departments of the Army, Navy, and Air Force. 2001. *Nutrition Standards and Education*. Ar 40-25/BUMEDINST 1011.6/AFI 44-141. Washington, DC: U.S. Department of Defense Headquarters.

Valberg LS. 1980. Plasma ferritin concentration: Their clinical significance and relevance to patient care. *Can Med Assoc* 122(11):1240–1248.

Valimaki MJ, Karkkainen M, Lamberg-Allardt C, Laitinen K, Alhava E, Heikkinen J, Impivaara O, Makela P, Palmgren J, Seppanen R, et al. 1994. Exercise, smoking, and calcium intake during adolescence and early adulthood as determinants of peak bone mass. Cardiovascular Risk in Young Finns Study Group. *Br Med J* 309(6949):230–235.

Van Loan MD, Sutherland B, Lowe NM, Turnlund JR, King JC. 1999. The effects of zinc depletion on peak force and total work of knee and shoulder extensor and flexor muscles. *Int J Sport Nutr* 9(2):125–135.

Van Rij AM, Hall MT, Dohm GL, Bray J, Pories WJ. 1986. Changes in zinc metabolism following exercise in human subjects. *Biol Trace Elem Res* 10:99–105.

Velin P, Dupont D, Daoud A. 1989. Nutritional copper deficiency: Apropos of a case. *Ann Pediatr (Paris)* 36(4):269–274.

Vendeland SC, Beilstein MA, Yeh JY, Ream W, Whanger PD. 1995. Rat skeletal muscle selenoprotein W: cDNA clone and mRNA modulation by dietary selenium. *Proc Natl Acad Sci* 92(19):8749–8753.

Verde T, Shephard RJ, Corey P, Moore R. 1982. Sweat composition in exercise and in heat. *J Appl Physiol* 53(6):1540–1545.

Verdon F, Burnand B, Stubi CL, Bonard C, Graff M, Michaud A, Bischoff T, de Vevey M, Studer JP, Herzig L, Chapuis C, Tissot J, Pecoud A, Favrat B. 2003. Iron supplementation for unexplained fatigue in non-anaemic women: Double blind randomised placebo controlled trial. *Br Med J* 326(7399):1124.

Viteri FE, Torun B. 1974. Anaemia and physical work capacity. *Clin Haematol* 3(3):609–626.

Vukovich M, Specker B. 2006. Influence of physical activity on calcium and bone. In: Weaver CM and Heaney RP, eds. *Calcium in Human Health*. Totowa, NJ: Humana Press. Pp. 227–246.

Wada L, Turnlund JR, King JC. 1985. Zinc utilization in young men fed adequate and low zinc intakes. *J Nutr* 115(10):1345–1354.

Walker AF, De Souza MC, Vickers MF, Abeyasekera S, Collins ML, Trinca LA. 1998. Magnesium supplementation alleviates premenstrual symptoms of fluid retention. *J Womens Health* 7(9): 1157–1165.

Waller MF, Haymes EM. 1996. The effects of heat and exercise on sweat iron loss. *Med Sci Sports Exerc* 28(2):197–203.

Ward KM, Rajan SS, Wysong M, Radulovic D, Clauw DJ. 1996. Phosphorus nuclear magnetic resonance spectroscopy: in vivo magnesium measurements in the skeletal muscle of normal subjects. *Magn Reson Med* 36(3):475–480.

Wary C, Brillault-Salvat C, Bloch G, Leroy-Willig A, Roumenov D, Grognet JM, Leclerc JH, Carlier PG. 1999. Effect of chronic magnesium supplementation on magnesium distribution in healthy volunteers evaluated by 31P-NMRS and ion selective electrodes. *Br J Clin Pharmacol* 48(5): 655–662.

Weaver CM. 2006. Clinical approaches for studying calcium metabolism and its telationship to disease. In: Weaver, C.M. and Heaney, R.P., eds. *Calcium in Human Health*. Totowa, NJ: Humana Press. Pp 65–81.

Weaver CM, Heaney RP. 2006. Appendix 2: Comparing sources for absorbable calcium and Appendix 4: Calcium checklist. In: Weaver CM, Heaney RP, eds. *Calcium in Human Health*. Totowa, NJ: Humana Press. Pp. 434, 436–437.

Weaver CM, Rajaram S. 1992. Exercise and iron status. *J Nutr* 122(3 Suppl):782–787.

Weaver CM, Teegarden D, Lyle RM, McCabe GP, McCabe LD, Proulx W, Kern M, Sedlock D, Anderson DD, Hillberry BM, Peacock M, Johnston CC. 2001. Impact of exercise on bone health and contraindication of oral contraceptive use in young women. *Med Sci Sports Exerc* 33(6):873–880.

Webb TE, Krill CE Jr, Oski Fa, Tsou KC. 1982. Relationship of iron status to urinary norepinephrine excretion in children 7–12 years of age. *J Pediatr Gastroenterol Nutr* 1(2):207–209.

Weglicki WB, Phillips TM, Freedman AM, Cassidy MM, Dickens BF. 1992. Magnesium-deficiency elevates circulating levels of inflammatory cytokines and endothelin. *Mol Cell Biochem* 110(2): 169–173.

Weigand E, Kirchgessner M. 1976a. Radioisotope dilution technique for determination of zinc absorption in vivo. *Nutr Metab* 20(5):307–313.

Weigand E, Kirchgessner M. 1976b. $^{65}$Zn-labeled tissue zinc for determination of endogenous fecal zinc excretion in growing rats. *Nutr Metab* 20(5):314–320.

Weight LM. 1993. 'Sports anaemia.' Does it exist? *Sports Med* 16(1):1–4.

Weight LM, Myburgh KH, Noakes TD. 1988a. Vitamin and mineral supplementation: Effect on the running performance of trained athletes. *Am J Clin Nutr* 47(2):192–195.

Weight LM, Noakes TD, Labadarios D, Graves J, Jacobs P, Berman PA. 1988b. Vitamin and mineral status of trained athletes including the effects of supplementation. *Am J Clin Nutr* 47(2): 186–191.

Weisman SM, Matkovic V. 2005. Potential use of biochemical markers of bone turnover for assessing the effect of calcium supplementation and predicting fracture risk. *Clin Ther* 27(3): 299–308.

Weller E, Bachert P, Meinck HM, Friedmann B, Bartsch P, Mairbaurl H. 1998. Lack of effect of oral Mg-supplementation on Mg in serum, blood cells, and calf muscle. *Med Sci Sports Exerc* 30(11):1584–1591.

Wheeler EF, el-Neil H, Willson JO, Weiner JS. 1973. The effect of work level and dietary intake on water balance and the excretion of sodium, potassium and iron in a hot climate. *Br J Nutr* 30(1):127–137.

Whiting SJ. 1995. The inhibitory effect of dietary calcium on iron bioavailability: A cause for concern? *Nutr Rev* 53(3):77–80.

WHO (World Health Organization). 1996. Selenium. In: *Trace Elements In Human Nutrition and Health*. Geneva, Switzerland: WHO. Pp. 105–122.

WHO and CDC (U.S. Centers for Disease Control and Prevention). 2005. *Assessing the Iron Status of Populations*. Geneva, Switzerland: WHO.

Wilkinson EA, Hawke CI. 1998a. Does oral zinc aid the healing of chronic leg ulcers? A systematic literature review. *Arch Dermatol* 134(12):1556–1560.

Wilkinson EAJ, Hawke C. 1998b. Oral zinc for arterial and venous leg ulcers. *The Cochrane Database of Systematic Reviews* 4(CD001273):DOI: 10.1002/14651858.CD001273.

Williams JA, Wagner J, Wasnich R, Heilbrun L. 1984. The effect of long-distance running upon appendicular bone mineral content. *Med Sci Sports Exerc* 16(3):223–227.

Willis MS, Monaghan SA, Miller ML, McKenna RW, Perkins WD, Levinson BS, Bhushan V, Kroft SH. 2005. Zinc-induced copper deficiency: A report of three cases initially recognized on bone marrow examination. *Am J Clin Pathol* 123(1):125–131.

Winfield AC, Moore J, Bracker M, Johnson CW. 1997. Risk factors associated with stress reactions in female Marines. *Mil Med* 162(10):698–702.

Winters-Stone KM, Snow CM. 2004. One year of oral calcium supplementation maintains cortical bone density in young adult female distance runners. *Int J Sport Nutr Exerc Metab* 14(1):7–17.

Woitge HW, Friedmann B, Suttner S, Farahmand I, Muller M, Schmidt-Gayk H, Baertsch P, Ziegler R, Seibel MJ. 1998. Changes in bone turnover induced by aerobic and anaerobic exercise in young males. *J Bone Miner Res* 13(12):1797–1804.

Wolman SL, Anderson GH, Marliss EB, Jeejeebhoy KN. 1979. Zinc in total parenteral nutrition: Requirements and metabolic effects. *Gastroenterology* 76(3):458–467.

Wood C, Watson RR. 1984. Interrelationships among nutritional staus, cellular immunity, and cancer. In: Watson RR, ed. *Nutrition, Disease Resistance, and Immune Function*. New York: Marcel Dekker. Pp. 53–69.

Wood RJ, Zheng JJ. 1997. High dietary calcium intakes reduce zinc absorption and balance in humans. *Am J Clin Nutr* 65(6):1803–1809.

Xia Y, Hill KE, Byrne DW, Xu J, Burk RF. 2005. Effectiveness of selenium supplements in a low-selenium area of China. *Am J Clin Nutr* 81(4):829–834.

Xu GL, Wang SC, Gu BQ, Yang YX, Song HB, Xue WL, Liang WS, Zhang PY. 1997. Further investigation on the role of selenium deficiency in the aetiology and pathogenesis of Keshan disease. *Biomed Environ Sci* 10(2–3):316–326.

Yaffe K, Clemons TE, McBee WL, Lindblad AS, Age-Related Eye Disease Study Research Group. 2004. Impact of antioxidants, zinc, and copper on cognition in the elderly: A randomized, controlled trial. *Neurology* 63(9):1705–1707.

Yang GQ, Zhu LZ, Liu SJ, Gu LZ, Wian PC, Huang JH, Lu MD. 1987. Human selenium requirements in China. In: Combs GF, Spallholz JE, Levander OA, Oldfield JE, eds. *Selenium in Biology and Medicine*. New York: Van Nostrand Reinhold. Pp. 589–607.

Yang G, Yin S, Zhou R, Gu L, Yan B, Liu Y, Liu Y. 1989a. Studies of safe maximal daily dietary Se-intake in a seleniferous area in China. Part II: Relation between Se-intake and the manifestation of clinical signs and certain biochemical alterations in blood and urine. *J Trace Elem Electrolytes Health Dis* 3(3):123–130.

Yang G, Zhou R, Yin S, Gu L, Yan B, Liu Y, Liu Y, Li X. 1989b. Studies of safe maximal daily dietary selenium intake in a seleniferous area in China. I. Selenium intake and tissue selenium levels of the inhabitants. *J Trace Elem Electrolytes Health Dis* 3(2):77–87.

Yeh JK, Aloia JF, Yasumura S. 1989. Effect of physical activity on calcium and phosphorus metabolism in the rat. *Am J Physiol* 256(1 Pt 1):E1–E6.

Yeh JK, Liu CC, Aloia JF. 1993. Effects of exercise and immobilization on bone formation and resorption in young rats. *Am J Physiol* 264(2 Pt 1):E182–E189.

Zhu YI, Haas JD. 1998. Altered metabolic response of iron-depleted nonanemic women during a 15-km time trial. *J Appl Physiol* 84(5):1768–1775.

Zittermann A, Sabatschus O, Jantzen S, Platen P, Danz A, Stehle P. 2002. Evidence for an acute rise of intestinal calcium absorption in response to aerobic exercise. *Eur J Nutr* 41(5):189–196.

# 4

# Research Needs

Mineral inadequacy and depletion in military personnel can come from many sources. Military personnel who participate in training and operational exercises routinely decrease their food intake and, as a result, may consume inadequate amounts of minerals. Even in the absence of reduced food intake, highly-demanding physical activities may result in mineral depletion, because physical and environmental stressors can increase the turnover and losses of minerals. Dietary or blood biochemical markers of nutritional status may not always reveal mineral deficiencies, which may be explained by a lack of sensitive biochemical markers of mineral status, brief durations of restricted intakes, or mineral mobilization from stores into the blood with increased metabolic demands and loss of body weight. Also, determining the independent effect of restricted energy intakes on specific micronutrient impairments is difficult.

Throughout this report, the committee stresses the need to establish Military Dietary Reference Intakes specific for military personnel in situations of extreme weather, intense exercise, and other stressors that might alter the nutrient requirements for maintaining or improving health and physical and cognitive performance. The committee also recognizes that the appropriate data to establish mineral standards for the military are scarce. Thus, there is a great need to conduct controlled studies on mineral nutrition and physical performance, cognitive function, and behavior with military personnel in garrison training and in the field while the soldiers are engaged in support, training, and combat and in the context of moderating variables. These variables include gender, body composition, fitness, task, physical demand, extreme environmental conditions, sleep deprivation, food restriction, and psychological stressors (e.g., depression, anxiety, fear). For dietary intervention studies, it is critical that nutrient interactions are considered in the design and interpretation of results. Studies should be controlled for other potentially limiting nutrients.

The data from the recommended studies are needed to evaluate critically the adequacy of current rations provided to and consumed by soldiers, and, if needed, will provide a foundation for developing new rations. Such information also may be useful to better understand the determinants of food intake by soldiers (Hirsch and Kramer, 1993). Therefore, the committee urges that efforts be made to answer some of these research questions more accurately by generating data from experimental studies that more closely reflect the military environment. This report is concerned with military personnel in garrison training; therefore, the research questions are targeted at soldiers in that environment. However, similar research questions could (and should) be posed about mineral requirements in soldiers who face other extreme field environments, such as those encountered during sustained operations.

The committee agreed that ongoing research in a number of nutritional areas is critical and discussed several strategies for addressing unresolved problems relating to military nutrition. In fact, it examined the value of a cohort longitudinal study that would collect data on a broad array of nutritional indexes throughout the military careers of a cohort of recruits or enlisted soldiers and determined that even though the study might be of some value its feasibility is questionable, especially considering the tremendous use of resources when the relevance of the data collected is unclear. Also, resources may be tapped for other more pressing needs, making a longitudinal study a long-term, difficult goal to accomplish. A more useful, reasonable, and economical strategy would be to conduct focused studies with clearer objectives that are more comprehensible to commanders. In any event, the committee recommends that attention is paid to existing nutrition-related research questions in a manner best suited to military circumstances.

## ORGANIZATION AND PRIORITIZATION

This chapter focuses on research needs—organized according to prioritization criteria—that would assist the military with answering questions related to mineral requirements for soldiers in garrison training, including design details that might be helpful when developing a research agenda. In the following section on research priorities, the committee describes design details of two overall, cross-cutting studies (i.e., they apply to more than one mineral); the two studies are considered the highest priority, because they will provide critical information regarding mineral losses and mineral status of military personnel in garrison training. Then, the subsequent sections on specific minerals list and prioritize (the first study is the highest priority, the last is the lowest priority) the most important studies to pursue, according to the strength of the current available evidence. In some of those sections, the committee lists a category under the heading *Other Research Needs*; these are studies that address interesting research questions, but for which less evidence has been collected.

The committee recognizes the high cost of the studies proposed; therefore, if resources are slim or there are other pressing needs—in addition to addressing the two highest-priority studies—the following research questions for specific minerals should be explored:

- Does iron supplementation prevent iron deficiency? What is the best strategy to prevent iron deficiency?
- How does physical activity influence calcium requirements?
- Does iron intake above the levels recommended in this report have beneficial effects in cognitive functions?
- Does magnesium intake above the levels recommended in this report offer protection from sleep deprivation disturbances?
- Does zinc intake above levels recommended in this report result in improved physical and cognitive performance?

## RESEARCH PRIORITIES

### 1. Study the Effects of Military Garrison Training on Mineral Losses and Performance

**A study is needed to assess the effects of environmental, physical, and psychological stressors encountered by military personnel—including heat, physical activity, and possibly sleep restriction—on the mineral losses and resulting effects on physical and mental performance using modern analytical capabilities. This study also should determine how much of each mineral is required to replenish losses and to optimize performance.**

It is expected that the primary increases in mineral losses during garrison training will be through sweat and urine, but endogenous fecal losses also may occur, either increasing with the stressful conditions or possibly decreasing to compensate for the sweat and urinary losses. Consequently, the committee suggests using a model environment that emulates conditions similar to military garrison training (the committee also suggests that, even though sustained operations are not the focus of this report, using a model environment similar to those conditions could assess the related effects). Following are the details of a proposed study that will provide answers to questions about mineral requirements during garrison training (see Figure 4-1). An account of the general design is followed by descriptions of the dietary interventions, exercise interventions, and sleep distortion intervention; outcome measurements related to sweat losses, physical performance, and cognitive performance also are described or referenced.

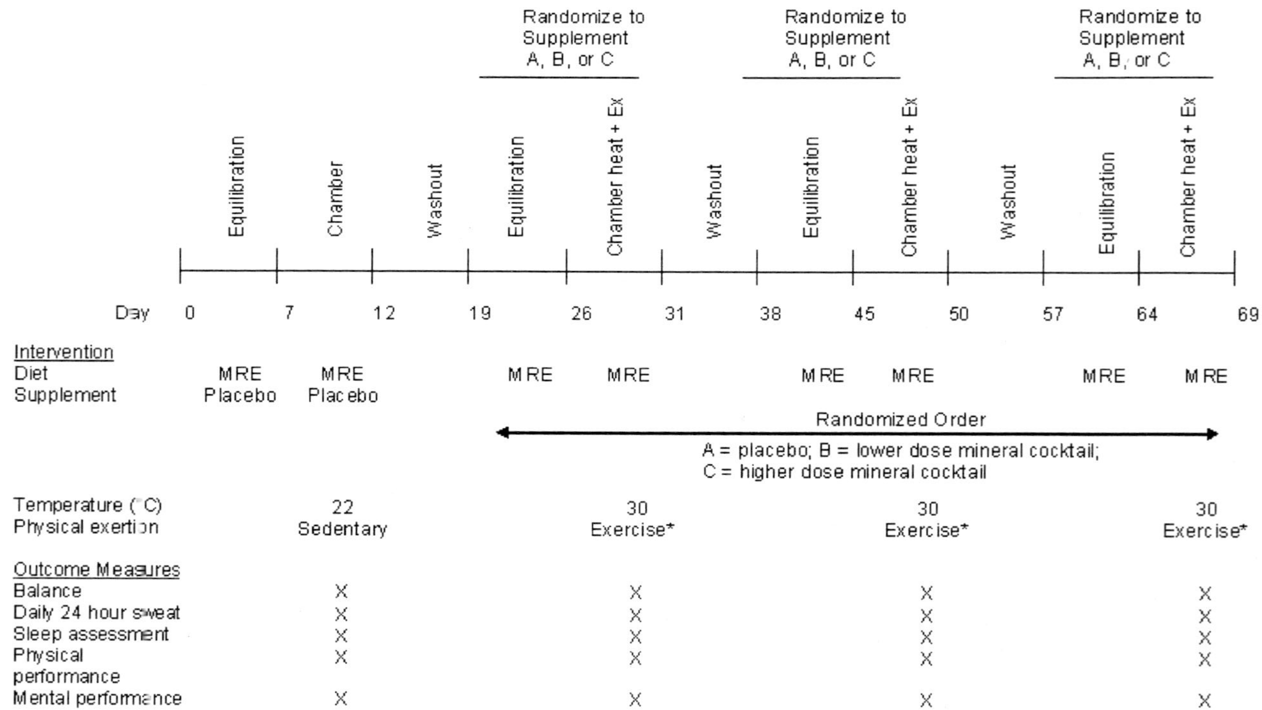


**FIGURE 4-1** Proposed study to determine the effect of sweat and physical exertion on mineral losses and physical and mental performance.

NOTE: Ex = exercise; MRE = Meal, Ready-to-Eat.

*Exercise for ≥ 4 hours/day with 40–50 lb load.

*General Design*

A proposed study design to determine the effect of sweat and physical exertion on mineral losses and on physical and mental performance is illustrated in Figure 4-1. Study subjects should represent the genders and age ranges of soldiers in the military population. Each subject would participate in a baseline phase (versus a stress phase with heat and heavy exercise) while consuming a controlled diet, based on either the current typical meals, ready to eat (MREs) or on the mineral values of the nutritional standards of operational rations (NSORs) [e.g., based on Recommended Dietary Allowance (RDA) for military garrison training], and would receive all subsequent treatments in randomized order while being subjected to heat and the physical demands typically experienced by military personnel. Controlled conditions would be achieved using an environmental chamber with supervised physical activity. Because training and operational exercises may involve significant reductions in total sleep and disruptions of the normal sleep–wake cycle, both of which reliably result in severe decrements in cognitive function and mood (Belenky et al., 1994; Lieberman et al., 2005), sleep restriction or disruption could be considered as an additional intervention.

*Dietary Interventions*

For all dietary interventions, studies should be controlled for other potentially limiting nutrients. One of the dietary periods during the stress phase should be identical to the baseline diet to determine the effect of heat and exercise on increases in mineral losses. There are several options for the dietary treatments. If the baseline dietary intake consists of typical MREs (usually with mineral levels higher than the NSOR), then other dietary treatments could include a lower and higher level of key minerals in "mineral cocktails" that include calcium, magnesium, iron, zinc, copper, and selenium. If the MRE diet does not meet the NSOR for any of the minerals, the lower dose of the intervention should be brought to at least the NSOR level.

An alternative design is that the baseline diet could be set on the NSOR values, and the intervention could consist of one or two higher doses of minerals. In any case, the higher dose of minerals in the cocktail should not exceed the Tolerable Upper Intake Level (UL) for any nutrient. A one-week adaptation to each dietary intake is reasonable since the initial mineral status of subjects is not one of deficiency. Washout periods between treatments should be at least seven days.

*Exercise Intervention*

The exercise intervention should mimic garrison training (or the military situation of interest). The amount of energy expended in physical activity per day for a male in garrison training can be estimated from Tharion et al. (2005).

The total energy expenditure is estimated at 16.5 MJ/day (~ 3,900 kcal/day). For a 70-kg man, the resting metabolic rate should be about 1,680 kcal/day and the digestion and metabolism of food is approximately 10 percent of the food's energy content. Assuming energy intake is equal to energy expended (IOM, 2002/2005), a little more than 1,800 kcal/day will be expended in physical activity. Using metabolic equivalent values (multiples of an individual's resting oxygen uptakes) to determine the kilocalories burned, walking at 3.5 mph on a level surface is the equivalent of about 4 kcal/min, and adding a 40-lb (18.14 kg) load should increase the energy expenditure by 1–2 kcal/min (Ainsworth et al., 2000); thus, the amount of energy expended from continuous exercise would be 300–360 kcal/h or about 3,000–3,600 kcal/day. Therefore, the exercise intervention to employ in the study could be walking (possibly using a treadmill) at 3.5 mph carrying a 40-lb (18.14 kg) load. The work can be intermittent so as to provide a recovery period between exercise bouts. An environmental temperature of approximately 30°C and 70 percent of relative humidity would simulate summer conditions in the southeastern United States.

*Sleep Deprivation Intervention*

If sleep deprivation is a concern and included in the intervention, then ensuring that the soldiers are reasonably well rested before participating in the study is critical. A representative scenario could be achieved during the five-day intervention phase by limiting sleep to 4 h/day (prolonged-moderate restriction), a single 24-hour episode without sleep (acute-severe restriction), or a combination of the two. This intervention's effectiveness can be verified by assessments of slow-wave activity in the electroencephalogram (EEG), sustained attention, and mood states. Sleep disruption (i.e., intermittent interruptions of sleep) and shifting the sleep–wake cycle (i.e., circadian disruption) are alternatives for restricting total sleep time that better represent real situations. The Committee on Military Nutrition Research (CMNR) [IOM, 2004] recently reviewed the impact of sleep loss and disruption on cognitive performance in the military and the currently available measures for assessing sleepiness in military settings.

*Measurement of Mineral Losses*

This experimental design provides evaluation of a dose–response effect of minerals on ameliorating mineral losses due to heat and sweat and can be used to evaluate a dose–response effect of minerals on physical and mental performance. Daily, 24-hour whole-body sweat analysis during each period will best quantify mineral losses and, if conducted over several days (e.g., five days), will indicate adaptation due to acclimatization. Analyzing sweat losses during one extended period (two to three weeks) to determine longer-term adaptation also could be valuable. The wash-down procedure for dermal collections is described by

Palacios et al. (2003). Because the increased sweat losses associated with high temperatures and heavy work are likely to occur without additional cellular losses, the mineral losses in sweat should be evaluated with and without procedures to exclude cellular debris, as described by Brune et al. (1986).

Complete balance data are needed to evaluate all routes of potential loss as well as the mineral intakes needed to correct the losses. A quantitative fecal marker should be used (e.g., polyethylene glycol, chromium, or $^{57}Cr$). Stable isotopic tracers could be used to determine interactions among minerals on absorption of calcium, zinc, and iron.

### *Cognition and Behavior Measurements*

Outcome measures in all study phases (including baseline) could include assessments of sleep patterns, mood states, and cognitive function (e.g., attention, memory, decision-making, and psychomotor skills).

A wide variety of potentially useful biochemical, physiological, and behavioral markers for mental performance in military personnel were identified and reviewed briefly in a recent IOM report, *Monitoring Metabolic Status* (IOM, 2004). Future research on mineral requirements to maintain and optimize cognitive function and behavior should include careful review and consideration of the markers in designs modeling the full range of complexities and demands common to research in military settings. This battery of tests should be developed in collaboration with Dr. Harris Lieberman (Lieberman, 2005; see Lieberman in Appendix B).

The methods used to monitor and evaluate the effects of nutrition on cognitive function and behavior are similar regardless of the particular mineral nutrient of interest. Because successful performance of mental tasks typically involves the coordinated operation of several distinct cognitive and psychomotor processes, assessing the effects of an experimental intervention also involves measuring performance in several cognitive and psychomotor tasks—tasks emphasizing sensation (i.e., the processes involved in detecting stimuli); attention [i.e., the processes of focusing on (selective) and allocating resources (intensive) to one aspect of the external or internal environment]; perception (i.e., the processes of interpreting or attaching meaning to stimuli); learning and memory (i.e., the processes of acquiring, storing, and retrieving information); reasoning (i.e., the processes of concept formation, problem solving, and decision making); and response selection and execution. An individual's knowledge base (e.g., general information, rules, and specific past events) is a critical component of cognitive function and, thus, also could be evaluated. Task failure can result from the breakdown of any one or more of the outlined component processes.

The many other factors that directly or indirectly affect mental performance may need to be addressed by ensuring that they are comparable among all treatment and control groups, included as covariates in statistical analyses, or manipulated as part of the intervention. Important moderating factors to consider when assessing mental performance in military personnel are motor skills (including the availability and limitations on the skills required to execute the behavior being recorded), training, and stressors. Improvements in task (physical or mental) performance result in part from the fact that some components in the process have become less effortful and more automated with training. Automating task performance, usually achieved through repetition, requires fewer resources to successfully complete the task but small, important errors may go unnoticed for a longer period of time than if the task were not automated. The proposed study might include an assessment of whether and how quickly complex tasks relevant to the military are automated, and how this relationship is mediated by environmental, physical, and psychological stressors.

Mental performance also is affected by chronic as well as physical and psychological states and stressors, which must be taken into account. Stressors directly related to physical and environmental factors common in the military include exercise-induced physical exhaustion, sleep restriction, food restriction, and extreme temperatures. Psychological states to be studied include mood states—such as anxiety, depression, hostility, and vigor—which also should be evaluated as outcomes in determining the effects of high-demand activities common on mental performance.

### *Measurements of Physical Performance*

The most important physical performance measurements are for aerobic and muscular endurance. There are many different tests that could measure these two variables, and the military should select the ones that have been proven to reflect the reality of military environments and physical performance demands. Because endurance exercise tests to exhaustion can be highly variable (Vogel, 1994), researchers recommend that an exercise time trial, where time will be the outcome measure, be used to determine aerobic endurance. A 15-km time trial on a cycle ergometer could be used to measure aerobic endurance as long as the study is conducted in a laboratory facility (Hinton et al., 2000). This test will require the subjects to first complete a maximal oxygen uptake ($VO_2max$) test, where $VO_2max$ and associated responses (maximal heart rate or ventilation) are measured. One test option is the bicycle test used by McArdle et al. (1973). An alternative time-trial method for measuring aerobic endurance in the field is a 20-km road march carrying a load (Vogel, 1994).

Several methods can be used for measuring muscular strength and endurance. The preferred methods measure dynamic strength using isotonic muscle contractions in lifting weights to determine the one repetition maximal weight or an isokinetic dynamometer to determine the peak torque at different velocities (Howley and Franks, 1997). When an isokinetic dynamometer is available, muscular endurance can be measured by having subjects repeat maximal contractions for 60 seconds (Vogel, 1994) and determining the rate of fatigue (the difference between peak and minimum torque). Alternative methods of measuring muscular endurance include subjects doing either as many push-ups as they can within a one-minute time period or the maximum number that they can do (Howley and Franks, 1997). As stated, among the available test options for evaluating performance, scenarios that most closely simulate and measure military physical performance activities are optimal (Vogel, 1994).

## 2. Determine Mineral Status and Food and Dietary Intakes

**The committee recommends that the military conducts periodic surveys to determine the mineral intakes and status of soldiers at various times from entry to training, deployment, or combat, especially for calcium and iron. If mineral status cannot be measured, then the intake levels, at least should be surveyed.**

The following paragraphs describe potential studies to address calcium intake and iron status determinations.

### *Iron*

**Justification.** Approximately 11–14 percent of women in the United States are iron deficient, according to the latest dietary survey (IOM, 2001). It is likely that the prevalence of iron deficiency among women joining the military is similar to that of women in the general population, although this fact is unproven. The committee concluded that women's iron status is an important criterion in determining the necessity of a strategy for increasing iron intake. If a strategy is needed, it is critical to identify the most efficient one for decreasing the deficiencies.

In addition to the potential iron deficiencies that may exist on entry into military service, an increase in iron requirements caused by active training could raise the prevalence of women's iron deficiency to > 50 percent; in fact, some women may become anemic. The adverse consequences on immune function, emotional and cognitive performance, and physical capacity may limit the effectiveness of women's training and performing duties. There are no systematic data available at this time on the true prevalence of iron deficiency and anemia in female troops either at service entry or during active military duty.

The committee concluded that, in addition to a study on the feasibility of monitoring women's status on entry into military service, surveillance programs should be established to monitor iron status at the end of all intensive training phases as well as periodically thereafter during military service, including during garrison training.

**Question.** What is the prevalence of iron deficiency and anemia in females in the military at service entry and during active service, including garrison training?

**Study design.** The study design is straightforward. The sampling should be statistically valid to represent military personnel's ages and races. Samples should be collected at the start of training or deployment as well as regularly throughout active duty to monitor the stability of the iron (or other minerals) nutritional status.

**Outcome measurements.** The outcome measures for iron status should include a complete blood count (CBC) (i.e., hemoglobin [Hb], hematocrit, platelets, etc.) plus serum ferritin, soluble serum transferrin receptor (sTfR), and perhaps erythrocyte protoporphyrin concentration (see Chapter 3).

*Calcium*

**Justification.** Calcium could be important for optimizing military performance by potentially helping to prevent stress fractures during training or combat and to modulate emotional health. Unfortunately, there is no biomarker that can indicate calcium nutrition status; instead, an indication of its status can be suggested from the total dietary intake. Researchers should conduct periodic surveys of calcium intake from food beverages, dietary supplements, and calcium-containing medications (e.g., antacids).

Very little is known currently about dietary supplement use among enlisted military personnel in garrison training; however, there is anecdotal evidence that it is common, probably at a level higher than in the U.S. general population and similar to the athletic community. Using mineral supplements—such as multivitamin mineral supplements and single supplements (e.g., calcium and iron)—is fairly common and often contributes to total nutrient intakes that might otherwise be inadequate. In addition to anecdotal evidence, researchers are using surveys—including an anticipated 2005 edition of the Health Behaviors survey through the Department of Defense Military Health System and pre- and post-deployment surveys on the use of dietary supplements (Corum, 2004)—to gauge dietary supplement use in the military. It is imperative that military health services and commanders be provided with the results.

Continuing the periodic surveys of food intake is important; however, given the use of dietary supplements, these surveys no longer provide enough information to describe accurately the total dietary intake of minerals by military personnel in the field, and the food surveys need to include questions on dietary supplement use. The assessment of total dietary intakes for many nutrients requires that food and beverage, as well as dietary supplements and certain medications containing nutrients (e.g., calcium-containing antacids), be included in the surveys, since sizeable numbers of enlisted personnel use nutrient-containing dietary supplements and over-the-counter medications containing calcium. Determining the content of calcium in rations is necessary for assessing intakes; however, food composition tables often may not reflect accurately that information for military rations. Therefore, to gain useful estimates of actual calcium intakes, composite military diets should be analyzed by atomic absorption spectrophotometry using acid-digested food samples. The same process, incurring only minimal additional resources, could be used to determine intake levels from rations for copper, magnesium, selenium, and zinc.

Coordinating survey activities within the military is important to avoid duplication of activities and to conserve limited resources. Because of the concerns relevant to iron and calcium, a more thorough knowledge of related supplement use among military personnel is a priority.

**Question.** What is the dietary intake of calcium from food, dietary supplements, and calcium-containing medications?

**Study design and outcome measurements.** Design and outcome measures for calcium status should include dietary surveys on food, dietary supplements, and medications containing calcium.

### *Other Research Needs*

- In addition to minerals, other dietary supplement products of unknown or unproven efficacy may be taken by enlisted personnel with the hope that they will improve performance or weight loss, or both. Although not a part of the current task, the committee acknowledges that the dietary intake surveys should extend to other supplements, including performance-enhancing supplements. The anecdotal evidence and the limited number of available surveys should provide insight as to which supplements the surveys should include.
- Among the various strategies for increasing nutrient intakes from foods, the use of dietary supplements may be warranted for some individuals, particularly women (e.g., to increase iron intake to adequate levels and folic acid intake, among women of child-bearing age, to minimize the risk of spina bifida in newborns) and individuals on weight-loss diets (e.g., to increase mineral intakes to adequate levels on hypocaloric regimens). Research is needed to determine the best strategy for increasing necessary dietary intakes.
- There is still a need for research that addresses the most appropriate ways to disseminate to professionals as well as to soldiers nutrition-related information on food and dietary supplements, including the findings from the CMNR studies.

## RESEARCH NEEDS

### Calcium

#### *Calcium Losses*

**Justification.** Daily, whole-body calcium losses through sweat and excreta under conditions relevant to military personnel are poorly understood. Sweat loss due to heat and physical exertion is the most probable route of excess loss. A short-term study could increase substantially the understanding of potential calcium losses that military personnel could experience as well as of the levels of calcium for correcting those losses.

**Question.** What is the effect of environmental, physical, and psychological stressors and other conditions relevant to the military, including heat and physical activity, on daily, whole-body calcium losses?

**Study design and outcome measurements.** See section on research priority 1, *Study the Effects of Military Garrison Training on Mineral Losses and Performance* for discussion on study design and outcome measurements (see also Figure 4-1).

*Calcium Dietary Intake Levels*

See section on research priority 2, *Determine Mineral Status and Food and Dietary Intakes.*

*Physical Activity and Calcium Metabolism*

**Justification.** A positive interaction between physical activity and calcium intake on bone has been demonstrated during growth and in postmenopausal women. However, the interaction of dietary calcium and physical activity on bone accrual or maintenance, especially in age groups and lifestyles relevant to the military, is unknown. Calcium needs may be altered with vigorous exercise.

**Question.** How does physical activity influence the calcium requirements in military personnel?

**Study design.** Calcium balance and kinetic studies on a range of calcium intakes (e.g., 500 to 2,000 mg/day) should be included in a crossover design, with and without exercise, that simulates garrison training conditions. Alternatively, the calcium balance studies discussed in research priority 1, *Study the Effects of Military Garrison Training on Mineral Losses and Performance* could be used to determine calcium losses under conditions relevant to the military population, so that requirements using the factorial approach could be modified accordingly.

**Outcome measurements.** The objective is to determine whether exercise shifts the curve representing the relationship between calcium intake and calcium retention resulting in a new threshold intake—a criterion for determining calcium requirements used by the Dietary Reference Intakes panel (IOM, 1997). This approach has been discussed by Weaver and Liebman (2002). Determination of the kinetic parameters would enable quantitative evaluation of calcium metabolism parameters perturbed by exercise including absorption, endogenous secretion, urinary and fecal excretion, bone-formation rates, and bone-resorption rates. These methods also have been described (Jackman et al., 1997; Wastney et al., 2000; Weaver, 2006), but they have not been applied to the exercise versus nonexercise conditions.

### *Calcium's Role in Weight Loss and Bone Loss*

**Justification.** It is unknown whether weight loss induces bone loss in physically active men or premenopausal women. In postmenopausal women, weight loss is associated with bone loss unless calcium intake is at levels that exceed the Adequate Intake (AI).

**Question.** Does weight loss induce bone loss in physically active men or premenopausal women?

**Study design.** Military men and women should be assigned randomly to placebo (soldiers on typical military diets, no calcium supplementation) versus supplemented (1,200–1,700 mg/day of calcium, diet plus supplemented) groups under conditions that lead to weight loss, including rigorous garrison training and reduced caloric consumption. Supplementation likely will result in total dietary calcium intakes of at least 1,600 mg/day, which has been shown to protect bone loss during weight loss (Jensen et al., 2001; Ricci et al., 1998; Riedt et al., 2005).

**Outcome measurements.** Bone-loss reduction would be measured by bone density (IOM, 2004).

### *Calcium and Oral Contraceptives*

**Justification.** Oral contraceptives, especially in physically active women, have been associated with reduced bone density in premenopausal, civilian women (See Chapter 3). Women who met the AI for calcium did not experience a negative interaction between exercise and oral contraceptives. However, the potential protective effect of calcium has not been tested rigorously, especially under the physical activity stress experienced by military women.

**Question.** Can dietary calcium counteract the negative interaction of exercise and oral contraceptives on women's bones?

**Study design.** The design incorporates a factorial study of oral contraceptives use (use versus nonuse) by exercise level (low versus high) and by calcium intake (no supplements versus supplements) in military women participating in rigorous garrison training. Subjects in the control group should be on a diet that provides calcium levels of < 800 mg/day, and subjects in the supplementation group should be provided with total dietary calcium intakes of > 1,000 mg/day.

**Outcome measurements.** Bone-density changes are the primary outcome measure. Use of bone imaging such as dual-energy X-ray absorptiometry (IOM, 2004) would help determine if exercise can protect against loss of bone strength due to lower calcium intakes in women who do not use oral contraceptives.

*Excess Calcium and Kidney Stone Risk*

**Justification.** The Institute of Medicine (IOM) Committee on Optimization of Nutrient Composition of Military Rations for Short-Term, High-Stress Situations recommended that assault rations for sustained operations contain calcium levels in the range of 750–850 mg/day, which is lower than the AI for the general population (1,000 mg/day) (IOM, 2006). The concern about a potential increased risk of renal kidney stones due to excessive calcium intake under the typical conditions of sustained operations (low fluid consumption, excessive sweat, and stress) justified the lower range. In civilians, kidney stone risk is reduced with calcium intakes greater than the AI; thus, the increased risk of kidney stone formation needs to be examined before the lower-calcium-range recommendation for military personnel in sustained operations can be implemented.

**Question.** Does calcium intake exceeding 850 mg/day increase the risk of kidney stones under sustained operations conditions (i.e., assault missions)?

**Study design.** A dose–response study using < 850–1,500 mg/day of calcium under assault-like conditions should be conducted as part of the reseach priority 1, *Study the Effects of Military Garrison Training on Mineral Losses and Performance.*

**Outcome measurements.** Outcome measurements will test hypercalciuria, hypocitraturia, urinary pH, and urine volume.

*Calcium and Cognition and Behavior*

**Justification.** Evidence from studies with civilians, primarily women with premenstrual distress, suggests that increasing calcium intake may improve mood states and mitigate symptoms associated with menstrual distress in women. There have been no studies on calcium nutrition and cognition and behavior with military personnel, and all civilian studies were conducted under minimal stress conditions. Thus, there is a need to determine the relationship between calcium intakes and mood states, particularly depression, in military personnel during garrison training conditions.

**Question.** Is there an effect between calcium intake and mood states, including depression, premenstrual syndrome (PMS), and premenstrual disphoric syndrome (PMDD), that could affect performance?

**Study design.** The study initially could run for two weeks, similar to the overall study in research priority 1, *Study the Effects of Military Garrison Training on Mineral Losses and Performance*, but include dietary intake supplementation of approximately 1,200 mg/day, which has been demonstrated to improve mood states in civilians with PMS (Thys-Jacobs et al., 1998). Lower supplementation levels (e.g., 500 mg/day) also could be tested. If there is no indication of mood improvement within two weeks, then supplementation and mood assessments should continue for a minimum of two months and preferably for four to six months (or, for women, for up to six menstrual cycles). Women suffering from PMS or PMDD [as diagnosed by the American Psychiatric Association's

*Diagnostic and Statistical Manual of Mental Disorders DSM-IV* (1994) or other diagnosis manuals or guidance tests] should be the study subjects.

**Outcome measurements.** The Profile of Mood States-Bipolar Form (POMS-BI) (Lorr and McNair, 1984) is recommended for efficiently measuring multiple mood states in the proposed study, because it has been used successfully in many previous studies with military personnel and has been validated thoroughly through extensive use with the general population as well as with mental health outpatients (Lorr and McNair, 1984; McNair et al., 2003; Nyenhuis et al., 1999). The POMS-BI is a self-report measure of bipolar mood states that has been designed specifically to assess mood changes before and after treatment and in response to experimental manipulations. The form yields scores on six bipolar subscales: composed–anxious, agreeable–hostile, elated–depressed, confident–unsure, energetic–tired, and clearheaded–confused. An overall measure of mood disturbance also can be calculated. Validated short versions of the POMS are available if the respondent burden is too great (Curran et al., 1995; Shacham, 1983).

The Menstrual Distress Questionnaire (MDQ) (Moos, 1968) has been used extensively to assess premenstrual and menstrual symptoms in civilian women and would be appropriate for use with female participants in the proposed study if used prospectively (i.e., daily ratings; Today Form). The MDQ is a self-report measure of the presence and severity of physical and psychological symptoms. Symptoms are grouped into eight factors: pain, water retention, autonomic reactions, negative affect, impaired concentration, behavior change, arousal, and control. Measurement of intervention effects on menstrual symptomatology requires that female participants complete (before they begin the study) a menstrual history that also assesses the participants' knowledge and beliefs of premenstrual symptom disorders (Marvan and Escobedo, 1999).

### *Other Research Needs*

If resources are available, assessments of cognitive and psychomotor function and of sleep quantity and quality could be included in the proposed study of calcium and mood states and menstrual symptomatology; alternatively, studies conducted to assess the effects of other minerals on cognitive and psychomotor function and on sleep quantity and quality could be broadened to include calcium. However, research on calcium's nutritional role in these other areas of function should be considered a low priority because there are no experimental data that indicate calcium intake or status, if within reasonable limits, directly affect mental performance or sleep.

## Copper

### *Copper Losses*

**Justification.** Copper losses in military personnel are unknown because the previously reported data do not address military conditions. Therefore, it is important to conduct balance studies under the stress (i.e., environmental, physical, and psychological) of military situations that would determine copper concentration in whole-body sweat losses and total-body copper losses, including urinary losses. A short-term study could substantially increase the understanding both the potential copper losses that military personnel could experience and the copper levels that might be required to correct those losses.

**Question.** What is the effect of environmental, physical, and psychological stressors and other conditions relevant to the military, including heat and physical activity, on daily, whole-body copper losses?

**Study design and outcome measurements.** See research priority 1, *Study the Effects of Military Garrison Training on Mineral Losses and Performance* for the recommended study design and outcome measurements (also see Figure 4-1).

*Copper Dietary Intake Levels*

**Justification.** The amount of copper consumed by military personnel is unknown. Because copper intakes were listed previously in the RDAs only as estimated safe and adequate daily dietary intakes for the general population, copper dietary intakes by military personnel in garrison training should be calculated and analyzed.

**Question.** How much copper is consumed by the military personnel under garrison training?

**Study design.** Recognizing that food composition tables often are inaccurate with respect to estimating the copper contents of foods in military rations, estimates of copper intake using existing food composition data tables would be approximate at best. Therefore, composite military diets should be analyzed for copper to estimate actual copper intakes. Copper intake from dietary supplements also should be determined. This copper diet analysis could be done jointly with the calcium analysis described in research priority 2, *Determine Mineral Status and Food and Dietary Intakes.*

**Outcome measurements.** Results should measure the amount of copper in military personnel's diets and rations using existing food composition data or copper analysis by atomic absorption spectrophotometry using acid-digested samples and AOAC International methods for sample preparation.

## Iron

*Iron Losses*

**Justification.** Daily, whole-body iron losses through sweat and excreta under conditions relevant to military personnel are poorly understood. Sweat losses due to heat and physical exertion are the most probable route of excess losses. A short-term study could substantially increase both the understanding of the potential iron losses that military personnel could experience and the levels of iron that might be necessary to correct those losses.

**Question.** What is the effect of environmental, physical, and psychological stressors and other conditions relevant to the military, including heat and physical activity, on daily, whole-body iron losses?

**Study design and outcome measurements.** See research priority 1, *Study the Effects of Military Garrison Training on Mineral Losses and Performance* for the recommended study design and outcome measurements (also see Figure 4-1).

*Prevalence of Iron Deficiency in Women*

See research priority 2, *Determine Mineral Status and Food and Dietary Intakes*.

*Iron and Cognition and Behavior*

**Justification.** Existing data indicate that iron deficiency, even without anemia, may impair attention, learning, and memory. Further, several putative mechanisms for describing the effects of iron on brain function and cognition have been identified. However, previous studies were conducted under laboratory (i.e., minimal stress) conditions and, with one exception, only in civilian populations. Thus, there is a need to determine the relationship between iron intake and status and cognitive function and behavior in military personnel under garrison training conditions.

**Question.** Could increasing iron intake for soldiers—who experience conditions that include sleep deprivation and high physical stress and exhaustion—benefit cognitive function (particularly memory) and affect military performance?

**Study design.** The following study design is suggested: a randomized, stratified, intervention placebo-controlled trial of iron deficient anemic (as determined by a combination of iron status indicators, see Chapter 3), iron deficient (< 12 μg/L of serum ferritin), and control groups subjected randomly to receive either iron supplements or a placebo (typical soldiers diets, no supplement). One or more levels of supplementation (e.g., 60 mg/day or 30 and 60 mg/day of iron) could be provided. The trial should likely last for at least two months or for the length of the training and should be replicated, if possible, in several locations or camps. Conditions should represent the physical, environmental, psychological, and sleep stressors common in military settings.

**Outcome measurements.** Outcomes for iron status would be determined by alterations in a combination of indicators such as Hb, sTfR, ferritin, body iron, serum transferring saturation (TSAT), and erythrocyte protoporphyrin concentration (see Chapter 3). Outcomes for cognitive and behavioral variables could be analyzed by a principal components analysis approach or other multivariant analysis (including measurements of learning, memory, attention, executive functions and depression, anxiety scales interlaced with specific cognitive tasks already in use by the U.S. Army Research Institute of Environmental Medicine during periods of high physical stress and exhaustion as well as in the ideal laboratory conditions).

The battery described by Lieberman et al. (2005, Lieberman, 2005; see Lieberman in Appendix B), with minor additions, is recommended for use in the proposed study because it is comprised of standardized and validated tasks that measure critical cognitive processes and psychomotor skills, also it has been used successfully in previous studies with military personnel. Included in the battery is a visual scanning task that measures sustained attention or vigilance; a matching-to-sample task that measures short-term memory and pattern recognition; a repeated acquisition task that measures motor learning, attention, and short-term memory; a grammatical reasoning task that measures logical reasoning; and a four-choice reaction-time task that measures psychomotor function. Data from several of these tasks are suitable for signal detection analysis as well as for traditional statistical analysis for intervention effects.

This battery, which is based on tasks requiring responses to visual stimuli, could be enhanced by including tasks that require responses to auditory stimuli, such as Bakan's auditory vigilance task (Bakan, 1959), and by extending the reaction-time task to include a single-choice condition for measuring simple motor fatigue. Finally, this battery of cognitive tasks will address directly the possible impact of iron nutrition on memory function.

Intervention effects on mood states, particularly depression and anxiety, can be determined by administering the POMS-BI. Alternatively, if a measure specific to depression is desired so that cognitive and somatic aspects of depression can be evaluated independently, then researchers recommend using a standardized and validated test, such as the Beck Depression Inventory II (Beck et al., 1996), in conjunction with the POMS-BI.

### *Supplement Use and Prevention of Iron Deficiency*

**Justification.** Iron supplementation can be a highly effective approach to treating iron deficiency, but iron can be toxic in large amounts. Hence, it is important to determine if supplementation is a viable route for protecting women who participate in heavy training from a decrease in iron status. Studies in the exercise literature demonstrate that small doses of ferrous sulfate can be effective in eliminating the decline in iron status that occurs with heavy training (Brownlie et al., 2002; Hinton et al., 2000). It is important to determine if iron supplements are necessary or if fortified foods or dietary recommendations, or both, can effect a change.

**Question.** Can supplemental iron and dietary intervention approaches alleviate the drop in iron status of female soldiers during garrison training or even during field missions?

**Study design.** The intervention could be a single pill, fortified foods plus a dietary recommendation, dietary recommendations, or a combination of supplementation plus fortification and dietary recommendations. Female recruits would be assigned randomly to the four intervention groups as well as to a placebo group (no intervention).

Further evaluation is needed to assess the possible advantage of routine iron supplementation for all female soldiers versus iron supplementation only for those who are iron deficient after screening, so stratification may be necessary.

**Outcome measurements.** Traditional iron status measures such as ferritin, sTfR, TSAT, erythrocyte protoporphyrin concentration, and CBC would be measured as an index of the test subjects' iron status (see Chapter 3). Dietary intake data (obtained by either a questionnaire or weighed food intakes), dietary supplement use, and measures of iron status would provide evidence of each intervention's effectiveness.

*Other Research Needs*

- Perform field testing of current filter paper technology to evaluate the feasibility of iron status biomarkers (i.e., ferritin or sTfR) as indicators of iron nutrition during long deployments.
- Develop methods to test field-friendly feel cognitive tasks (e.g., finger-tapping, memory tasks, etc.) that can be used without computers as a means of assessing of alterations in cognitive functioning.

## Magnesium

*Magnesium Losses*

**Justification.** Daily, whole-body magnesium losses through sweat and excreta under conditions relevant to military personnel are poorly understood. Sweat losses due to heat and physical exertion are the most probable route of magnesium losses. A short-term study could increase substantially the understanding of the potential magnesium losses that military personnel could experience and the magnesium levels that might be necessary to correct those losses.

**Question.** What is the effect of environmental, physical, and psychological stressors and other conditions relevant to the military, including heat and physical activity, on daily, whole-body magnesium losses?

**Study design and outcome measurements.** See research priority 1, *Study the Effects of Military Garrison Training on Mineral Losses and Performance* for information on the recommended study design and outcome measurements (also see Figure 4-1).

*Magnesium and Cognition and Behavior*

**Justification.** Although there are no data specific to military personnel that address a possible relationship between magnesium nutrition and sleep, experimental studies with civilians have shown that magnesium is involved in regulating brain activity (Penland, 1995), plasma markers of magnesium status change with sleep deprivation (Takase et al., 2004), and magnesium supplementation decreases sleep disturbances, at least in the elderly (Held et al., 2002). Civilian studies also have demonstrated that magnesium nutrition may be related to depression (Murck, 2002). Further, several putative mechanisms for effects of magnesium on brain function relevant to sleep, cognition, and behavior have been identified. Given that sleep deprivation and disruption could occur common during military training and especially during sustained operations and produce severe decrements in cognitive function and mood states (Belenky et al., 1994; Lieberman et al., 2005), there is a need to determine whether increasing magnesium intake will improve sleep, protect against the effects of sleep deprivation, or regulate mood states of military personnel in garrison training and during sustained operations.

**Question.** Does increased magnesium intake improve sleep, protect against sleep deprivation, and regulate mood states of military personnel?

**Study design.** This study can be conducted as part of the priority research 1. Study the Effects of Military Garrison Training on Mineral Losses and Performance, in which the dietary treatments consist of MREs supplemented with 0, 150, 300 mg/day of magnesium. These amounts were used in previous civilian studies and pose minimal risk of exceeding the UL when combined with typical dietary intakes. Assessments of sleep quantity and quality and of mood states should be conducted during the five-day periods of intervention with physical, environmental, and psychological stressors.

**Outcome measurements.** The gold standard for measuring sleep architecture is polysomnography (PSG), which includes measurements of brain electrical activity (by electroencephalography), eye movements (by electrooculargram), and muscle tone (by electromyogram) was reviewed by the report *Monitoring Metabolic Status* (IOM, 2004). Data collected during the PSG can be analyzed spectrally and collated to permit identification and quantification of sleep stages and, thus, sleep patterns and should be used in the proposed laboratory simulation where there will be no practical equipment constraints. Wrist-worn actigraphy would be the recommended practical alternative to PSG in a field study. Assessment of slow-wave (1–3.9 Hz delta and 4–7.9 Hz theta) activity in the EEG can be used to determine physiological changes in brain arousal and sleep quantity. Analysis of the PSG should be complemented by performing a sleep latency test (Wesensten, 2004) and administering a subjective measure of sleepiness (IOM, 2004), to assess sleep quality.

Intervention effects (Lorr and and McNair, 1984) on mood states, particularly depression, can be determined by administering the POMS-BI (see section above *Calcium and Cognition and Behavior*). Alternatively, if a measure specific to depression is desired so that cognitive and somatic aspects of depression can be evaluated independently, then using a standardized and validated test, such as the Beck Depression Inventory (Beck et al., 1996), in conjunction with the POMS-BI is recommended. Electrophysiological measurements are likely to respond to changes in magnesium status and when resources permit, should be included as outcome measures.

The consequences of sleep deprivation and disruption on mental performance can be determined by administering a battery of cognitive tasks, including those that assess attention (particularly vigilance), perception (including pattern recognition), learning and memory, reasoning, and decision making. Effects on psychomotor performance can be determined with single and multiple-choice reaction-time tasks. The battery described by Lieberman et al. (2005), with minor additions, is recommended for use in the proposed study (see the section on research needs for iron). The Committee on Military Nutrition Research (IOM, 2004) recently reviewed the impact of sleep loss and disruption on cognitive performance in the military and the currently available measures for assessing sleepiness in military settings.

### *Magnesium Dietary Intake Levels*

**Justification.** The amount of magnesium consumed by military personnel is unknown, and there are only estimates of magnesium content in military rations, calculated mostly from food composition databases. In order to verify if the dietary intake level of magnesium is adequate the level in the diets, including dietary supplements, should be determined.

**Question.** How much magnesium is consumed by military personnel under garrison training?

**Study design.** Food composition tables often are inaccurate to estimate the magnesium contents of foods in military rations, and estimates of magnesium intake using existing food composition data tables are approximate at best. Therefore, composite military diets should be analyzed (by atomic absorption spectrophotometry using acid-digested samples) for magnesium to gain useful estimates of actual magnesium intakes. Researchers also should determine the frequency with which military personnel use supplements containing appreciable amounts of magnesium. This analysis could be done jointly with the calcium analysis described in research priority 2. *Determine Mineral Status and Food and Dietary Intakes.*

**Outcome measurements.** Measures will reflect the amount of magnesium in the military diets and rations using existing food composition data and actual magnesium analysis.

## Selenium

### *Selenium Losses*

**Justification.** Daily, whole-body selenium losses through sweat and excreta in conditions relevant to military personnel are poorly understood. Sweat losses due to heat and physical exertion are the most probable route of excess losses. A short-term study could increase substantially the understanding of the potential selenium losses that military personnel could experience and the levels of selenium that might be necessary to correct those losses.

**Question.** What is the effect of conditions relevant to the military, including heat and physical activity, on daily, whole-body selenium losses?

**Study design and outcome measurements.** See the study design in research priority 1, *Study the Effects of Military Garrison Training on Mineral Losses and Performance.*

### *Selenium and Immune Function*

**Justification.** There are data that suggest that selenium deprivation can impair immune function.

**Question.** Does selenium supplementation of nondeficient subjects improve immune function?

**Study design.** Military men and women should be placed randomly in placebo groups (soldiers eating typical diets, using no supplementation) and in a group taking a selenium supplement of 200 μg/day. The total dietary intake would fall below the IOM UL for selenium (400 μg/day).

**Outcome measurements.** Following four weeks of supplementation, immune status improvements would be measured by postvaccination immune responses [e.g., antibody production and T-cell number and function (phytohemagglutinin and pokeweed mitogen) studies].

### *Selenium Dietary Intake Levels*

**Justification.** The amount of selenium consumed by military personnel is unknown, and there are only estimates of the selenium content in military rations, calculated mostly from food composition databases. In order to verify if the dietary intake level of selenium is adequate the level in the diets, including dietary supplements, should be determined.

**Question.** How much selenium is consumed by the military personnel under garrison training?

**Study design.** Food composition tables often are inaccurate for estimating the selenium contents of military rations, estimates of selenium intake using existing food composition data tables are approximate at best. Therefore, composite military diets should be analyzed (by atomic absorption spectrophotometry using acid-digested samples) for selenium to gain useful estimates of actual selenium intakes. Researchers also should determine the frequency with which military personnel use supplements containing appreciable amounts (> 50 μg/day) of selenium. This selenium diet analysis could be done jointly with the calcium analysis described in research priority 2, *Determine Mineral Status and Food and Dietary Intakes.*

**Outcome Measurements.** The measures should reflect the amount of selenium in military diets and rations using existing food composition data and actual selenium analysis.

*Selenium and Cognitive Function*

**Justification.** Data from several civilian studies have shown that increasing selenium intake may improve mood states, including depression, anxiety, and confusion (see Chapter 3). There have been no studies of selenium nutrition and cognition and behavior with military personnel, and civilian studies were conducted under minimal stress conditions. Thus, there is a need to determine the relationship between selenium intake and status and mood states in military personnel engaged in support, training, and combat operations and in the context of moderating variables, including physical, environmental, and psychological stressors.

**Question.** Does increasing the selenium intakes of soldiers undergoing military garrison training improve their mood states, particularly depression, and therefore affect military performance?

**Study design.** The research question can be addressed as part of research priority 1, *Study the Effects of Military Garrison Training on Mineral Losses and Performance*. The dietary treatment should consist of MREs supplemented with 0, 50, and 100 μg/day of selenium. These amounts were used in previous civilian studies and pose minimal risk of exceeding the UL for selenium (400 μg/day) when combined with typical dietary intakes. If there is no indication of mood improvement after two weeks of supplementation, then supplementations and mood assessments should continue for a minimum of 2 months and preferably 4–6 months.

**Outcome measurements.** The POMS-BI (Lorr and McNair, 1984) is recommended for use to efficiently measure multiple mood states (see section above *Calcium and Cognition and Behavior*).

*Other Research Needs*

- Screen major water sources for selenium content.

## Zinc

*Zinc Losses*

**Justification.** The increase in zinc requirement for military personnel under garrison training conditions is based primarily on data that show increased sweat losses under conditions of heat exposure and exertion. Such increases are based on experiments lasting up to 12 days, with few subjects, and without measurements that could assess possible adaptation in the intestinal absorption or endogenous excretion of zinc (See Chapter 3). A short-term study could increase substantially the understanding of the potential zinc losses that military personnel could experience and the levels of zinc that might be necessary to correct those losses.

**Question.** Is there long-term adaptation in sweat losses or adaptation in other aspects of zinc balance that counteract the short-term increase in sweat losses with heat exposure and exertion?

**Study design.** See the study design in research priority 1, *Study the Effects of Military Garrison Training on Mineral Losses and Performance.*

**Outcome measurements.** The measures will address zinc levels in diet, stools, urine, and sweat (elemental balance). Isotopic measurements of zinc absorption and endogenous intestinal excretion are recommended.

### *Zinc Supplementation and Physical Performance*

**Justification.** Physical and mental performance measurements can provide the best evidence for setting dietary recommendations, especially since there are no reliable biochemical indexes of marginal zinc status. Performance data to justify increases in zinc intake need to be updated as newer, more sensitive measurements become available. An improvement in dynamic isokinetic strength was observed with 135 mg/day of zinc tablets (composition unknown) for 14 days (Krotkiewski et al., 1982); this outcome should be tested with zinc supplemented in more moderate amounts, such as 10–15 mg/day. Assuming that baseline intakes from MREs will be approximately 10–15 mg/day (placebo), a supplementation of 10–15 mg/day will amount to a total dietary intake of 20 and 30 mg/day for women and men, respectively, which is below the IOM UL of 40 mg/day.

**Question.** Does zinc supplementation enhance physical functions that may positively influence a soldier's performance?

**Study design.** The randomized, placebo-controlled trials in the study design for Research Priority 1. *Study the Effects of Military Garrison Training on Mineral Losses and Performance* could be followed to test physical performance with moderate amounts of supplemental zinc (e.g., 10–15 mg/day) added to placebo dietary intakes (approximately 10–15 mg/day) for approximately two weeks. For efficiency, zinc may be tested along with other nutrient supplements, with positive results leading to further testing for identification of the effective nutrients.

**Outcome measurements.** Measures should address dynamic isokinetic strength, similar to that measured by Krotkiewski et al. (1982). Additional sensitive outcome measurements should be used as new testing conditions become available (see measurements of physical performance in Research Priority 1, *Study the Effects of Military Garrison Training on Mineral Losses and Performance*).

*Zinc and Cognition and Behavior*

**Justification.** Although there are no previous studies of military personnel, data from the few available civilian studies suggest that zinc nutrition may have a role in cognitive function, particularly memory and mood states (e.g., depression). However, previous studies were conducted under laboratory conditions (i.e., minimal stress). Several putative mechanisms for effects of zinc on brain function and cognition have been identified. Thus, there is a need to determine the relationship between zinc intake and status and cognitive function and behavior in military personnel engaged in support, training, and combat operations and in the context of moderating variables, including physical, environmental, and psychological stressors.

**Question.** Does increasing the zinc intakes of soldiers undergoing military garrison training benefit cognitive function, particularly memory, or mood states (e.g., depression), and therefore affect military performance?

**Study design.** The research question can be addressed as part of the overall Research Priority 1, *Study the Effects of Military Garrison Training on Mineral Losses and Performance.* The dietary treatment should consist of MREs supplemented with 0, 10, and 20 mg/day of zinc. These amounts were used in previous civilian studies, including three conducted on children, and pose minimal risk of exceeding the IOM UL (40 mg/day) when combined with typical dietary intakes.

**Outcome measurements.** The battery described by Lieberman et al. (2005) (see section above *Iron and Cognition and Behavior*) is recommended to assess the relationship between zinc nutrition and mental performance. Possible effects of zinc on mood states, including depression, can be assessed with the POMS-BI, as described previously (see section above *Calcium and Cognition and Behavior*). Alternatively, if a measure specific to depression is desired so that the cognitive and somatic aspects of depression can be evaluated independently, then using a standardized and validated test, such as the Beck Depression Inventory II (Beck et al., 1996), in conjunction with the POMS-BI is recommended.

*Zinc Dietary Intake Levels*

**Justification.** The amount of zinc consumed by military personnel is unknown, and there are only estimates of zinc content in military rations, calculated mostly from food composition databases. In order to verify if the dietary intake level of zinc is adequate the level in the diets, including dietary supplements, should be determined.

**Question.** How much zinc is consumed by military personnel under garrison training?

**Study design.** Food composition tables often may not accurately reflect the zinc contents in the military rations, estimates of zinc intake using existing food composition data tables are approximate at best. Therefore, composite military diets should be analyzed (by atomic absorption spectrophotometry using acid-digested samples) for zinc to gain useful estimates of actual zinc intakes. Researchers also should determine the frequency with which military personnel use supplements containing appreciable amounts of zinc. This zinc diet analysis could be done jointly with the calcium analysis described in Research Priority 2, *Determine Mineral Status and Food and Dietary Intakes.*

## REFERENCES


Ainsworth BE, Haskell WL, Whitt MC, Irwin ML, Swartz AM, Strath SJ, O'Brien WL, Bassett DR Jr, Schmitz KH, Emplaincourt PO, Jacobs DR Jr, Leon AS. 2000. Compendium of physical activities: An update of activity codes and MET intensities. *Med Sci Sports Exerc* 32(9 Suppl): S498–S504.

American Psychiatric Association. 1994. *Diagnostic and Statistical Manual of Mental Disorders: DSM-IV.* 4th ed. Washington, DC: American Psychiatric Association.

Bakan P. 1959. Extraversion-introversion and improvement in an auditory vigilance task. *Br J Psychol* 50:325–332.

Beck AT, Steer RA, Brown GK. 1996. *BDI-II Beck Depression Inventory: Manual.* 2nd ed. San Antonio, TX: Psychological Corporation.

Belenky G, Penetar DM, Thorne D, Popp K, Leu J, Thomas M, Sing H, Balkin T, Wesensten N, Redmond D. 1994. The effects of sleep deprivation on performance during continuous combat operations. In: Institute of Medicine, Marriott BM, ed. *Food Components to Enhance Performance: An Evaluation of Potential Performance-Enhancing Food Components for Operational Rations.* Washington, DC: National Academy Press. Pp.127–135.

Brownlie T 4th, Utermohlen V, Hinton PS, Giordano C, Haas JD. 2002. Marginal iron deficiency without anemia impairs aerobic adaptation among previously untrained women. *Am J Clin Nutr* 75(4):734–742

Brune M, Magnusson B, Persson H, Hallberg L. 1986. Iron losses in sweat. *Am J Clin Nutr* 43(3): 438–443.

Corum SJC. 2004. Dietary supplement use in the military: Do Army health care providers know enough? *AMEDD* PB 8-04-1/2/3:36–38.

Curran SL, Andrykowski MA, Studts JL. 1995. Short form of the Profile of Mood States (POMS-SF): Psychometric information. *Psychol Assess* 7(1):80–83.

Held K, Antonijevic IA, Kunzel H, Uhr M, Wetter TC, Golly IC, Steiger A, Murck H. 2002. Oral $Mg^{2+}$ supplementation reverses age-related neuroendocrine and sleep EEG changes in humans. *Pharmacopsychiatry* 35(4):135–143.

Hinton PS, Giordano C, Brownlie T, Haas JD. 2000. Iron supplementation improves endurance after training in iron-depleted, nonanemic women. *J Appl Physiol* 88(3):1103–1111.

Hirsch ES, Kramer FM. 1993. Situational influences on food intake. In: Institute of Medicine, Marriott BM, ed. *Nutritional Needs in Hot Environments: Applications for Military Personnel in Field Operations.* Washington, DC: National Academy Press. Pp. 215–243.

Howley ET, Franks BD. 1997. *Health Fitness Instructor's Handbook.* Champaign, IL: Human Kinetics

IOM (Institute of Medicine). 1997. *Dietary Reference Intakes for Calcium, Phosphorus, Magnesium, Vitamin D, and Fluoride.* Washington, DC: National Academy Press.

IOM. 2001. *Dietary Reference Intakes. Vitamin A, Vitamin K, Arsenic, Boron, Chromium, Copper, Iodine, Iron, Manganese, Molybdenum, Nickel, Silicon, Vanadium, and Zinc.* Washington, DC: National Academy Press.

IOM. 2002/2005. *Dietary Reference Intakes for Energy, Carbohydrate, Fiber, Fat, Fatty Acids, Cholesterol, Protein, and Amino Acids.* Washington, DC: The National Academies Press.

IOM. 2004. *Monitoring Metabolic Status. Predicting Decrements in Physiological and Cognitive Performance.* Washington, DC: The National Academies Press.

IOM. 2006. *Nutrient Composition of Rations For Short-Term, High-Intensity Combat Operations.* Washington, DC: The National Academies Press.

Jackman LA, Millane SS, Martin BR, Wood OB, McCabe GP, Peacock M, Weaver CM. 1997. Calcium retention in relation to calcium intake and postmenarcheal age in adolescent females. *Am J Clin Nutr* 66(2):327–333.

Jensen LB, Kollerup G, Quaade F, Sorensen OH. 2001. Bone minerals changes in obese women during a moderate weight loss with and without calcium supplementation. *J Bone Miner Res* 16(1):141–147.

Krotkiewski M, Gudmundsson M, Backstrom P, Mandroukas K. 1982. Zinc and muscle strength and endurance. *Acta Physiol Scand* 116(3):309–311.

Lieberman HR. 2005 (June 15). *Evaluating Nutritional Effects on Cognitive Function in Warfighters: Lessons Learned.* Paper presented at the Institute of Medicine Workshop on The Mineral Requirements for Cognitive and Physical Performance of Military Personnel, Washington, DC: Institute of Medicine Committee on Mineral Requirements for Cognitive and Physical Performance of Military Personnel.

Lieberman HR, Bathalon GP, Falco CM, Kramer FM, Morgan CA, Niro P. 2005. Severe decrements in cognitive function and mood induced by sleep loss, heat, dehydration, and undernutrition during simulated combat. *Biol Psychiatry* 57(4):422–429.

Lorr M, McNair DM. 1984. *Manual Profile of Mood States BI-Polar Form (POMS-BI).* San Diego, CA: Educational and Industrial Testing Service.

Marvan ML, Escobedo C. 1999. Premenstrual symptomatology: Role of prior knowledge about premenstrual syndrome. *Psychosom Med* 61(2):163–167.

McArdle WD, Katch FI, Pechar GS. 1973. Comparison of continuous and discontinuous treadmill and bicycle tests for max $VO_2$. *Med Sci Sports* 5(3):156–160.

McNair DM, Heuchert JWP, Shilony E. 2003. *Profile of Mood States: Bibliography 1964–2002.* North Tonawanda, NY: Multi-Health Systems.

Moos RH. 1968. The development of a menstrual distress questionnaire. *Psychosom Med* 30(6):853–867.

Murck H. 2002. Magnesium and affective disorders. *Nutr Neurosci* 5(6):375–389.

Nyenhuis DL, Yamamoto C, Luchetta T, Terrien A, Parmentier A. 1999. Adult and geriatric normative data and validation of the profile of mood states. *J Clin Psychol* 55(1):79–86.

Palacios C, Wigertz K, Weaver CM. 2003. Comparison of 24 hour whole body versus patch tests for estimating body surface electrolyte losses. *Int J Sport Nutr Exerc Metab* 13(4):479–488.

Penland JG. 1995. Quantitative analysis of EEG effects following experimental marginal magnesium and boron deprivation. *Magnes Res* 8(4):341–358.

Ricci TA, Chowdhury HA, Heymsfield SB, Stahl T, Pierson RN Jr, Shapses SA. 1998. Calcium supplementation suppresses bone turnover during weight reduction in postmenopausal women. *J Bone Miner Res* 13(6):1045–1050.

Riedt CS, Cifuentes M, Stahl T, Chowdhury HA, Schlussel Y, Shapses SA. 2005. Overweight postmenopausal women lose bone with moderate weight reduction and 1 g/day calcium intake. *J Bone Miner Res* 20(3):455–463.

Shacham S. 1983. A shortened version of the Profile of Mood States. *J Pers Assess* 47(3):305–306.

Takase B, Akima T, Satomura K, Ohsuzu F, Mastui T, Ishihara M, Kurita A. 2004. Effects of chronic sleep deprivation on autonomic activity by examining heart rate variability, plasma catecholamine, and intracellular magnesium levels. *Biomed Pharmacother* 58(Suppl 1):S35–S39.

Thairon WJ, Lieberman HR, Montain SJ, Young AJ, Baker-Fulco CJ, DeLany JP, Hoyt RW. 2005. Energy requirements of military personnel. *Appetite* 44(1):47–65.

Thys-Jacobs S, Starkey P, Bernstein D, Tian J. 1998. Calcium carbonate and the premenstrual syndrome: Effects on premenstrual and menstrual symptoms. Premenstrual Syndrome Study Group. *Am J Obstet Gynecol* 179(2):444–452.

Vogel JA. 1994. Evaluation of physical performance. In: Institute of Medicine, Marriott BM, ed. *Food Components to Enhance Performance: An Evaluation of Potential Performance-Enhancing Food Components for Operational Rations*. Washington, DC: National Academy Press. Pp. 113–126.

Wastney ME, Martin BR, Peacock M, Smith D, Jiang XY, Jackman LA, Weaver CM. 2000. Changes in calcium kinetics in adolescent girls induced by high calcium intake. *J Clin Endocrinol Metab* 85(12):4470–4475.

Weaver CM. 2006. Clinical approaches for studying calcium metabolism and its relationship to disease. In: Weaver CM, Heaney RP, eds. *Calcium in Human Health*. Totowa, NJ: Humana Press. Pp. 65–93.

Weaver CM, Liebman M. 2002. Biomarkers of bone health appropriate for evaluating functional foods designed to reduce risk of osteoporosis. *Br J Nutr* 88(Suppl 2):S225–S232.

Wesensten N. 2004. Biomarkers for brain hypometabolism due to sleep deprivation. In: Institute of Medicine, *Monitoring Metabolic Status. Predicting Decrements in Physiological and Cognitive Perfomance*. Washington, DC: The National Academies Press. Pp. 381–391.

# 5

# Answers to the Military's Questions

This chapter summarizes answers to the specific questions that were posed to the committee. In an attempt to summarize the answers, descriptions of critical issues are merely reviewed. For more details and in-depth discussions of the critical issues the reader is referred to Chapters 2, 3, and 4 where full discussions, including explanations of inconsistent results or needs for further research for promising areas are included. Therefore, for each question and to avoid redundancy, only a summary of the issues already addressed in other chapters are presented here; the specific recommendations for each question are also included.

## QUESTIONS 1 AND 2

**1. Which dietary minerals are likely to have an impact on human performance? Are these minerals provided in adequate amounts in the meals, ready to eat (MREs) and the current first strike rations (FSRs)?**

**2. Is there a potential for any significant deficiency in essential minerals when soldiers subsist on (a) MREs during garrison training (i.e., intense training and one-day missions) or (b) FSRs during combat missions (i.e., repeated cycles of three- to seven-day combat missions, with two- to three-day recovery periods that include garrison dining)?**

Questions 1 and 2 are closely related and will be addressed together. Based on the military's information on mineral status and performance levels (Friedl, 2005; see Friedl in Appendix B) and the commmittee's experience with the functions, metabolism, and nutrient intake requirements, six minerals—calcium, copper, iron, magnesium, selenium, and zinc—were deemed important for military performance.

The committee used information (the mineral composition for 3 different MREs containing 24 menus each and 3 different FSRs menus) provided by the U.S. Army Research Institute of Environmental Medicine to evaluate the selected minerals' content adequacy in the operational rations (see Appendix C). Content adequacy can be evaluated considering groups (i.e., is the mineral content adequate for the population?) or individuals (i.e., is the mineral content adequate for each individual?). Because the committee had no data on the distribution of mineral intakes for military garrison training, the mineral content of menus for the population could not be evaluated. Instead, the recommended $RDA_{MGT}$ and $AI_{MGT}$ (Recommended Dietary Allowance and Adequate Intake for military garrison training, respectively) were used as benchmarks to evaluate mineral content adequacy of the various rations for individuals. (see Question 4 for the process on arriving at the new $RDA_{MGT}$ and $AI_{MGT}$).

For this exercise, the committee assumed that women will consume two MREs and men will consume three MREs. The average mineral content levels for each MRE or FSR were used to assess adequacy; in other words, three MREs or two MREs need to meet (without exceeding the Tolerable Upper Intake Levels [ULs]), at the minimum, the specific $RDA_{MGT}$ and $AI_{MGT}$ recommended by this committee for men and women, respectively. The content of one FSR needs to be within the recommended range for assault rations (IOM, 2006). However, consideration should be given to the fact that, although the average content might be adequate, some menus within each ration seem to be low in specific minerals (e.g., calcium). It was assumed for this study that the mix of menu choices eaten daily are sufficient to meet the average level of the minerals of interest. However, individuals' repeated selection of MREs that have low levels of particular minerals presents a risk of developing mineral deficiencies. The committee recommends, therefore, that menus on the low end of the mineral content range be revised to meet the recommended intake levels for both men and women.

On average most mineral content in rations will meet the committee's recommendations (see Table 5-1, Chapter 3 for details). The exceptions are the iron content for women ($RDA_{MGT}$ = 24 mg/day versus an average of 18 mg in two MREs) and the zinc content for men ($RDA_{MGT}$ = 15 mg/day versus an average of about 14 mg in three MREs) and women ($RDA_{MGT}$ = 11 mg/day versus an average of about 9 mg in two MREs). The mineral content of the FSRs appears to meet the recommendations of the current committee, except for calcium, whose average content in the FSRs (673 mg) is slightly lower than recommended in the Institute of Medicine (IOM) report, *Nutrient Composition of Rations for Short-Term, High Intensity Combat Operations* (750 mg, see Table 5-1) (2006).

The committee concluded that more research is needed on calcium intake and any associated risk of kidney-stone formation before lowering the range of calcium in assault rations below the AI of 1,000 mg/day.

The level of specific mineral intakes depends not only on the mineral content of the rations but also on the rations' composition (i.e., interaction with

**TABLE 5-1** Mineral Intakes: Institute of Medicine Dietary Reference Intakes, Current Military Dietary Reference Intakes, Recommended Intakes for Garrison Training ($EAR_{MGT}$, $RDA_{MGT}$, or $AI_{MGT}$), and Recommended Levels for Assault Rations

| Nutrient | IOM RDA or AI | MDRI | $RDA_{MGT}$ or $AI_{MGT}$ | Levels For Assault Rations* |
|---|---|---|---|---|
| Calcium (mg) | | | | |
| Male | 1,000 | 1,000 | 1,000 | 750–850 |
| Female | 1,000 | 1,000 | 1,000 | |
| Copper (µg) | | | | |
| Male | 900 | ND | 1,800 | 900–1,600 |
| Female | 900 | ND | 1,500 | |
| Iron (mg) | | | | |
| Male | 8 | 10 | 14 | 8–18 |
| Female | 18 | 15 | 24 | |
| Magnesium (mg) | | | | |
| Male | 420 | 420 | 420 | 400–550 |
| Female | 320 | 320 | 320 | |
| Selenium (µg) | | | | |
| Male | 55 | 55 | 55 | 55–230 |
| Female | 55 | 55 | 55 | |
| Zinc (mg) | | | | |
| Male | 11 | 15 | 15 | 11–25 |
| Female | 8 | 12 | 11 | |

NOTE: AI = Adequate Intake; EAR = Estimated Average Requirement; MDRI = Military Dietary Reference Intake; MGT = military garrison training; ND = not determined; RDA = Recommended Dietary Allowance.
*IOM (2006).

other components), food consumption behavior (e.g., do soldiers eat 100 percent of the rations?), and ration selection. Therefore, the committee concluded that surveys on actual mineral intake or status—especially for calcium and iron—need to be conducted for the adequacy of the rations' mineral content to be evaluated and that for food composition analysis should continue to be performed.

## QUESTION 3

**3. During garrison training, do weight loss diets (energy or macronutrient restricted) have the potential to lead to deficiencies of specific essential minerals?**

The principal determinant of mineral balance in healthy individuals who are physically active is that there be an adequate intake of all essential nutrients.

This situation would be the usual condition for soldiers in garrison training who eat prepared foods or rations that have intakes meeting the military's dietary reference intake (MDRI) requirements (U.S. Departments of the Army, Navy, and Air Force, 2001). Under some field conditions, particularly during operations in training or active combat, weight loss primarily caused by inadequate intakes in relation to increases in energy expenditure is common. However, under other conditions weight constancy or even weight gain is common (as is reported to be characteristic of the current operations in Iraq).

Mineral status during weight loss depends significantly on the severity of caloric deprivation, macronutrient composition of the diet, and mineral intake. The most severe caloric deficiency is due to total fasting, which would never be intended during military operations. Without energy or mineral intake but with adequate fluid intake, mineral balances would be negative for all of the minerals under consideration, including calcium, magnesium, phosphorus, sodium, potassium, zinc, selenium, copper, and iron. Such a regimen can be tolerated in obese individuals for many months so long as there is sufficient fat and water, and very obese individuals have tolerated fasting (receiving only noncaloric liquids) for up to 249 days (Bloom, 1959; Runcie and Thomson, 1970; Thomson et al., 1966). Even though there would be substantial lean-tissue loss (approximately one-quarter to one-third of the weight loss) as well as bone loss and reduced exercise capacity, death from protein-calorie malnutrition likely would occur only when there was lean-tissue loss representing about one-half of the lean tissue or about 40 percent of the initial body weight (Henry, 1990). Dysphoria, postural hypotension, and changes in mood are frequent in the early stages of starvation, but after initial adaptation to a fasting state (which occurs over the first week or so), substantial deficits in physical performance are not found until approximately a 10-percent weight loss is reached. For normal-weight individuals (the expectation is that most individuals found in military settings would be of normal weight), total fasting is much less well tolerated, even initially. Mortality would happen probably within 6–11 weeks, and physical performance would be very poor in the later weeks. Death would take place due to an absence of stored fat sufficient to meet the energy deficit; this claim is based on the experience of the Irish Republican Army hunger strikers in Northern Ireland (Leiter and Marliss, 1982). Thus, death usually would occur because of an acute lack of energy caused by depleted body energy stores.

A less severe, but still hypocaloric, diet would be described as one that provides some intake but less, often far less, than about 50 percent of caloric needs. A substantial experience with such diets occurred in the 1970s when liquid protein diets based on collagen were used as the principal source of protein and calories, leading to multiple mineral deficiencies. A number of deaths occurred in obese individuals consuming such regimens for periods of at least several months; the deaths were thought to be due to a combination of lean tissue loss and mineral deficiencies, particularly of potassium, copper, and phosphorus

(Amatruda et al., 1983; Isner et al., 1979; Klevay, 1979). Subsequently, similar degrees of caloric deprivation—but with adequate mineral and high biologic value protein intake, as found in semistarvation ketogenic diets—were effective for short-term weight loss of considerable degree without causing undue safety concerns in obese individuals (Palgi et al., 1985). These cases of caloric deprivation emphasize the importance of protein composition and mineral intake under the related conditions. However, the use of this type of regimen for military purposes was discontinued—except for unanticipated combat situations—after experience with a severely hypocaloric diet, which met less than 50 percent of the energy needs during Ranger training, led to substantial and unacceptable clinical deficits associated with greater than 10-percent weight loss (Moore et al., 1992).

Caloric deficits of about 1,000–1,500 kilocalories that still provide greater than 50 percent of caloric needs are well tolerated clinically for weight loss in the overweight and obese as well as during short-term military operations (IOM, 2006). Similar diets used for intentional weight loss on an outpatient basis rarely lead to a 10-percent weight loss, frequently because of a lack of compliance, and thus, lead to unchanged or even improved physical performance. In military combat settings, where other food sources are unavailable, it would be good clinical policy to avoid prolonged periods of hypocaloric feeding, which could lead to weight losses greater than 10 percent.

The principal variables, in terms of mineral balance, of these mildly hypocaloric diets are the macronutrient content (particularly if high or low in protein) and the mineral content. The minerals of greatest interest are calcium, magnesium, and zinc, since the likely duration of use intended in a military context makes substantial imbalances for iron, copper, and selenium of little clinical relevance, particularly when these minerals are provided daily in MDRI quantities. Of the three minerals of greatest interest, magnesium is the least likely to present a clinical problem, because the body can reduce urinary magnesium losses to minute levels, even without limiting magnesium intake. Zinc is of greater concern because of its importance in immune function and the potential for occurrence of diarrheal illness in military operations [as mentioned in Hamer (2005) and in Hamer in Appendix B, diarrhea is a risk factor for zinc losses]. If however there is an absence of diarrhea and if zinc is consumed at MDRI quantities, then the net zinc lost due to weight loss on a hypocaloric diet reflects net nitrogen loss. Thus, minimization of net nitrogen loss would be the greater concern when compared with zinc loss.

Studies of elemental balance in underweight subjects have demonstrated that lean tissue has a fixed ratio of nitrogen to potassium, phosphorus, and sodium, and the three latter must all be provided in minimal amounts for lean tissue to be maintained (Rudman et al., 1975). However, these amounts are met easily by each of the minerals' RDA. Calcium balance under these conditions is dependent on phosphorus and sodium, since bone-mineral repletion can not occur in the absence of these elements (Rudman et al., 1975). Thus, the most important variable is a relatively high protein intake of 1.2–1.5 g/kg (IOM, 2006); benefits of a high-protein diet include a reduction in hunger (when compared with an isocaloric diet high in carbohydrates) as well as a number of metabolic benefits related to insulin action (Noakes et al., 2005). Bone turnover was increased with both the high-protein and high-carbohydrate diets and included an increase in both serum osteocalcin and urinary collagen cross-link excretion, markers of bone resorption (Noakes et al., 2005).

The iron status (also of both diets) was well maintained and indicated no changes in hemoglobin, even though dietary iron reached RDA levels only in the high-protein diet (Noakes et al., 2005). This finding is in contrast to that of Kretsch et al. (1998) where research indicated that obese women consuming a diet providing approximately 50 percent of estimated calories led to a significant reduction in hemoglobin and hematocrit and a reduction in cognitive ability related to sustained attention. The difference in findings may be linked to the iron status at the beginning of the diet period, which appeared to be better in the former study, and perhaps as well to the higher protein intake particularly in the high-protein group (Kretsch et al., 1998; Noakes et al., 2005). The protein intake in the Kretsch et al. (1998) study was not regulated and, thus, was likely to be less than 1 g/kg.

A number of studies have demonstrated the importance of higher protein intakes to improve preservation of lean tissue during weight loss when the protein is substituted with isocaloric amounts of carbohydrate (Baba et al., 1999; Farnsworth et al., 2003; Piatti et al., 1994). However, similar benefits in terms of hunger reduction and improvement in lipid metabolism can be achieved if the carbohydrates are provided in larger quantities as long as those used have a low glycemic index (Pereira et al., 2004). Nonetheless, for the maximal preservation of body protein with weight loss, protein intakes of 1.2–1.5 g/kg would need to be present. When the dietary protein is in this range, whether the protein is mostly from high-calcium dairy products (2,400 mg/day) or from mixed-protein and moderate calcium products (500 mg/day of calcium), the effects on fasting insulin, lipids, blood pressure, and fibrinolysis and endothelial function (i.e., metabolic parameters) are independent of diet (Bowen et al., 2005). A study from the same group did show, however, that the lower calcium intake caused a larger increase in urinary deoxypyridinoline as a marker of bone breakdown and an increase in osteocalcin in the mixed-protein diet, only suggesting a benefit for the high-dairy protein with its higher calcium in reducing bone turnover (Bowen et al., 2004).

Calcium is the principal mineral of concern regarding weight loss diets, because its metabolism may be altered by dietary composition. Evidence shows that weight loss—in overweight and obese subjects as well as in postmenopausal women consuming their usual calcium intake—is associated with a loss in bone mass (Hannan et al., 2000; Ricci et al., 2001) and an increase in fracture risk (Langlois et al., 1996). Although many minerals are essential for bone health and function, the risk of calcium inadequacy in the diet is higher than risks of other deficiencies. Because of its role in bone health and potential alterations in metabolism if intake is inadequate, calcium is the principal mineral of concern regarding weight loss diets. In overweight postmenopausal women, weight loss resulting from moderately hypocaloric intakes leads to reduced calcium absorption, but net positive calcium balance can be achieved with 1.8 g/day of calcium as compared to 1.0 g/day (Cifuentes et al., 2004). A follow-up study demonstrated that calcium supplementation at 1.7 g/day minimizes bone loss during weight loss in overweight postmenopausal women (Riedt et al., 2005). An earlier study on obese postmenopausal women also showed that calcium supplementation of 1 g/day reduced urinary collagen pyridinium crosslinks, osteocalcin, and parathormone during weight loss (Ricci et al., 1998). The effect was not observed in obese premenopausal women (Shapses et al., 2001).

The relationships between weight loss, level of protein intake, calcium intake, and bone health have not been studied in physically active premenopausal women, a population that would be relevant to the military. However, to safeguard against potential bone deficiency during weight loss higher protein intakes and calcium intakes of at least 1 g/day—with, perhaps, even greater benefit if intakes are in the 1,500–1,700 mg/day range—are recommended. These recommended intake levels should be tested on young adults who are intentionally dieting for weight loss; if weight loss is a consequence of the training itself and the reduced energy intakes found in military scenarios, then, the high protein/high calcium intake should be tested in not obese, or even overweight soldiers.

With regard to weight loss and its impact on the other essential minerals—including magnesium, zinc, selenium, copper, and iron—there is little evidence to show that there is either (1) a reduced efficiency of use, and thus a need for increased mineral intakes, or (2) a reduced need for mineral intakes during periods of modest hypocaloric intakes (1,000–1,500 kcal/day) that provide at least 50 percent of daily caloric needs. Hence, providing the essential minerals in the amounts proposed in this report should be sufficient to maintain optimal function during weight loss.

## QUESTION 4

**4. Do the high-performance activities of soldiers cause excessive mineral loss, thereby raising the mineral dietary requirements?**

There is evidence to believe that exercise-related mineral loss, occurring mainly through the sweat but also through feces and urine, might be significant. However, many of the studies addressing mineral secretion and exercise cannot be applied to the military environment, or have design flaws, or both. Nonetheless, because of the number of studies suggesting that the losses are real, the committee has increased the requirements for iron, copper, and zinc, based on the best available data and on their expertise and reasonable judgements (see

Table 5-1). Chapter 3 details the recommendations. These values should be considered provisional and should be reconsidered after new studies (following the design recommendations in Chapter 4) become available.

The data for copper are variable partially due to differences in sweat collection and copper quantification methods. Based on the best data available, the committee concluded that male soldiers in garrison training will lose at least 500 μg/day of copper (female soldiers will lose at least 350 μg/day) through sweat.

The data on iron, with regard to sweat losses, come from civilian studies and vary considerably. However, the committee concluded that sweat losses might be significant during exercise and need to be considered when establishing iron requirements. The committee believes soldiers could lose as much as 1 mg/day of iron (0.6 mg/day for women) through sweat.

Likewise, studies on zinc increases in the sweat generated by exercise reveal that as much as 2.0 mg/day and 1.3 mg/day, for men and women, respectively, could be lost because of garrison training conditions.

Calcium requirements may also be higher under the stress of physical activity and environmental conditions normally experienced by military personnel in garrison training. There is evidence indicating that factors like increased sweat losses, loss of bone mass with oral contraceptives, or increased losses with weight loss could raise the requirements. Other factors encountered during training, however, such as the beneficial effects of exercise on bone metabolism, may compensate for those losses. All these various factors that affect calcium and bone metabolism act concomitantly and the overall impact of garrison training on requirements is still uncertain. The committee concluded that there is not enough evidence to change the calcium dietary requirements for soldiers in garrison training but urged researchers to conduct appropriate studies that could address this issue.

In all cases, acclimatization to heat and exercise is likely to occur, but questions regarding the extent of acclimatization remain unanswered. In addition, new models (designed according to Chapter 4's recommendations) that better simulate military garrison training conditions need to be developed, and the resulting data on mineral losses must be collected. There was not enough data to assess whether or not physical activity would increase urinary or fecal mineral losses. However, there are suggestions to this effect (i.e., substantial fecal iron losses could occur with extreme exercise); research in this area also is warranted (see Chapter 4).

Nutrient standards for military personnel in garrison training or in operations should be derived as indicated in Box 5-1. Based on the sweat loss findings, the committee adjusted the IOM Estimated Average Requirements (EARs) and calculated new EARs and RDAs ($EARs_{MGT}$ and $RDAs_{MGT}$) for copper, iron, and zinc (see Table 5-1). The committee recommends using the current IOM AI level of calcium for the general population as the $AI_{MGT}$ until more research becomes available (see Table 5-1).

**BOX 5-1**
**Establishing Nutrient Standards for Military Personnel**

Recommendation: Nutrient standards for military personnel in garrison training should be derived as follows:

1. $EAR_{MGT}$ : Modify the current IOM EAR by adjusting for the variable of interest (e.g., level of sweat losses).
2. $RDA_{MGT}$ : Add 2 × SD (standard deviation) of the $EAR_{MGT}$, to ensure that 97–98 percent of soldiers will have adequate intake.

There were not enough data addressing the impact of sweat losses on magnesium and selenium levels to recommend an increase in dietary intake (see Chapter 3 for details). Research on sweat, urinary, and fecal losses under military garrison training conditions also is warranted (see Chapter 4). The committee recommends using the current IOM RDAs for magnesium and selenium for the general population as the $RDA_{MGT}$ until more research becomes available (see Table 5-1).

## QUESTION 5

**5. Is there any scientific evidence that mineral supplements (individually or in combination) improve soldiers' performance?**

There is no definitive evidence that specific mineral supplementation in amounts greater than those recommended as dietary requirements will improve soldiers' physical or cognitive performance. Therefore, the committee has not recommended the intake of supplements to this effect. There are, however, scientific studies that strongly suggest the potential for improved performance and are summarized below (see Chapter 3 for details).

A positive relationship between physical activity and calcium intake on bone density has been demonstrated in postmenopausal women and children, although not in age groups or lifestyles relevant to the military (Lau et al., 1992; Prince et al., 1991; Specker, 1996; Specker and Binkley, 2003). However, related research with premenopausal women has shown mixed results (Recker et al., 1992; Valimaki et al., 1994). The type of exercise may influence bone turnover as well as dietary intake. In research conducted on cadets, only males showed that milk consumption positively influences bone health; there was also a significant impact on cortical thickness related to milk consumption and exercise (Nieves, 2005; see Nieves in Appendix B). Calcium also appears to improve mood states, especially premenstrual distress syndrome (PMS) and depression (Penland and Johnson, 1993; Thys-Jacobs et al., 1989). Although results are encouraging for calcium to relieve negative mood states, this has been done only with civilians and nonstressful situations; this suggestion needs to be demonstrated under the environmental and stressful conditions of garrison training. The reader is referred to Chapter 3 for more details.

Although the few studies performed in the military population do not suggest a relationship between iron status and cognition and mood states, there is sufficient evidence from studies in the civilian population that supports an association between iron status and improved cognitive functions and behavior (e.g., Bruner et al., 1996; Groner et al., 1986, see Chapter 3). Some of these conclusions come from studies on iron deficiency. One of the pieces of evidence comes from a 16-week intervention study using women who, as part of the study, were provided with iron supplements (see Beard and Murray Kolb in Appendix B). After 16 weeks, some women had improved their iron status independently of the iron supplementation. There was a strong association between the women who reached the highest iron status (due to iron supplementation or other reasons) and improved measurements of attention, learning skills, and memory functions. Although one cannot ensure that iron supplementation will have a beneficial effect in all cases, it appears that improved iron status, possibly beyond the current recommended 15 μg/L of ferritin (level at which iron stores are present), may have beneficial effects in cognitive functions relevant for the military.

Studies conducted to determine the effects of iron supplementation on mood states also indicate that depression can be alleviated by treating iron deficiency (Beard et al., 2005; Corwin et al., 2003). Although there is no doubt that the data are promising, all of the studies linking cognition and behavior with iron status have been done with civilians. Therefore, the committee concluded that before requirements for iron are increased with the objective of improving cognitive performance or mood states, more research is needed focusing on the subjects and environment of interest to the military.

A few studies also have been performed on the potential relationship between magnesium nutrition and improved effects of sleep deprivation that might affect future recommendations for military personnel. The association between selenium and zinc and mood states also has garnered interest. The data for these relationships, though, are still preliminary and, thus, merely suggestive.

Taken all the research together, the committee concluded there is no scientific evidence to raise the recommendations for minerals with the objective of improving physical or cognitive performance or behavior. The committee also determined that it would be worthwhile to allocate enough resources for answering questions on the potential effects of supplemental calcium on physical performance and mood states, supplemental iron on cognitive functions, and supplemental magnesium on sleep deprivation effects and mood states. In addition, the relationship between supplemental zinc and cognition and mood states, as well as supplemental selenium and improvement of mood states, also could be considered (see Chapter 4).

## QUESTION 6

**6. Are the Military Dietary Reference Intakes (MDRIs) for dietary minerals reflective of the Institute of Medicine (IOM) Dietary Reference Intakes (Recommended Dietary Allowances [RDAs] or Adequate Intakes [AIs])? Should the MDRIs follow the IOM RDA or AIs or should differences persist because of the specific needs of soldiers?**

The MDRIs have been developed as a variant of the IOM Dietary Reference Intakes (DRIs) to account for the different environments and physical activity encountered by soldiers and to plan appropriate nutrient intakes and rations for them. The MDRIs and the nutritional standards for operational rations (NSORs) were established most recently in 2001 and were based on the IOM DRIs that were current at that time (U.S. Departments of the Army, Navy, and Air Force, 2001). Many of the MDRI values are similar to the DRIs, with the notable exception of sodium. The current MDRIs for minerals are the same as the IOM RDAs or AIs.

There are reasons, however, to establish reference nutrient intakes that would apply specifically to the military population and help them to maintain a nutrient balance. First, the military population is different from civilians in terms of anthropometric criteria—that is, military personnel are slightly different in height, weight, and body fat and are generally more physically fit—and performance activity levels (typically higher in soldiers). Mineral values in the MDRIs should reflect the differences in anthropometry and in the mineral losses caused by high-performance activity.

Second, the military lifestyle includes unique circumstances that are rarely encountered by civilians. These circumstances include multiple physical and psychological stressors (e.g., intense and continuous exercise while carrying heavy weight, sleep deprivation, stressful combat situations, extreme weather conditions) that can alter a soldier's physiology.

The third reason for establishing military-specific nutrient requirements is to optimize the health and performance of enlisted men and women. The criteria for establishing requirements for the general population by the IOM has been to maintain health, so most of the data would ideally come from balance studies. However, one of the military's main objectives is to succeed in operations that demand ultimate physical and cognitive performance—consequently, if performance benefits are demonstrated, then the military would recommend higher nutrient levels. As science emerges regarding the unique nutrient needs of military personnel, additional adjustments will be necessary to meet those needs.

The MDRIs should continue to reflect the IOM DRIs, with modifications made to specific nutrient requirements if sufficient scientific evidence demonstrates related needs and benefits. Also, the MDRIs can be used as guidelines for rations development for the individual soldier.

The IOM DRIs can be used for dietary assessment and planning to guarantee a low prevalence of inadequate nutrient intakes (IOM, 2000, 2003). To plan menus or rations for a large group, planners should know the EAR (and its distribution) of the target population, not only the mean and standard deviation, but also the percentile intake levels. However, when planning diets for individuals, using only the RDAs or AIs is appropriate and sufficient (IOM, 2003). The MDRIs could be used to plan and assess menus for military personnel in the same way that the IOM DRIs are used for civilians.

The difficulty in assessing the nutritional adequacy of menus for soldiers in garrison training is, as mentioned previously, that determinations will depend not only on the mean or median intakes but also on the range of the intake distribution, which is unknown for the military population. Instead, MDRIs could be used by cafeteria menu planners as a useful benchmark for what levels of nutrients are needed in foods on the menus. The IOM report *Applications in Dietary Planning* (IOM, 2003) should serve as a guide for using the MDRIs to plan the diets of military personnel. For the present, food-service managers should guarantee that cafeteria food is nutritionally diverse (contains selections from all food groups) and adequate, so that the options offered are likely to meet an individual's MDRI. To assist in the design of cafeteria food choices, food-service managers should include dietitians and nutritionists who are capable of applying nutrition guides, such as the *Dietary Guidelines for Americans* (http://www.healthierus.gov/dietaryguidelines/) and *MyPyramid* (http://www.mypyramid.gov/), that will meet the military's needs.

Although the nutrient intake levels for soldiers who eat rations are unknown, it can be assumed safely that they will not vary too much if all of the rations issued are consumed. When planning, rations should meet the new military MDRIs ($RDA_{MGT}$ or $AI_{MGT}$) for minerals. In situations where gender differences exist, rations should contain the highest recommended amounts, but those amounts should remain lower than the UL for the age range. Hence, the current NSORs based on MDRIs are established to represent the minimal levels of nutrients in operational rations. When adjusted as described, $RDA_{MGT}$ (and $AI_{MGT}$) would be the basis of NSORs and would provide adequate levels for military personnel in garrison training.

The committee supports the use of NSORs—modified accordingly as new scientific data become available—as minimum levels of nutrients in operational rations. The NSORs might vary depending on specific military situations; for instance, NSORs for military garrison training and for sustained operations may differ.

## QUESTION 7

**7. How do changes in drinking water sources during military deployment affect the balance of essential dietary minerals (e.g., U.S. public water supply versus bottled water versus field purification water)?**

The military's great efforts to educate soldiers on the need for water consumption have resulted in an improved conciousness regarding water intake.

Consequently, water could become a method to deliver minerals. By virtue of the diverse water sources processed for the military, water could be a source of mineral intake variation with potential consequences on military performance. However, due to purification processes, it appears that the mineral content of the water for consumption is fairly low and would not contribute significantly to dietary intakes of minerals.

The military provides soldiers with water from sources that meet the standards for chemical and microbiological levels. During foreign deployments, drinking water may come from local water supplies and undergo additional treatments such as filtration and chlorination for bacterial control and removal of dissolved solids. For example, currently deployed soldiers consume mineral water that is produced at eight different sites and inspected by the military for bacteria, contaminants, and mineral content. In order for the water to be shipped to the soldiers, the mineral content has to be as low as what is found in U.S. commercially available mineral water; minerals are added in some cases (e.g., calcium is added to improve the taste). Soldiers also have access to nonbottled water that is essentially mineral free because it has been filtered through reverse osmosis purification units. The bioavailability of each mineral from water would depend on the salt form in the water. However, scant research exists to suggest that water can be a source of essential minerals.

Considering the typical water consumption volumes of approximately 3 L/day, the committee concluded that due to processes applied to fresh water for human consumption, differences in mineral content of water are not such that will affect the total intake levels of minerals by military personnel and do not contribute to the balance of essential dietary minerals. The committee concluded that the addition of calcium and magnesium to water consumed by military personnel is warranted only when improving the taste is the desirable outcome. There is no evidence to suggest that the addition of substantial levels of calcium and magnesium would be an efficient strategy to meet nutritional standards; in addition, there is little research on bioavailability of minerals from water. Additional cost evaluation of using water as a vehicle for minerals should be conducted if it is to be considered for implementation.

## REFERENCES

Amatruda JM, Biddle TL, Patton ML, Lockwood DH. 1983. Vigorous supplementation of a hypocaloric diet prevents cardiac arrhythmias and mineral depletion. *Am J Med* 74(6):1016–1022.

Baba NH, Sawaya S, Torbay N, Habbal Z, Azar S, Hashim SA. 1999. High protein vs high carbohydrate hypoenergetic diet for the treatment of obese hyperinsulinemic subjects. *Int J Obes Relat Metab Disord* 23(11):1202–1206.

Beard JL, Hendricks MK, Perez EM, Murray-Kolb LE, Berg A, Vernon-Feagans L, Irlam J, Isaacs W, Sive A, Tomlinson M. 2005. Maternal iron deficiency anemia affects postpartum emotions and cognition. *J Nutr* 135(2):267–272.

Bloom WL. 1959. Fasting as an introduction to the treatment of obesity. *Metabolism* 8(3):214–220.

Bowen J, Noakes M, Clifton PM. 2004. A high dairy protein, high-calcium diet minimizes bone turnover in overweight adults during weight loss. *J Nutr* 134(3):568–573.

Bowen J, Noakes M, Clifton PM. 2005. Effect of calcium and dairy foods in high protein, energy-restricted diets on weight loss and metabolic parameters in overweight adults. *Int J Obes (Lond)* 29(8):957–965.

Bruner AB, Joffe A, Duggan AK, Casella JF, Brandt J. 1996. Randomised study of cognitive effects of iron supplementation in non-anaemic iron-deficient adolescent girls. *Lancet* 348(9033): 992–996.

Cifuentes M, Riedt CS, Brolin RE, Field MP, Sherrell RM, Shapses SA. 2004. Weight loss and calcium intake influence calcium absorption in overweight postmenopausal women. *Am J Clin Nutr* 80(1):123–130.

Corwin EJ, Murray-Kolb LE, Beard JL. 2003. Low hemoglobin level is a risk factor for postpartum depression. *J Nutr* 133(12):4139–4142.

Farnsworth E, Luscombe ND, Noakes M, Wittert G, Argyiou E, Clifton PM. 2003. Effect of a high-protein, energy-restricted diet on body composition, glycemic control, and lipid concentrations in overweight and obese hyperinsulinemic men and women. *Am J Clin Nutr* 78(1): 31–39.

Friedl KE. 2005 (June 13). *Concerns About the Effects of Military Environments on Mineral Metabolism and Consequences of Marginal Deficiencies to Performance.* Paper presented at the Institute of Medicine Workshop on Mineral Requirements for Cognitive and Physical Performance of Military Personnel, Washinton, DC. Institute of Medicine Committee on Mineral Requirements for Cognitive and Physical Performance of Military Personnel.

Groner JA, Holtzman NA, Charney E, Mellits ED. 1986. A randomized trial of oral iron on tests of short-term memory and attention span in young pregnant women. *J Adolesc Health Care* 7(1):44–48.

Hamer DH. 2005 (June 14). *Mineral Intake Needs and Infection Diseases.* Paper presented at the Institue of Medicine Workshop on The Mineral Requirements for Cognitive and Physical Performance of Military Personnel, Washington, DC: Institute of Medicine Committee on Mineral Requirements for Cognitive and Physical Performance of Military Personnel.

Hannan MT, Felson DT, Dawson-Hughes B, Tucker KL, Cupples LA, Wilson PW, Kiel DP. 2000. Risk factors for longitudinal bone loss in elderly men and women: The Framingham Osteoporosis Study. *J Bone Miner Res* 15(4):710–720.

Henry CJ. 1990. Body mass index and the limits of human survival. *Eur J Clin Nutr* 44(4):329–335.

IOM (Institute of Medicine). 2000. *Dietary Reference Intakes. Applications in Dietary Assessment.* Washington, DC: National Academy Press.

IOM. 2003. *Dietary Reference Intakes. Applications in Dietary Planning.* Washington, DC: The National Academies Press.

IOM. 2006. *Nutrient Composition of Rations for Short-Term, High-Intensity Combat Operations.* Washington, DC: The National Academies Press.

Isner JM, Sours HE, Paris AL, Ferrans VJ, Roberts WC. 1979. Sudden, unexpected death in avid dieters using the liquid-protein-modified-fast diet. Observations in 17 patients and the role of the prolonged QT interval. *Circulation* 60(6):1401–1412.

Klevay LM. 1979. Copper deficiency with liquid protein diets? *N Engl J Med* 300(1):48.

Kretsch MJ, Fong AK, Green MW, Johnson HL. 1998. Cognitive function, iron status, and hemoglobin concentration in obese dieting women. *Eur J Clin Nutr* 52(7):512–518.

Langlois JA, Harris T, Looker AC, Madans J. 1996. Weight change between age 50 years and old age is associated with risk of hip fracture in white women aged 67 years and older. *Arch Intern Med* 156(9):989–994.

Lau EM, Woo J, Leung PC, Swaminathan R, Leung D. 1992. The effects of calcium supplementation and exercise on bone density in elderly Chinese women. *Osteoporos Int* 2(4):168–173.

Leiter LA, Marliss EB. 1982. Survival during fasting may depend on fat as well as protein stores. *J Am Med Assoc* 248(18):2306–2307.

Moore RJ, Friedl KE, Kramer TR, Martinez-Lopez LE, Hoyt RW, Tulley RE, DeLany JP, Askew EW, Vogel JA. 1992. *Changes in Soldier Nutritional Status & Immune Function During the Ranger Training Course.* Technical Report T13-92. Natick, MA: U.S. Army Medical Research and Development Command.

Nieves JW. 2005 (June 14). *Physical Activity and Nutrition: Effects on Bone Turnover, Bone Mass, and Stress Fractures.* Paper presented at the Institue of Medicine Workshop on The Mineral Requirements for Cognitive and Physical Performance of Military Personnel, Washington, DC. Institute of Medicine Committee on Mineral Requirements for Cognitive and Physical Performance of Military Personnel.

Noakes M, Keogh JB, Foster PR, Clifton PM. 2005. Effect of an energy-restricted, high-protein, low-fat diet relative to a conventional high-carbohydrate, low-fat diet on weight loss, body composition, nutritional status, and markers of cardiovascular health in obese women. *Am J Clin Nutr* 81(6):1298–1306.

Palgi A, Read JL, Greenberg I, Hoefer MA, Bistrian BR, Blackburn GL. 1985. Multidisciplinary treatment of obesity with a protein-sparing modified fast: Results in 668 outpatients. *Am J Public Health* 75(10):1190–1194.

Penland JG, Johnson PE. 1993. Dietary calcium and manganese effects on menstrual cycle symptoms. *Am J Obstet Gynecol* 168(5):1417–1423.

Pereira MA, Swain J, Goldfine AB, Rifai N, Ludwig DS. 2004. Effects of a low-glycemic load diet on resting energy expenditure and heart disease risk factors during weight loss. *J Am Med Assoc* 292(20):2482–2490.

Piatti PM, Monti F, Fermo I, Baruffaldi L, Nasser R, Santambrogio G, Librenti MC, Galli-Kienle M, Pontiroli AE, Pozza G. 1994. Hypocaloric high-protein diet improves glucose oxidation and spares lean body mass: Comparison to hypocaloric high-carbohydrate diet. *Metabolism* 43(12): 1481–1487.

Prince RL, Smith M, Dick IM, Price RI, Webb PG, Henderson NK, Harris MM. 1991. Prevention of postmenopausal osteoporosis. A comparative study of exercise, calcium supplementation, and hormone-replacement therapy. *N Engl J Med* 325(17):1189–1195.

Recker RR, Davies KM, Hinders SM, Heaney RP, Stegman MR, Kimmel DB. 1992. Bone gain in young adult women. *J Am Med Assoc* 268(17):2403–2408.

Ricci TA, Chowdhury HA, Heymsfield SB, Stahl T, Pierson RN Jr, Shapses SA. 1998. Calcium supplementation suppresses bone turnover during weight reduction in postmenopausal women. *J Bone Miner Res* 13(6):1045–1050.

Ricci TA, Heymsfield SB, Pierson RN Jr, Stahl T, Chowdhury HA, Shapses SA. 2001. Moderate energy restriction increases bone resorption in obese postmenopausal women. *Am J Clin Nutr* 73(2):347–352.

Riedt CS, Cifuentes M, Stahl T, Chowdhury HA, Schlussel Y, Shapses SA. 2005. Overweight postmenopausal women lose bone with moderate weight reduction and 1 g/day calcium intake. *J Bone Miner Res* 20(3):455–463.

Rudman D, Millikan WJ, Richardson TJ, Bixler TJ 2nd, Stackhouse J, McGarrity WC. 1975. Elemental balances during intravenous hyperalimentation of underweight adult subjects. *J Clin Invest* 55(1):94–104.

Runcie J, Thomson TJ. 1970. Prolonged starvation—a dangerous procedure? *Br Med J* 3(720): 432–435.

Shapses SA, Von Thun NL, Heymsfield SB, Ricci TA, Ospina M, Pierson RN Jr, Stahl T. 2001. Bone turnover and density in obese premenopausal women during moderate weight loss and calcium supplementation. *J Bone Miner Res* 16(7):1329–1336.

Specker BL. 1996. Evidence for an interaction between calcium intake and physical activity on changes in bone mineral density. *J Bone Miner Res* 11(10):1539–1544.

Specker B, Binkley T. 2003. Randomized trial of physical activity and calcium supplementation on bone mineral content in 3- to 5-year-old children. *J Bone Miner Res* 18(5):885–892.

Thomson TJ, Runcie J, Miller V. 1966. Treatment of obesity by total fasting for up to 249 days. *Lancet* 2(7471):992–996.

Thys-Jacobs S, Ceccarelli S, Bierman A, Weisman H, Cohen MA, Alvir J. 1989. Calcium supplementation in premenstrual syndrome: A randomized crossover trial. *J Gen Intern Med* 4(3): 183–189.

U.S. Departments of the Army, Navy, and Air Force. 2001. *Nutrition Standards and Education.* AR 40-25/BUMEDINST 10110.6/AFI 44-141. Washington, DC: U.S. Department of Defense Headquarters.

Valimaki MJ, Karkkainen M, Lamberg-Allardt C, Laitinen K, Alhava E, Heikkinen J, Impivaara O, Makela P, Palmgren J, Seppanen R, Vuori I . 1994. Exercise, smoking, and calcium intake during adolescence and early adulthood as determinants of peak bone mass. *Br Med J* 309(6949):230–235.

# A

# Workshop Agenda

**Mineral Dietary Requirements for Military Performance**

**Committee on Mineral Requirements for Cognitive and Physical Performance of Military Personnel**

**Food and Nutrition Board**

**Institute of Medicine**

**The National Academies**

The National Academies, 2101 Constitution Avenue NW, Washington, DC
*June 13–15, 2005*

**June 13, 2005**

**1:00 p.m.** **WELCOME AND INTRODUCTORY REMARKS**
*Robert M. Russell, Committee Chair*

**1:10** **INTRODUCTION TO COMBAT RATIONS**
(Moderator: Wayne Askew, Committee on Military Nutrition Research)

1:15 History of Committee for Military Nutrition Research
*John W. Erdman, Chair*

| | |
|---|---|
| 1:35 | Overview of Committee's Task and Workshop Goals<br>*Andrew J. Young, U.S. Army Research Institute of Environmental Medicine, Natick, Massachusetts* |
| 1:55 | Physiological Demands and Nutritional Needs of Military Personnel<br>*Karl E. Friedl, U.S. Army Research Institute of Environmental Medicine, Natick, Massachusetts* |
| 2:15 | Development of Military Dietary Reference Intakes and Mineral Content of Military Rations<br>*Carol J. Baker-Fulco, U.S. Army Research Institute of Environmental Medicine, Natick, Massachusetts* |
| 2:45 | Discussion |
| 3:15 | Break |
| **3:30** | **MINERAL METABOLISM**<br>(Moderator: Gerald Combs Jr., Committee on Mineral Requirements for Cognitive and Physical Performance of Military Personnel) |
| 3:35 | Bioavailability of Iron, Zinc and Copper as Influenced by Host and Dietary Factors<br>*Janet R. Hunt, USDA-ARS Grand Forks Human Nutrition Research Center, Grand Forks, North Dakota* |
| 3:55 | Absorption Mechanisms and Metabolism of Iron, Zinc, and Copper<br>*Cathy W. Levenson, Florida State University, Tallahassee* |
| 4:15 | Absorption Mechanisms, Bioavailability, and Metabolism of Calcium and Magnesium<br>*Connie M. Weaver, Purdue University, West Lafayette, Indiana* |
| 4:35 | Drinking Water as a Source of Mineral Nutrition<br>*Gerald F Combs, Jr., USDA-ARS Grand Forks Human Nutrition Research Center, Grand Forks, North Dakota* |
| 4:55 | Discussion on Mineral Metabolism |
| 6:00 | End of Day |

**June 14, 2005**

| | |
|---|---|
| 8:30 a.m. | Breakfast |
| **9:00** | **MINERAL METABOLISM**<br>(Moderator: Gerald Combs Jr., Committee on Mineral Requirements for Military Personnel) |
| 9:05 | Assessment of Zinc, Copper and Magnesium Status<br>*Carl L. Keen, University of California at Davis* |
| **9:25** | **STRESS FACTORS AFFECTING HOMEOSTASIS**<br>(Moderator: Mike Sawka, *U.S. Army Research Institute of Environmental Medicine*) |
| 9:30 | Environmental Stressors during Military Operations<br>*Mike N. Sawka, U.S. Army Research Institute of Environmental Medicine, Natick, Massachusetts* |
| 9:50 | Mineral Sweat Losses during Exercise<br>*Emily M. Haymes, Florida State University, Tallahassee* |
| 10:10 | Weight Loss and Mineral Status<br>*Steven B. Heymsfield, Merck & Co. Inc., Rahway, New Jersey* |
| 10:30 | Protein Metabolism and Mineral Requirements<br>*Henry C. Lukaski, USDA-ARS Grand Forks Human Nutrition Research Center, Grand Forks, North Dakota* |
| 10:50 | Break |
| 11:10 | Discussion of Stress Factors Affecting Homeostasis |
| 12:00 | Lunch |

**POTENTIAL BENEFITS OF MINERALS**

| | |
|---|---|
| **1:00** | **MINERALS AND THE IMMUNE SYSTEM**<br>(Moderator: Esther Sternberg, Committee on Military Nutrition Research) |

| | |
|---|---|
| 1:05 | Interactive Influences of Physical Activity and Psychological Stress on Immune Function<br>*Monika Fleshner, University of Colorado, Boulder* |
| 1:25 | Mineral Metabolism during Infection<br>*David H. Hamer, Boston University and Tufts University, Boston, Massachusetts* |
| 1:45 | Minerals and Prevention of Infectious Diseases<br>*David H. Hamer, Boston University and Tufts University, Boston, Massachusetts* |
| 2:05 | Effects of Exercise and Mineral Nutrition on Immune Function<br>*Mark Davis, University of South Carolina* |
| 2:35 | Zinc, Copper, and Immune Function<br>*Sue S. Percival, University of Florida, Gainesville* |
| 2:55 | Break |
| 3:15 | Selenium and Immune Function<br>*John F. Sheridan, Ohio State University, Columbus* |
| 3:35 | Discussion of Minerals and the Immune System |
| **4:30** | **INJURY AND OPTIMIZATION OF RECOVERY**<br>(Moderator: Connie Weaver, Committee on Mineral Requirements for Cognitive and Physical Performance of Military Personnel) |
| 4:35 | Muscle Injury (Inflammation also?) and Recovery: Description of Process and Role of Minerals<br>*Joseph G. Cannon, Medical College of Georgia, Augusta* |
| 4:55 | Physical Activity and Nutrition Effects on Bone Turnover, Bone Density and Stress Fractures<br>*Jeri W. Nieves, Helen Hayes Hospital, West Haverstraw, New York* |
| 5:15 | Discussion of Minerals and Recovery from Injury |
| 6:00 | End of Day |

## June 15, 2004

8:00 a.m. Breakfast

## POTENTIAL BENEFITS OF MINERALS (continued)

**8:30** **MINERALS AND COGNITION AND BEHAVIOR**
(Moderator: James Penland, Committee on Mineral Requirements for Military Personnel)

8:35 Evaluating Nutritional Effects on Cognitive Function in Warfighters: Lessons Learned
*Harris R. Lieberman, U.S. Army Research Institute of Environmental Medicine, Natick, Massachusetts*

8:55 Iron and Cognitive Performance
*John L. Beard, Pennsylvania State University, University Park*

9:15 Zinc and Behavior
*James G. Penland USDA-ARS Grand Forks Human Nutrition Research Center, Grand Forks, North Dakota*

9:35 Break

9:55 Discussion of Minerals and Cognition and Behavior

**10:30** **MINERALS AND PHYSICAL PERFORMANCE**
(Moderator: Melinda Manore, Committee on Military Nutrition Research)

10:50 Zinc and Magnesium Requirements: Effects on and During Exercise
*Henry C. Lukaski, USDA-ARS Grand Forks Human Nutrition Research Center, Grand Forks, North Dakota*

11:10 Iron and Physical Performance-Thermogenesis, Energetic Efficiency
*Jere D. Haas, Cornell University, Ithaca, New York*

11:30 Discussion of Minerals and Physical Performance

12:00 End of Workshop

# B

# Workshop Papers

## Concerns About the Effects of Military Environments on Mineral Metabolism and Consequences of Marginal Deficiencies to Performance

*Karl E. Friedl*
*U.S. Army Research Institute of Environmental Medicine, Natick, Massachusetts*

### OVERVIEW

#### Statement of the Problem

Mineral requirements to sustain soldier performance in stressful conditions have been considered in military nutrition studies for many decades but rarely as the primary focus of the studies (Johnson, 1986; Sauberlich, 1984). These studies, which were often underpowered, only descriptive, or not designed to address specific hypotheses in this area, raised questions that remained unresolved. The primary concern is the inability to-date to determine if there is a problem related to mineral metabolism (especially iron, calcium, zinc, and magnesium) that impairs health and performance in some soldiers in any field conditions. This should be considered from at least the following two perspectives: (a) does the military environment produce somewhat unique derangements or specifically change mineral intake requirements that affect performance? and (b) are marginally deficient individuals (regardless of the reason for their deficiency) impaired relative to the demands of military performance? Answers to these questions are also important as they will help the Army address persistent suggestions about using mineral supplemention for soldiers that arise from health advocates and interested entrepreneurs.

## Military Stressors

Key stressors in the military environment include thermoregulatory challenges, hard work and exercise, inadequate rest and energy intakes, and psychological stress. Inadequate food intake is a problem in field environments, where soldiers typically underconsume by 25 percent of their energy requirements, and it can be worsened by the loss of appetite in hot or hypoxic environments; underconsumption is also a consequence of strictly enforced body fat standards, possibly with a larger effect on service women than men because women are more likely to exceed the standards and restrict their food intake. High sweat rate and water turnover is an important feature of hot work environments. Psychological stressors range from trauma (e.g., exposure to traumatic injuries and death, exposures to populations living in poverty and ruin, and feelings of helplessness in some peacekeeping operations) and anxiety (e.g., worry about personal safety and family separation), to information overload (e.g., managing complex data from multiple sources). The extent to which these exposures are manifested in various stress responses depend on the resilience of the individual as well as leadership, unit cohesion, and other stress mitigators.

Some unique environments and exposures (e.g., cold, altitude, enclosed environments, blast overpressure in field artillery units, noise and toxic chemicals around military vehicles and aircraft, radiofrequency radiation in communications centers) may also have to be considered when recommending optimal mineral intakes. A previous Committee on Military Nutrition Research (CMNR) concluded that none of these special environments had been adequately characterized as producing higher oxidative stress burdens to soldiers than that for the healthy active U.S. population (IOM, 1999).

## Health and Performance Outcomes

Soldiers are likely to be involved in demanding physical tasks that require strength and endurance; most physical tasks require lifting and carrying heavy loads. There are also significant mental demands that come with increased speed, complexity, and lethality of modern warfare; in this regard, every individual soldier may be called upon for rapid decision making and judgment calls, may require fine psychomotor performance (e.g., marksmanship), spatial mapping ability, pattern recognition, etc. Mood and motivation are important underlying aspects of soldier mental performance at all times. Even momentary lapses in mental and physical performance may have catastrophic effects in today's military environment.

Practical tests that adequately reflect militarily-relevant performance have been elusive but various test paradigms have provided useful measures in military studies, such as repeated box lifts (strength endurance), simulated sentry duty (vigilance, judgment, psychomotor performance), and simulated mission control center (multiple cognitive domains). The Army is increasingly turning to realistic training simulators that include electronic "combat" games and new markmanship trainers; these systems can also be converted to research tools that unobtrusively assess performance.

In addition to cognition abilities, a fully responsive immune system is critical to maintain the health and optimal health needed to face the demands of military lifestyle. Regardless of how good our vaccines may be, soldiers are not likely to be protected against all the endemic and deliberate infectious threats that may determine success or failure of a mission, nor will they have equipment and drugs to fully prevent inflammatory responses to physical demands and other physical and chemical threats. This highlights one more broad outcome of interest to the Army, optimizing a soldier's resistance to disease and injury. Some of the host defense systems that determine immunological and inflammatory responses appear to be importantly affected by mineral status.

## RANGER TRAINING AS A STRESS MODEL

In the early 1990s, the Army had concerns about the high prevalence of infectious illnesses (pneumococcal pneumonia and soft tissue infections such as cellulitis) occurring in healthy young men undergoing 65 days of Ranger training with multiple stressors, including extreme food and sleep restriction and hot humid conditions. This concern led to a request to determine if we could just provide "an iron pill or a vitamin" to prevent soldiers from getting sick while subjected to the same high level of stressful training. Initially we conducted a descriptive study to quantify the stressors (1,000 kcal/day energy deficits; 3.6 hr/day sleep) and their effects; this was followed by a study that increased feeding by only 400 kcal/day, which was associated with marked improvement in immune function and reduction in infection rates (Kramer et al., 1997). Most of the men lost all of their fat reserves and the main adverse outcomes due to the semistarvation were in the cognitive and immune function (Friedl, 2003; Friedl et al., 2001). In addition, soldiers were hyperphagic and had sleep disturbances for several weeks after the course but were fully recovered six months later.

During the initial planning of these experiments, we worried repeatedly about what would happen to iron and hematological parameters in association with the extreme privation. It was assumed that at some point hemoglobin and hematocrit would become low enough that it would not be safe or ethical to continue to draw blood from the test volunteers. This never happened and the significant changes in iron status that were observed occurred in the first few weeks of the course and corrected by the end of the course (Figure B-1). The observed changes were ascribed to acute phase responses, with no changes in iron, zinc, or copper status between baseline and the end of the course (Moore et al., 1993; Shippee et al., 1993). One possible explanation for the absence of a progressive decline in iron status is that periodic re-feeding that occurred at the end of each two week phase through the four training phases of this course replenished any deficiencies (sampling was done at the end of each phase of restriction and before the re-feeding began). The loss of muscle mass in this study would have also provided a steady supply of minerals and nutrients into the circulation. These findings matched those in the 1973 biomedical studies of Ranger training, with comparable weight loss and also no significant changes in hematological parameters and iron status across the training period. Thus, we did not detect overt mineral deficiencies in one of the most stressful models we could ethically study. However, only iron was targeted for study a priori and periodic re-feeding provided a less challenging intermittent replenishment.

## MILITARY QUESTIONS

### Is There a Problem (#1)?: Stress of Initial Entry Training and Iron Status in Young Women

Iron became a subject of interest after a 1979 study identified deficiencies in female West Point cadets; this was observed again in the decennial 1989 study, despite the high prevalence of mineral and vitamin supplement use (Friedl et al., 1991; Kretsch et al., 1986). The observation was attributed to "just part of the stress of West Point," rather than being considered a medical concern, a treatable condition, or an important performance issue. However, in 1993, a comprehensive study of womens' health and performance in the last gender-segregated Army basic training class also suggested a high incidence of iron deficiency anemia compared to the U.S. population (Westphal et al., 1995). We noted inadequate intakes of several minerals compared to established RDAs, a slight worsening of iron status through the course, and a correspondence between poor iron status and physical fitness test run time (Westphal et al., 1995). Several subsequent studies attempted to followup on these findings as part of the 1994 Defense Women's Health Research Program (DWHRP). One followed a select population of new female officers, comparing iron and hematological status to treadmill measured aerobic performance at the beginning and end of their officer basic course. This group was uniformly well nourished and fit, and offered no significant correlation between measures of iron and hematological status and aerobic performance (Cline et al., 1998); this sample was probably not representative of the majority of female soldiers. The second study was a cross sectional examination of three populations of female soldiers, with iron and hematological

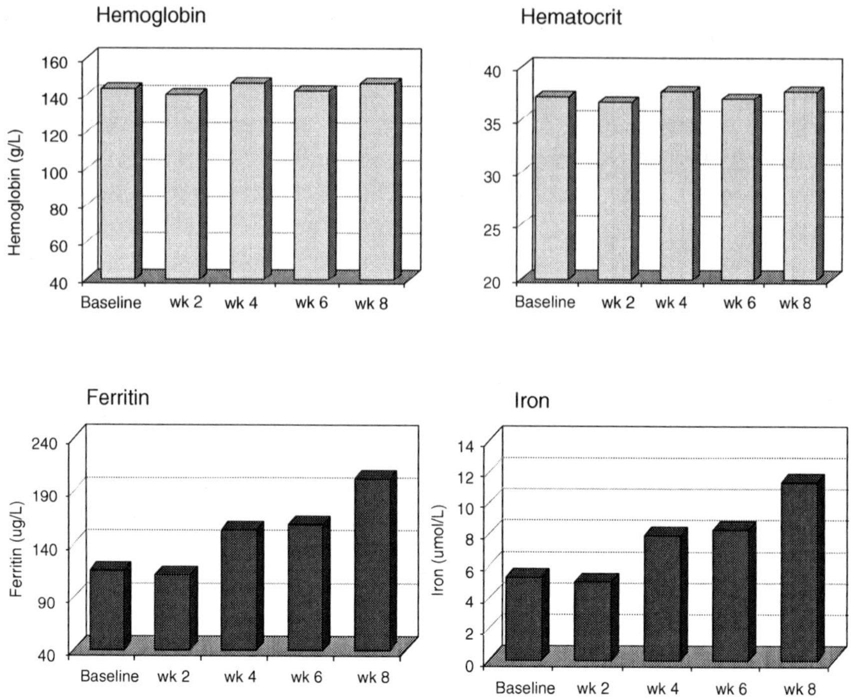


**FIGURE B-1** Changes in iron status indicators status during Ranger training under severe food restriction and other stressors.
SOURCE: Moore et al. (1993).

data that suggested a worsening status through their initial training (IOM, 1995). The cross sectional design presented a significant weakness in this study, and because of different locations, feeding regimens, and stressors, it was difficult to draw conclusions about the nature of this apparent decline in health status. A clinical study investigated the prevalence of iron deficiency in women referred to a military gastroenterology clinic, concluding that the majority of asymptomatic iron deficiency anemia cases, including several already diagnosed by specialists as having excess blood loss related to menstrual flow, actually had a high prevalence of significant endoscopy findings (Kepzyk et al., 1999). A fourth study funded in the DWHRP examined the benefits to neurocognitive performance from zinc and iron repletion in marginal deficiency. In preliminary analyses, many cognitive and psychometric tests were apparently improved (Sandstead, 2001); however, the results have not yet been reported.

## Is There a Problem (#2)?: Calcium Requirements and Bone Health

Calcium intakes have been given more attention in military studies in the past decade because of research initiatives on prevention of stress fractures, particularly in female recruits. As part of the DHWRP, the CMNR convened a special review of women's body composition, nutrition and health which included a major review of stress fractures in the military (IOM, 1998). The subsequent Bone Health and Military Medical Readiness (BHMMR) research program was shaped by the recommendations from this review and from the DRI report on calcium, vitamin D, and related nutrients (IOM, 1997).

One important DWHRP project demonstrated that energy deficit, not intense exercise, was a key determinant of menstrual disturbances (Loucks and Thuma, 2003), refuting earlier concepts of a "female athlete triad" of intense exercise, menstrual abnormalities and osteoporosis. This was consistent with findings that high functioning women, such as Olympic athletes, exercising intensively but not restricting their diet had normal rates of oligomenorrhea. As a follow up effort supported by the BHMMR, experimental manipulations of the energy deficit that exceeded thresholds and caused alterations in LH (luteinized hormone) pulsatility, produced changes in bone mineral metabolism consistent with demineralization (Ihle and Loucks, 2004).

Another important study, currently underway, is testing the hypothesis that 2,000 mg of calcium along with 800 IU of Vitamin D can substantially reduce the acute occurrence of stress fracture in a study of 5,200 young women during eight weeks of recruit training at the Great Lakes Naval Base. Part of the hypothesis and assumptions are that young women still have not attained peak bone mass, recruit training stimulates new bone formation, calcium intakes are normally low in this population, and substantial sweat calcium losses occur in this training (Lappe, 2003).

Special populations such as submariners living for extended periods in closed environments and away from sunlight have reduced plasma levels of 25-(OH) Vitamin D and special challenges in calcium metabolism (Sack et al., 1986). Two studies in progress in the BHMMR program are defining Vitamin D needs in relation to ethnicity and skin pigmentation, following up on a research gap identified in the review of calcium, vitamin D, and related nutrients (IOM, 1997).

## Are We Missing a Performance Enhancing Benefit (Or Are Some Supplements a Health or Performance Risk)?

Some military studies have raised questions about the effects of stressors on mineral requirements and/or effects of supplementation on mitigation of stress responses. For example, as part of an important series of starvation and limited intake studies to determine minimum requirements for 10-day patrols, the 1968

Panama study measured intakes and losses for sodium, potassium, calcium, and magnesium, including sweat and urine excretion rates (Consolazio et al., 1979). The authors concluded that magnesium intakes were deficient but there was no biomedical evidence of a decline in magnesium levels. In a study at the Uniformed Services University of Health Sciences (USUHS), magnesium balance in anaerobic exercise was considered. Another study tested specific performance benefits of zinc combined with Vitamin E on exhaustive running in women, based on hypothesized antioxidant actions, but found no effect of acute dosing (Singh et al., 1999). However, there has been no concerted effort through a carefully planned program of studies to determine benefits and risks of mineral supplements in military populations.

Most service members report using supplements of some kind; this is currently being resurveyed to improve estimates of specific supplement use. Young soldiers are at high risk for the use of supplements with putative performance enhancement because of the ready availability of these products in military commissaries and stores, and because of perceptions that military training and operational demands somehow drive a higher intake requirement, as well as the strategically seeded suggestions of performance enhancement in popular fitness magazines and the prevalent belief that such claims could not be made if they were not true (Friedl et al., 1992). A potentially important question that has never been addressed in military research studies is whether or not higher than usual intakes of certain supplements, including minerals, produce a deficiency state from withdrawal that is likely to occur when soldiers leave them behind for a field exercise or operational deployment. Another concern would be individual and population bases of upper limits of intakes, such as the obvious problem of iron overload if supplements are provided across military groups, for men and women or to all women regardless of their iron status.

## SUMMARY

Constant discoveries of new roles of minerals in integrated physiological processes, where a mineral deficiency may have far reaching consequences on stress responses and susceptibility to disease makes this an important and relevant line of inquiry for military medical research. The key question that has never been properly addressed in military or other relevant studies is "can we achieve a sizeable improvement in mental or physical functioning, especially in stressful operational or training conditions, by improving the mineral status of young men and women in the military?" This area of investigation has been hindered by the absence of (1) practical and validated tools to definitely assess outcomes including neuropsychological outcomes and changes in disease susceptibility, (2) adequate indices of mineral status, not confused by stress states including acute phase responses, and (3) clear indications of health and performance deficiencies.

Research conducted under the special performance demands and conditions in which soldiers have to operate will not be addressed elsewhere and needs to be conducted by the Army. In fact, there is no other federal agency with a primary focus on biomedical aspects of performance; more typically the research is focused purely on health outcomes. This work is primarily centered at the U.S. Army Research Institute of Environmental Medicine in the Military Nutrition Division in collaboration with the Pennington Biomedical Research Center and with scientific guidance from the Institute of Medicine's CMNR.

The key question(s) can also be framed by a pragmatic question: Should the Department of Defense consider the addition of a mineral supplement pack in every ration with instructions on use for "health and performance optimization," or perhaps other strategies on the use of whole foods?

## DISCLAIMER

The opinions and assertions in this paper are those of the authors and do not necessarily reflect the official views of the Department of the Army.

## REFERENCES

Cline AD, Patton JF, Tharion WJ. 1998. Assessment of the relationship between iron status, dietary intake, performance, and mood state of female Army officers in a basic training population. Technical Report T98-24, September 1998. AD A351 973. Natick, MA: U.S. Army Research Institute of Environmental Medicine.

Consolazio CF, Johnson HL, Nelson R. 1979. The relationship of diet to the performance of the combat soldier. Minimal calorie intake during combat patrols in a hot humid environment (Panama). Letterman Army Institute of Research Report No. 76. October 1979.

Friedl KE. 2003. Military nutritional immunology. In: Hughes DA, Darlington LG, Bendich A, eds. *Diet and Human Immune Function*. Totowa, NJ: Humana Press, Inc. Pp. 381–396.

Friedl KE, Marchitelli LJ, Sherman DE, Tulley R. 1991. Nutritional Assessment of Cadets at the U.S. Military Academy: Part 1. Anthropometric and Biochemical Measures. Technical Report No. T4-91, November 1990. ADA231918. Natick, MA: U.S. Army Research Institute of Environmental Medicine.

Friedl KE, Moore LJ, Marchitelli LJ. 1992. Physiology of nutritional supplements. "Steroid replacers": Let the athlete beware! *Natl Strength Conditioning Assoc J* 14:14–19.

Friedl KE, Mays MZ, Kramer TR, Shippee RL. 2001. Acute recovery of physiological and cognitive function in U.S. Army Ranger students in a multistressor field environment. In: *The Effect of Prolonged Military Activities in Man—Physiological and Biochemical Changes—Possible Means of Rapid Recuperation*. Technical Report RTO-MP-042. Neuilly-sur-Seine Cedex, France: North Atlantic Treaty Organization.

Ihle R, Loucks AB. 2004. Dose-response relationships between energy availability and bone turnover in young exercising women. *J Bone Miner Res* 19:1231–1240.

IOM (Institute of Medicine). 1995. *A Review of Issues Related to Iron Status in Women during U.S. Army Basic Combat Training*. Letter Report to BG Russ Zajtchuk, December 19, 1995.

IOM. 1997. *Dietary Reference Intakes for Calcium, Phosphorus, Magnesium, Vitamin D, and Fluoride*. Washington, DC: National Academy Press.

IOM. 1998. *Reducing Stress Fracture in Physically Active Military Women*. Washington, DC: National Academy Press.

IOM. 1999. *Letter Report to the Office of the Surgeon General United States Army on Antioxidants and Oxidative Stress in Military Personnel*. Washington, DC: Institute of Medicine.

Johnson HL. 1986. Practical military implications of fluid and nutritional imbalances for performance. In: *Predicting Decrements in Military Performance Due to Inadequate Nutrition*. Washington DC: National Academy Press. Pp. 55–68.

Kepczyk T, Cremins JE, Long BD, Bachinski MB, Smith LR, McNally PR. 1999. A prospective, multidisciplinary evaluation of premenopausal women with iron deficiency anemia. *Am J Gastroenterol* 94:109–115.

Kramer TR, Moore RJ, Shippee RL, Friedl KE, Martinez-Lopez L, Chan MM, Askew EW (1997). Effects of food restriction in military training on T-lymphocyte responses. *Int J Sportsmed* 18:S84–S90.

Kretsch MJ, Conforti PM, Sauberlich HE. 1986. Nutrient intake evaluation of male and female cadets at the United States Military Academy, West Point, New York. Technical Report LAIR-218. April 1986. ADA168120. San Francisco, CA: Letterman Army Institute of Research.

Lappe JM. 2003. Efficacy of calcium and Vitamin D supplementation for the prevention of stress fracture in female Naval recruits. Annual Report. Grant # DAMD17-01-1-0807. ADA419678. October 2003. Omaha, NE: Creighton University.

Loucks AB, Thuma JR. 2003. Luteinizing hormone pulsatility is disrupted at a threshold of energy availability in regularly menstruating women. *J Clin Endocr Metab* 88:297–311.

Moore RJ, KE Friedl, RT Tulley, EW Askew. 1993. Maintenance of iron status in healthy men during an extended period of stress and physical activity. *Am J Clin Nutr* 58:923–927.

Sack DM, Holick M, Bondi KR. 1986. Calcium and Vitamin D metabolism in submariners—carbon dioxide, sunlight, and absorption considerations. Technical Report NSMRL-1037. January 1986. ADA166292. Groton, CT: Naval Submarine Medical Research Laboratory.

Sandstead HH. 2001. Repletion of zinc and iron deficiencies improve cognition of premenopausal women. Final Report. Grant DAMD17-95-C-5112. December 2001. Galveston, TX: University of Texas Medical Branch.

Sauberlich HE. 1984. Implications of nutritional status on human biochemistry, physiology and health. *Clin Biochem* 17:132–142.

Shippee RL, Friedl KE, Tulley R, Christensen E, Arsenault J. 1993. Changes in plasma iron, copper, and zinc concentrations of young males during 8 weeks of extreme physiological and psychological stress. *J Am Coll Nutr* 12:614 (abstract).

Singh A, Papanicolaou DA, Lawrence LL, Howel EA, Chrousos GP, Deuster PA. 1999. Neuroendocrine responses to running in women after zinc and vitamin E supplementation. *Med Sci Sports Exerc* 31:536–542.

Westphal KA, Friedl KE, Sharp MA, King N, Kramer TR, Reynolds KL, Marchitelli LJ. 1995. Health, performance, and nutritional status of U.S. Army women during basic combat training. Technical Report No. T96-2. May 1995. ADA302042. Natick, MA: U.S. Army Research Institute of Environmental Medicine.

# Derivation of the Military Dietary Reference Intakes and the Mineral Content of Military Rations

*Carol J. Baker-Fulco*
*U.S. Army Research Institute of Environmental Medicine,*
*Natick, Massachusetts*

This paper presents the nutritional standards for military rations and the mineral composition of military field rations. In addition, it summarizes the findings of a few studies that have estimated mineral intakes of soldiers in the field and in garrison. This paper focuses on operational rations, which are rations intended for military operations, whether combat or field training. A ration is one day's food supply for a group or an individual. The type of ration provided is based upon the unit's mission, tactical scenario, location, and availability of food service equipment and personnel. The operational rations examined in this paper are the Meal, Ready-to-Eat (MRE); Meal, Cold Weather (MCW); one of the Unitized Group Rations (UGR), the Heat-and-Serve (H&S); and the First Strike Ration (FSR).

## DESCRIPTIONS OF OPERATIONAL RATION

The MRE is the standard individual operational ration and consists of heat-processed entrees and other food components that require no preparation. Each meal contains an entrée/starch, crackers, a spread (cheese, peanut butter, jam or jelly), a dessert or snack, beverages, and an accessory packet that contains coffee, tea or cider and condiments. The MRE is issued at three menu bags per day for a complete ration with an average of 3,900 kcal. For variety, there are twenty-four different meal menus in the inventory.

The MCW is a higher calorie ration intended for arctic feeding. This ration contains freeze-dried, cooked entrees and other low-moisture foods that will not freeze. Meal bags for each of the twelve menus contain the entrée and a variety of spreads and crackers, cookies, sports bars, nuts, candy, and powdered drink mixes. The MCW is issued at three menu bags per day for a provision of roughly 4,500 kcal. The MCW menus are identical to those of the Food Packet, Long Range Patrol (LRP) which is a restricted ration issued as one menu bag per day during special operations when weight and volume of the ration are critical factors.

Another restricted calorie ration considered in this report is the FSR. The FSR is a new, individual combat ration developed for forward deployed ground forces engaged in high-intensity operations. This ration is smaller and lighter than a full day's ration of MREs and is comprised of foods that can be eaten "on the move." The FSR as currently configured provides about 2,800 kcal.

The UGR is a group of rations in which all the components for 50 complete meals are packaged as one unit to streamline the ordering and delivery process. There are seven breakfast and fourteen lunch and dinner menus for each type of UGR; however, the lunch meal is often a MRE. The UGR-Heat & Serve (UGR-H&S) is comprised of shelf-stable, ready-to-eat entrees, starches, vegetables, and desserts packaged in short, rectangular plastic trays. It is the more common (hot) group feeding ration for the field and is used when neither cooking nor refrigeration are possible. Each meal, including the mandatory supplement of milk, provides an average of 1,400 kcal. UGR menus may be enhanced with cold breakfast cereal, bread, fresh fruits and salad. There are other UGR options that comprise perishable and frozen ingredients (UGR-A) or are cook-prepared from canned and dehydrated foods (UGR-B), but these will not be discussed in this paper.

## MILITARY DIETARY AND RATION STANDARDS

Nutritional standards for operational and restricted rations (NSOR), i.e., what the rations must contain, are presented in the tri-service regulation, Nutritional Standards and Education, which for the Army is Army Regulation (AR) 40-25 (U.S. Departments of the Army, Navy, and Air Force, 2001). The NSORs are based on the Military Dietary Reference Intakes (MDRI) presented in the same regulation (see Table B-1). The MDRIs are, in turn, based on the Dietary Reference Intakes (DRIs) (IOM, 1997, 1998, 2000a) or earlier Recommended Dietary Allowances (RDA) (National Research Council, 1989). Since the current regulation was prepared prior to the 2001 DRI publication (IOM, 2001)—which updated the RDAs for iron, iodine and zinc, and established DRIs for chromium, copper, manganese and molybdenum—current MDRIs are based on the 1989 RDAs for iron, iodine, and zinc, and there are no MDRIs for chromium, copper, manganese and molybdenum. A soon to be drafted change to the regulation will update the MDRIs and include additional MDRIs based on the more recent IOM publications.

The MDRIs are applicable to healthy, 17 to 50 year old, physically active military men and non-lactating, non-pregnant women. This age range covers the majority of military personnel on active or reserve duty. The 17 to 50 year age range incorporates three of the age classes for which DRIs have been set (14 to 18, 19 to 30, and 31 to 50 years) and three of the age classes used in the 10th edition of the RDA (15 to 18, 19 to 24, and 25 to 50 years). For most nutrients, the MDRI is the highest gender-specific reference value or RDA. However, the MDRIs for calcium, phosphorus, and iron for males and calcium, phosphorus, and magnesium for females, are not based on the highest reference intake or allowance, which is for 14 to 18 year old individuals. Only 2–3 percent of the military population is 17 to 18 years old; thus, inflating the MDRIs to meet the needs of relatively so few individuals is not warranted. The regulation advises

**TABLE B-1** Military Nutritional Allowances and Ration Standards for Minerals

| | | MDRIs | | NSORs | |
|---|---|---|---|---|---|
| Nutrient | Unit | Men | Women | Operational | Restricted |
| Energy: | | | | | |
| Light activity | kcal | 3,000 | 2,200 | | |
| **Moderate activity** | kcal | **3,250** | 2,300 | | |
| **Heavy activity** | kcal | **3,950** | 2,700 | **3,600** | 1,500 |
| Exceptionally-heavy | kcal | 4,600 | 3,150 | | |
| Calcium | mg | 1,000 | 1,000 | 1,000 | 500 |
| Fluoride | mg | 4.0 | 3.1 | 4.0 | 2.0 |
| Iodine | μg | 150 | 150 | 150 | 75 |
| Iron | mg | 10 | 15 | 15 | 8 |
| Magnesium | mg | 420 | 320 | 420 | 210 |
| Phosphorus | mg | 700 | 700 | 700 | 350 |
| Potassium | mg | 3,200 | 2,500 | 3,200 | 2,000 |
| Selenium | μg | 55 | 55 | 55 | 28 |
| Sodium* | mg | 5,000 | 3,600 | 5,000–7,000 | 2,500–3,500 |
| Zinc | mg | 15 | 12 | 15 | 8 |

NOTE: MDRI = Military Dietary Reference Intake; NSOR = Nutritional Standard for Operational Rations.

*Sodium recommendations are based on 1,400–1,700 milligrams of sodium per 1,000 kcal of energy consumed. The MDRI values in the table represent the midpoints of the ranges calculated using energy intakes for moderate activity of 3,250 kcal for men and 2,300 kcal for women.

SOURCE: U.S. Departments of the Army, Navy, and Air Force (2001).

persons planning menus or diets for groups with a large proportion of 17 to 18 year olds to consider the higher requirements of that age group. The military population in general tends to be a little heavier and more active then the American population, thus the military energy allowances are higher than the DRI values.

In addition to prescribing the dietary allowances and standards for operational rations (full rations and restricted rations), AR 40-25 prescribes the length of time that certain rations can be used as a sole source of nutrition. The MRE can be fed for up to 21 days, while restricted rations are limited to 10 days.

There are nutritional standards for nutritionally complete and restricted operational rations. The full ration standards are based directly on the MDRIs. For most nutrients, the ration standard is the higher of the two gender-specific MDRIs. The energy standard is based on the estimated average energy requirement for moderate to heavy physical activity, to provide for the extended workdays and high levels of activity typical of operational settings (combat or training). Although there are groups that will have energy requirements much higher than 3,600 kcal, this is a practical standard, given that many warfighters have lower energy needs and that there is less time or inclination to eat as the intensity and duration of activity increase.

The NSORs are minimum content standards at the time of consumption except for sodium. The MDRIs and NSORs for sodium are much higher than the DRIs (1,500 mg) (IOM, 2005) or other dietary guidelines for the general population because of the potential for military personnel to sustain high sodium losses in sweat in hot environments or strenuous activity (CMNR, 1991).

Restricted rations are used when operational conditions and missions require troops to subsist for short periods on nutritionally-inadequate rations. Such scenarios include long-range patrol, assault and reconnaissance, and other situations where resupply is tactically unfeasible. The restricted ration standards for most nutrients are set at 50 percent of the respective standards for operational rations, rounding up to the same number of digits used to express the NSOR. This convention is mainly based on the work of Consolazio and colleagues from the 1960s that suggests that nutrient intakes at 50 percent of RDA levels for no more than 10 days do not measurably affect health or performance (Consolazio, 1976). Intakes at these levels maintain bodily functions and prevent rapid depletion of body stores.

## MINERAL CONTENT OF OPERATIONAL RATIONS

### Calculated Menu Data

The ration composition data presented here are from the Combat Feeding Directorate, Natick (i.e., the ration developers) and derive from a variety of sources. Most of the data are values calculated using Genesis R&D nutrition and labeling software and database (ESHA Research, Salem, OR). The ration developers in Combat Feeding calculate the nutrient composition of their prototype formulations, while the contracted manufacturers calculate the nutrient content of their products according to their, often-different, proprietary formulations. Chemically analyzed data are mostly limited to macronutrients or select nutrients (such as sodium) that may be stipulated in the procurement contracts. Data for the commercial items in the ration are taken from the USDA Survey Nutrient Database as maintained in the Genesis or Food Processor applications or the USDA National Nutrient Database for Standard Reference.

Ration composition data for some minerals (e.g., copper or selenium) are missing or very incomplete and do not provide reasonable estimates of ration provisions and, thus, are not presented here. The data presented in Table B-2 and Table B-3 are estimated average values of all menus in a particular ration system and do not reflect the variability due to different manufacturers or to ingredient sources and growing conditions. There are currently 24 menus in the MRE line, 12 menus in the MCW, and 7 breakfast menus and 14 lunch and dinner menus in the UGR. For the MRE, the values are averages of the three contracted ration assemblers which are also the manufacturers of the major ration components.

**TABLE B-2** Calculated Mean Mineral Content of Meals in Meal-Based Rations

| | Ca (mg) | I* (μg) | Fe (mg) | Mg (mg) | P (mg) | K (mg) | Na* (mg) | Se (μg) | Zn (mg) |
|---|---|---|---|---|---|---|---|---|---|
| *⅓ NSOR* | *333* | *50* | *5* | *140* | *233* | *1,067* | *<2,333* | *18.3* | *5* |
| MRE XXII | 511 | — | 7.9 | 114 | 643 | 1,048 | 2,046 | 10.1 | 4.2 |
| MRE XXIII | 527 | — | 8.6 | 130 | 646 | 1,027 | 2,051 | 11.9 | 4.2 |
| MRE XXIV | 557 | — | 9.0 | 141 | 691 | 1,084 | 2,181 | 12.5 | 4.7 |
| MCW | 475 | 62 | 10.9 | 201 | — | 1,666 | 3,078 | 53.2 | 6.1 |
| UGR B'fast | 467 | 49 | 7.2 | 111 | 456 | 1,747 | 2,580 | 9.2 | 6.9 |
| UGR Dinner | 472 | — | 9.7 | 190 | 590 | 1,873 | 2,465 | 16.0 | 7.6 |

NOTE: The UGR menu data is for the 2003 production year. Ca = Calcium; I = Iodine; Fe = Iron; Mg = Magnesium; P = Phosphorus; K = Potassium; Na = Sodium; Se = Selenium; Zn = Zinc. NSOR = Nutritional Standard for Operational Rations; MRE = Meal, Ready-to-Eat; MCW = Meal, Cold Weather; UGR = Unitized Group Ration; B'fast = Breakfast.
*Values for iodine and sodium do not include content of salt packet.

Table B-2 presents mineral contents of average meals in current meal-based rations to include the past three production years of MREs, the MCW, and UGR menus for 2003. The UGRs are typically provided as a hot breakfast and a hot dinner with a MRE for "lunch." The first row of the table presents the ration standards for the corresponding minerals divided by three as comparison figures for a meal.

Although calcium was a nutrient of concern in earlier versions of field rations, it is not so in current rations. The levels of calcium, as of phosphorus,

**TABLE B-3** Mean Mineral Content of First Strike Ration Compared to Standards

| | Ca (mg) | I* (μg) | Fe (mg) | Mg (mg) | P (mg) | K (mg) | Na* (mg) | Se (μg) | Zn (mg) |
|---|---|---|---|---|---|---|---|---|---|
| *NSOR* | *100* | *150* | *15* | *420* | *700* | *3,200* | *>5,000* | *55* | *5* |
| *Restricted Ration* | *500* | *75* | *8* | *210* | *350* | *2,000* | *>2,500* | *28* | *8* |
| FSR | 679 | 53 | 17.4 | 393 | 1,167 | 2,356 | 4,244 | 115 | 12.1 |

NOTE: Ca = Calcium; I = Iodine; Fe = Iron; Mg = Magnesium; P = Phosphorus; K = Potassium; Na = Sodium; Se = Selenium; Zn = Zinc. NSOR = Nutritional Standard for Operational Rations; FSR = First Strike Ration
*Values for iodine and sodium do not include content of salt packet.

surpass the requirement by substantial amounts. The mineral content (especially calcium) of the UGR menus reflects the contribution of the mandatory milk at both meals but not the optional dry cereal or bread. The wheat snack bread, crackers, cheese spreads, and dairy shakes in the MRE each provide more than 150 mg calcium per serving. The iron content of all meals is relatively high, yielding nutrient densities of 6.9 mg/1,000 kcal, 7.1 mg/1,000 kcal, and 7.5 mg/1,000 kcal for MRE XXIV, MCW, and UGR dinner, respectively. The iodine values do not include iodine provided by the salt packet. The salt in the accessory pack is required to be iodized; however, salt used as an ingredient in ration components is specifically not iodized due to concerns about taste and acceptability. Table B-2 shows that the magnesium content of MREs has increased and now meets the NSOR. This improvement is due to the inclusion of more bean and nut items. The apparently low magnesium content (compared to $^{1}/_{3}$ NSOR) of the UGR breakfast would be offset by the UGR dinner plus a MRE. The potassium level of the MRE is just meeting the NSOR while the sodium content of the MRE is about twice that of potassium, still within the range of the NSOR. The average UGR meals contain much higher levels of potassium and sodium than MREs. The sodium content of both the estimated average UGR breakfast and dinner exceeds the maximum sodium content standard (see Table B-2). Much of the sodium is contained in the entrées. In the MRE, 39 percent of the sodium comes from the entrée, while 44 percent of the sodium in the UGR dinner is in the entrée.

Selenium in the MREs appears to be lower than the NSOR (Table B-2), but this is mostly because there is no selenium data for many MRE components. The selenium data for the MCW and UGR are much more complete and show that these rations would be expected to provide ample amounts of this mineral. The very generous content of selenium in the MCW is from the egg dishes that are present in 3 of the 12 menus. The zinc content of the MRE has improved but remains below the NSOR (see Table B-2). The calculated zinc content of MRE XXIV is at 94 percent of the NSOR, while the zinc level of the MCW is 122 percent and that of the UGR is 168 percent of the NSOR. The zinc provision of rations is predominately from the beef containing entrées, which in the MRE are in 8 to 9 of the 24 menus. If beef-based entrées were removed from the MRE, the average for the menu line would be closer to three and a half milligrams of zinc per meal.

The MCW is relatively high in sodium and potassium (as well as protein), compared to the NSOR and its predecessor, the Ration, Cold Weather (RCW), which was specifically designed to contain modest amounts of these nutrients to moderate water requirements. The mineral content of the MCW is so generous because this ration is composed of three restricted rations, the LRP. As the NSORs for restricted rations for most nutrients are half the standards for full operational rations, three LRP ration packets per day provide minerals well above the full ration standards.

**TABLE B-4** Mineral Content of Additional Ration Components

| | Amt | Ca (mg) | I (μg) | Fe (mg) | Mg (mg) | P (mg) | K (mg) | Se (μg) | Na (mg) | Zn (mg) |
|---|---|---|---|---|---|---|---|---|---|---|
| MRE Salt | 4g | 0.96 | 40 | 0 | 0.08 | 0 | 0.32 | — | 1,550 | 0 |
| Pouch Bread | 51g | 75 | 0 | 1.64 | 13 | 53 | 67 | — | 593 | 0.38 |

NOTE: Ca = Calcium; I = Iodine; Fe = Iron; Mg = Magnesium; P = Phosphorus; K = Potassium; Na = Sodium; Se = Selenium; Zn = Zinc. MRE = Meal, Ready-to-Eat.

Table B-3 shows the estimated levels of minerals in the First Strike Ration in comparison to the nutritional standards for full operational rations as well as the standards for restricted rations. Although the First Strike Ration is technically a restricted calorie ration because it provides less than 3600 kcal, as currently formulated it provides 2800 to 2900 kcal. Because this ration is composed of mostly nutrient-dense foods, it greatly exceeds the nutritional standards for restricted ration and, in many cases, meets the standards for full operational rations.

The ration standards for and the ration contents of sodium presented do not include sodium provided in salt packets. There is a salt packet in the accessory packet of every MRE, FSR, and LRP menu. The mineral composition of this individual salt packet is shown in Table B-4. The packet contains four grams of salt; in contrast, most commercial salt packets contain less than one gram of salt. The large salt packet provides for the preparation of antiseptic salt water solutions and for high sodium intakes during periods of heat acclimation, if needed. Field study data indicate that consumption of the salt packet is limited.

Although no longer a mandatory supplement, bread is a frequently provided enhancement to the UGR. Table B-4 also shows the estimated mineral contents of shelf-stable white bread which is called pouch bread. Other UGR enhancements (data not shown) are assorted, bowl-pack cold cereals at breakfast (potentially providing significant amounts of copper, iron, magnesium, and zinc) and fresh fruit and salad at dinner (significant sources of iron, magnesium, potassium and other trace elements). When dry cereal is served, an additional ½ pint of milk must be provided, adding significant quantities of calcium and phosphorus as well as magnesium, potassium, and zinc to the menu. The milk may be ultra-high temperature (UHT), soy, or fresh.

### Laboratory Analyses of Ration Components

The data discussed in the previous section were calculated values provided by the Combat Feeding Directorate. In order to assess whether those values are over- or under-estimates of actual content, we had select components of MRE

XXIII chemically analyzed. We purchased MREs from each of the three assemblers and sent 32 items (18 of the 24 entrées plus 14 side dishes and snacks—see Table B-5 for list) to a food analysis laboratory (Woodson Tenet Laboratories Division, Eurofins Scientific Inc, Des Moines, IA). The selection of ration items to analyze was based on consideration of the quality of existing data, the popularity of the item, the number of times the item appears in the entire menu line, and an expected significant mineral composition. In addition, we did not analyze components that were slated to be dropped from the MRE menu line within the next two procurement cycles. The analyses included proximates (data not shown) and the minerals calcium, iron, magnesium, phosphorus, potassium, and zinc. The selection of minerals to assay was limited to nutrients for which Combat Feeding was compiling data. Thus, we did not assay copper because Combat Feeding does not report values for this nutrient. Although Combat Feeding has started to request selenium data, we did not assay selenium because we would have had to analyze almost all menu components to fill the gaps in missing data.

Figures B-2 to B-7 present the comparison of the lab values with the calculated or estimated values as per Combat Feeding. For calcium (Figure B-2), although there are some significant differences for individual products, on average there is no significant difference between the lab data and Combat Feeding data. The average of the analytical values for iron content was significantly less (28 percent less) than the average of the estimated values (Figure B-3). This was unexpected given that iron is one of the nutrients required on nutrition facts labels. Per U.S. food labeling laws, nutrients such as minerals that are added as

**TABLE B-5** MRE Components Chemically Analyzed

| Entrées | Side Dishes and Snacks |
|---|---|
| BBQ Pork Rib | Western Beans |
| Beef Enchiladas | Beef Snack Strips |
| Beef Patty | Minestrone Stew |
| Beef Ravioli | Cheese Spread (2 flavors) |
| Beef Stew | Dairy Shake (3 flavors) |
| Beefsteak w/ Mushrooms | Mashed Potatoes |
| Meat Loaf w/ Gravy | Crackers (2 flavors) |
| Roast Beef | Clam Chowder |
| Chicken w/ Salsa | Wheat Snack Bread |
| Chili and Macaroni | Pound Cake (composite of flavors) |
| Grilled Chicken Breast | |
| Manicotti w/ Vegetables | |
| Spaghetti w/ Meat Sauce | |
| Jambalaya | |
| Chicken w/ Cavatelli | |
| Cheese Tortellini | |
| Chicken Tetrazzini | |

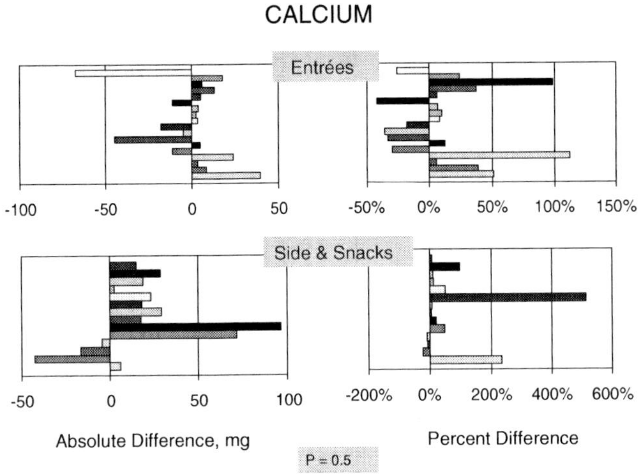


**FIGURE B-2** Differences between analytical values and calculated values for the calcium content of 18 entrees and 14 side dishes or snacks in MREs. Each bar represents an individual ration component. The two panels on the left show absolute differences; the two right panels show percent differences. Values negative if calculated > analytical; values positive if analytical > calculated.
NOTE: Axes are not to same scale.

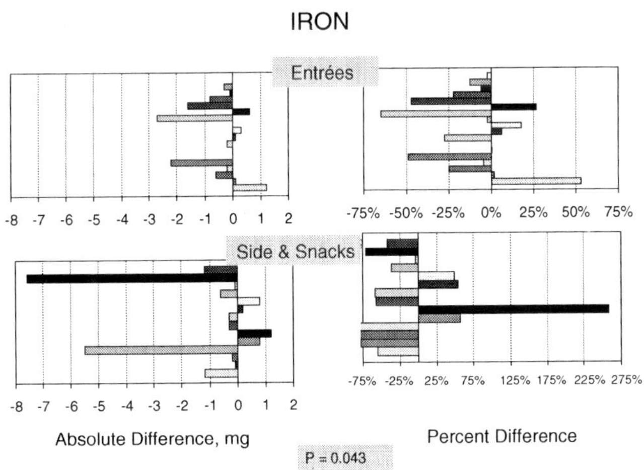


**FIGURE B-3** Differences between analytical values and calculated values for the iron content of 18 entrees and 14 side dishes or snacks in MREs. Each bar represents an individual ration component. The two panels on the left show absolute differences; the two right panels show percent differences. Values negative if calculated > analytical; values positive if analytical > calculated.
NOTE: Axes are not to same scale.

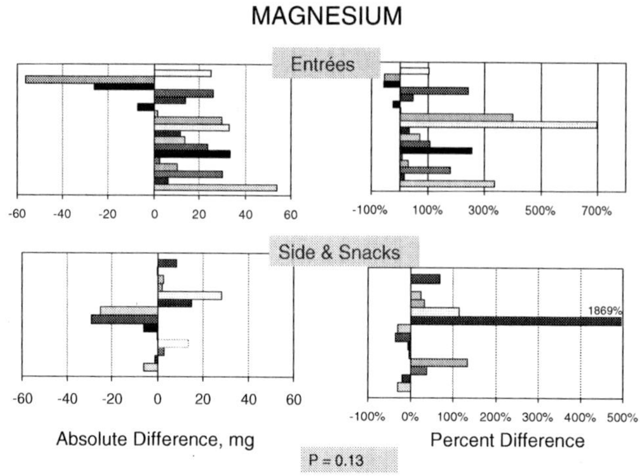


**FIGURE B-4** Differences between analytical values and calculated values for the magnesium content of 18 entrees and 14 side dishes or snacks in MREs. Each bar represents an individual ration component. The two panels on the left show absolute differences; the two right panels show percent differences. Values negative if calculated > analytical; values positive if analytical > calculated.
NOTE: Axes are not to same scale.

enrichments or fortificants must be present at levels *at least* equal to the value declared on the label. For naturally occurring minerals, except sodium, the actual nutrient content must be at least equal to 80 percent of the value declared. Therefore, we would expect the ration manufacturers to provide iron content values that support their label declarations (which are usually minimum content claims) and, thus, find the actual contents to be greater. Given that the calculated iron content of MRE menus is quite generous (7.9–9.0 mg per meal), an actual content 25–30 percent less than expected is not of concern. For magnesium (Figure B-4), although there is no statistically significant difference between the averages of the lab values and the calculated values, most of the measured contents of the individual items were higher than calculated. The average potassium content (Figure B-5) of the components analyzed was much higher than expected by the calculated values, while the measured content of sodium (Figure B-6) was much lower than the calculated values indicated. For zinc (Figure B-7), the lab values were on average higher than the calculated values. Entrées are the greatest contributors of zinc in the ration and these are the items for which we found the greatest differences between analytical and calculated values. In general, the

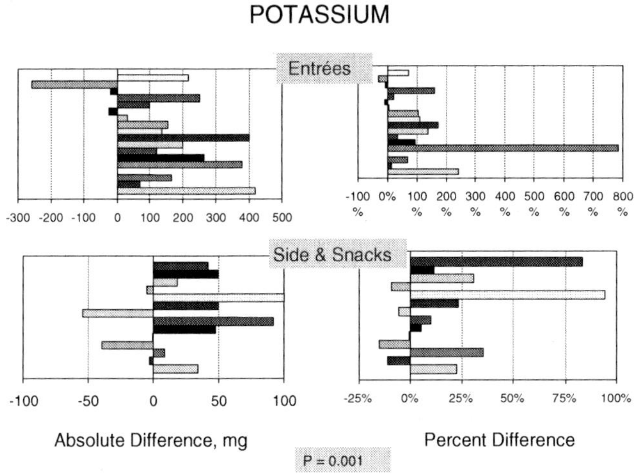


**FIGURE B-5** Differences between analytical values and calculated values for the potassium content of 18 entrees and 14 side dishes or snacks in MREs. Each bar represents an individual ration component. The two panels on the left show absolute differences; the two right panels show percent differences. Values negative if calculated > analytical; values positive if analytical > calculated.
NOTE: Axes are not to same scale.

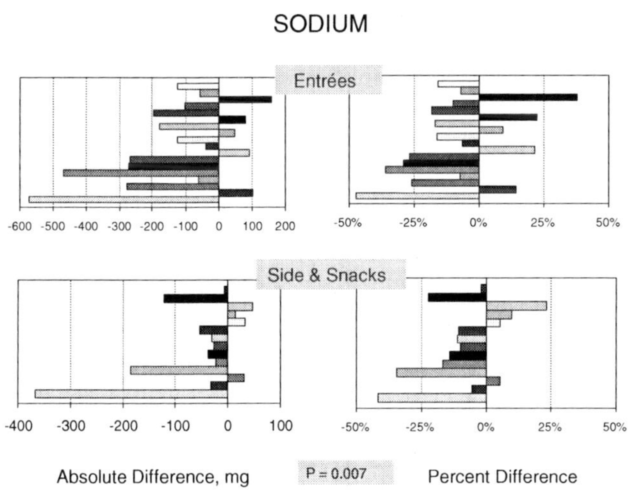


**FIGURE B-6** Differences between analytical values and calculated values for the sodium content of 18 entrees and 14 side dishes or snacks in MREs. Each bar represents an individual ration component. The two panels on the left show absolute differences; the two right panels show percent differences. Values negative if calculated > analytical; values positive if analytical > calculated.
NOTE: Axes are not to same scale.

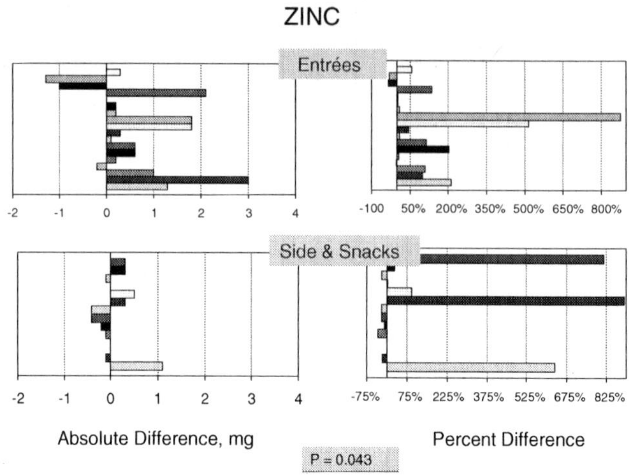


**FIGURE B-7** Differences between analytical values and calculated values for the zinc content of 18 entrees and 14 side dishes or snacks in MREs. Each bar represents an individual ration component. The two panels on the left show absolute differences; the two right panels show percent differences. Values negative if calculated > analytical; values positive if analytical > calculated.
NOTE: Axes are not to same scale.

analytical data indicate that the menu analyses based on calculated values are reasonably accurate for calcium and magnesium, but overestimate iron and sodium and underestimate the actual contents of zinc and potassium.

## MINERAL INTAKE OF MILITARY PERSONNEL

Because food is only nutritious if consumed, it is important to consider actual nutrient intakes when assessing the adequacy of a feeding system. Table B-6 outlines mean mineral intakes of a group of 30 Army Rangers consuming MREs during a 7-day field training exercise in 1996 (Military Nutrition Division, USARIEM, unpublished data). The last column of the table shows the approximate nutrient content of the rations provided. Although mineral provision would have been adequate, intakes were relatively low for calcium, magnesium, and potassium. Energy intake during this study was 2,435 ± 547 kcal, which is approximately 64 percent of the total energy content of the rations provided. In contrast, calcium intake was only about 43 percent of the ration content while magnesium, potassium, and zinc intakes were 50–60 percent of that provided.

Figures B-8 through B-10 present the results of three different field and garrison studies with the data shown as proportions of the study samples with

**TABLE B-6** Mineral Intakes of Army Rangers Consuming MREs (1996)

| | Unit | Mean ± SD | DRI | ~Provision |
|---|---|---|---|---|
| Calcium | mg | 639 ± 212 | 1,000 | 1,500 |
| Iron | mg | 15.1 ± 3.7 | 8 | 21 |
| Magnesium | mg | 265 ± 61 | 400–420 | 480 |
| Phosphorus | mg | 1,451 ± 387 | 700 | 2,300 |
| Potassium | mg | 2,041 ± 484 | 4,700 | 3,800 |
| Sodium | mg | 4,423 ± 1,301 | 2,300 | 5,000* |
| Zinc | mg | 11.7 ± 2.5 | 11 | 20 |

*Excluding salt packet.
SOURCE: Military Nutrition Division, USARIEM (unpublished data).

mean dietary intakes less than the Estimated Average Requirement (EAR) and the proportions meeting the RDA or Adequate Intake (AI) level. The prevalence of inadequate dietary intakes in a population is estimated from the proportion of the population with intakes below the median requirement (i.e., EAR). RDAs and AIs are dietary intake goals for individuals that are likely to meet or exceed their requirements. Thus, individual intakes at RDA or AI levels indicate little likelihood of inadequacy (IOM, 2000b). On the other hand, usual intakes less than the RDA or AI cannot be interpreted to mean an individual's intake was inadequate. As there was insufficient scientific evidence upon which to set an EAR and, thus, a RDA for calcium, intakes can be only compared to an AI, which is a level of calcium intake associated with adequate calcium retention.

Figure B-8 shows the results of a study conducted with combat support hospital staff in 1997 to evaluate the then current MRE and a test ration which was slightly higher in carbohydrate and lower in fat than the standard MRE ration and included novel ration items and packaging concepts (Baker-Fulco et al., 2002). Be aware that the concept ration was not designed to be nutritionally complete. Few men or women met their individual dietary intake goal for calcium; indeed, the majority of men and women reported calcium intakes less than 70 percent of the AI. Substantial proportions of both men and women had likely inadequate dietary intakes of magnesium and zinc. The low magnesium intake is of particular concern, as almost 60 percent of men and 75 percent of women had dietary intakes less than the EAR. Although the incidence of low zinc intakes was less than that for magnesium, about 20 percent of the men and more than 40 percent of the women consumed less than the EAR for zinc. Almost all subjects, including women, had apparently adequate iron intakes. Primarily because women consumed less energy than men, greater proportions of women than men ($p < 0.01$) failed to meet intake criteria for calcium, iron, magnesium, and zinc (Baker-Fulco et al., 2002).

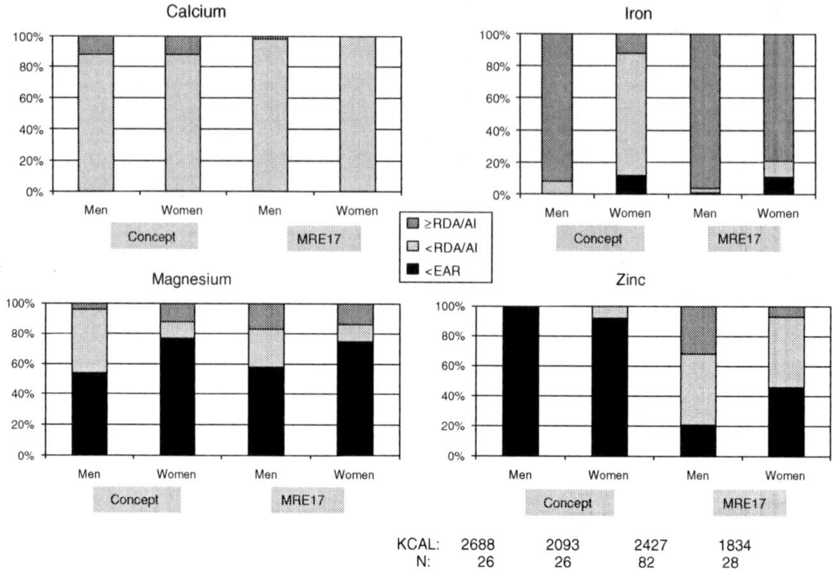


**FIGURE B-8** Proportion of combat support hospital staff with mineral intakes at specific Dietary Reference Intake levels while consuming MREs. Subjects consumed one of two rations, a Concept test ration or the standard MRE XVII. Mean energy intake and sample size of each ration and gender group is shown below the bottom right panel. NOTE: RDA = Recommended Dietary Allowance; AI = Adequate Intake; EAR = Estimated Average Requirement. The prevalence of inadequate dietary intakes in a population is estimated from the proportion of the population with intakes below the EAR. Individual intakes at or exceeding RDA or AI levels are likely adequate.

Figure B-9 presents the results of a 1998 garrison study with 146 Army Rangers which would reflect their dietary status prior to a field deployment (Military Nutrition Division, USARIEM, unpublished data). The majority of their food intake came from outside food sources. The self-reported 3-day food record data suggest that slightly over 40 percent of these Rangers were at risk of a low magnesium intake, while only 12 percent had a zinc intake less than the EAR. More than 75 percent of the Rangers reported diets that meet the RDA (11 mg) for zinc and, in fact, half reported zinc intakes that meet or exceed the higher MDRI (15 mg). Prevalences of inadequate intakes of calcium, iron, and potassium appear low. This was the first study for which the food composition data for copper was sufficient to be able to estimate copper intakes; the data suggest the prevalence of inadequate copper intake by Rangers is low with only 5 percent reporting copper intakes less than the EAR. Ninety percent of the Rangers reported sodium intakes in excess of the AI level.

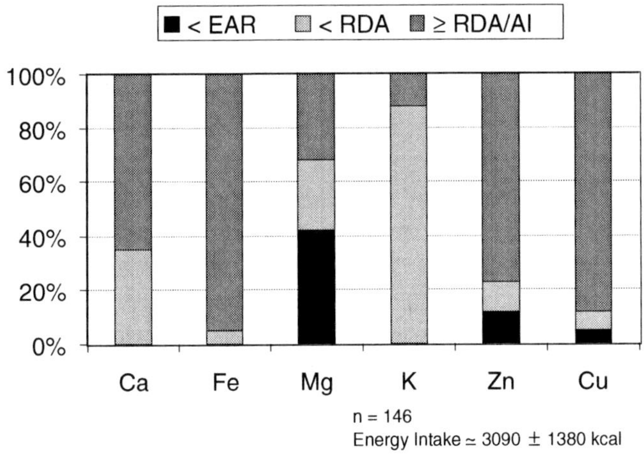


**FIGURE B-9** Proportion of Army Rangers in garrison with mineral intakes at specific Dietary Reference Intake levels. Sample size and mean energy intake are shown below the chart.

NOTE: RDA = Recommended Dietary Allowance; AI = Adequate Intake; EAR = Estimated Average Requirement. The prevalence of inadequate dietary intakes in a population is estimated from the proportion of the population with intakes below the EAR. Individual intakes at or exceeding RDA or AI levels are likely adequate.

Similar results were found in a 9-day garrison study conducted with 40 Special Forces Soldiers eating predominately in a military dining facility (Figure B-10) (Tharion et al., 2004). Dietary intake data were collected by a visual estimation method for foods consumed in the dining facility; outside food intake was collected by self-reported food record. Except for magnesium, the prevalence of inadequate intakes of the reported minerals was nil. Magnesium intakes of 16 of the 40 SF Soldiers were less than the EAR. The entire study sample achieved dietary intakes at RDA levels for iron, zinc, and copper. However, only 63 percent of the study sample achieved the higher MDRI goal for zinc. Dietary intake of all subjects exceeded the AI for sodium.

## CONCLUSIONS

The absolute contents of minerals in operational rations, with the exception of selenium, meet ration standards. However, the concentrations (i.e., nutrient densities) of calcium, magnesium, and zinc are insufficient to ensure low prevalences of inadequate intakes. There are inadequate data on which to evaluate the adequacy of the nutrient densities of copper and selenium. The sodium content

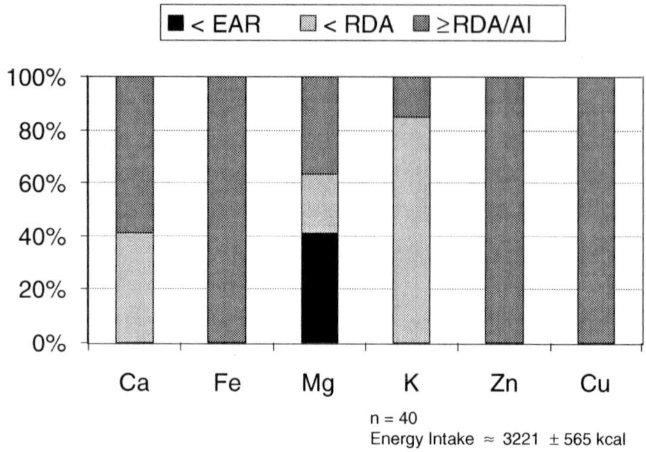


**FIGURE B-10** Proportion of Special Forces Soldiers in garrison with mineral intakes at specific Dietary Reference Intake levels. Sample size and mean energy intake are shown below the chart.
NOTE: RDA = Recommended Dietary Allowance; AI = Adequate Intake; EAR = Estimated Average Requirement. The prevalence of inadequate dietary intakes in a population is estimated from the proportion of the population with intakes below the EAR. Individual intakes at or exceeding RDA or AI levels are likely adequate.

of operational rations is likely higher than necessary while the content of potassium is less than desirable.

Ongoing laboratory analyses of additional MRE items as well as components from other operational rations are needed to reliably calculate mineral composition of ration menus. Additional field studies are also needed to determine energy and nutrient intakes of soldiers subsisting on operational rations so that appropriate target nutrient densities can be established. Field studies also provide food selection and consumption data to help identify the best food vehicles for fortification. Reliable laboratory biomarkers of mineral status are needed so that status of soldiers before deployment and changes in status during deployment can be assessed. This information is critical to the evaluation of product reformulations and revised menus.

## REFERENCES

Baker-Fulco CJ, Kramer FM, Johnson J, Lesher LL, Merrill E, DeLany J. 2002. *Dietary Intakes of Female and Male Combat Support Hospital Personnel Subsisting on Meal-Focused or Standard Versions of the Meal, Ready-to-Eat*. Technical Report T-02/23. Natick, MA: USARIEM.

CMNR (Committee on Military Nutrition Research). 1991. *Military Nutrition Initiatives*. Washington, DC: Institute of Medicine Publication IOM-91-05.

Consolazio CF. 1976. The impact of low caloric feeding during exercise. In: *Food for the Armed Forces*. Technical Report NRDC TR 76-42-OTD. Natick, MA: Natick Research and Development Center. Pp. 61–94.
IOM (Institute of Medicine). 1997. *Dietary Reference Intakes for Calcium, Phosphorus, Magnesium, Vitamin D, and Fluoride*. Washington, DC: National Academy Press.
IOM. 1998. *Dietary Reference Intakes for Thiamin, Riboflavin, Niacin, Vitamin $B_6$, Folate, Vitamin $B_{12}$, Pantothenic Acid, Biotin, and Choline*. Washington, DC: National Academy Press.
IOM. 2000a. *Dietary Reference Intakes for Vitamin C, Vitamin E, Selenium, and Carotenoids*. Washington, DC: National Academy Press.
IOM. 2000b. *Dietary Reference Intakes for Applications in Dietary Assessment*. Washington, DC: National Academy Press.
IOM. 2001. *Dietary Reference Intakes for Vitamin A, Vitamin K, Arsenic, Boron, Chromium, Copper, Iodine, Iron, Manganese, Molybdenum, Nickel, Silicon, Vanadium, and Zinc*. Washington, DC: National Academy Press.
IOM. 2005. *Dietary Reference Intakes for Water, Potassium, Sodium, Chloride, and Sulfate*. Washington, DC: The National Academies Press.
National Research Council. 1989. *Recommended Dietary Allowances*. 10th Edition. Washington, DC: National Academy Press.
Tharion WJ, Baker-Fulco CJ, Bovill ME, Montain SJ, Delany JP, Champagne CM, Hoyt RW, Lieberman HR. 2004. Adequacy of garrison feeding for Special Forces soldiers during training. *Military Medicine* 169(6):483–490.
U.S. Departments of the Army, Navy, and Air Force. 2001. *Nutrition Standards and Education*. AR 40-25/BUMEDINST 10110.6/AFI 44-141. Washington, DC: U.S. Department of Defense Headquarters.

# Bioavailability of Iron, Zinc, and Copper as Influenced by Host and Dietary Factors

*Janet R. Hunt*
*USDA-ARS Grand Forks Human Nutrition Research Center,*
*Grand Forks, North Dakota*

## INTRODUCTION

To determine the mineral intake that will support or enhance performance of military personnel, the bioavailability of the minerals must be considered, in addition to the quantity of the mineral required for biological function. Bioavailability describes the biological utilization of a mineral as consumed, and is affected both by dietary and host factors. This paper briefly summarizes information on the bioavailability of iron, zinc, and copper, emphasizing topics of particular application to setting nutritional guidelines for feeding the military.

## IRON BIOAVAILABILITY

Body iron is mainly controlled at the point of intestinal absorption rather than excretion (McCance and Widdowson, 1937), and iron bioavailability is largely determined by the factors that affect intestinal absorption. Absorbed iron must replace approximately 1 mg of obligatory iron losses daily in men and postmenopausal women, and up to an additional 2.5 mg daily in menstruating women (Institute of Medicine, 2001). Iron absorption is substantially influenced by both host and dietary factors.

Dietary factors that influence absorption include the form of dietary iron (either heme or nonheme), as well as dietary constituents consumed concurrently that help keep nonheme iron reduced and soluble.

Heme iron, the protoporphyrin iron complex that enters intestinal mucosal cells intact, is absorbed more efficiently than nonheme iron. Heme iron accounts for ~40 percent of the iron in meat, poultry, and fish flesh, and constitutes 0–2.5 mg of the dietary iron consumed daily. Absorption of heme iron is enhanced by unidentified factors in meat, poultry, or fish (Layrisse et al., 1968; Martinez-Torres and Layrisse, 1971) and inhibited by calcium (Hallberg et al., 1991) when consumed in the same meal (Box B-1).

Nonheme iron describes the remaining iron in foods, which has been found to form a chemically exchangeable iron pool in the intestinal lumen (Cook et al., 1972). Absorption of this nonheme iron is affected by other dietary constituents consumed in the same meal (Box B-1), that influence the solubility and reduced (ferrous) valence state. Meat, poultry, and fish (Layrisse et al., 1968; Martinez-Torres and Layrisse, 1971) and ascorbic acid (Cook and Monsen, 1977; Hallberg et al., 1986) enhance nonheme iron absorption in a dose-dependent manner, and are especially effective in the presence of inhibitors such as phytic acid and

**BOX B-1**
**Food Components that Enhance or Inhibit Iron Absorption, When Consumed Concurrently**

**Heme Iron Absorption**

| Enhancers | Inhibitors |
|---|---|
| • Meat, poultry, fish | • Calcium |

**Non-heme Iron Absorption**

| Enhancers | Inhibitors |
|---|---|
| • Meat, poultry, fish | • Phytic acid |
| • Ascorbic acid | • Polyphenols/tannins (tea and coffee) |
| • Alcohol | • Soy protein |
| • Retinol? | • Egg |
| • Carotene? | • Calcium |
| • Other organic acids? | • Antacids |

**Interactions**

- Ascorbic acid or meat, poultry, and fish—enhancing effects are greater with phytate or polyphenols

polyphenols (Hallberg et al., 1989; Hallberg and Hulthen, 2000). Alcohol enhances nonheme iron absorption, possibly by enhancing gastric acid secretion which promotes the reduced valence state (Hallberg and Hulthen, 2000). Carotenes been reported as enhancers of nonheme iron absorption (Garcia-Casal et al., 1998; Layrisse et al., 2000). Reports of enhancement by retinoids are inconsistent (Garcia-Casal et al., 1998; Layrisse et al., 2000; Walczyk et al., 2003). Citric, malic, and tartaric acids enhance nonheme iron absorption at a high (100-fold) molar ratio (Gillooly et al., 1983), which may not be practically relevant.

Inhibitors of nonheme iron absorption include phytic acid (inositol hexaphosphate, the main food form of inositol phosphates) in whole grains, legumes, lentils, and nuts (Gillooly et al., 1983; Hallberg et al., 1989); iron-binding polyphenols, such as flavonoids, phenolic acids, and their polymerization products, in tea, coffee, red wines, and a variety of other cereals, vegetables, and spices (Brune et al., 1989; Gillooly et al., 1983; Hallberg and Hulthen, 2000); soy protein (apparently independent of the phytic acid in soy), (Hurrell et al., 1992); and eggs (Callender et al., 1970; Hallberg and Hulthen, 2000; Hurrell, 2003). Calcium inhibits the absorption of both nonheme as well as heme iron (Cook et al., 1991; Hallberg et al., 1991). Zinc in a 1:5 iron:zinc molar ratio reduces iron absorption when given with water, but not with a meal (Rossander-Hulten et al., 1991). Supplemental zinc in equimolar quantities may inhibit iron absorption (Crofton et al., 1989) and impair the iron status of women with low iron reserves (Donangelo et al., 2002). Extensive research on dietary iron bioavailability has helped quantify dose effects and interactions, and algorithms have been developed to calculate the iron bioavailability of diets (Hallberg and Hulthen, 2000; Reddy et al., 2000), but these need further validation.

Host factors that influence iron absorption include iron stores, erythropoiesis, hypoxia, pregnancy, and inflammation (Finch, 1994; Miret et al., 2003). Iron absorption is inversely related to iron status (Cook, 1990; Hallberg et al., 1997; Lynch et al., 1989; Roughead and Hunt, 2000; Taylor et al., 1988). With serum ferritin concentrations from 300 to ~5 μg/L, heme iron absorption can differ by nearly 3-fold, from approximately 20 to 50 percent, and the efficiency of nonheme iron absorption (from a high bioavailability diet) is influenced to a greater extent, from less than 1 to over 35 percent. Recent high iron intake reduces nonheme (Hoglund, 1969) but not heme iron absorption, independent of detectable changes in serum ferritin (Roughead and Hunt, 2000). The genetic mutation associated with hemochromatosis in people from Northern Europe results in increased absorption of both heme and nonheme iron (Lynch et al., 1989). About 10 percent of those populations are heterozygous for the same mutation, but this does not appear to increase iron absorption (Hunt and Zeng, 2004; Roe et al., 2005). However, additional genetic as well as environmental factors may influence an increasing occurrence of high serum ferritin with age, especially in adult men (IOM, 2001). Chronic inflammation is associated with anemia (e.g., anemia of chronic disease) which may partly be the result of reduced iron absorption

(Weber et al., 1988). Control of these host factors affecting iron absorption appears to involve the polypeptide hepcidin, which is secreted from the liver in response to high iron stores or infectious stimuli, and both down-regulates intestinal iron absorption and stimulated macrophage iron uptake, reducing serum iron (Ganz, 2003). Inflammatory stress from heavy exercise and exertion may initiate a sequence of increased IL(interleukin)-6 production (Margeli et al., 2005), followed by production of hepcidin (Nemeth et al., 2004), and possibly reduced iron absorption, although the latter has not been clearly demonstrated.

Gender does not directly influence iron absorption: men and women with the same iron status absorb iron similarly. However, women of child-bearing ages have considerably lower iron status than men: the 5th, 50th, and 95th percentiles for serum ferritin are 9, 37, and 124 for U.S. women and 42, 118, and 263 for men, respectively (IOM, 2001). In the U.S., iron deficiency in women of childbearing age is more common among minorities (8–10 percent in White, non-Hispanics vs. 15–19 percent in Black, non-Hispanics and 19–22 percent in Mexican Americans) and those with low income (Looker and Cogswell, 2002; Looker et al., 1997). Because of their reduced iron status, menstruating women absorb nonheme iron about twice as efficiently as men (Hunt, 2003b). Women with low iron stores can absorb 25–30 percent of the iron from a diet with high bioavailability, or as much as 3–4 mg iron daily. However, absorption by such women can be substantially reduced by factors that decrease dietary iron bioavailability, such as low meat intake, high phytic acid, and tea consumption (Hunt, 2003b).

Iron absorption can vary at least 15-fold relative to body iron stores, and 6-to-10-fold relative to dietary bioavailability, from diets with similar total iron content. However, these substantial differences in iron absorption, as measured with isotopic tracers, are slow to influence clinical indices of body iron status. In controlled trials of weeks or months duration, serum ferritin was unresponsive to differences in ascorbic acid (Cook et al., 1984; Garcia et al., 2003; Hunt et al., 1994; Malone et al., 1986; Monsen et al., 1991) calcium (Minihane and Fairweather-Tait, 1998; Sokoll and Dawson-Hughes, 1992), or several dietary factors affecting iron absorption by 4-to-6-fold (Hunt, 2003b; Hunt and Roughead, 2000; Hunt and Roughead, 1999). Dietary changes apparently require months or years to influence body iron stores, but such differences have been observed with cross-sectional studies of vegetarians, who consistently have lower iron stores than omnivores (Hunt, 2003a). Likewise, serum ferritin was positively associated with ingestion of heme iron, supplemental iron, dietary vitamin C, and alcohol and negatively associated with coffee drinking, in a cross-sectional study of elderly subjects (Fleming et al., 1998).

Changes in iron status are also relatively gradual with iron supplementation: serum ferritin increased by 4–5 μg/L with 20 mg iron as $FeSO_4$ daily for 6 weeks (Hinton et al., 2000), and 10–12 μg/L with 50 mg iron as $FeSO_4$ daily (with meals) for 12 weeks (Roughead and Hunt, 2000). Women with low iron stores were unable to maintain the difference in serum ferritin achieved with 12 weeks supplementation for 12 weeks after supplements were discontinued (Roughead and Hunt, 2000). These data suggest that to improve the iron status of women with low iron stores (serum ferritin < 20 μg/L) within several weeks, supplemental doses of 20–50 mg nonheme iron/day may be required on a continuing basis. Somewhat more positive results occurred with supplements containing 11 percent of the iron in the heme form: 9 or 27 mg daily iron increased serum ferritin by ~5 (a nonsignificant difference) or 12 μg/L ($p < 0.05$), respectively, and increased hemoglobin values from ~136 to 142 g/L ($p < 0.05$) in women with low iron stores (Fogelholm et al., 1994). These changes occurred within 1 month, with little change in 5 more months of supplementation (Fogelholm et al., 1994).

A ranking of the bioavailability to humans of iron salts used for fortification is likely determined by iron valence and solubility (ferrous sulfate, ferrous succinate, ferrous lactate, ferrous fumarate, ferrous glycine sulphate, ferrous glutamate, ferrous gluconate, > ferrous citrate, ferrous tartrate, ferrous pyrophosphate > ferric sulphate, ferric citrate) (Brise and Hallberg, 1962). Chelated forms of iron such as sodium iron ethylendiaminetetraacetic acid (NaFeEDTA) or ferrous bis-glycinate are highly bioavailable and in comparison to iron salts, are less influenced by inhibitors such as phytic acid (Bovell-Benjamin et al., 2000; Hurrell, 2002). Iron fortification sources such as ferric pyrophosphate, ferric orthophosphate and elemental iron powders are relatively inert in dry foods, minimizing adverse chemical reactions that may impair food color, taste, and shelf-life, but also reducing iron absorption relative to salts such as ferrous sulfate. Some micronization and emulsification technologies appear to improve the bioavailability of ferric pyrophosphate (Fidler et al., 2004) and may be useful with other iron forms. The bioavailability of elemental iron powders, composed of relatively pure iron metal with a zero valence state, is inversely related to particle size, surface area, and solubility, and differs according to specific production processes; the bioavailability to replete anemic rats is greatest for carbonyl, followed by electrolytic, and then the several reduced iron powders (Swain et al., 2003). However, the bioavailability of elemental iron powders is difficult to determine sensitively in humans because the commercial powders cannot be isotopically labeled.

## ZINC BIOAVAILABILITY

Both zinc absorption and excretion adaptively adjust to control body zinc in animals with zinc intakes from marginal to luxuriant (Hunt et al., 1987; Weigand and Kirchgessner, 1976a; Weigand and Kirchgessner, 1976b). Humans absorb zinc more efficiently when dietary zinc is low (Lee et al., 1993; Taylor et al., 1991; Wada et al., 1985), but this at least partly reflects the immediate effect of the amount ingested, rather than a long-term adaptation to changed zinc intake (Sandström and Cederblad, 1980; Sandström et al., 1980). As more zinc is ingested, absorptive efficiency decreases considerably, but the absolute amount absorbed increases.

Several dietary factors may influence human zinc absorption (Lonnerdal, 2000). The zinc content and phytate content, or phytate-to-zinc molar ratio are primary factors, and these are applied in a dietary algorithm for estimating fraction zinc absorption from adult diets (International Zinc Nutrition Consultative Group [IZiNG], 2004). Most of the zinc in Western diets is derived from animal foods, with beef supplying about a quarter of dietary zinc (Subar et al., 1998), which is highly bioavailable. Plant sources such as legumes, whole grains, nuts and seeds are also rich in zinc, which is less bioavailable because these sources are also high in phytic acid, a zinc chelator (Harland and Oberleas, 1987). Mixed or refined diets have phytate:zinc molar ratios of 4–18, whereas unrefined cereal based diets can range from 18 to 30 (IZiNCG, 2004). Although phytic acid in unrefined foods reduces fractional zinc absorption, the higher zinc content of these foods may make these foods preferable to more refined products. For example, nearly 50 percent more zinc was absorbed from a serving of whole wheat, compared with white bread (0.22 versus 0.15 mg, respectively), because the zinc content of the whole wheat bread more than compensated for a less efficient absorption of zinc (16.6 compared to 38.2 percent, respectively) (Sandström et al., 1980).

Zinc bioavailability is enhanced by dietary protein when zinc content is constant (Sandström et al., 1980), but this may differ with specific sources of protein (Davidsson et al., 1996), and the practical importance of protein may be confounded by the food zinc content, which correlates directly with protein content. Women tested with diets high or low in meat (replacing refined carbohydrates) absorbed zinc with similar efficiency, so the amount absorbed was proportional to the nearly 2-fold difference in dietary zinc content (Hunt et al., 1995).

Calcium has been proposed to reduce zinc absorption, but tests are equivocal with calcium either reducing (Wood and Zheng, 1997) or not influencing human zinc absorption (Dawson-Hughes et al., 1986; Lonnerdal et al., 1984; Spencer et al., 1984). Calcium is more likely to inhibit zinc absorption in the presence of phytic acid, by forming insoluble complexes (Fordyce et al., 1987). However, this 3-way interaction has not been clearly demonstrated in humans (Lonnerdal, 2000), and was not observed when calcium was added to a soy-based infant formula (Lonnerdal et al., 1984), or when dairy products (sources of protein as well as calcium) were added to whole wheat bread, a source of phytic acid (Sandström et al., 1980).

Other divalent cations could interfere with zinc absorption by competing for transport sites. Iron reduces zinc absorption when administered using supplemental amounts of inorganic salts (iron:zinc molar ratios of 25:1), but zinc absorption is unaffected in the presence of a food matrix or with more moderate ratios of iron and zinc (iron:zinc molar ratios of 2.5:1) (Lonnerdal, 2000;

Sandström et al., 1985; Solomons and Jacob, 1981; Whittaker, 1998). Supplementing diets with 2 mg copper did not affect zinc absorption by young or elderly adults (August et al., 1989).

Because women generally consume less food, including less dietary zinc, the efficiency of zinc absorption from typical diets is likely to be somewhat greater for women than men. For instance, using experimental diets based on representative U.S. diet surveys, women absorbed 29 ± 8 percent, or 2.3 mg zinc from a diet containing 7.8 mg zinc and 1,570 kcal, and men absorbed 22 ± 4 percent, or 3.1 mg zinc from a diet containing 14.0 mg and 2,545 kcal (Hunt et al., 1992).

It is difficult to evaluate the impact of zinc bioavailability on zinc nutrition since there are no sensitive clinical indices of marginal zinc status. Plasma zinc does not correlate with zinc absorption measurements (Hunt et al., 1995) and has been relatively insensitive to several weeks of severe dietary zinc restriction (Johnson et al., 1993; Wada et al., 1985). However, iron supplementation reduced plasma zinc in a study of pregnant Peruvian women (O'Brien et al., 1999). Plasma zinc was also reduced in research volunteers several weeks after changing to a vegetarian diet (Hunt et al., 1998; Srikumar et al., 1992), and was correlated inversely with dietary phytate:zinc molar ratios in adolescent girls consuming lacto-ovo-vegetarian diets (Donovan and Gibson, 1995), but usually has not differed between vegetarians and non-vegetarians in cross-sectional studies (Anderson et al., 1981; Donovan and Gibson, 1995; Kies et al., 1983; Krajcovicova-Kudlackova et al., 1995; Latta and Liebman, 1984). Because of lower zinc absorption, people consuming vegetarian diets, especially with phytate:zinc molar ratios exceeding 15, may require 20 to 50 percent more zinc than nonvegetarians (Hunt et al., 1998; IOM, 2001).

Zinc sulfate and zinc oxide are relatively inexpensive and are the forms of zinc most commonly used for food fortification (IZiNCG, 2004). Although zinc sulfate is much more soluble in water than zinc oxide, the two forms have been found equally well absorbed when used to fortify wheat products (de Romana et al., 2003; Herman et al., 2002). In addition to these two forms, zinc chloride, zinc gluconate, and zinc stearate are generally recognized as safe by the U.S. Food and Drug Administration.

## COPPER BIOAVAILABILITY

Much less information is available about the bioavailability of copper. Good food sources include organ meats, seafood, nuts, seeds, whole grains, and chocolate. Absorptive efficiency is inversely proportional to dietary copper content. For example, young men consuming diets containing 0.8, 1.7, or 7.5 mg/day absorbed 12, 36, and 56 percent of the dietary copper (Turnlund et al., 1989). Similarly, the greater copper content of an experimental vegetarian diet was associated with a lower fractional apparent absorption, but more total copper absorbed, despite a 3-fold greater phytic acid content compared to a nonvegetarian diet (Hunt and Vanderpool, 2001). Copper absorption was not reduced by supplemental ascorbic acid (Jacob et al., 1987) or by phytic acid or cellulose (Turnlund et al., 1985).

Compared with men, women tended to absorb copper from similar meals slightly more efficiently, which may compensate for a typically lower dietary copper intake (Johnson et al., 1992). Copper absorption was not different between young and elderly adults (Johnson et al., 1992; Turnlund et al., 1988).

High zinc intakes can reduce copper absorption (IOM, 2001), and zinc supplements have been used to treat Wilson's disease, an inherited disease that results in copper toxicity (Brewer et al., 1983).

## CONCLUSIONS

The bioavailability as well as the content of iron, zinc and copper should be considered when planning military diets. The bioavailability of these nutrients is generally high in North American diets, but bioavailability can be reduced by food choices such as the selection of a vegetarian diet. Biochemical indices are available to assess iron, but not zinc or copper nutritional status. Approximately 20 percent of menstruating women have low iron stores, and iron deficiency is more prevalent in minorities and those of low income. To address iron deficiency in these women, food-based approaches, including food fortification, are likely to require months or years to influence iron status, and would unnecessarily increase bioavailable iron for men. Iron supplementation should be evaluated for these specific women, or perhaps for all military women.

## REFERENCES


Anderson BM, Gibson RS, Sabry JH. 1981. The iron and zinc status of long-term vegetarian women. *Am J Clin Nutr* 34:1042–1048.

August D, Janghorbani M, Young VR. 1989. Determination of zinc and copper absorption at three dietary Zn-Cu ratios by using stable isotope methods in young adult and elderly subjects. *Am J Clin Nutr* 50:1457–1463.

Bovell-Benjamin AC, Viteri FE, Allen LH. 2000. Iron absorption from ferrous bisglycinate and ferric trisglycinate in whole maize is regulated by iron status. *Am J Clin Nutr* 71(6):1563–1569.

Brewer GJ, Hill GM, Prasad AS, Cossack ZT, Rabbani P. 1983. Oral zinc therapy for Wilson's disease. *Ann Intern Med* 99(3):314–319.

Brise H, Hallberg L. 1962. Absorbability of different iron compounds. *Acta Med Scand* 171 (Suppl): 23–38.

Brune M, Rossander L, Hallberg L. 1989. Iron absorption and phenolic compounds: Importance of different phenolic structures. *Eur J Clin Nutr* 43(8):547–557.

Callender ST, Marney SR, Jr., Warner GT. 1970. Eggs and iron absorption. *Br J Haematol* 19(6): 657–665.

Cook JD. 1990. Adaptation in iron metabolism. *Am J Clin Nutr* 51:301–308.

Cook JD, Monsen ER. 1977. Vitamin C, the common cold, and iron absorption. *Am J Clin Nutr* 30:235–241.

Cook JD, Layrisse M, Martinez-Tores C, Walker R, Monsen E, Finch CA. 1972. Food iron absorption measured by an extrinsic tag. *J Clin Invest* 51:805–815.

Cook JD, Watson SS, Simpson KM, Lipschitz DA, Skikne BS. 1984. The effect of high ascorbic acid supplementation on body iron stores. *Blood* 64:721–726.

Cook JD, Dassenko SA, Whittaker P. 1991. Calcium supplementation: Effect on iron absorption. *Am J Clin Nutr* 53(1):106–111.

Crofton RW, Gvozdanovic D, Gvozdanovic S, Khin CC, Brunt PW, Mowat NA, Aggett PJ. 1989. Inorganic zinc and the intestinal absorption of ferrous iron. *Am J Clin Nutr* 50(1):141–144.

Davidsson L, Almgren A, Sandstrom B, Juillerat M, Hurrell RF. 1996. Zinc absorption in adult humans: The effect of protein sources added to liquid test meals. *Br J Nutr* 75(4):607–613.

Dawson-Hughes B, Seligson FH, Hughes VA. 1986. Effects of calcium carbonate and hydroxyappetite on zinc and iron retention in postmenopausal women. *Am J Clin Nutr* 44:83–88.

de Romana DL, Lonnerdal B. 2003. Absorption of zinc from wheat products fortified with iron and either zinc sulfate or zinc oxide. *Am J Clin Nutr* 78(2):279–283.

Donangelo CM, Woodhouse LR, King SM, Viteri FE, King JC. 2002. Supplemental zinc lowers measures of iron status in young women with low iron reserves. *J Nutr* 132(7):1860–1864.

Donovan UM, Gibson RS. 1995. Iron and zinc status of young women aged 14 to 19 years consuming vegetarian and omnivorous diets. *J Am Coll Nutr* 14(5):463–472.

Fidler MC, Walczyk T, Davidsson L, Zeder C, Sakaguchi N, Juneja LR, Hurrell RF. 2004. A micronised, dispersible ferric pyrophosphate with high relative bioavailability in man. *Br J Nutr* 91(1):107–112.

Finch C. 1994. Regulators of iron balance in humans. *Blood* 84:1697–1702.

Fleming DJ, Jacques PF, Dallal GE, Tucker KL, Wilson PW, Wood RJ. 1998. Dietary determinants of iron stores in a free-living elderly population: The Framingham Heart Study. *Am J Clin Nutr* 67:722–733.

Fogelholm M, Suominen M, Rita H. 1994. Effects of low-dose iron supplementation in women with low serum ferritin concentration. *Eur J Clin Nutr* 48(10):753–756.

Fordyce EJ, Forbes RM, Robbins KR, Erdman JW Jr. 1987. Phytate X calcium/zinc molar ratios: Are they predictive of zinc bioavailability? *J Food Sci* 52(2):440–444.

Ganz T. 2003. Hepcidin, a key regulator of iron metabolism and mediator of anemia of inflammation. *Blood* 102(3):783.

Garcia OP, Diaz M, Rosado JL, Allen LH. 2003. Ascorbic acid from lime juice does not improve the iron status of iron-deficient women in rural Mexico. *Am J Clin Nutr* 78(2):267–273.

Garcia-Casal MN, Layrisse M, Solano L, Baron MA, Arguello F, Llovera D, Ramirez J, Leets I, Tropper E. 1998. Vitamin A and beta-carotene can improve nonheme iron absorption from rice, wheat, and corn by humans. *J Nutr* 128:646–650.

Gillooly M, Bothwell TH, Torrance JD, MacPhail AP, Derman DP, Bezwoda WR, Mills W, Charlton RW, Mayet F. 1983. The effects of organic acids, phytates and polyphenols on the absorption of iron from vegetables. *Br J Nutr* 49(3):331–342.

Hallberg L, Hulthen L. 2000. Prediction of dietary iron absorption: An algorithm for calculating absorption and bioavailability of dietary iron. *Am J Clin Nutr* 2000 (Erratum) 72:1242.

Hallberg L, Brune M, Rossander L. 1986. Effect of ascorbic acid on iron absorption from different types of meals. Studies with ascorbate rich foods and synthetic ascorbic acid given in different amounts with different meals. *Human Nutr: Appl Nutr* 40A:97–113.

Hallberg L, Brune M, Rossander L. 1989. Iron absorption in man: Ascorbic acid and dose-dependent inhibition by phytate. *Am J Clin Nutr* 49:140–144.

Hallberg L, Brune M, Erlandsson M, Sandberg AS, Rossander-Hulton L. 1991. Calcium: Effect of different amounts on nonheme- and heme-iron absorption in humans. *Am J Clin Nutr* 53: 112–119.

Hallberg L, Hulten L, Gramatkovski E. 1997. Iron absorption from the whole diet in men: How effective is the regulation of iron absorption? *Am J Clin Nutr* 66:347–356.

Harland BF, Oberleas D. 1987. Phytate in foods. *Wld Rev Nutr Diet* 52:235–259.

Herman S, Griffin IJ, Suwarti S, Ernawati F, Permaesih D, Pambudi D, Abrams SA. 2002. Co-fortification of iron-fortified flour with zinc sulfate, but not zinc oxide, decreases iron absorption in Indonesian children. *Am J Clin Nutr* 76(4):813–817.

Hinton PS, Giordano C, Brownlie T, Haas JD. 2000. Iron supplementation improves endurance after training in iron-depleted, nonanemic women. *J Appl Physiol* 88(3):1103–1111.

Hoglund S. 1969. Studies in iron absorption VI. Transitory effect of oral administration of iron on iron absorption. *Blood* 34(4):505–510.

Hunt JR. 2003a. Bioavailability of iron, zinc, and other trace minerals from vegetarian diets. *Am J Clin Nutr* 78(3 Suppl):633S–639S.

Hunt JR. 2003b. High-, but not low-bioavailability diets enable substantial control of women's iron absorption in relation to body iron stores, with minimal adaptation within several weeks. *Am J Clin Nutr* 78(6):1168–1177.

Hunt JR, Roughead ZK. 1999. Nonheme iron absorption, fecal ferritin excretion, and blood indexes of iron status in women consuming controlled lactoovovegetarian diets for 8 wk. *Am J Clin Nutr* 69:944–952.

Hunt JR, Roughead ZK. 2000. Adaptation of iron absorption in men consuming diets with high or low iron bioavailability. *Am J Clin Nutr* 71(1):94–102.

Hunt JR, Vanderpool RA. 2001. Apparent copper absorption from a vegetarian diet. *Am J Clin Nutr* 74(6):803–807.

Hunt JR, Zeng H. 2004. Iron absorption by heterozygous carriers of the HFE C282Y mutation associated with hemochromatosis. *Am J Clin Nutr* 80(4):924–931.

Hunt JR, Johnson PE, Swan PB. 1987. Influence of usual zinc intake and zinc in a meal on 65Zn retention and turnover in the rat. *J Nutr* 117:1427–1433.

Hunt JR, Mullen LK, Lykken GI. 1992. Zinc retention from an experimental diet based on the U.S. FDA Total Diet Study. *Nutr Res* 12:1335–1344.

Hunt JR, Gallagher SK, Johnson LK. 1994. Effect of ascorbic acid on apparent iron absorption by women with low iron stores. *Am J Clin Nutr* 59:1381–1385.

Hunt JR, Gallagher SK, Johnson LK, Lykken GI. 1995. High- versus low-meat diets: Effects on zinc absorption, iron status, and calcium, copper, iron, magnesium, manganese, nitrogen, phosphorus, and zinc balance in postmenopausal women. *Am J Clin Nutr* 62(3):621–632.

Hunt JR, Matthys LA, Johnson LK. 1998. Zinc absorption, mineral balance, and blood lipids in women consuming controlled lactoovovegetarian and omnivorous diets for 8 wk. *Am J Clin Nutr* 67:421–430

Hurrell RF. 2002. Fortification: Overcoming technical and practical barriers. *J Nutr* 132(4 Suppl): 806S–812S.

Hurrell RF. 2003. Influence of vegetable protein sources on trace element and mineral bioavailability. *J Nutr* 133(9):2973S–2977S.

Hurrell RF, Juillerat MA. 1992. Soy protein, phytate, and iron absorption in humans. *Am J Clin Nutr* 56(3):573–578.

International Zinc Nutrition Consultative Group (IZiNCG). 2004. Chapter 1: Overview of zinc nutrition. Assessment of the risk of zinc deficiency in populations and options for its control. *Food and Nutrition Bulletin* 25:S99–S129.

IOM (Institute of Medicine). 2001. *Dietary Reference Intakes for Vitamin A, Vitamin K, Arsenic, Boron, Chromium, Copper, Iodine, Iron, Manganese, Molybdenum, Nickel, Silicon, Vanadium, and Zinc*. Washington, DC: National Academy Press.

Jacob RA, Skala JH, Omaye ST, Turlund JR. 1987. Effect of varying ascorbic acid intakes on copper absorption and ceruloplasmin levels of young men. *J Nutr* 117(12):2109–2215.

Johnson PE, Milne DB, Lykken GI. 1992. Effects of age and sex on copper absorption, biological half-life and status in humans. *Am J Clin Nutr* 56(5):917–925.

Johnson PE, Hunt CD, Milne DB, Mullen LK. 1993. Homeostatic control of zinc metabolism in men: Zinc excretion and balance in men fed diets low in zinc. *Am J Clin Nutr* 57(4):557–565.

Kies C, Young E, McEndree L. 1983. Zinc bioavailability from vegetarian diets. Influence of dietary fiber, ascorbic acid, and past dietary practices. In: Inglett GE, ed. *Nutritional Bioavailability of Zinc*. Washington, DC: American Chemical Society. Pp. 115–126.

Krajcovicova-Kudlackova M, Simoncic R, Babinska K, Bederova A, Brtkova A, Magalova T, Grancicova E. 1995. Selected vitamins and trace elements in blood of vegetarians. *Ann Nutr Metab* 39(6):334–339.

Latta D, Liebman M. 1984. Iron and zinc status of vegetarian and nonvegetarian males. *Nutr Rep Int* 30(1):141–149.

Layrisse M, Martinez-Torres C, Roche M. 1968. Effect of interaction of various foods on iron absorption. *Am J Clin Nutr* 21:1175–1183.

Layrisse M, Garcia-Casal MN, Solano L, Baron MA, Arguello F, Llovera D, Ramirez J, Leets I, Tropper E. 2000. New property of vitamin A and beta-carotene on human iron absorption: Effect on phytate and polyphenols as inhibitors of iron absorption. *Arch Latinoam Nutr* 50(3): 243–248.

Lee DY, Prasad AS, Hydrick-Adair C, Brewer G, Johnson PE. 1993. Homeostasis of zinc in marginal human zinc deficiency—Role of absorption and endogenous excretion of zinc. *J Lab Clin Med* 122(5):549–556.

Lonnerdal B. 2000. Dietary factors influencing zinc absorption. *J Nutr* 130(5):1378S–1383S.

Lonnerdal B, Cederblad A, Davidsson L, Sandstrom B. 1984. The effect of individual components of soy formula and cows' milk formula on zinc bioavailability. *Am J Clin Nutr* 40(5):1064–1070.

Looker AC, Cogswell ME. 2002. Iron deficiency—United States, 1999–2000. *MMWR Weekly* 51(40): 897–899.

Looker AC, Dallman PR, Carrol MD, Gunter EW, Johnson CL. 1997. Prevalence of iron deficiency in the United States. *JAMA* 277(12):973–976.

Lynch SR, Skikne BS, Cook JD. 1989. Food iron absorption in idiopathic hemochromatosis. *Blood* 74:2187–2193.

Malone HE, Kevany JP, Scott JM, O'Broin SD, O'Connor G. 1986. Ascorbic acid supplementation: Its effects on body iron stores and white blood cells. *Irish J Med Sci* 155:74–79.

Margeli A, Skenderi K, Tsironi M, Hantzi E, Matalas AL, Vrettou C, Kanavakis E, Chrousos G, Papassotiriou I. 2005. Dramatic elevations of interleukin-6 and acute phase reactants in athletes participating in the ultradistance foot race spartathlon: Severe systemic inflammation and lipid and lipoprotein changes in protracted exercise. *J Clin Endocrinol Metab* 90(7):3914–3918.

Martinez-Torres C, Layrisse M. 1971. Iron absorption from veal muscle. *Am J Clin Nutr* 24:531–540.

McCance RA, Widdowson EM. 1937. Absorption and excretion of iron. *Lancet* 2:680–684.

Minihane AM, Fairweather-Tait SJ. 1998. Effect of calcium supplementation on daily nonheme-iron absorption and long-term iron status. *Am J Clin Nutr* 68:96–102.

Miret S, Simpson RJ, McKie AT. 2003. Physiology and molecular biology of dietary iron absorption. *Annu Rev Nutr* 23:283–301.

Monsen, ER, Labbe RF, Lee W, Finch CA. 1991. Iron balance in healthy menstruating women: Effect of diet and ascorbate supplementation. In: *Trace Elements in Man and Animals (TEMA-7.* Dubrovnic, Yugoslavia: University of Zagreb, Institute for Medical Research and Occupational Health. Pp. 6.2–6.3.

Nemeth E, Rivera S, Gabayan V, Keller C, Taudorf S, Pederson BK, Ganz T. 2004. IL-6 mediates hypoferremia of inflammation by inducing the synthesis of the iron regulatory hormone hepcidin. *J Clin Invest* 113(9):1271–1276.

O'Brien KO, Zavaleta N, Caulfield LE, Yang DX, Abrams SA. 1999. Influence of prenatal iron and zinc supplements on supplemental iron absorption, red blood cell iron incorporation, and iron status in pregnant Peruvian women. *Am J Clin Nutr* 69(3):509–515.

Reddy MB, Hurrell RF, Cook JD. 2000. Estimation of nonheme-iron bioavailability from meal composition. *Am J Clin Nutr* 71(4):937–943.

Roe MA, Heath AL, Oyston SL, Macrow C, Hoogewerff JA, Foxall R, Dainty JR, Majsak-Newman G, Willis G, Fairweather-Tait SJ. 2005. Iron absorption in male C282Y heterozygotes. *Am J Clin Nutr* 81(4):814–821.

Rossander-Hulten L, Brune M, Sandstrom B, Lonnerdal B, Hallberg L. 1991. Competitive inhibition of iron absorption by manganese and zinc in humans. *Am J Clin Nutr* 54:152–156.

Roughead ZK, Hunt JR. 2000. Adaptation in iron absorption: Iron supplementation reduces nonheme-iron but not heme-iron absorption from food. *Am J Clin Nutr* 72(4):982–989.

Sandström B, Cederblad A. 1980. Zinc absorption from composite meals II. Influence of the main protein source. *Am J Clin Nutr* 33:1778–1783.

Sandström B, Arvidsson B, Cederblad A, Bjorn-Rasmussen E. 1980. Zinc absorption from composite meals I. The significance of wheat extraction rate, zinc, calcium, and protein content in meals based on bread. *Am J Clin Nutr* 33:739–745.

Sandström B, Davidsson L, Cederblad A, Lonnerdal B. 1985. Oral iron, dietary ligands and zinc absorption. *J Nutr* 115:411–414.

Sokoll LJ, Dawson-Hughes B. 1992. Calcium supplementation and plasma ferritin concentrations in premenopausal women. *Am J Clin Nutr* 56:1045–1048.

Solomons NW, Jacob RA. 1981. Studies on the bioavailability of zinc in humans: Effects of heme and nonheme iron on the absorption of zinc. *Am J Clin Nutr* 34:475–482.

Spencer H, Kramer L, Norris C, Osis D. 1984. Effect of calcium and phosphorus on zinc metabolism in man. *Am J Clin Nutr* 40:1213–1218.

Srikumar TS, Johansson GK, Ockerman PA, Gustafsson JA, Akesson B. 1992. Trace element status in healthy subjects switching from a mixed to a lactovegetarian diet for 12 mo. *Am J Clin Nutr* 55:885–890.

Subar AF, Krebs-Smith SM, Cook A, Kahle LL. 1998. Dietary sources of nutrients among U.S. adults, 1989 to 1991. *J Am Dietet Assoc* 98:537–547.

Swain JH, Newman SM, Hunt JR. 2003. Bioavailability of elemental iron powders to rats is less than bakery-grade ferrous sulfate and predicted by iron solubility and particle surface area. *J Nutr* 133(11):3546–3552.

Taylor CM, Bacon JR, Aggett PJ, Bremner I. 1991. Homeostatic regulation of zinc absorption and endogenous losses in zinc- deprived men [published erratum appears in *Am J Clin Nutr* 1992 Aug;56(2):462]. *Am J Clin Nutr* 53(3):755–763.

Taylor P, Martinez-Torres C, Leets I, Ramirez J, Garcia-Casal MN, Layrisse M. 1988. Relationships among iron absorption, percent saturation of plasma transferrin and serum ferritin concentration in humans. *J Nutr* 118(9):1110–1115.

Turnlund JR, King JC, Gong B, Keyes WR, Michel MC. 1985. A stable isotope study of copper absorption in young men: Effect of phytate and alpha-cellulose. *Am J Clin Nutr* 42:18–23.

Turnlund JR, Reager RD, Costa, F. 1988. Iron and copper absorption in young and elderly men. *Nutr Res* 8:333–343.

Turnlund JR, Keyes WR, Anderson HL, Acord LL. 1989. Copper absorption and retention in young men at three levels of dietary copper by use of the stable isotope 65Cu. *Am J Clin Nutr* 49: 870.

Wada L, Turnlund JR, King JC. 1985. Zinc utilization in young men fed adequate and low zinc intakes. *J Nutr* 115(10):1345–1354.

Walczyk T, Davidsson L, Rossander-Hulthen L, Hallberg L, Hurrell RF. 2003. No enhancing effect of vitamin A on iron absorption in humans. *Am J Clin Nutr* 77(1):144–149.

Weber J, Were JM, Julius HW, Marx JJ. 1988. Decreased iron absorption in patients with active rheumatoid arthritis, with and without iron deficiency. *Ann Rheum Dis* 47(5):404–409.

Weigand E, Kirchgessner M. 1976a. 65Zn-labeled tissue zinc for determination of endogenous fecal zinc excretion in growing rats. *Nutr Metab* 20:314–320.

Weigand E, Kirchgessner M. 1976b. Radioisotope dilution technique for determination of zinc absorption in vivo. *Nutr Metab* 20:307–313.
Whittaker P. 1998. Iron and zinc interactions in humans. *Am J Clin Nutr* 68(2 Suppl):442S–446S.
Wood RJ, Zheng JJ. 1997. High dietary calcium intakes reduce zinc absorption and balance in humans. *Am J Clin Nutr* 65:1803–1809.

# Functional Metabolism of Copper, Zinc, and Iron

*Cathy W. Levenson*
*Florida State University, Tallahassee*

## INTRODUCTION

The metabolism of copper, zinc, and iron occurs in every organ, tissue, and cell type of the human body. The molecular, biochemical, and physiological roles that these nutrients play are so fundamental that these metals are essential not just for optimal physiological performance, but for sustaining life itself. Any attempt to understand the effects that military service, and the inherent physical and emotional demands of training and combat, would have on metal metabolism must first address the actual roles of these metals and how they function in the metabolic processes that regulate physiological function.

## METAL TRANSPORT

After intestinal absorption of dietary copper, zinc, and iron, these essential nutrients are transported through the serum to specific organs. For example, both copper and zinc appear to be transported through the serum for delivery to tissues via albumin as well as other small molecular weight ligands including serum amino acids and peptides such as glutathione (Lovstad, 2004; Stewart et al., 2003). Interestingly, the majority of serum copper, at least 65 percent in humans, is associated with the enzyme ceruloplasmin. While the enzymatic activity of this protein requires copper, and is thus frequently used as a copper status indicator, this protein does not appear to play a significant role in the transport and delivery of copper to tissues. Instead, the primary role of this powerful serum antioxidant appears to be its role in iron metabolism (Sharp, 2005).

While the binding of copper and zinc to serum albumin and peptides is relatively non-specific, iron, in contrast, has a specialized transport system. The protein responsible for the transport and delivery of iron to tissues is transferrin. At the cellular level, target tissues take up iron via a receptor-mediated endocytotic mechanism that is specifically regulated by the availability of iron (Levenson and Tassabehji, 2004). Increases in iron availability decrease the abundance of the transferrin receptor and limit cellular iron uptake. However, in periods of low dietary iron availability ferritin levels are decreased and translation and synthesis of the transferrin receptor is increased in an attempt to maximize cellular iron uptake (Levenson and Tassabehji, 2004).

## FUNCTIONAL METABOLISM OF COPPER

### Immune System

In the military setting, it is clear that optimal immune function is essential. Exposure to a variety of novel bacterial, both intestinal and cutaneous, is an accepted part of military life, particularly in international theaters. Close living quarters increase the risk of transmission of bacterial and viral infection. Copper, zinc, and iron are all essential for immune function (reviewed in Failla, 2003). In the case of copper, a number of studies have reported neutropenia resulting from copper deficiency, the most recent of which was published just this year (Nagano et al., 2005). Other work on the functional metabolism of copper in the immune system has shown that copper deficiency impairs the activity of the cytokine interleukin-2 (IL-2) in human T-lymphocytes (Hopkins and Failla, 1997), and suppresses monocyte differentiation (Huang et al., 2001).

### Red Blood Cells

Iron is carried to the bone marrow for incorporation into developing erythrocytes by the serum transport protein transferrin. However, the ability of iron to bind to this protein is dependent of the ferrioxidase activity of the copper-dependent enzyme ceruloplasmin. Without copper and ceruloplasmin activity, iron is trapped in the ferrous state. Unable to bind to transferrin, iron delivery is prevented, resulting in symptoms consistent with iron deficiency including microcytic, hypochromic anemia. Unfortunately, misdiagnosis of copper deficiency as iron deficiency and treatment with iron supplements could result in iron overload. Thus, understanding the functional metabolism and interactions of these two nutrients is important as anemia would clearly impair physical performance in military personnel.

While primary dietary copper deficiency is likely to be very rare, it is important to note that high levels of zinc intake inhibit copper absorption. This in turn can lead to neurotropenia, reduced ceruloplasmin activity, defective iron transport, and microcytic, hypochromic anemia (Willis et al., 2005). A recent report showed that supplementation with 100 mg zinc/day resulted in marked anemia and severe neutropenia associated with copper deficiency (Irving et al., 2003). Thus, while it is important that dietary zinc be adequate to meet the increased needs of military personnel, it is important that diets not be supplemented with zinc at levels that would induce copper deficiency.

## Muscle

Clearly optimal physical performance in military personnel is dependent on optimal muscle metabolism including substrate utilization, mitochondrial oxidation, and ATP synthesis. This is true both for both skeletal muscle and mitochondria-rich cardiac muscle. It has been known for some time that the trace metal copper is essential for the activity of cytochrome *c* oxidase, an essential mitochondrial enzyme used in the synthesis of ATP (Rossi et al., 1998). More recent work has suggested that copper may also regulate synthesis of other members of the mitochondrial electron transport chain such as ATP synthase (Medeiros and Wildmon, 1997). Additionally, the copper-dependent enzymes lysyl-oxidase, which is responsible for collagen cross-linking, and Cu, Zn-superoxide dismutase, a cytosolic free radical scavenger, are both needed for normal muscle function.

## Brain and Nervous System

The role of copper in neuronal metabolism and neurological function is complex. First, the brain synthesizes ceruloplasmin. Unlike ceruloplasmin that is synthesized in the liver for export into the serum, the ceruloplasmin in the brain is anchored in cell membranes where it functions in iron metabolism. The absence of ceruloplasmin activity results in brain iron toxicity (Xu et al., 2004). Other copper dependent enzymes in the brain and nervous system include dopamine beta-monooxygenase, that is responsible for the conversion of the neurotransmitter dopamine into norepinephrine. Norepinephrine is in turn converted into epinephrine, or adrenaline. Interestingly, the actual effect of copper deficiency is complex, as dietary copper deficiency in rats produced elevated dopamine beta-monooxygenase activity (Prohaska and Brokate, 2001). Regardless of the exact mechanism, these data show that copper deficiency would likely disrupt the normal "fight or flight" response to stress that is associated with catecholamine production, and would come into play during both combat and training settings.

Peptidylglycine alpha-amidating monooxygenase (PAM) is also copper dependent (Prohaska et al., 1995). This enzyme, found both intracellularly as well as in the serum, is responsible for the post-translational modification, maturation and activation of a wide variety of neurohormones including vasopressin that regulates water balance and blood pressure, gastrin and cholecystokinin (CCK) in the gastrointestinal system, calcitonin that regulates bone calcium deposition, thryotropin, substance P, and neuropeptide Y (NPY) (Eipper et al., 1993). While all of these hormones play vital roles, of particular interest to the stress of combat is the role that NPY may play. Our data show that NPY is regulated by copper in the central nervous system (Rutkoski et al., 1999), and that synthesis of this peptide in the adrenal gland is an important part of the physiological response and adaptation to psychological stress (Levenson and Moore, 1998).

## FUNCTIONAL METABOLISM OF IRON

### Red Blood Cells

The role of iron in hemoglobin function and oxygen transport is well known. Clearly the delivery of oxygen to muscle, particularly in times of peak demand, is essential for optimal muscle performance. Dietary iron deficiency leads to microcytic, hypochromic anemia. When dietary iron is limited, erythrocyte hemoglobin synthesis is reduced, both because iron is an essential part of the porphyrin ring structure of hemoglobin, and because iron deficiency impairs the activity of at least one enzyme in the heme synthetic pathway. Additionally, we know that iron deficiency, and the resulting decrease in hemoglobin concentration, results in increased division of pro-erythrocytes in the bone marrow, leading to decreased erythrocyte diameter and volume, and impairing oxygen delivery capability.

### Muscle

For many years the fatigue and irritability associated with dietary iron deficiency were attributed to the anemia discussed above. While reduced oxygen delivery can certainly contribute to these symptoms, there is a growing appreciation for the role of iron in skeletal and cardiac muscle. Iron is required for the electron transport chain in the mitochondrial that is responsible for ATP synthesis. Iron deficiency reduces mitochondrial cytochrome c, cytochrome oxidase, glycerol-3-phosphate dehydrogenase activity, and respiratory capacity (McLane et al., 1981). Furthermore, it appears that the fatigue associated with iron deficiency can be corrected with iron supplements, even in the absence of anemia (Brutsaert et al., 2003). An understanding of the role of iron in functional muscle metabolism is important, particularly for females who may have lower iron stores. This also illustrates the need to evaluate iron status not simply by hemoglobin or hemtocrit, but rather by other measures that may be more reflective of total body iron status such as total iron binding capacity (TIBC) and serum ferritin.

### Brain and Nervous System

Like copper, iron is not only an essential nutrient, but, in high concentrations, is toxic. For many years evidence has been mounting that suggests a role for iron accumulation in the death and destruction of dopaminergic neurons of the substantia nigra. Damage to these catecholaminergic neurons results in abnormal motor behavior, balance disturbances, tremors, and cognitive declines most frequently associated with Parkinson's disease (Zecca et al., 2004). Iron accumulation has also been associated with Fredrick's ataxia and Alzheimer's disease (Zecca et al., 2004). While the long term avoidance of these disorders is important for both military personnel and the general population, the most recent epidemiological data suggest that high intakes of dietary iron alone do not cause Parkinson's disease. For example, when the diets of Parkinson's patients and age-matched controls were compared, it was found that dietary iron intakes were not different (Logroscino et al., 1998). However, it should be noted that there was an association between high dietary fat intake and Parkinson's disease that was exacerbated by high dietary iron levels, suggesting that iron-induced oxidative processes maybe a significant part of Parkinson's etiology (Logroscino et al., 1998). These data highlight the need to examine overall dietary intake, not just metal intake, for risk assessment.

Clearly, there are many iron dependent processes in the brain. While there are data suggesting that chelation of iron may provide protection from Parkinson's disease (Kaur et al., 2003), newly emerging data show that dietary iron deficiency may contribute to increased risk of gait and balance disorders resulting from damage to dopaminergic neurons (Levenson et al., 2004). Mice fed an iron deficient diet for six weeks had significantly lower striatal dopamine concentrations and poorer motor behavior scores than those fed an iron adequate control diet (Levenson et al., 2004). Other work has revealed that iron restriction impairs dopamine metabolism (Erikson et al., 2000), disrupts dopamine receptor function (Nelson et al., 1997), and induces programmed cell death mechanisms in dopaminergic neurons (Levenson et al., 2004). Future work will be needed to understand the potential risk that iron deficiency poses for normal neuronal function. But for now it is clear that adequate iron status, as measured by TIBC and not just the presence of anemia, should be maintained.

## FUNCTIONAL METABOLISM OF ZINC

### Biochemical Functions

The physiological functions of zinc can largely be attributed to the catalytic and structural roles of zinc bound to specific proteins. For example, zinc is known to be required for the catalytic activity of approximately 100 mammalian enzymes. Zinc dependent enzymes, such as glyceraldehyde dehydrogenase, lactate dehydrogenase, and DNA and RNA polymerases, are so ubiquitous that there is virtually no metabolic cycle that is not dependent on zinc. The biochemical role of zinc is also illustrated by the existence of hundreds, if not thousands, of zinc-finger proteins that act as DNA-binding transcription factors to regulate gene expression. Zinc-finger proteins, that coordinate zinc in their structure through cysteines and histidines, also act as RNA binding proteins as well as participate in protein-protein interactions that regulate cellular function and metabolism.

Because of the vast number of biochemical and molecular functions, it is not surprising that the functional metabolism of zinc is important. For example, cellular proliferation and differentiation that take place upon immune system activation are both dependent on zinc and appear to be disrupted in zinc deficiency. Secretion of a number of important cytokines such as IL-2, interferon-gamma, and tumor necrosis factor alpha are reduced by dietary zinc deficiency (Fraker et al., 2000). Furthermore, tissue growth, including the growth of new muscle tissue and wound healing, is dependent on adequate dietary zinc (Andrews and Gallagher-Allred, 1999).

## Brain and Nervous System

Zinc is needed for many aspects of brain and nervous system function including neuronal differentiation, synaptic activity, receptor modulation and function, and neuronal survival. It is well accepted that the central nervous system, particularly the hypothalamus, is responsible for regulation of appetite and feeding behaviors. Adequate food intake is essential not only to maintain energy balance and body weight, but also to insure adequate micronutrient intake. Our lab (Evans et al., 2004) as well as many others, has shown that when fed a zinc-restricted diet, rats develop a profound anorexia within approximately one week Given a choice between dietary carbohydrate, protein and fat, zinc deficient rats virtually eliminate carbohydrate intake (Rains and Shay, 1995). While the cellular and molecular mechanisms responsible for these observations are still being investigated (Levenson, 2003), it is interesting to speculate what effect dietary zinc has on human feeding behavior. While human food intake and selection is too complex to attribute to a single factor, it has been hypothesized that zinc deficiency may play a role in the development of some cases of human anorexia nervosa (Tannhauser, 2002). There is also evidence that zinc deficiency results in decreased taste acuity in humans (Russell et al., 1983), a problem that could easily contribute to reduced food intake. Thus, given the increased energy requirements of combat troops and the usual decrease in apetite due to a variety of stressors during military life, maintaining adequate zinc nutriture appears to be important. However, the data regarding the involvement of zinc in food behavior of humans is not well understood.

There is also a growing body of literature, spanning the last two decades, suggesting a link between clinical depression and zinc deficiency (for recent reviews see Nowak et al., 2005 and Levenson, 2006). For example, not only has it been shown that patients suffering from major depression have lower serum zinc levels, but the severity of the zinc deficiency can also be correlated with the severity of the depression (Maes et al., 1994). Patients whose symptoms are resistant to treatment have even lower serum zinc levels than those who respond to conventional pharmacological treatments (Maes et al., 1999). Zinc has also successfully been used as an adjunct to antidepressant treatment. In a double-blind trial, treatment with tricyclic antidepressants or selective serotonin reuptake inhibitors was significantly enhanced when supplemented with zinc compared with a placebo (Levenson, 2006; Nowak et al., 2003). While there are many causes of depression, including genetics, there is no dispute that stressful environments and situations, both acute and chronic, are a significant factor in the development of depression and depression-like disorders (Wurtman, 2005). Given the emerging evidence that dietary zinc may play a role in the development of depression, every effort should be made to maintain the zinc status of individuals exposed to stressful living and working conditions.

## CONCLUSIONS

An examination of the functional metabolism of the copper, zinc, and iron shows that each of these nutrients is a vital and essential regulator of the immune system, muscle metabolism and performance, red blood cell function, and the brain and nervous system. The role of trace metals in the metabolism of these different organ systems is particularly important during periods of physical and psychological stress associated with combat and training of military personnel.

## REFERENCES

Andrews M, Gallagher-Allred C. 1999. The role of zinc in wound healing. *Adv Wound Care* 2: 137–138.

Brutsaert TD, Hernandez-Cordero S, Rivera J, Viola T, Hughes G, Haas JD. 2003. Iron supplementation improves progressive fatigue resistance during dynamic knee extensor exercise in iron-depleted, nonanemic women. *Am J Clin Nutr* 77:441–448.

Eipper BA, Milgram SL, Husten EJ, Yun HY, Mains RE. 1993. Peptidylglycine alpha-amidating monooxygenase: A multifunctional protein with catalytic, processing, and routing domains. *Protein Sci* 2:489–497.

Erikson KM, Jones BC, Beard JL. 2000. Iron deficiency alters dopamine transporter functioning in rat striatum. *J Nutr* 130:2831–2837.

Evans SA, Overton JM, Alshingiti A, Levenson CW. 2004. Regulation of metabolic rate and substrate utilization by zinc deficiency. *Metabolism* 53:727–732.

Failla ML. 2003. Trace elements and host defense: recent advances and continuing challenges. *J Nutr* 133:1443S–1447S.

Hopkins RG, Failla ML. 1997. Copper deficiency reduces interleukin-2 (IL-2) production and IL-2 mRNA in human T-lymphocytes. *J Nutr* 127:257–262.

Huang ZL, Failla ML, Reeves PG. 2001. Differentiation of human U937 promonocytic cells is impaired by moderate copper deficiency. *Exp Biol Med* (Maywood) 226:222–228.

Irving JA, Mattman A, Lockitch G, Farrell K, Wadsworth LD. 2003. Element of caution: A case of reversible cytopenias associated with excessive zinc supplementation. *CMAJ* 169:129–131.

Kaur D, Yantiri F, Rajagopalan S, Kumar J, Mo JQ, Boonplueang R, Viswanath V, Jacobs R, Yang L, Beal MF, DiMonte D, Volitaskis I, Ellerby L, Cherny RA, Bush AI, Andersen JK. 2003. Genetic or pharmacological iron chelation prevents MPTP-induced neurotoxicity in vivo: A novel therapy for Parkinson's disease. *Neuron* 37:899–909.

Levenson CW. 2003. Zinc regulation of food intake: New insights on the role of neuropeptide Y. *Nutr Rev* 61:247–249.

Levenson CW. 2006. Zinc: The new antidepressant? *Nutr Rev* 64(1):39–42.

Levenson CW, Moore JB. 1998. Response of rat adrenal neuropeptide Y and tyrosine hydroxylase mRNA to acute stress is enhanced by long-term voluntary exercise. *Neurosci Lett* 242: 177–179.

Levenson CW, Tassabehji NM. 2004. Iron and ageing: An introduction to iron regulatory mechanisms. *Ageing Res Rev* 3:251–263.

Levenson CW, Cutler RG, Ladenheim B, Cadet JL, Hare J, Mattson MP. 2004. Role of dietary iron restriction in a mouse model of Parkinson's disease. *Exp Neurol* 190:506–514.

Lovstad RA. 2004, A kinetic study on the distribution of Cu(II)-ions between albumin and transferrin. *Biometals* 17:111–113.

Maes M, D'Haese PC, Scharpe S, D'Hondt P, Cosyns P, De Broe ME. 1994. Hypozincemia in depression. *J Affect Disord* 31:135–140.

Maes M, De Vos N, Demedts P, Wauters A, Neels H. 1999. Lower serum zinc in major depression in relation to changes in serum acute phase proteins. *J Affect Disord* 56:189–194.

McLane JA, Fell RD, McKay RH, Winder WW, Brown EB, Holloszy JO. 1981, Physiological and biochemical effects of iron deficiency on rat skeletal muscle. *Am J Physiol* 241:C47–C54.

Nagano T, Toyoda T, Tanabe H, Nagato T, Tsuchida T, Kitamura A, Kasai G. 2005. Clinical features of hematological disorders caused by copper deficiency during long-term enteral nutrition. *Intern Med* 44:554–559.

Nelson C, Erikson K, Pinero DJ, Beard JL. 1997. In vivo dopamine metabolism is altered in iron-deficient anemic rats. *J Nutr* 127:2282–2288.

Nowak G, Siwek M, Dudek D, Zieba A, Pilc A. 2003. Effect of zinc supplementation on antidepressant therapy in unipolar depression: A preliminary placebo-controlled study. *Pol J Pharmacol* 55:1143–1147.

Nowak G, Szewczyk B, Pilc A. 2005. Zinc and depression. An update. *Pharmacol Rep* 57:713–718.

Prohaska JR, Brokate B. 2001. Dietary copper deficiency alters protein levels of rat dopamine beta-monooxygenase and tyrosine monooxygenase. *Exp Biol Med* (Maywood) 226:199–207.

Prohaska JR, Bailey WR, Lear PM. 1995. Copper deficiency alters rat peptidylglycine alpha-amidating monooxygenase activity. *J Nutr* 125:1447–1454.

Rains TM, Shay NF. 1995. Zinc status specifically changes preferences for carbohydrate and protein in rats selecting from separate carbohydrate-, protein-, and fat-containing diets. *J Nutr* 125: 2874–2879.

Rossi L, Lippe G, Marchese E, De Martino A, Mavelli I, Rotilio G, Ciriolo MR. 1998. Decrease of cytochrome c oxidase protein in heart mitochondria of copper-deficient rats. *Biometals* 11:207–212.

Russell RM, Cox ME, Solomons N. 1983. Zinc and the special senses. *Ann Intern Med* 99:227–239.

Rutkoski NJ, Fitch CA, Yeiser EC, Dodge J, Trombley PQ, Levenson CW. 1999. Regulation of neuropeptide Y mRNA and peptide concentrations by copper in rat olfactory bulb. *Brain Res Mol Brain Res* 65:80–86.

Sharp P. 2004. The molecular basis of copper and iron interactions. *Proc Nutr Soc* 63:563–569.

Stewart AJ, Blindauer CA, Berezenko S, Sleep D, Sadler PJ. 2003. Interdomain zinc site on human albumin. *Proc Natl Acad Sci* 100:3701–3706.

Tannhauser PP. 2002. Anorexia nervosa: A multifactorial disease of nutritional origin? *Int J Adolesc Med Health* 14:185–191.

Willis MS, Monaghan SA, Miller ML, McKenna RW, Perkins WD, Levinson BS, Bhushan V, Kroft SH. 2005. Zinc-induced copper deficiency: a report of three cases initially recognized on bone marrow examination. *Am J Clin Pathol* 123:125–131.

Xu X, Pin S, Gathinji M, Fuchs R, Harris ZL. 2004. Aceruloplasminemia: an inherited neurodegenerative disease with impairment of iron homeostasis. *Ann N Y Acad Sci* 1012:299–305.

Zecca L, Youdim MB, Riederer P, Connor JR, Crichton RR. 2004. Iron, brain ageing and neurodegenerative disorders. *Nat Rev Neurosci* 5:863–873.

# Absorption Mechanisms, Bioavailability, and Metabolism of Calcium and Magnesium

*Connie M. Weaver*
*Purdue University, West Lafayette, Indiana*

## INTRODUCTION

The essentiality of calcium for many vital functions has led to important discoveries regarding its metabolism and bioavailability from food and supplement sources. Many of the changes in bone occur during early years and therefore much of the research to answer metabolism and requirement questions has been conducted in children and young adults. The onset of osteoporosis in the elderly and adverse consequences has also spurred research on preventative measures to minimize it. Among the U.S. population, calcium intake inadequacy is common, especially among women.

The role of magnesium in bone health is also well recognized and deficiencies have adverse consequences in bone formation (brittle bones), endocrine function, possibly also disrupting mood states and sleep regulation. However, magnesium deficiencies due to dietary inadequacy in the U.S. population are not common although they can occur as comorbidity to other conditions such as malabsorption or renal disfunction.

Soldiers face a variety of stressors that go from intense physical activity to the psychological stressors such as anxieties or sleep disturbances. Under military situations, whether training or in combat, these stress factors may influence the metabolism of calcium or magnesium or both, resulting in daily requirements that might be different than those for the general U.S. population. In addition, typical operational rations may be inadequate regarding the levels of these two minerals or they might be designed in a way that lowers their bioavailability. This paper describes factors that influence the metabolism and absorption of magnesium or calcium and potential risks of deficiency among military population in training or combat.

## FUNCTION AND CONSEQUENCES OF DEFICIENCY

Calcium and magnesium are the two most important minerals for bone development and maintenance that are at risk for being deficient in the diet. The proportion of the total body's calcium in bone is 99 percent for and 60 percent for magnesium. Calcium exists as hydroxyapatite in crystals and as amorphous calcium phosphate. Magnesium is important to bone quality by controlling crystal growth of hydroxyapatite to prevent formation of brittle bone. Accumulation of bone mass during growth and protection of loss later in life directly and linearly predicts risk of fracture (Heaney et al., 2000).

Aside from the structural functions of calcium and magnesium in bone, they are also important in sustaining other living tissues. Calcium serves as a second messenger and stabilizes key proteins. Magnesium is a co-factor for numerous enzymes and is especially associated with those involved in energy metabolism.

Calcium is under homeostatic regulation to maintain serum concentrations within a narrow range. Serum magnesium decreases during depletion, but not dependably. Thus, serum levels are not considered good indicators of status for either mineral. If serum levels are not maintained by adequate intakes from the diet, the skeleton serves as a large reserve. Chronic bone resorption due to inadequate intake of calcium is associated with decreased peak bone mass and increased skeletal fragility depending on the lifestage (Heaney et al., 2000; Heaney and Weaver, 2003).

## HOMEOSTATIC REGULATION

Maintenance of serum calcium at approximately 2.5 mmol/L occurs because of coordinated actions at the gut, kidney, and skeleton in response to the hormonal regulation through the PTH-vitamin D axis (Figure B-11) (Weaver and Heaney, 2006a). When serum calcium levels fall due to dietary deficiency, calcium absorption increases, tubular reabsorption increases, and bone resorption is elevated. Daily calcium transfer in average young adult women is illustrated in Figure B-12.

In contrast to calcium, there is no identified hormonal regulation of magnesium (Rude and Shils, 2006). Daily magnesium transfer is illustrated in Figure B-13 (Rude and Shils, 2006). The main site of magnesium regulation is the kidney. The kidney is very efficient at conserving magnesium during periods of low intake to maintain homeostasis. During periods of dietary deficiency, urinary excretion can decrease to 1 mEq/day. At the other extreme, almost all of an intravenously administered magnesium load is excreted in the urine within 24 hours.

## ABSORPTION MECHANISMS

For both calcium and magnesium, absorption occurs predominantly in the small intestine. For both ions, absorption occurs by both saturable transcellular absorption that is physiologically regulated and nonsaturable paracellular absorption that is dependent on concentrations in the lumen (Weaver and Heaney, 2006a). Absorption for both calcium and magnesium increases while fractional absorption decreases with increasing dose as shown for calcium in Figure B-14 for calcium (Fine et al., 1991; Heaney et al., 1990). The range in absorption efficiency is great for both minerals, i.e., 5 to 75 percent, but average magnesium absorption is higher than calcium.

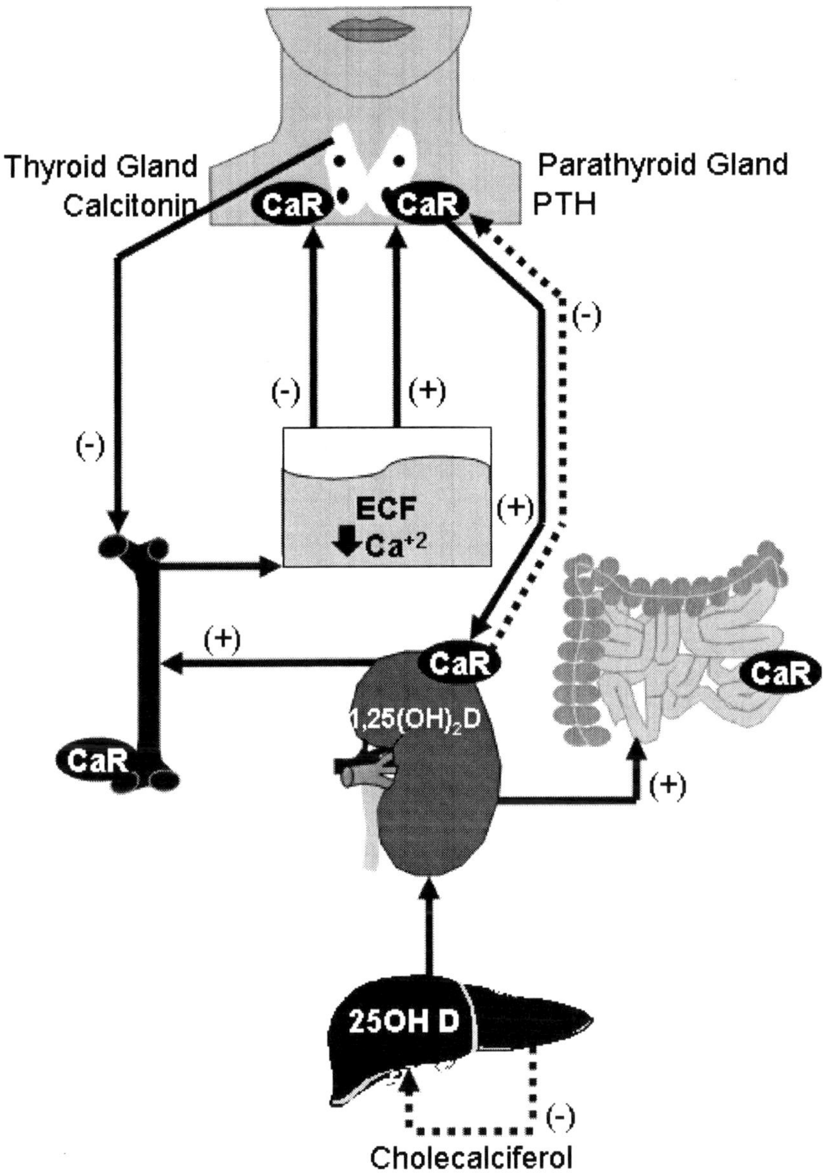


**FIGURE B-11** Homeostatic regulation of calcium. Copyright C.M. Weaver, 2005.

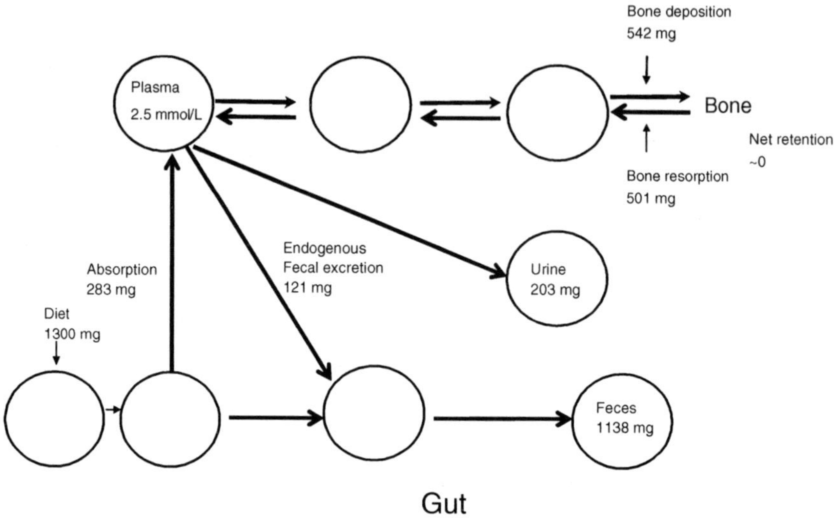


**FIGURE B-12** Daily mass calcium transfer in adult women total body 1–1.2 kg. Copyright C.M. Weaver, 2005.

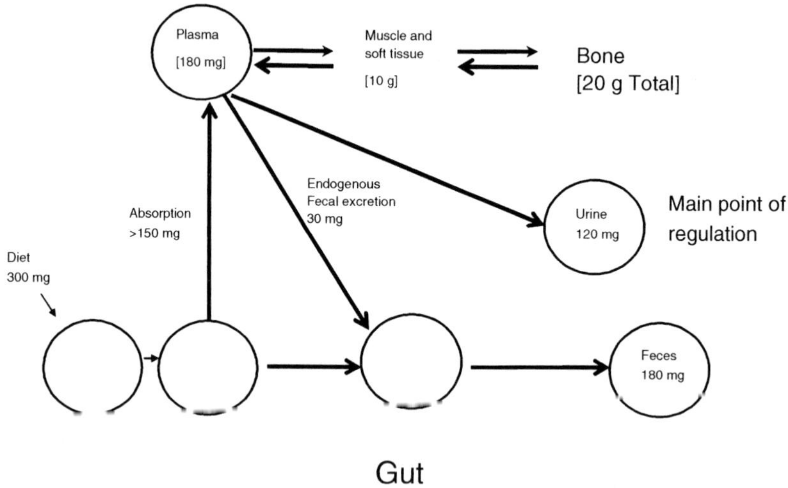


**FIGURE B-13** Daily mass magnesium transfer and [body pools] total body 28–40 g. Copyright C.M. Weaver, 2005.

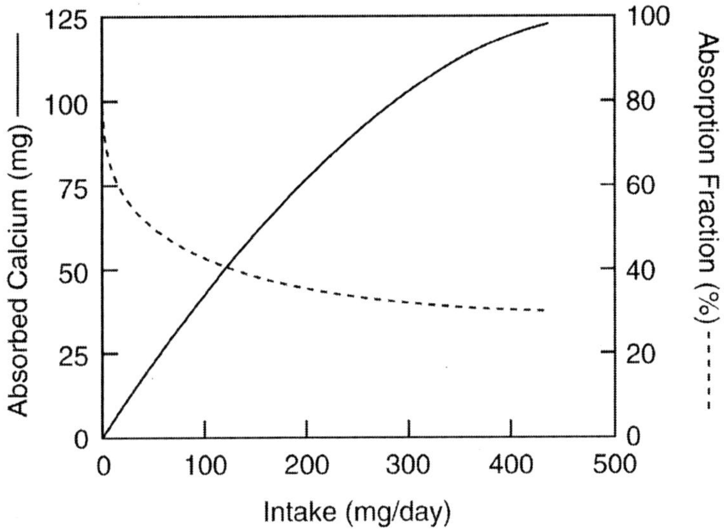


**FIGURE B-14** Effect of load on calcium absorption.
SOURCE: Weaver, 2001. Used with permission.

## BIOAVAILABILITY

Most of the major sources of calcium from foods and supplements and some fortified foods have been evaluated using sensitive isotopic tracer techniques and intrinsically labeled foods and salts. Because different applications of isotopic tracer techniques produce different absolute values for calcium absorption (Wastney et al., in press), it is important to use a common referent in bioavailability studies so that relative bioavailability among various sources can be established. For foods, the referent is typically milk, and for salts, it is calcium carbonate. A comparison of bioavailability from major sources of calcium is given in Table B-7. The most potent inhibitor of calcium absorption is oxalate. However, foods that contain oxalate vary in the degree of calcium bioavailability, from the low calcium bioavailability in spinach to soy foods with calcium bioavailability comparable to milk. Phytate is a modest inhibitor of calcium absorption. Enhancers of calcium absorption have received much study, but there is no known universally consistent enhancing ingredient. Some ingredients enhance calcium absorption in single studies, but the effect disappears during chronic feeding due to adaptation, i.e., lactulose and whey (Brommage et al., 1993; Zhao et al., in press). Vegetables from the Brassica family have superior bioavailability to most other sources, but the nature of this enhancement has been elusive.

**TABLE B-7** Comparing Sources for Absorbable Calcium

| Source | Serving Size (g) | Calcium Content (mg/serving) | Estimated Absorption Efficiency (%)[a] | Absorbable Ca/serving[b] (mg) | Servings Needed to Equal 1 Cup Milk |
|---|---|---|---|---|---|
| **Foods** | | | | | |
| Milk | 240 | 300 | 32.1 | 96.3 | 1.0 |
| Beans, pinto | 86 | 44.7 | 26.7 | 11.9 | 8.1 |
| Beans, red | 172 | 40.5 | 24.4 | 9.9 | 9.7 |
| Beans, white | 110 | 113 | 21.8 | 24.7 | 3.9 |
| Bok Choy | 85 | 79 | 53.8 | 42.5 | 2.3 |
| Broccoli | 71 | 35 | 61.3 | 21.5 | 4.5 |
| Cheddar Cheese | 42 | 303 | 32.1 | 97.2 | 1.0 |
| Cheese Food | 42 | 241 | 32.1 | 77.4 | 1.2 |
| Chinese Cabbage Flower Leaves | 85 | 239 | 39.6 | 94.7 | 1.0 |
| Chinese Mustard Green | 85 | 212 | 40.2 | 85.3 | 1.1 |
| Chinese Spinach | 85 | 347 | 8.36 | 29 | 3.3 |
| Kale | 85 | 61 | 49.3 | 30.1 | 3.2 |
| Spinach | 85 | 115 | 5.1 | 5.9 | 16.3 |
| Sugar Cookies | 15 | 3 | 91.9 | 2.76 | 34.9 |
| Sweet Potatoes | 164 | 44 | 22.2 | 9.8 | 9.8 |

| | | | | | |
|---|---|---|---|---|---|
| Rhubarb | 120 | 174 | 8.54 | 10.1 | 9.5 |
| Whole Wheat Bread | 28 | 20 | 82.0 | 16.6 | 5.8 |
| Wheat Bran Cereal | 28 | 20 | 38.0 | 7.54 | 12.8 |
| Yogurt | 240 | 300 | 32.1 | 96.3 | 1.0 |
| **Fortified Foods** | | | | | |
| Tofu, Calcium Set | 126 | 258 | 31.0 | 80.0 | 1.2 |
| Orange Juice with Calcium Citrate Malate | 240 | 300 | 36.3 | 109 | 0.88 |
| Soy Milk with Tricalcium Phosphate | 240 | 300 | 24 | 72 | 1.3 |
| Bread with Calcium Sulfate | 16.8 | 300 | 43.0 | 129 | 0.74 |
| **Calcium Salts** | | | | | |
| Calcium Carbonate | | 200 | 41.2 | 82.6 | |
| | | 300 | 34.2 | 102.6 | |
| Calcium Citrate | | 300 | 37.9 | 113.7 | |
| Calcium Citrate Malate | | 250 | 37.3 | 93.3 | |
| Calcium Glycerophosphate | | 300 | 27.1 | 81.3 | |

[a]Adjusted for load using the equation for milk (fractional absorption = 0.889–0.0964 in load) then adjusting for the ration of calcium absorption of the test food relative to milk tested at the same load, the absorptive index.

[b]Calculated as calcium content × fractional absorption.

SOURCE: Weaver and Heaney, in press.

In contrast to calcium, very little is known about magnesium bioavailability. One study measured magnesium absorption from vegetables intrinsically labeled with stable isotopes of magnesium and found true absorption ranged from 52 percent to 62 percent (Schwartz et al., 1984). Absorption was lower in bran-rich sources, presumably due to the inhibition in absorption by the phytate. Several magnesium salts have been evaluated for magnesium absorption using a urinary elimination approach. Magnesium oxide has much lower absorption than the citrate, lactate, or hydroxide salts (Bohmer et al., 1990; Lindberg et al., 1990). Bioavailability of the chloride, lactate, and aspartate salts was similar (Firoz and Graber, 2001). Enteric-coated magnesium chloride has a much lower absorption than magnesium acetate (Fine et al., 1991).

In general, ensuring that magnesium and calcium are sufficient in the diets is of larger concern than the issue of bioavailability because the impact is larger given that manipulations designed to alter bioavailability are usually modest. Both nutrients are consumed in amounts below the recommended intakes in adults (IOM, 1997); the intake inadequacies are more severe for the calcium intake of women (50th percentile of 19–30 year old is 612 mg/day versus an AI of 1,000 mg).

## DIETARY INTERACTIONS

A schematic of nutrients which affect calcium metabolism and the points of regulation is given in Figure B-15. The most important dietary interaction for calcium is with sodium. Dietary sodium increases urinary calcium loss because of the co-transport of calcium and sodium in the kidney. In adolescent girls, this effect was greater in whites than blacks (Wigertz et al., 2005). Dietary protein increases urinary calcium loss, but does not increase net calcium loss from the body and bone resorption is not increased (Kerstetter et al., 2005; Roughead et al., 2003). Dietary protein can increase bone mass which has been associated with increased serum IGF-1 levels (Dawson-Hughes, 2003). The loss in the urine with increased protein intake appears to be offset by increased calcium absorption (Kerstetter et al., 2005). A diet rich in fruits and vegetables is thought to reduce urinary calcium loss, presumably through effects on acid-base balance. This effect is thought to be at least partially related to potassium content. Because active calcium absorption is vitamin D dependent, vitamin D status influences calcium absorption. It also influences bone resorption (Weaver and Heaney, 2006b).

## INFLUENCE OF PHYSICAL ACTIVITY

There have been several studies on the interaction of calcium intake and physical activity on bone health. These are reviewed in the calcium section of Chapter 3 of

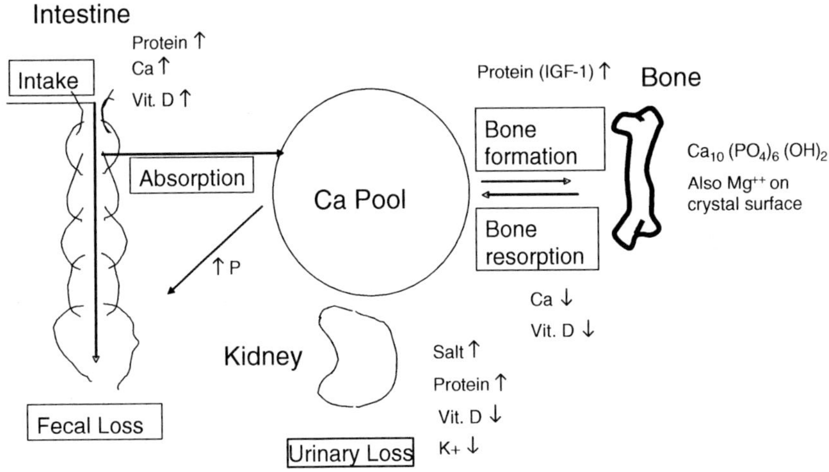


**FIGURE B-15** Summary of diet effects on calcium metabolism. Copyright C.M. Weaver, 2005.

this report. There have been few studies on the impact of physical activity on calcium and magnesium requirements or metabolism (Weaver, 2000). It is plausible that weight bearing exercise could counteract a marginally deficient diet in calcium for bone strength because it can increase bone geometry (Specker and Binkley, 2003). On the other hand, physical activity could increase mineral losses from the body which could increase their requirement. The most likely route of loss is dermal, especially during situations of high heat and humidity. Our understanding of dermal losses is covered in this report (See Haymes, 2005 in this Appendix).

## SUMMARY

Calcium and magnesium are two minerals frequently at risk for deficiency in the diet. These minerals are important for bone health as well as for many other functions. They may be at greater risk of loss during physical activity through sweat loss. The dietary component that most negatively affects calcium retention is sodium. This effect is greater in whites than blacks. Achieving adequate intakes are more important than concerns over bioavailability or dietary interactions because of the larger impact on nutrition for these two minerals.

## REFERENCES

Bohmer T, Roseth A, Holm H, Weberg-Teigen S, Wahl L. 1990. Bioavailability of oral magnesium supplementation in female students evaluated from elimination of magnesium in 24-hour urine. *Magnesium and Trace Elements* 9:272–278.

Brommage R, Binacua C, Antille S, Carrie AL. 1993. Intestinal calcium absorption in rats is stimulated by dietary lactulose and other resistant sugars. *J Nutr* 123:2186–2194.

Dawson-Hughes B. 2003. Interaction of dietary calcium and protein in bone health in humans. *J Nutr* 133:852S–854S.

Fine KD, Santa Ana CA, Porter JL, Fordtran JS. 1991. Intestinal absorption of magnesium from food and supplements. *J Clin Invest* 88:396–402.

Firoz M, Graber M. 2001. Bioavailability of U.S. commercial magnesium preparations. *Magnesium Research* 14:257–262.

Heaney RP, Weaver CM. 2003. Calcium and Vitamin D. In: Bilezikian JP, ed. *Endocrinology and Metabolism Clinic of North America: Osteoporosis* 32:181–194. Philadelphia, PA: Elsevier Science.

Heaney RP, Weaver CM, and Fitzimmsons ML. 1990. The influence of calcium load on absorption fraction. *Am J Clin Nutr* 5(11):1135–1138.

Heaney RP, Abrams S, Dawson-Hughes B, Looker A, Marcus R, Matkovic V, Weaver CM. 2000. Peak Bone Mass. *Osteoporosis Intl* 11:985–1009.

IOM (Institute of Medicine). 1997. Dietary Reference Intakes for Calcium, Phosphorus, Magnesium, Vitamin D, and Fluoride. Washington, DC: National Academy Press.

Kerstetter JE, O'Brien KO, Caseria DM, Wall DE, Insogna KL. 2004. The impact of dietary protein on calcium absorption and kinetic measures of bone turnover in women. *J Clin Endoc Metab* 90(1):26–31.

Lindberg JS, Zobitz MM, Poindexter JR, Pak CYC. 1990. Magnesium bioavailability from magnesium citrate and magnesium oxide. *J Amer Coll Nutr* 9:48–55.

Roughead K, Johnson LK, Lykken GI, Hunt JR. 2003. Controlled high meat diets do not affect calcium retention or indices of bone status in healthy postmenopausal women. *J Nutr* 133:1020–1026.

Rude RK. 2006. Magnesium. In: Shils ME, Shike M, Ross AC, Caballero B, Cousins RJ, eds. *Modern Nutrition in Health Disease*. 10th Ed. Lippincott Williams & Wilkins.

Rude R, Gruber H. 2004. Magnesium deficiency and osteoporosis: Animal and human observations. *J Nutr Biochem* 15:710–716.

Rude RKG, Wei LY, Frausto A, Mills BG. 2003. Magnesium deficiency: Effect on bone and mineral metabolism in the mouse. *Calcified Tissue Int* 72:32–41.

Schwartz R, Spencer H, Welsh JJ. 1984. Magnesium absorption in human subjects from leafy vegetables intrinsically labeled with stable $^{28}$Mg. *Amer J Clin Nutr* 39:571–576.

Specker B, Binkley T. 2003. Randomized trial of physical activity and calcium supplementation on bone mineral content in 3- to 5-year old children. *J Bone Miner Res* 18:885–892.

Wastney ME, Zhao Y, Weaver CM. 2006. Kinetic Studies. In: Weaver CM, Heaney RP, eds. *Calcium and Human Health*. Humana Press.

Weaver CM, Heaney RP. 2006a. Calcium. In: Shils ME, Shike M, Ross AC, Caballero B, Cousins RJ, eds. *Modern Nutrition in Health Disease*. 10th Ed. Lippincott Williams & Wilkins.

Weaver CM, Heaney RP. 2006b. Food Sources, Supplements, and Bioavailability. In: Weaver CM, Heaney RP, eds. *Calcium and Human Health*. Humana Press.

Wigertz K, Palacios C, Jackman LA, Martin BR, McCabe LD, McCabe GP, Peacock M, Pratt JH, Weaver CM. 2005. Racial differences in calcium retention in response to dietary salt in adolescent girls. *Am J Clin Nutr* 81:845–850.

Zhao Y, Martin BR, Wastney ME, Schollum L, Weaver CM. 2005. Acute versus chronic effects of whey proteins on calcium absorption in growing rats. *Exp Biol Med* 230(8):536–542.

# Drinking Water as a Source of Mineral Nutrition

*Gerald F. Combs, Jr.*
*USDA-ARS Grand Forks Human Nutrition Research Center,*
*Grand Forks, North Dakota*

## INTRODUCTION

This paper describes the content of minerals in drinkable water and explores the possibility that consumption of water during foreign deployments of the military personnel can substantially increase the daily intake of essential minerals. The diverse sources of water consumption might result in substantial variations on water mineral levels. Consumption of water could then be factored in when planning levels of these minerals in meals for individuals or populations. It is possible to use water as a vehicle to deliver minerals the intakes of which are otherwise inadequate. The applicability of this strategy to military populations is explored. Also, the relevance of obtaining water from various sources is addressed; the importance of this variability in the context of provision of a wide range of mineral levels is discussed.

## MINERALS IN NATURAL WATER SUPPLIES

The mineral contents of lakes and rivers vary with climate, local geology, the type and extent of local agriculture and extent of urbanization (Bowen, 1979) (Table B-8). In temperate areas, calcium is the dominant mineral element in fresh water, while rivers draining arid areas tend to be rich in sodium (Na) and chlorine (Cl), and tropical rivers, being more dilute in general, tend to contain greater concentrations of iron (Fe) and silicon (Si). Thus, fresh water supplies can provide nutritionally important amounts of calcium (Ca), magnesium (Mg), Fe, manganese (Mn). Industrialized countries have used municipal water as a vehicle for providing fluorine. In a few locales, surface run-off from selenium-rich soils has been found to contain biologically significant amounts of that element; but such cases are few and most water supplies are very low in selenium (Se). Few water supplies contain appreciable amounts of copper (Cu); however, the use of copper piping between municipal reservoirs and consumers' taps can increase the amounts of the element if the water is soft. For example, Angino (1979) found 16 percent of U.S. tap water samples to contain at least 0.2 mg Cu per L, and 6 percent to contain 0.5 mg Cu per L. Drinking water in Boston and Seattle has been estimated to provide 0.46 (Sparrow et al., 1982) and 1.3–2.2 mg Cu daily (Sharrett et al., 1982), respectively.

River waters typically contain fairly large amounts of organic matter that can act as ligands for such trace elements as Cu, Fe, Mn, molybdenum (Mo), nickel (Ni), and zinc (Zn). However, the hydrolysis and formation of chelates

**TABLE B-8** Nutritionally Essential Mineral Elements in Fresh- and Sea-Water

| Element | Freshwater Mean (range) [amount per L] | Freshwater Probable Species | Seawater Mean (range) [amount per L*] | Seawater Probable Species* |
|---|---|---|---|---|
| B | 15 (7–500) μg | $B(OH)_3$ | 4.44 mg | $B(OH)_3$ |
| Ca | 15 (2–120) mg | $Ca^{+2}$ | 412 mg | $Ca^{+2}$ |
| Cl | 7 (1–35) mg | $Cl^-$ | 19.35 g | $Cl^-$ |
| Cr | 1 (0.1–6) μg | $Cr(OH)_3$, $CrO_4^{-2}$ | 0.3 (0.2–50) μg | $Cr(OH)_3$, $CrO_4^{-2}$ |
| Cu | 3 (0.2–30) μg | $CuOH^+$, org. complexes | 0.25(0.05–12) μg | $CuOH^+$, $CuCO_3$ |
| F | 100 (50–2,700) μg | $F^-$ | 1.3 mg $L^{-1}$ | $F^-$, $MgF^+$ |
| Fe | 500 (10–1,400) μg | Colloidal | 2 (0.03–70) μg | Colloidal, $Fe(OH)_2^+$ |
| I | 2 (0.5–7) μg | $I^-$ | 60 (50–70) μg | $I^-$, $IO_3^-$, $CH_3I$ |
| K | 2.2 (0.5–10) mg | $K^+$ | 399 mg | $K^+$ |
| Mg | 4 (0.4–6) mg | $Mg^{+2}$ | 1.29 g | $Mg^{+2}$ |
| Mn | 8 (0.02–130) μg | $Mn^{+2}$ | 0.2 (0.03–21) μg | $Mn^{+2}$, $MnCl^+$, colloidal |
| Mo | 0.5 (0.03–10) μg | $MoO_4^{-2}$ | 10 (4–10) μg | $MoO_4^{-2}$ |
| Na | 6 (0.7–25) mg | $Na^+$ | 10.77 g | $Na^+$ |
| Ni | 0.5 (0.02–27) μg | $Ni^{+2}$ | 0.56(0.13–43) μg | $Ni^{+2}$, $NiCO_3$ |
| P | 20 (1–300) μg | $H_2PO_4^-$ | 60 (60–88) μg | $HPO_4^{-2}$, $MgPO_4^-$ |
| Se | 0.2 (0.2–1) μg | $SeO3^{-2}$ | 0.2 (0.052–0.2) μg | $SeO3^{-2}$, $SeO4^{-2}$ |
| Zn | 15 (0.2–100) μg | $Zn^{+2}$, org. complexes | 0.03 μg | $Zn^{+2}$, $ZnOH^+$ |

SOURCE: *Bowen (1979).

may be relatively slow processes, taking days to years to form turbid solutions; such reactions may not have come to equilibrium before river water enters the ocean so that many minerals enter ocean waters in forms that are poorly available for biological utilization.

The concentrations of the dominant minerals in seawater [Na, potassium (K), Mg, Ca] vary somewhat, but the mixing of the oceans results in each being in a fairly stable ratio with Cl (Bowen, 1979) (Table B-8). Concentrations of minor mineral constituents with relatively short residence times, however, can vary according to depth or location, or both. Some [Ca, phosphorus (P), Si] are markedly depleted in the upper layers due to removal by plankton or biological precipitation; others (Cu, Fe, Mn, Se, Zn) can be relatively high in surfaces waters fed by river inputs from mineralized areas or industrialized communities. Soluble forms of minerals can exist in cationic ($Ca^{+2}$, $Cu^{+2}$, $Fe^{+2}$, $Fe^{+3}$, $K^{+}$, $Mg^{++}$, $Mn^{++}$, $Na^{+}$, $Ni^{+}$, $Zn^{++}$) and anionic ($B_4O_7^{-2}$, $Cr_2O_7^{-2}$, $F^{-}$, $I^{-}$, $MoO_4^{-2}$, $PO_4^{-2}$, $SeO_3^{-2}$, $SeO_4^{-2}$) species; in ocean water they exist bound to various ligands (e.g., to hydroxyl or ketone ligands for B, Cr, Cu, Fe, I, Mo, P, Se, Si, Zn; to chlorine ligands for Mn; or to carbonate ligands for Cu, Ni, Zn). Insoluble forms of minerals precipitate as sediments; those near the mouths of rivers typically contain large amounts of Al and Fe as insoluble hydroxides. The main types of sediments in ocean waters include $CaCO_3$ from the re-dissolved skeletons of marine organisms, silica from the re-dissolved skeletons of diatoms and other organisms, and Fe-containing, aluminosilicate red clays derived from continental rocks. Colloidal hydroxides of Fe, Mn and Se are known to form at the pH of seawater. Such polymers can scavenge polyvalent elements. Because their formation is dependent on redox potential, the relatively low concentrations of dissolved $O_2$ at lower depths (< 1 mg $L^{-1}$) results in Fe and Mn being reduced to their soluble ions ($Fe^{+2}$, $Mn^{+2}$) that are absorbed on colloidal hydroxides.

## ENTERIC ABSORPTION OF MINERALS FROM WATER

The absorption and post-absorptive utilization of minerals depends on its chemical form as well as the presence or absence in the gut of factors of dietary origin that can affect those processes. For example, water-born Se (selenite, selenate) is passively absorbed at somewhat lower efficiencies (60–80 percent) than the selenoaminoacids in foods (90–95 percent) that are actively transported across the gut (Combs and Combs, 1986). The utilization of non-heme Fe can be markedly improved by including in the diet sources of ascorbic acid (e.g., oranges) or meats both of which promote the utilization of non-heme Fe (Gordon and Godber, 1989). In similar fashion, the presence of citrate or histidine in the gut can enhance the absorption of ingested Zn, and dietary ascorbate can enhance the antagonistic effect of Fe on Cu utilization (Salovaara et al., 2002; Swain et al., 2002).

There is no reason to think that minerals consumed in drinking water are not subject to the same determinants of bioavailability that affect their utilization from in foods. However, for the most part the bioavailability of minerals from water has not been broadly studied. Some of the determinants known to affect bioavailability of minerals from foods are constituents of the foods consumed: phytate, phosphorus and triglycerides can each reduce the lumenal solubility and, hence, the absorption of Ca; calcium absorption is also decreased by increasing levels of oxalic acic (see also Weaver 2005 in this Appendix). Phytate and other non-fermentable fiber components can and reduce the absorption of Zn, Mg, Fe and P. Other determinants relate to either foods or water: sulfides can react with Cu to form insoluble CuS; minerals that share transporters can be mutually inhibitory for absorption, eg., sulfite and selenite, Cd and Zn, Zn and Cu, Ca and Fe; the bioavailability of the divalent cations ($Ca^{++}$, $Fe^{++}$, $Cu^{++}$, $Zn^{++}$) can be enhanced by certain chelating substances (e.g., unidentified factors in meats, ascorbic acid in fruits) and pro-biotic factors (e.g., inulin and other fructo-oligosaccharides) (see Boeckner et al., 2001; Pallauf and Rimbach, 1997).

For these reasons, the utilization of minerals from drinking water may depend as much on the contents of inhibitor and promoter substances also present in the gut as it does on the chemical form(s) of minerals consumed in the water. In general, the bioavailability of water-borne Fe may be improved by minimizing foods containing phytates and polyphenols and by including meats and sources of ascorbic acid. Similarly, the utilization of water-born Ca should be optimized by minimizing oxalate-containing vegetables (e.g., spinach, rhubarb, beet greens, chard); and the utilization of water-born Ca, Fe, Mg, P, or Zn may be enhanced using diets low in unrefined (> 90 percent extraction), unfermented cereal grains and high-phytate products (see also Hunt 2005 in this Appendix).

## MINERALS IN PROCESSED WATER

The processing of water, by distillation or reverse osmosis, is widely practiced, including for U.S. military needs, and is rapidly growing as the principle source of new fresh water worldwide. In addition to procuring water for human consumption according to the EPA standards, these methods yield water of high purity and, thus, very low mineral content. Such water is highly corrosive which may result in minerals leaching in water such as zinc and iron but depending on the nature of the pipe. To minimize concerns about human toxicity with the potential leaching of heavy metals water processors typically add back selected mineral salts in a step referred to as "stabilization." As a whole, this purification/reconstitution process can result in mineral contents differing widely between the water product and the original source. Few commercially bottled waters not labeled as "mineral water" on the American market contain appreciable amounts of minerals.

In 2003, the World Health Organization (WHO) convened an expert panel to review the evidence of health effects associated with drinking and cooking water mineral content (WHO, 2004). The panel reviewed more than 80 observational studies conducted in 1957–2003; most, but not all, showed inverse relationships of the hardness of water supplies and the risk of cardiovascular disease (particularly, ischemic heart disease) (Calderon and Craun, in press; Craun and Calderon, in press; Monarca et al., 2003; Monarca et al., in press; Nardi et al., 2003). While the panel was unable to determine whether that relationship involved Ca, Mg or the combination of those elements, the primary contributors to hardness, it pointed out that low Mg intakes have been shown to increase supraventricular beats in humans (Klevay and Milne, 2003). The panel also cited evidence that the consumption of water with high levels of Ca does not increase, but may reduce the risk of calcium oxalate urinary stones (Donato et al., 2003), unless calcium supplements were taken separate from consumption of dietary oxalate from food (Curhan et al., 1993, 1997, 2004). There are no data, however, to suggest that water-borne minerals are utilized any differently from the same minerals in foods.

Available data for Ca and Mg indicate that these minerals are, in fact, widely under-consumed. The Institute of Medicine (1997) estimated that the median daily intakes of 19–30 year old Americans were: 61 percent (females) and 95 percent (males) of Adequate Intake (AI) levels for Ca, and 66 percent (females) and 82 percent (males) of Recommended Dietary Allowance (RDA) levels for Mg.

Data on intake of minerals by military personnel is scant. The few studies that have collected such data reported that magnesium intakes from foods may be insufficient for much of the population and also that women, in general, may be at a higher risk of mineral deficiencies because they tend to consume less food. Therefore, water-borne minerals can contribute to the mineral nutrition of such individuals, particularly under conditions requiring high fluid intakes.

## WATER CONSUMPTION

Water, the largest single constituent of the body, is tightly regulated and must be maintained within 1–2 percent balance to sustain thermoregulation and physical work capacity (IOM, 2004). This is accomplished by consuming water in proportion to body water losses. Because water losses are subject to environmental factors, water requirements can vary widely (Grandjean et al., 2003; IOM, 2004). Water is lost from the body through urine (typically, 1–2 L/day), feces (approximately 100 ml/day), insensible respiratory, trans-epidermal and evaporative losses (cumulatively, approximately 450 ml/day), and sweat. Sweat losses vary considerably (1–8 + L/day) according to environmental temperature and humidity, and to endogenous heat production during physical activity; under extreme conditions, individuals can produce as much as 3–4 L/hour. In 2003, the IOM set Adequate Intake (AI) for water (2.7 L/day for females, 19–30 years, and 3.7 L/day for males, 19–30 years, assuming that approximately 20 percent would come from foods) (IOM, 2004). Water from food can vary from 0.5–1 L/day; the

**TABLE B-9** Potential Nutritional Contributions of Minerals Occurring in Freshwater Supplies

| Element | Daily Need (19–30 y male) | Reported Water Mineral (/L), Mean (range)[a] | % Daily Need (range) Met, by Rate of Water Consumption | |
|---|---|---|---|---|
| | | | 2 L/day | 4 L/day |
| Ca | 1,000 mg[b] | 15 (2–120) mg | 3 (0.4–24) | 6 (1–48) |
| Cl | 2,300 mg[b] | 7 (1–35) mg | 1 (0.1–3) | 1 (0.2–6) |
| Cr | 35 μg[b] | 1 (0.1–6) μg | 6 (1–34) | 12 (2–64) |
| Cu | 9 mg[c] | 3 (0.2–30) μg | 1 (0.02–7) | 1 (0.1–13) |
| F | 4 mg[b] | 100 (50–2,700) μg | 5 (3–135) | 10 (6–270) |
| Fe | 8 mg[c] | 500 (10–1,400) μg | 13 (0.3–35) | 25 (1–70) |
| I | 150 μg[c] | 2 (0.5–7) μg | 3 (1–9) | 5 (3–19) |
| K | 4,700 mg[b] | 2.2 (0.5–10) mg | 0.1 (0.02–0.4) | 0.2 (0.04–1) |
| Mg | 400 mg[b] | 4 (0.4–6) mg | 2 (0.2–3) | 4 (0.4–6) |
| Mn | 2.3 mg[b] | 8 (0.02–130) μg | 1 (<0.01–11) | 1 (<0.01–23) |
| Mo | 45 mg[c] | 0.5 (0.03–10) μg | <0.01 (<0.01–0.04) | <0.01 (<0.01–0.1) |
| Na | 1,500 mg[b] | 6 (0.7–25) mg | 1 (0.1–3) | 2 (0.2–7) |
| P | 700 mg[c] | 20 (1–300) μg | 6 (0.3–86) | 11 (0.6–171) |
| Se | 55 μg[c] | 0.2 (0.2–1) μg | 1 (1–4) | 1 (1–7) |
| Zn | 11 mg[c] | 15 (0.2–100) μg | 0.3 (<0.01–2) | 1 (<0.01–4) |

SOURCE: [a]Bowen (1979); [b]Adequate Intake from IOM (1997, 2001, 2004); [c]Recommended Dietary Allowance from IOM (1997, 2000, 2001).

balance of daily water need must be met by consuming fluids. Thus, under practical circumstances, total fluid requirements can range from 2–16 L/day (IOM, 2004; Sawka and Montain, 2003) (Figure B-16). Reports from the military point to water consumption of about 3 L/day when soldiers are under garrison training (J. Kent and S. Corum, personal communication, U.S. Army, August 24, 2005) or 4–5 L/day when they are in sustained operations (IOM, 2005).

| 6 L/day | 8 L/day | 10 L/day | 12 L/day | 14 L/day | 16 L/day |
|---|---|---|---|---|---|
| 9 | 12 | 15 | 18 | 19 | 21 |
| (1–72) | (2–96) | (2–120) | (2–140) | (3–168) | (4–190) |
| 2 | 3 | 4 | 5 | 5 | 6 |
| (0.2–10) | (0.3–13) | (0.5–19) | (1–22) | (1–25) | (1–26) |
| 18 | 24 | 30 | 36 | 42 | 24 |
| (3–98) | (4–128) | (5–162) | (6–192) | (7–226) | (8–256) |
| 2 | 3 | 3 | 4 | 5 | 6 |
| (0.1–20) | (0.2–27) | (0.2–33) | (0.2–40) | (0.3–47) | (0.4–54) |
| 15 | 20 | 25 | 30 | 35 | 40 |
| (8–400) | (12–540) | (15–670) | (16–800) | (20–940) | (24–1,040) |
| 38 | 50 | 63 | 76 | 88 | 100 |
| (1–105) | (1–140) | (2–175) | (2–210) | (2–245) | (2–280) |
| 8 | 10 | 13 | 16 | 18 | 10 |
| (4–28) | (6–38) | (7–47) | (8–56) | (10–66) | (12–76) |
| 0.3 | 0.4 | 1 | 1 | 1 | 1 |
| (0.1–1) | (0.1–2) | (0.1–2) | (0.2–2) | (0.2–3) | (0.2–4) |
| 6 | 8 | 10 | 12 | 14 | 16 |
| (1–9) | (1–12) | (1–15) | (2–18) | (2–21) | (2–24) |
| 2 | 2 | 3 | 4 | 4 | 4 |
| (<0.01–34) | (<0.01–46) | (<0.01–57) | (<0.01–68) | (0.01–80) | (0.01–96) |
| 0.01 | 0.01 | 0.01 | 0.02 | 0.02 | 0.02 |
| (0.01–0.1) | (0.01–0.2) | (0.01–0.2) | (0.02–0.2) | (0.02–0.3) | (0.02–0.4) |
| 2 | 3 | 4 | 4 | 6 | 6 |
| (0.3–10) | (0.4–13) | (0.5–17) | (0.6–20) | (0.7–23) | (1–26) |
| 17 | 22 | 23 | 34 | 34 | 44 |
| (1–257) | (1–342) | (2–428) | (2–514) | (3–600) | (2–684) |
| 2 | 3 | 3 | 4 | 5 | 6 |
| (2–11) | (2–14) | (3–18) | (4–22) | (4–25) | (4–28) |
| 1 | 1 | 1 | 2 | 2 | 2 |
| (<0.01–5) | (<0.01–7) | (<0.01–9) | (0.02–10) | (0.03–13) | (0.03–14) |

## IMPLICATIONS OF USING PROCESSED DRINKING WATER

The mineral nutritional value of drinking water depends on both its mineral content and level of consumption. The use of "hard" waters can provide significant amounts of Ca, Mg, Mn, and Fe, although the latter is likely to be present in colloidal forms of limited direct nutritional value. Under circumstances of high water consumption (e.g., > 6 L/day), many natural waters can also be significant sources of Cr, F, Fe, I, and P; in fact, some water sources can provide RDA

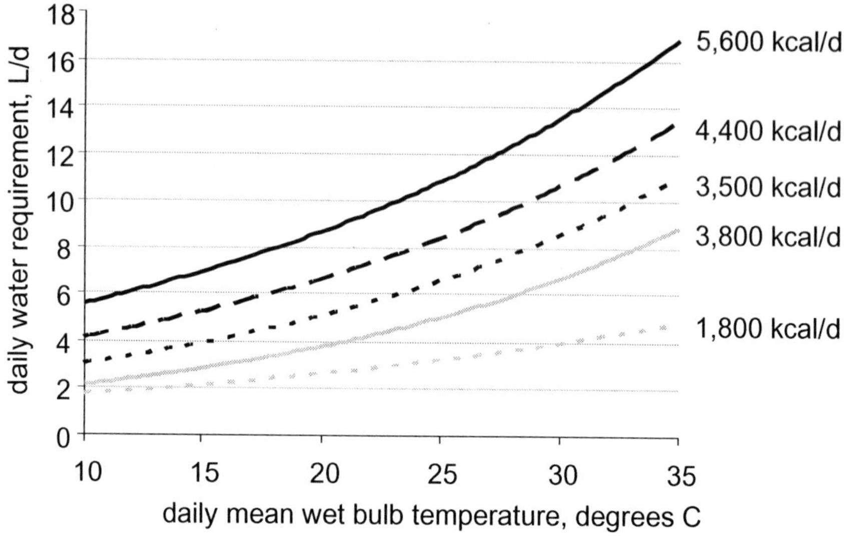


**FIGURE B-16** Daily water requirement as a function of environmental temperature and total energy expenditure.
SOURCE: Sawka and Montain (2001). Used with permission from the International Life Sciences Institute.

levels of those minerals (Table B-9). However, most processed waters are very poor sources of minerals unless they have been re-mineralized during "stabilization." In many cases, processed drinking water, including commercially bottled water may provide little, if any, essential nutrients. Variability of mineral levels among waters for consumption in military settings does not appear to be a factor to be considered when estimating amounts of minerals needed in operational rations or menus.

Drinking water represents, however, a potential vehicle for delivering essential minerals to troops many of whom will have high fluid intakes during hot weather duty. This presents opportunities for the military to develop mineral content standards for drinking water produced or purchased for troop consumption. Such standards could be useful in ensuring adequate intakes of key minerals not easily achieved by dietary means.

## REFERENCES


Angino, EE. 1979. Geochemistry of drinking water as affected by distribution and treatment. In: Angino EE, Sandstead HH, Comstock GW, Corbett RG, Strong JP, Voors AW, eds. *Geochemistry of Water in Relation to Cardiovascular Disease*. Washington, DC: National Academy Press.

Boeckner LS, Schnepf MI, Tungland BC. 2001. Inulin: A review of nutritional and health implications. *Adv Food Nutr Res* 43:1–63.

Bowen HJM. 1979. *Environmental Chemistry of the Elements.* New York: Academic Press. Pp. 13–29.

Calderon R, Craun GF. The association of cardiovascular disease risks with water hardness: A review of the epidemiological studies published from 1957–1979. In: Cotruvo J, Fawell J, eds. *Nutrients in Drinking Water and the Potential Health Consequences of Long-Term Consumption of Demineralized and Remineralized and Altered Mineral Content Drinking Waters* Washington, DC: ILSI Press; In press.

Combs Jr, GF, Combs SB. 1986. *The Role of Selenium in Nutrition and Health.* Academic Press, New York, Pp. 179–182.

Craun G, Calderon R. The association of cardiovascular disease risks with water hardness: Interpreting the epidemiological evidence. In: Cotruvo J, Fawell J, eds. *Nutrients in Drinking Water and the Potential Health Consequences of Long-Term Consumption of Demineralized and Remineralized and Altered Mineral Content Drinking Waters* Washington, DC: ILSI Press; In press.

Curhan GC, Willett WC, Rimm EB, Stampfer MJ. 1993. A prospective study of dietary calcium and other nutrients and the risk of symptomatic kidney stones. *N Engl J Med* 328(12):833–838.

Curhan GC, Willett WC, Speizer FE, Spiegelman D, Stampfer MJ. 1997. Comparison of dietary calcium with supplemental calcium and other nutrients as factors affecting the risk for kidney stones in women. *Ann Intern Med* 126(7):497–504.

Curhan GC, Willett WC, Knight EL, Stampfer MJ. 2004. Dietary factors and the risk of incident kidney stones in younger women: Nurses' Health Study II. *Arch Intern Med* 164(8):885–891.

Donato F, Monarca S, Premi S, Gelatti U. 2003. Durezza dell'acqua potablie e mallatie cronico-degenerative. Parte III. Patologie tumorali, urolitiasi, malformazioni fetali, deterioramento delle funzioni cognitive nell'anziano, diabete mellito ed eczema atopico. *Ann Ig* 15:57–70.

Gordon DT, Godber JS. 1989. The enhancement of nonheme iron bioavailability by beef protein in the rat. *J Nutr* 119:446-452.

Grandjean AC, Reimers KJ, Buyckx ME. 2003. Hydration: Issues for the 21st century. *Nutr Rev* 61:261–271.

IOM (Institute of Medicine). 1997. *Dietary Reference Intakes for Calcium, Phosphorus, Magnesium, Vitamin D and Fluoride.* Washington, DC: National Academy Press.

IOM. 2000. *Dietary Reference Intakes for Vitamin C, Vitamin E, Selenium and Carotenoids.* Washington, DC: National Academy Press.

IOM. 2001. *Dietary Reference Intakes for Vitamin A, Vitamin K, Arsenic, Boron, Chromium, Copper, Iodine, Iron, Manganese, Molybdenum, Nickel, Silicon, Vanadium and Zinc.* Washington, DC: National Academy Press.

IOM. 2004. *Dietary Reference Intakes for Water, Potassium, Sodium, Chloride and Sulfate.* Washington, DC: The National Academies Press.

Klevay LM, Milne DB. 2003. Low dietary magnesium increases supraventricular ectopy. *Am J Clin Nutr* 57:550–554.

Monarca S, Donato F, Zerbini I. In press. *Drinking water hardness and cardiovascular diseases.* In: Cotruvo J, Fawell J, eds. *Nutrients in Drinking Water and the Potential Health Consequences of Long-Term Consumption of Demineralized and Remineralized and Altered Mineral Content Drinking Waters* Washington, DC: ILSI Press.

Monarca S, Zerbini I, Simonati C, Gelatti U. 2003. Durezza dell'acqua potablie e mallatie cronico-degenerative. Parte II. Malattie cardiovasculari. *Ann Ig* 15:41–56.

Nardi G, Donato F, Monarca S, Gelatti U. 2003. Durezza dell'acqua potablie e mallatie cronico-degenerative. Parte I. Analisi dell recherché epidemiologiche. *Ann Ig* 15:35–40.

Pallauf J, Rimbach G. 1997. Nutritional significance of phytic acid and phytase. *Arch Tierernahr* 50:301–319.

Salovaara S, Sandberg AS, Andlid T. 2002. Organic acids influence iron uptake in the human epithelial cell line Caco-2. *J Agric Food Chem* 50:6233–6238.

Sawka MN, Montain SJ. 2001. Fluid and electrolyte balance: Effects on thermoregulation and exercise in the heat. In: Bowman BA, Russell RM, eds. *Present Knowledge in Nutrition*. 8th edition. Washington, DC: ILSI Press.

Sharrett AR, Carter AP, Orheim RM, Feinleib M. 1982. Daily intake of lead, cadmium, copper, and zinc from drinking water: The Seattle Study of Trace Metal Exposure. *Environ Res* 28: 456–475.

Sparrow D, Silbert JE, Weiss ST. 1982. The relationship of pulmonary function to copper concentrations in drinking water. *Am Rev Respir Dis* 126:312–315.

Swain JH, Tabatabai LB, Reddy MB. 2002. Histidine content of low-molecular-weight beef proteins influences nonheme iron bioavailability in Caco-2 cells. *J Nutr* 132:245–251.

WHO (World Health Organization). 2004. *Nutrient Minerals in Drinking-Water and the Potential Health Consequences of Consumption of Demineralized and Remineralized and Altered Mineral Content Drinking-Water: Consensus of the Meeting*. [Online]. Available: http://www.who.int/water_sanitation_health/dwq/nutconsensus/en/print.html [accessed January 31, 2006].

# Assessment of Zinc, Copper, and Magnesium Status: Current Approaches and Promising New Directions

*Carl L. Keen and Janet Y. Uriu-Adams*
*University of California-Davis*

## INTRODUCTION

It is intuitively well understood that optimal nutritional status can favorably impact health and performance. However, the extent to which marginal deficiencies of essential micro- and macro-nutrients might affect the performance of typically healthy individuals, including military personnel who are presumably consuming well-balanced diets is less appreciated. Even in well developed countries, marginal deficiencies of several essential nutrients including zinc, copper, and magnesium are common. The frequency of these deficiencies can increase under stressful conditions. For example, military personnel undergoing energy restriction, sleep deprivation, and physical, environmental, and psychological stress during combat are at risk for suboptimal nutrition due to reduced nutrient intake, as well as stress-induced alterations in mineral metabolism and homeostasis. Deficiencies of these minerals can impair daily activities and functions, reduce the rate of wound healing and recovery from injuries, and increase the risk for infections due to a compromised immune function. Given the above, the assessment of an individual's nutritional status is clearly a high priority within the military. However, these assessments are often challenging as many methods currently in use lack both precision and accuracy. This paper will address the current biomarkers used to assess zinc, copper, and magnesium status, as well as the limitations of these assessments. The potential for using novel metabolic profiles such as metabolomics, metallomics or breathomics as new and promising methods for nutrient status assessment will also be discussed.

## CAUSES OF MINERAL DEFICIENCIES

Mineral deficiencies can arise through multiple mechanisms (Keen et al., 2003a). Primary deficiencies are those that occur as a result of low dietary intakes of the micronutrient. Recent reports of mineral intakes show that zinc, copper and magnesium are low in select populations even in developed countries (Briefel et al., 2000; Champagne et al., 2004; Ford and Mokdad, 2003; Olivares et al., 2004; Tarasuk et al., 2005). However, a simple inspection of an individual's dietary intake provides limited information regarding their nutritional status as multiple factors (genetic, disease, drugs, physiological, and environmental stressors) can cause secondary, or 'conditioned' mineral deficiencies. Genetic factors including mutant genes, polymorphisms, and multiple gene defects can result in abnormal zinc and copper metabolism. For example, acrodermatitis enteropathica (characterized by zinc deficiency), is caused by mutations in the ZIP4 zinc transporter (Wang et al., 2002). Menke's disease (copper deficiency) and Wilson's disease (copper toxicity) are due to mutations in the copper-transporting ATPases, ATP7A and ATP7B, respectively (Harris, 2000). Interactions between minerals and food components including phytates, fiber, vitamins, and other minerals can reduce mineral absorption and result in a mineral deficiency in an individual despite their having a seemingly "adequate" level of intake of the mineral. A substantial body of literature has documented that drugs and certain chemicals or toxicants can produce a secondary mineral deficiency by chelating metals and decreasing their absorption, increasing their excretion, or both. Disease-associated changes in micronutrient metabolism have been noted in diabetes. This is of particular concern given the increase in the frequency of diabetes that is being seen in numerous populations. Similarly, physiological stress, infection, or conditions of inflammation such as cardiovascular disease and obesity, can produce an acute phase response, and a subsequent re-distribution of minerals in body tissues. Lastly, excessive loss of micronutrients from sweat has been noted, a concern for individuals undergoing physical exertion, particularly under harsh environmental conditions. Urinary and fecal mineral losses during intense exercise can also be larger than during resting periods.

### Nutritional Biomarkers

There is an essential need for an accurate evaluation of an individual's mineral status. Ideally, the biomarker(s) used would be highly sensitive, and highly specific. These markers would be substances that reflect the activity of an enzyme or process that is directly or indirectly impacted by a deficiency of the specific nutrient. That is, during a nutrient deficiency, the product, or precursor, of an enzymatic reaction or process is increased, or decreased, in the blood, urine, or breath. Moreover, significant changes in the concentration of the biomarker should occur prior to extensive tissue damage.

There are several issues that must be considered before choosing a nutritional biomarker (Box B-2). Some center around methodology such as whether the method is reliable and reproducible, whether the assay is robust enough to detect small changes over background, the length of time it takes to perform the assay (i.e., minutes, hours, or days), the risks for false positives or negatives, whether the assay can be performed in the field versus in a hospital or laboratory, and issues regarding the stability of the biomarker prior to analysis (e.g., transport and storage issues). Other key concerns relate to the interpretation of the results. For any biomarker that is used for nutritional status assessment, it is important to establish reference ranges for various populations, as well as the within-person and between-person variance. In cases where the individual vari-

**BOX B-2**
**Questions in Choosing a Nutritional Biomarker**

Is the method reliable and reproducible?

Do appropriate reference ranges exist for the population being studied?

Is the assay robust enough (signal to noise) to be of practical value?

Can the assay be done within a short time period?

Is the within-person and between-person variance known?

If the variance between individuals is larger than the within-person variance, do we need to maintain longitudinal records for each individual?

Is there a high risk for false positives, or false negatives?

Are there issues of timing relative to dietary exposure: recent versus usual intakes, acute versus chronic exposure?

Is the type of measurement a direct measure (static indicator) or functional assay?

Does the subject need to fast prior to the collection of a sample?

What is the stability of the marker? (Can the sample be easily transported?)

Does an acute change in the "marker" reflect an immediate risk, or the potential for risk?

ance is larger than the within-person variance, it might be necessary to establish longitudinal records for each individual. It would be important to determine whether fasting prior to the collection of a sample affects the biomarker, as well as whether the biomarker value can accurately distinguish between recent intake versus usual intakes, and between acute versus chronic exposure. Moreover, the questions of whether an acute change in the biomarker reflects an immediate risk, or the potential for risk, should be determined.

## Zinc

Over 200 diverse metalloproteins that are involved in carbohydrate, protein, lipid, and nucleic acid metabolism require zinc as a cofactor. Zinc can act at the catalytic site as well as having stabilizing or regulatory effects. Currently, zinc status is typically assessed by measuring the zinc concentration in easily accessible pools such as plasma, serum, or hair, or blood cells such as erythrocytes or lymphocytes (Hambidge, 2003; IOM, 2002b). The activity of zinc-dependent enzymes such as angiotensin converting enzyme (ACE) or extracellular superoxide dismutase (SOD) has also been used. Zinc-regulated genes such as metallothionein have been proposed to be useful as indices of zinc status (Cao and Cousins, 2000; Liuzzi and Cousins, 2004). The measurement of certain hormones and growth factors such as growth hormone and insulin-like growth factor (IGF) have also been proposed to be sensitive to zinc status, however, these markers show less sensitivity. The majority of the above markers are to a large extent reflective of the zinc status of the blood pool. In this regard it is important to note that approximately 91 percent of body zinc in a normal adult is found in muscle, bone, and liver while blood represents less than 0.1 percent of total body zinc (King and Keen, 1994). Moreover, of the 0.1 percent of zinc that is in blood, only 12–22 percent of that is present in plasma. Thus, plasma represents a very small fraction of total body zinc. Numerous factors can decrease plasma or serum zinc concentrations including pregnancy, oral contraceptive use, and infection or stress which precipitate an acute phase response, while other factors can increase plasma and serum zinc concentrations including fasting, or muscle injury where tissue breakdown occurs. Additionally, circadian rhythms can affect plasma and serum zinc concentrations and, thus, the time of day the sample is taken must be taken into account when evaluating the results. Given the above, it has been suggested that a suite of markers, as opposed to single markers, be used to more accurately ascertain zinc status. It is well known that zinc deficiency can result in hypogeusia (taste impairment). A report by Takeda et al. (2004) found that in patients with zinc deficiency-related hypogeusia, serum zinc was within the normal range, however, the ratio of ACE activity (apo-ACE/holo-ACE) was a more sensitive indicator of zinc status than serum zinc. The discovery of the ZnT (SLC30/CDF) and ZIP (Zrt/IRT-like proteins) families of zinc transporters involved in the regulation, export, and import of zinc in a variety of tissues has prompted the question of whether the protein or mRNA of these proteins could be used as biomarkers for zinc status. Using quantitative real-time RT-PCR, it has been shown that modest dietary zinc supplementation in humans (15 mg Zn/day for 10 days) increased metallothionein and ZnT1 mRNA, and decreased Zip3 mRNA in dried spots of whole blood indicating that these targets were responsive to zinc supplementation (Aydemir et al., 2006). In addition, since zinc deficiency increases oxidative stress, it has been suggested that perhaps a signature of oxidative stress markers might be used to assess zinc status (see below).

## Copper

Copper is an essential mineral that is involved in numerous electron transfer reactions due to the metal's redox cycling capability. Copper deficiency can adversely affect energy production, glucose and cholesterol metabolism, iron metabolism, hematopoietic and immune systems, oxidative defense system, neuropeptide synthesis and processing, and heart and vessel integrity and function (Keen et al., 2003b; Uriu-Adams and Keen, 2005). While severe copper deficiency is uncommon, marginal copper deficiency may be prevalent even in developed countries (IOM, 2002a; Uriu-Adams and Keen, 2005). Exercise, infection, inflammation, diabetes and hypertension, and the consumption of zinc supplements can adversely affect copper metabolism (IOM, 2002a; Uriu-Adams and Keen, 2005) and precipitate a sub-clinical copper deficiency.

Currently, copper status is commonly assessed by analyzing the concentration of copper in plasma, serum, or blood cells such as platelets and leukocytes (IOM, 2002a). The concentration or activity of the copper-binding protein, ceruloplasmin (Cp) in plasma, or the oxidant defense enzyme, superoxide dismutase (SOD) in erythrocytes is commonly assessed. However, given that Cp is an acute phase protein that is induced by physiological stressors such as inflammation, infection and disease, the risk for a false negative is high with respect to the identification of a "conditioned" copper deficiency. Similarly, an inflammatory response can make the interpretation of oxidative defense markers problematic. Thus, as with zinc, it has been suggested that more than one copper status index should be used to assess status. The activity of numerous copper-dependent enzymes such as cytochrome-c oxidase, lysyl oxidase, diamine oxidase, and peptidylglycine a-amidating monoxygenase in blood or cells to assess copper status has been reported (Hambidge, 2003). Indices of immune status (number or bactericidal activity of neutrophils) have also been used. A recent report shows that the protein expression of CCS (copper chaperone for Cu/Zn superoxide dismutase) in erythrocytes and liver was increased in rats made mildly copper deficient by feeding diets that were moderately high in zinc (Iskandar et al., 2005). It will be important to test whether CCS protein expression can be used as a sensitive biomarker to assess copper status in humans. As copper deficiency increases oxidative stress, identification of a signature oxidative stress marker for copper deficiency could be helpful (see below).

## Magnesium

Magnesium, an abundant intracellular divalent cation, is involved in numerous metabolic processes and is a cofactor for over 300 enzymes. The biochemical abnormalities of magnesium deficiency include hypokalemia and hypocalcemia which can lead to clinical manifestations of muscle cramps, tetany, and tremors, arrhythmias, cardiomyopathy, convulsion, and death. A number of studies suggest that magnesium intake is inadequate which could lead to compromised magnesium status (IOM, 1997). About 75 percent of magnesium intake is obtained from milk, meat, eggs, vegetables, fruits, grains, and nuts. However, over the past decade, magnesium intake has decreased due in part to increased consumption of refined and processed foods, which generally have low magnesium content. In addition, food components such as phytates, phosphorus, calcium, protein, and fat can affect magnesium absorption. While severe magnesium deficiency is not thought to be a common occurrence in humans, low concentrations of plasma magnesium are commonly reported. For example, low magnesium is observed in people with diabetes or asthma, in alcoholics, in patients with cancer, malabsorption syndromes or renal disease, in burn patients and the elderly, as well as in individuals who exercise (Britton et al., 1994; IOM, 1997).

Currently, a number of measures are commonly used to assess magnesium nutriture including magnesium concentrations in plasma or serum, or erythrocytes or lymphocytes (IOM, 1997) although there is considerable debate about whether blood magnesium levels reflect overall magnesium status. Ionized magnesium in plasma or erythrocytes (measured by ion-selective electrodes) or free intracellular magnesium levels in erythrocytes (measured by nuclear magnetic resonance) have been suggested to be better indicators although these methods require rigorous validity testing and the establishment of functional cut-offs. Intravenous or parenterally administered magnesium loading (magnesium tolerance test) have also been used to assess magnesium status in adults. The intravenous method is invasive, and both methods require that the subject have normal renal function. Moreover, while the magnesium tolerance test has been used to detect magnesium depletion or risk of depletion, it does not appear to be sensitive to magnesium supplementation conditions in normal subjects with adequate magnesium status. For example, in healthy subjects, the mean retention of an administered magnesiun load did not change significantly after three months of magnesium supplementation (350 mg/day) (IOM, 1997). Additionally, the activity of magnesium-dependent enzymes (such as Na/K ATPase), or analyses of substances that have been noted to be affected by magnesium deficiency such as thromboxane B2, C-reactive protein, endothelin-1, and nitric oxide production have been suggested as possible biomarkers for magnesium (Franz, 2004). However, changes in these markers have been noted in other disease states and, thus, these are not exclusive for magnesium alone. As with other nutrients, multiple biomarker measurements may be needed for accurate assessment of status. Similar to zinc and copper, magnesium deficiency can increase oxidative stress. As discussed below, the use of signature oxidative stress markers may be a potential way to assess status.

## FUTURE METHODS OF NUTRIENT STATUS ASSESSMENT

### Metabolomics

Metabolomics, the measurement of comprehensive profiles of low-molecular-weight metabolites (Whitfield et al., 2004), is an exciting tool that can be employed to assess nutritional status. A recent key paper from the American Society for Nutritional Sciences Long Range Planning Committee addressed the "nutritional phenotype" in the age of metabolomics (Zeisel et al., 2005). In the future, human nutritional status may be defined and measured by integrating information obtained from genetic, transcriptomic, proteomic, and metabolomic profiles, as they respond to diet, disease, environmental, and behavioral or lifestyle factors. We are at the beginning stages of determining what metabolites are most relevant and important to nutrition, and what metabolomic profiles constitute the normal versus pathological phenotype. The linking of proteomic and metabolomic changes has been studied with regard to the vascular system as it relates to cardiovascular disease (Mayr et al., 2004). Similarly, metabolite profiling has been used in the fields of toxicology and drug discovery, in the identification of patients with coronary heart disease, and in the metabolism of components found in the diet (Whitfield et al., 2004). An exciting prospect for the future is whether characteristic profiles for individual minerals can be identified under different degrees of deficiency conditions. While it is still too early to know the extent to which metabolomics will be useful in characterizing an individual's acute, versus chronic, nutritional status, it is reasonable to predict that metabolomic approaches will be invaluable in the future tailoring of nutritional recommendations for individuals in conditions of physical stress. In our opinion, a high research priority should be the identification of metabolomic signatures for acute and chronic deficiencies, of the essential micro- and macro-molecules. It is important to note that the metabolomic signatures associated with both chronic and acute deficiencies are likely to be different for individuals in diverse geographical regions, particularly when considering the profiles of individuals at extreme temperatures or altitudes. Thus, results obtained from subjects in mild temperate zones, such as those in the typical research university, may not be appropriate for military personnel engaged in activities in extreme environments.

## Metallomics

Recently, bioinorganic speciation analysis of metal and metalloid species within a cell or tissue type (metallomics) has been described as a new method for examining the role of metals in health and disease (Szpunar, 2004; Szpunar, 2005). As minerals are essential for biochemical function, the determination of not only the concentration of an individual metal species but also its distribution among cellular compartments of different cell types and the identification of the cellular bio-ligand to which it is complexed could shed light on what happens when cells are exposed to external stimuli, disease, physiological stress or nutrient deprivation, or toxicity. In the future, once this method is validated, body fluids or tissue biopsies may undergo metallomics as a way to assess nutrient status. Similar to metabolomics, research in this area should be considered a high priority for the military.

## Breathomics

The odors found in breath have been used as a diagnostic tool for centuries. For example, the smell of fruity, rotten apples in the breath of diabetics has been used for centuries to diagnose diabetic ketoacidosis. Similarly, renal failure is associated with "urine-like" breath, while liver failure has been associated with fetor hepaticus. People with selenium deficiency have been noted to have breath that smells of garlic or alcohol. Dr. Michael Phillips and his team at New York Medical College have argued that breathomics may represent a rapid, noninvasive diagnostic tool for disease and wellness. This technique entails the trapping of metabolites (volatile organic compounds, VOCs) produced in the body either at basal levels or after a load test, from breath samples. After breath collection, the VOCs are released from the trap using automated thermal desorbers, separated by gas chromatography, and analyzed using mass spectrometry. The data collected are further analyzed by computer taking into account VOCs present in room air. There are several advantages of breath testing including that the breath collection apparatus is portable, and it is user-friendly and easy to operate. Importantly, there is minimal to no discomfort to patients. Finally, breath VOCs can be identified and quantified with picomolar sensitivity (10-12 mol/L). However, as with other "omic" technologies (e.g., metabolomics), the total number of different VOCs is greater than 3,000 making data interpretation somewhat problematic. With the above said, breathomics has been used to characterize different profiles of oxidative stress in patients with certain cancers, cardiovascular disease, diabetes, and preeclampsia (Moretti et al., 2004; Phillips et al., 2003; Phillips et al., 2004a; Phillips et al., 2004b).

Profiles of oxidative stress or damage markers in breath samples may also prove useful in assessing mineral deficiency-induced alterations to the oxidant defense system. An imbalance in the production and elimination of reactive oxygen species (ROS) by the oxidant defense system can result in oxidative stress and damage to macromolecules. For example, copper deficiency decreases the activity of CuZnSOD which results in increased superoxide anions. One consequence of the increased superoxide anion concentration is an increase in the formation of peroxynitrite leading to protein nitration (Beckers-Trapp et al., 2006). In zinc deficiency, oxidative stress results in lipid peroxidation and DNA damage (Olin et al., 1993; Oteiza et al., 1995). Similar findings have been noted in magnesium deficiency (Rayssiguier et al., 1993; Stafford et al., 1993). The peroxidation of lipids results in the production of lipid free radicals including non-volatile products such as conjugated dienes, lipid hydroperoxides, malondialdehyde and 4-hydroxynonenal, and volatile products such as alkanes and methylated alkanes. The volatile products can then be examined in breath samples. This technique has been used to detect lipid peroxidation in copper deficient rats as an index of whole body oxidative stress (Saari et al., 1990). It remains to be seen whether individual nutrient deficiencies can be precisely identified by specific profiles of markers of oxidative stress or damage. We would suggest that the characterization of breath "oxidative stress profiles" associated with acute and chronic nutritional deficiencies should be a high priority research area for the military. However, perhaps a more critical question is whether breath testing can also be a potential method for the rapid evaluation of an individual's response to food. For example, if one were interested in identifying antioxidant effects of certain foods, one could use an experimental design similar to a drug intervention study. Normal controls and disease group subjects, e.g., cardiovascular disease, would be dosed with the candidate food. Serial breath tests would be obtained and oxidative stress profiles could be assessed. With regard to health and disease, in theory, with relatively small advancements in technology, one could envision an initial breath test in the field, followed by an onsite analysis of the sample at a more comprehensive hospital. An individual's response to nutritional therapy could then be followed with respect to markers of oxidative stress and tissue damage and repair. The expedient assessment of oxidative damage and response of the individual to different conditions could represent a breakthrough in patient care even if the method ultimately is not sensitive enough to determine specific nutrient (e.g., zinc, copper, or magnesium) deficiencies.

## CONCLUSIONS

Most of the biomarkers commonly used for assessing zinc, copper, and magnesium status, particularly with respect to the identification of functional deficiencies, have low sensitivity and specificity. As a consequence, there can be a high risk for false negatives, as well as false positives. The use of multiple biomarkers for a given mineral may in part compensate for the above, however, problems still exist. Lab-on-a-chip technologies may soon allow for the rapid evaluation of multiple biomarkers that collectively provide information on a set of key nutrients. Evolving "omic" technologies will provide new assessment approaches that should allow for considerable improvements in our ability to correctly identify functional mineral deficiencies in short periods of time. With the identification of polymorphisms that increase an individual's risk for the development of, or susceptibility to, certain mineral deficiencies, consideration should be given to the development of individualized "omic" profiles that reflect their "optimal" status for nutrients of concern.

## ACKNOWLEDGEMENTS

This work was supported by National Institutes of Health grants HD-26777, HD01743, and AT-00652 and a gift from the International Copper Association.

## REFERENCES

Aydemir TB, Blanchard RB, Cousins FJ. 2006. Zinc supplementation of young men alters metallothionein, zinc transporter, and cytokine gene expression in leukocyte populations. *Proc Natl Acad Sci USA* 103:1699–1704.

Beckers-Trapp ME, Lanoue L, Keen CL, Rucker RB, Uriu-Adams JY. 2005. Abnormal development and increased 3-nitrotyrosine in copper-deficient mouse embryos. *Free Radical Biology and Medicine* 40(1):35–44.

Briefel RR, Bialostosky K, Kennedy-Stephenson J, McDowell MA, Ervin RB, Wright JD. 2000. Zinc intake of the U.S. population: Findings from the third National Health and Nutrition Examination Survey, 1988–1994. *J Nutr* 130:1367S–1373S.

Britton J, Pavord I, Richards K, Wisniewski A, Knox A, Lewis S, Tattersfield A, Weiss S.1994. Dietary magnesium, lung function, wheezing, and airway hyperreactivity in a random adult population sample. *Lancet* 344:357–362.

Cao J, Cousins RJ. 2000. Metallothionein mRNA in monocytes and peripheral blood mononuclear cells and in cells from dried blood spots increases after zinc supplementation of men. *J Nutr* 130:2180–2187.

Champagne CM, Bogle ML, McGee BB, Yadrick K, Allen HR, Kramer TR, Simpson P, Gossett J, Weber J. 2004. Dietary intake in the lower Mississippi delta region: Results from the Foods of our Delta Study. *J Am Diet Assoc* 104:199–207.

Ford ES, Mokdad AH. 2003. Dietary magnesium intake in a national sample of U.S. adults. *J Nutr* 133:2879–2882.

Franz KB. 2004. A functional biological marker is needed for diagnosing magnesium deficiency. *J Am Coll Nutr* 23:738S–741S.

Hambidge M. 2003. Biomarkers of trace mineral intake and status. *J Nutr* 133 (Suppl 3):948S–955S.

Harris ED. 2000. Cellular copper transport and metabolism. *Annu Rev Nutr* 20:291–310.

IOM (Institute of Medicine). 1997. Magnesium. In: *Dietary Reference Intakes for Calcium, Phosphorus, Magnesium, Vitamin D, and Fluoride*. Washington, DC: National Academy Press. Pp. 190–249.

IOM. 2002a. Copper. In: *Dietary Reference Intakes: Vitamin A, Vitamin K, Arsenic, Boron, Chromium, Copper, Iodine, Iron, Manganese, Molybdenum, Nickel, Silicon, Vanadium, and Zinc*. Washington, DC: National Academy Press. Pp. 224–257.

IOM. 2002b. Zinc. In: *Dietary Reference Intakes: Vitamin A, Vvitamin K, Arsenic, Boron, Chromium, Copper, Iodine, Iron, Manganese, Molybdenum, Nickel, Silicon, Vanadium, and Zinc.* Washington, DC: National Academy Press. Pp. 442–501.

Iskandar M, Swist E, Trick KD, Wang B, L'Abbe MR, Bertinato J. 2005. Copper chaperone for Cu/Zn superoxide dismutase is a sensitive biomarker of mild copper deficiency induced by moderately high intakes of zinc. *Nutr J* 4:35–44.

Keen CL, Clegg MS, Hanna LA, Lanoue L, Rogers JM, Daston GP, Oteiza P, Uriu-Adams JY. 2003a. The plausibility of micronutrient deficiencies being a significant contributing factor to the occurrence of pregnancy complications. *J Nutr* 133:1597S–1605S.

Keen CL, Hanna LA, Lanoue L, Uriu-Adams JY, Rucker RB, Clegg MS. 2003b. Developmental consequences of trace mineral deficiencies in rodents: Acute and long-term effects. *J Nutr* 133:1477S–1480S.

King JC, Keen CL. 1994. Zinc. In: Shils ME, Olson JA, Shike M, eds. *Modern nutrition in health and disease*. Philadelphia, PA: Lea & Febiger. Pp. 214–230.

Liuzzi JP, Cousins RJ. 2004. Mammalian zinc transporters. *Annu Rev Nutr* 24:151–172.

Mayr M, Mayr U, Chung YL, Yin X, Griffiths JR, Xu Q. 2004. Vascular proteomics: Linking proteomic and metabolomic changes. *Proteomics* 4:3751–3761.

Moretti M, Phillips M, Abouzeid A, Cataneo RN, Greenberg J. 2004. Increased breath markers of oxidative stress in normal pregnancy and in preeclampsia. *Am J Obstet Gynecol* 190:1184–1190.

Olin KL, Shigenaga MK, Ames BN, Golub MS, Gershwin ME, Hendrickx AG, Keen CL. 1993. Maternal dietary zinc influences DNA strand break and 8-hydroxy-2'-deoxyguanosine levels in infant rhesus monkey liver. *Proc Soc Exp Biol Med* 203:461–466.

Olivares M, Pizarro F, de Pablo S, Araya M, Uauy R. 2004. Iron, zinc, and copper: Contents in common Chilean foods and daily intakes in Santiago, Chile. *Nutrition* 20:205–212.

Oteiza PI, Olin KL, Fraga CG, Keen CL. 1995. Zinc deficiency causes oxidative damage to proteins, lipids and DNA in rat testes. *J Nutr* 125:823–829.

Phillips M, Cataneo RN, Ditkoff BA, Fisher P, Greenberg J, Gunawardena R, Kwon CS, Rahbari-Oskoui F, Wong C. 2003. Volatile markers of breast cancer in the breath. *Breast J* 9:184–191.

Phillips M, Boehmer JP, Cataneo RN, Cheema T, Eisen HJ, Fallon JT, Fisher PE, Gass A, Greenberg J, Kobashigawa J, Mancini D, Rayburn B, Zucker MJ. 2004a. Heart allograft rejection: Detection with breath alkanes in low levels (the HARDBALL study). *J Heart Lung Transplant* 23:701–708.

Phillips M, Cataneo RN, Cheema T, Greenberg J. 2004b. Increased breath biomarkers of oxidative stress in diabetes mellitus. *Clin Chim Acta* 344:189–194.

Rayssiguier Y, Gueux E, Bussiere L, Durlach J, Mazur A. 1993. Dietary magnesium affects susceptibility of lipoproteins and tissues to peroxidation in rats. *J Am Coll Nutr* 12:133–137.

Saari JT, Dickerson FD, Habib MP. 1990. Ethane production in copper-deficient rats. *Proc Soc Exp Biol Med* 195:30–33.

Stafford RE, Mak IT, Kramer JH, Weglicki WB. 1993. Protein oxidation in magnesium deficient rat brains and kidneys. *Biochem Biophys Res Commun* 196:596–600.

Szpunar J. 2004. Metallomics: A new frontier in analytical chemistry. *Anal Bioanal Chem* 378: 54–56.

Szpunar J. 2005. Advances in analytical methodology for bioinorganic speciation analysis: Metallomics, metalloproteomics and heteroatom tagged proteomics and metabolomics. *Analyst* 130: 442–465.

Takeda N, Takaoka T, Ueda C, Toda N, Kalubi B, Yamamoto S. 2004. Zinc deficiency in patients with idiopathic taste impairment with regard to angiotensin converting enzyme activity. *Auris Nasus Larynx* 31:425–428.

Tarasuk V, Dachner N, Li J. 2005. Homeless youth in Toronto are nutritionally vulnerable. *J Nutr* 135:1926–1933.

Uriu-Adams JY, Keen CL. 2005. Copper, oxidative stress, and human health. *Mol Aspects Med* 26:268–298.

Wang K, Zhou B, Kuo YM, Zemansky J, Gitschier J. 2002. A novel member of a zinc transporter family is defective in acrodermatitis enteropathica. *Am J Hum Genet* 71:66–73.

Whitfield PD, German AJ, Noble PJ. 2004. Metabolomics: An emerging post-genomic tool for nutrition. *Br J Nutr* 92:549–555.

Zeisel SH, Freake HC, Bauman DE, Bier DM, Burrin DG, German JB, Klein S, Marquis GS, Milner JA, Pelto GH, Rasmussen KM. 2005. The nutritional phenotype in the age of metabolomics. *J Nutr* 135:1613–1616.

# Environmental Stressors During Military Operations

*Robert Carter III, Samuel N. Cheuvront, Andrew J. Young, and Michael N. Sawka*
*U.S. Army Research Institute of Environmental Medicine,*
*Natick, Massachusetts*

## INTRODUCTION

U.S. fighting doctrine states that "U.S. Army forces must be prepared to fight and win on short notice anywhere in the world, from blistering deserts to frigid wastelands, in rain forests and mountains—and all types of terrain" and that soldiers are the most important and most vulnerable part of the war fighting system (Department of the Army, 2003). Military operations require soldiers to perform strenuous exercise for long hours and will push them to their physiologic limits, often with minimal logistical support so troops may find themselves under-equipped for the hostile environmental conditions. Harsh environments limit use of air support and crew-served vehicles, thereby placing a greater combat burden on dismounted soldiers who must sustain high metabolic rates to traverse rugged terrain and carry heavy loads. These environmental and work load conditions can impose significant adverse consequences on soldier performance and health.

## HEAT STRESS

Soldiers encounter heat stress from environmental conditions, body heat production and the clothing or equipment they wear. Heat stress increases sweat rate and circulatory responses to dissipate body heat (Mack and Nadel, 1996). When the climatic condition is warmer than skin, it also causes the body to gain heat from the climate, and, thus, increases the amount of heat the body must dissipate (Sawka et al., 1996). In addition, exercise increases metabolic rate above resting levels, and, thus, increase the rate at which heat must be dissipated to keep core temperature from increasing to dangerous levels. Climatic heat stress and physical exercise interact synergistically, and may push physiological systems to their limits (Sawka and Young, 2000).

If the body stores heat, skin and core temperature will increase. In response, the body initiates heat loss responses (sweating and increased skin blood flow). Unless heat stress exceeds the thermoregulatory system's capacity to dissipate heat, the heat loss responses will increase until they restore heat balance and core temperature stops increasing. However, if climate or clothing limits heat loss below the rate of heat production, then increases in sweating and skin blood flow will not restore heat balance but will only increase physiological strain.

Heat stress increases skin blood flow that elevates skin temperature (Rowell, 1986). Skin temperature generally increases with ambient temperature but remains below core temperature. When sweating does not occur, increasing skin blood flow will elevate skin temperature, and decreasing skin blood flow will lower skin temperature nearer to ambient temperature. Thus, heat loss by conduction, convection and radiation is controlled by varying skin blood flow, and thereby skin temperature.

Maintaining a high skin blood flow helps dissipate heat but strains the cardiovascular system during physical work in the heat. High skin blood flow is associated with pooling of blood in compliant skin and subcutaneous vascular beds. This pooling reduces cardiac filling and stroke volume, thus requiring a higher heart rate to maintain cardiac output (Rowell, 1986). For these conditions, the primary cardiovascular challenge is to have sufficient cardiac output to simultaneously support high skin blood flow for heat dissipation and high muscle blood flow for metabolism. To help compensate for reduced cardiac filling, sympathetic activity is increased to elevate myocardial contractility and to divert blood flow from the viscera to skin and muscle.

## Changes in Metabolism

Acute heat stress increases the metabolic rate to perform submaximal exercise, possibly because the rate of ATP utilization to develop a given muscle tension is increased as muscle temperature increases. Aerobic metabolism and muscle total adenine pool may decrease, while oxygen debt, blood and muscle lactate accumulation, skeletal muscle glycogen utilization and inosine 5-monophosphate concentration may all increase during exercise with higher muscle temperatures (Young, 1990). The increased glycogen utilization is probably mediated by elevated epinephrine and muscle hyperthermia. In addition, lactate uptake and oxidation by the liver (and probably non-exercising muscle) are impaired during exercise-heat stress. Elevated muscle temperature does not appear to alter oxidative adaptations or mitochondria biogenesis (Young, 1990).

Heat acclimatization usually lowers total metabolic rate during exercise due to reductions in aerobic and anaerobic components, but this effect is probably too small to reduce heat storage (Sawka et al., 2000). On the other hand, changes in substrate metabolism induced by heat acclimatization may help to improve endurance. Blood and muscle lactate accumulation and muscle glycogen depletion during exercise are often reduced following heat acclimatization.

### Changes in Body Fluids and Electrolytes

Sweating rate is dependent upon the environmental conditions, clothing worn, exercise intensity, and heat acclimatization state. Soldiers working in hot weather often have sweating rates of 0.3 to 1.2 L/hour (Sawka and Young, 2000). Persons performing more intense activity while wearing more clothing or equipment often have sweating rates of 1 to 2 L/hour (IOM, 2004). In comparison, athletes performing high intensity exercise in the heat commonly have sweating rates of 1.0 to 2.5 L/hour (Mack and Nadel, 1996). Fluid requirements will vary in relation to ambient temperature, clothing worn, acclimatization state, and physical activity levels (IOM, 2004). Daily fluid requirements might range (for sedentary to very active persons) from 2–4 L/day in temperate environments and from 4–12 L/day in hot environments (IOM, 2004). Figure B-17 demonstrates the distribution of daily sweating rates for soldiers performing military activities in desert and tropic climates.

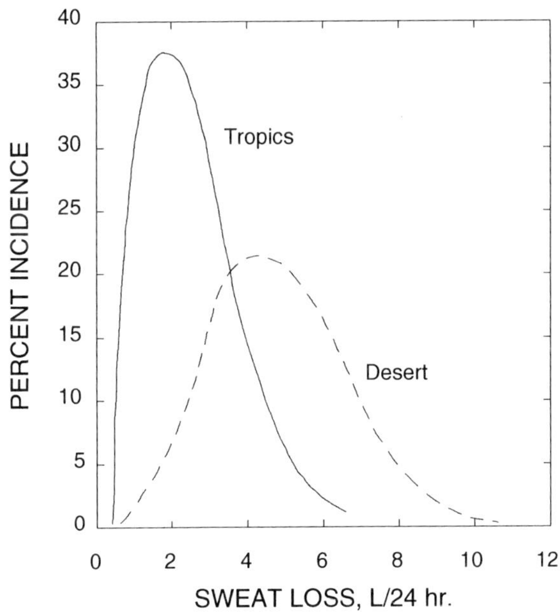


**FIGURE B-17** Distribution of daily sweating rates for active soldiers in desert and tropical climates. Percent incidence refers to the percentage of the subject population achieving the given daily sweat loss.
SOURCE: Molnar (1947).

Sweat is hypotonic to extracellular fluid and contains electrolytes, primarily sodium chloride and to a lesser extent potassium, which are lost in sweat. Sweat sodium concentration averages ~40 mEq/L (range 10–100 mEq /L) and varies depending upon diet, sweating rate, hydration status, and heat acclimatization state. Heat acclimatized persons have relatively low sodium concentrations (> 50 percent reduction) in sweat. Sweat potassium concentration averages 5 mEq/L (range 3–15 mEq/L), calcium averages 1 mEq/L (range 0.3–2 mEq/L) and magnesium averages 0.8 mEq/L (range 0.2–1.5 mEq/L). Electrolyte supplementation is not necessary, except for their first several days of heat acclimatization, as normal dietary sodium intake will cover the sweat losses as heat acclimatization occurs (IOM, 2004).

It is important that unacclimatizated soldiers replace their sweat and electrolyte losses while performing exercise in the heat. If sodium losses are not replaced, the extracellular fluid volume will also decrease in volume and, consequently, dehydration will occur. If sweat losses are not replaced then a body water deficit, or dehydration will occur. Both types of dehydration (hypertonic hypovolemia or isomotic hypovolemia) reduce physical exercise and cognitive performance and increases the potential for heat strain. The greater the water deficit the greater the adverse consequences mediated by dehydration.

## COLD STRESS

Human thermoregulatory adaptations to cold stress are modest and less understood than adaptations to chronic heat (Young, 1996). Cold stress environments include not only exposure to extremely low temperatures (for example, Arctic regions), but also cold-wet exposures (for example, rain, immersion) in warmer ambient temperatures (Toner and McArdle, 1996). In the cold, heat balance and requirements for shivering are dependent upon the severity of climatic cold stress, effectiveness of vasoconstriction as well as the intensity and mode of exercise (Sawka and Young, 2000).

Cold-induced vasoconstriction decreases blood flow to peripheral tissues and makes them susceptible to cold injury (O'Brien et al., 2005). Reduced muscle temperature degrades finger dexterity and muscular strength while reduced core temperature can degrade the ability to achieve maximal metabolic rates and submaximal endurance performance. Body composition is the most important physiological determinant of thermoregulatory tolerance to cold exposure. The clothing insulation required for warmth and comfort is much higher during rest and light activity than during strenuous activity and over insulation can cause heat stress that elicits sweating, wet clothing and dehydration. Each of those factors can have undesirable affects on soldier performance and cold injury susceptibility.

Cold exposure elicits a peripheral vasoconstriction resulting in a decrease in peripheral blood flow which reduces convective heat transfer between the body's core and shell (skin, subcutaneous fat, and skeletal muscle). During whole-body cold exposure, the vasoconstrictor response spreads throughout the body's peripheral shell. Vasoconstriction begins when skin temperature falls below about 35°C, and becomes maximal when skin temperature is about 31°C or less. The vasoconstrictor response to cold exposure retards heat loss and help to defend core temperature, but at the expense of a decline in temperature of peripheral tissue which also makes them susceptible to cold injury (O'Brien et al., 2005). In effect, insulation is increased effectively but skin temperature declines.

### Changes in Metabolism

In addition to vasoconstriction, another major mechanism elicited to defend body temperature during cold exposure is an increased metabolic heat production, from shivering, which helps offset heat losses. Muscle is generally the source of the increased metabolic heat production in humans and this heat production can be increased even further with exercise. Cold exposure can increase muscle energy metabolism during exercise and reduce exercise performance (Young et al., 1996). Blood lactate concentrations during exercise in cold may be higher than in temperate conditions depending on whether experimental conditions allow shivering to occur during exercise.

### Changes in Body Fluids and Electrolytes

Another physiological response sometimes elicited by cold exposure is diuresis. Termed cold-induced diuresis (CID), this response is actually secondary to the cold-induced vasoconstriction and resulting redistribution of body fluids from the peripheral to central circulation. Exercise minimizes cold-induced vasoconstriction and the reduction in peripheral blood flow suppresses or blunts CID. For this reason, and because the effect is self-limiting (i.e., CID diminishes as body water content falls), this response to cold is not of major physiological significance. CID elicits isoosmotic dehydration.

Clothing insulation needed for warmth and comfort in cold environments is much higher during rest and light activity than during strenuous activity. Therefore, if one begins exercising vigorously while wearing clothing selected for sedentary activities in the cold, sweating and the resultant drinking fluid requirements can increase substantially. Further, sweat can accumulate in clothing, compromising its insulative properties which will again be necessary when exercise stops. Adequate fluids must be ingested to replace these losses or dehydration will ensue. As observed by LeBlanc, man in the cold is not necessarily a cold man (Young, 1996).

## ALTITUDE STRESS

When soldiers ascend to higher altitudes, atmospheric oxygen pressure declines and reduced $O_2$ diffusion from the alveolus to blood causes a fall in arterial $O_2$ pressure ($PaO_2$), $O_2$ saturation of hemoglobin ($SaO_2$), and arterial $O_2$ content ($CaO_2$). Because of the relationship between $PaO_2$ and hemoglobin, significant decrements in resting $SaO_2$ do not emerge until the altitude exceeds ~2,400 m. Although the resting $SaO_2$ is well preserved up to ~2,400 m, the drop in $PaO_2$ decreases the diffusion of oxygen from the lungs to the blood and then from the blood to the cells. This decrease in oxygen diffusion rate becomes apparent during aerobic exercise as an arterial oxygen desaturation occurs at altitudes as low as 1,000 m. Thus, exercise performance deteriorates at altitudes slightly greater than 1,000 m, even though resting $SaO_2$ is near sea-level values. With altitudes higher than 1,000 m, the decrements in aerobic exercise performance are even more noticeable (Fulco et al., 1998).

## Changes in Body Fluids and Electrolytes

Soldiers ascending to high altitude normally experience diuresis and natriuresis that mediate a reduced total body water at a new equilibrium level. These responses are initiated within several hours of hypoxic exposure and occur continuously during altitude acclimatization (Sawka et al., 2000). As persons ascend to higher altitudes there are additional fluid and electrolyte losses. Total body water losses of ~1–7 percent have been reported. Renal function is well preserved during rest and exercise at high altitude. A hypoxia mediated stimulation of arterial chemoreceptor is believed to mediate the renal excretory responses by increasing overall flow and filtration fraction. High altitude exposure has profound affects on fluid regulatory hormones that help mediate dehydration. Atrial natriuretic peptide (a hormone released by walls of the cardiac atrium in response to high sodium concentration or stretching of the atria and acts to excrete sodium and water, and to cause vasodilation in the circulatory system) as well as glucocorticoid responses are elevated while aldosterone responses are blunted by high altitude exposure. In addition, high altitude exposure lessens vasopressin (an anti-diuretic hormone) responses at rest, by increasing the osmotic threshold for vasopressin release so that free water excretion is increased; high altitude also reduces thirst. During exercise at high altitude, vasopressin responses are decreased relative to the exercise intensity; however, the osmotic threshold is not changed. Other water losses, such as respiratory water loss at altitude is higher than respiratory water loss at sea level (Young et al., 1996). Persons ascending to high altitude will have plasma volume reductions that are proportional to the ascended altitude and exposure duration (Sawka et al., 2000). Plasma volume will be decreased ~10 percent at an altitude of 3,000 m.

An inappropriate thirst response coupled with increased water loss and a transient diuresis, can result in rapid dehydration when military operations are conducted at high altitude; this higher risk of dehydrations along with low oxygen pressure, may result in substantial decrements in military performance.

## ENERGY EXPENDITURE AND HEAT STRAIN

Daily energy expenditure is a function of the terrain, load carried, duration, and intensity of the work task. Table B-10 provides daily energy expenditures (measured by doubly labeled water) for military activities. Clearly, soldiers are active and average daily energy expenditures of > 4,400 kcal. Extreme military operational scenarios can demand daily energy expenditures > 6,000 kcal/day. Such energy expenditures would only be for "very elite" soldiers with an exceptionally demanding mission. Combat foot soldiers carry their own supplies at high energy expenditure costs. The loads they carry can be very heavy depending on what phase of a mission they are performing. A recent field study by Dean and Dupont (2003) in which soldier loads were measured during actual operations in Afghanistan revealed that soldiers in the traveling phase of a mission carried an average of 59.3 kg (131 lb).

A by product of muscular contraction is metabolic heat production that is transferred from the active muscle to blood and the body core. Since skeletal muscle contraction is ~20 percent efficient, and then ~80 percent of expended energy is released as heat that needs to be dissipated from the body to avoid heat

**TABLE B-10** Daily Energy Expenditures (Measured by Double-Labeled Water) of Military Activities

| Group | Activity | Kcal/day |
|---|---|---|
| Army Special Forces | Combat exercise, temperate | 3,400 |
| Army Engineers | Build road and airstrip at altitude | 3,549 |
| Army Transportation Company | Garrison | 3,568 |
| Marine Combat Engineers | Construction | 3,668 |
| Israeli Infantry | Combat exercise, summer | 3,937 |
| Army | Support hospital | 3,960 |
| Army Ranger | Training course | 4,010 |
| Army Ranger | Training course | 4,090 |
| Marine | Artillery exercise, desert | 4,115 |
| Marine | Combat exercise, winter | 4,198 |
| Army | Artillery exercise, winter | 4,253 |
| Israeli Infantry | Combat exercise, winter | 4,281 |
| Army Special Forces | Combat exercise, winter | 4,558 |
| Marine | Crucible, women | 4,679 |
| Australian Infantry | Jungle training | 4,750 |
| Army Special Forces | Assessment school | 5,183 |
| Army Ranger | Combat exercise | 5,185 |
| Norwegian Ranger | Training course | 6,250 |
| Marine | Crucible, men | 6,067 |
| Average | | 4,405 |

SOURCE: Departments of Army and Air Force (2003).

storage and increasing body temperature. Heat exchange between body and the environment is governed by biophysical properties dictated by surrounding air or water temperature; air humidity; air or water motion; solar, sky, and ground radiation; and clothing. These biophysical properties combined with the metabolic rate can result in either heat or cold strain.

## SUMMARY

Military operations can occur in harsh climates and extremely hostile environments with minimal logistical support. Environmental stresses can induce physiologic strain and reduce military performance. The alterations in metabolism, body fluids and electrolyte concentrations due to environmental exposures to heat, cold, or altitude can alter the mineral levels in body compartments due to alterations in sweat and urine output. The role of that these losses contribute to performance degradation is unclear but, if they are substantial and may affect performance or health, they need to be considered when recommending mineral intake for military operations or training under extreme environmental conditions.

## DISCLAIMER

The views, opinions and findings contained in this report are those of the authors and should not be construed as an official Department of Army position or decision, unless so designated by other official documentation. Approved for public release; distribution is unlimited.

## REFERENCES

Dean CE, Dupont F. 2003. *Modern Warrior's Combat Load. Dismounted Operations in Afghanistan.* April–May 2003. Letter Report. Ft. Leavenworth, KS: U.S. Army Center for Army Lessons Learned.

Departments of Army and Air Force. 2003. *Heat Stress Control and Heat Casualty Management.* Technical Bulletin Med 506. Washington, DC: Headquarters, Departments of Army and Air Force.

Fulco CS, Rock PB, Cymerman A. 1998. Maximal and submaximal exercise performance at altitude. *Aviat Space Environ Med* 69:793–801.

Institute of Medicine. 2004. Water. In: *Dietary Reference Intakes: Water, Potassium, Sodium, Chloride, and Sulfate.* Washington, DC: The National Academies Press.

Mack GW, Nadel ER. 1996. Body fluid balance during heat stress in humans. In: Fregly MJ, Blatteis CM, eds. *Handbook of Physiology, Section 4, Environmental Physiology.* New York: Oxford University Press. Pp. 187–214.

O'Brien C. 2005. Reproducibility of the cold-induced vasdilation response in the human finger. *J Appl Physiol* 98(4):1334–1340.

Rowell LB. 1986. *Human Circulation: Regulation during Physical Stress.* New York: Oxford University Press.

Sawka MN, Young AJ. 2000. Physical exercise in hot and cold climates. In: Garrett WE, Kirkendall DT, eds. *Exercise and Sport Science.* Philadelphia, PA: Lippincott, Williams and Wilkins. Pp. 385–400.

Sawka MN, Wenger CB, Pandolf KB. 1996. Thermoregulatory responses to acute exercise-heat stress and heat acclimation. In: Fregly MJ, Blatteis CM, eds. *Handbook of Physiology, Section 4, Environmental Physiology.* New York: Oxford University Press. Pp. 157–185.
Sawka MN, Convertino VA, Eichner ER, Schnieder SM, Young AJ. 2000. Blood volume: Importance and adaptations to exercise training, environmental stresses, and trauma/sickness. *Med. Sci Sports Exerc* 32:332–348.
Toner MM, McArdle WD. 1996. Human thermoregulatory responses to acute cold stress with special reference to water immersion. In: Fregly MJ, Blatteis CM, eds. *Handbook of Physiology, Section 4, Environmental Physiology.* New York, NY: Oxford University Press. Pp. 379–418.
U.S. Army Training and Doctrine Command. 2003. *Operations.* FM 100-5. Washington, DC: Headquarters, Department of the Army.
Young AJ. 1990. Energy substrate utilization during exercise in extreme environments. In: Pandolf KB and Hollozsy JO, eds. *Exercise and Sport Sciences Reviews.* Baltimore, MD: Williams and Wilkins. Pp. 65–117.
Young AJ. 1996. Homeostatic responses to prolonged cold exposure: Human cold acclimatization. In: Fregly MJ, Blatteis CM, eds. *Handbook of Physiology, Section 4, Environmental Physiology.* New York, NY: Oxford University Press. Pp. 419–438.
Young AJ, Sawka MN, Pandolf KB. Physiology of cold exposure. 1996. In: Marriott BM, Carlson SJ, eds. *Nutritional Needs in Cold and in High-Altitude Environments.* Washington, DC: National Academy Press. Pp. 127–147.

## Mineral Sweat Losses During Exercise

*Emily M. Haymes*
*Florida State University, Tallahassee*

The extreme environmental conditions during military operations or training may affect sweat losses of minerals and, therefore, those losses constitute a risk factor for mineral inadequacy and potential performance decrements and need to be considered when evaluating mineral requirements for military personnel. Although other physical or psychological stressors might also alter mineral metabolism, sweat due to exercise and high temperatures appears to be one major mechanism of substantial mineral losses. Although less frequently studied, fecal and urinary losses might also be of importance with intense physical activity and they are also reported in this paper when known.

Several studies have measured mineral concentration in sweat during and following exercise. The concentrations of calcium, magnesium, iron, and zinc have been found to vary widely in the sweat during exercise. Several factors appear to influence sweat mineral concentrations including the methods used to collect the sweat and site of sweat collection, the environmental conditions in which the sweat is collected, and duration of the exercise sweat collection. Much less is known about sweat losses of copper or other minerals. Because many studies have been conducted under different environmental situations or using various collection methods, the results of the studies presented show apparent discrepancies; in addition, because of the special extreme environments endured by military personnel, care should be taken when extrapolating these results to mineral losses of military personnel. Only the studies of prolonged exercise in the heat by Consolazio and colleagues (Consolazio et al., 1962, 1964) have measured sweat mineral losses in conditions that simulate those experienced by military personnel.

## FACTORS AFFECTING SWEAT MINERAL CONCENTRATIONS

The site of sweat collection influences the sweat concentration and can lead to inconsistent results if this factor is overlooked. Most of the studies that measured sweat mineral concentrations during exercise have used regional sites (e.g., back, arm) for sweat collection. Two studies that directly compared whole body sweat mineral content with regional site sweat collections using patches and arm bags found higher mineral concentrations in the sweat from the regional sites (Jacob et al., 1981; Palacios et al., 2003). The conclusion from these studies is that the use of regional sites to project whole body mineral loss led to overestimation of total body sweat mineral losses.

The environment, and particularly environment temperature and humidity, influences sweat losses of iron and zinc, being lower during exercise in warm environments compared to cooler temperatures (Tipton et al., 1993; Waller and Haymes, 1996). Because sweat rates are higher in warm environments, the decrease in sweat mineral concentration appears to be due to sweat dilution. The total amount of sweat iron and zinc lost was the same in the two environments.

Another factor that cannot be overlooked when considering sweat losses is acclimatization, that is, the physiological adaptation to the environment that occurs over days or weeks. For instance, sweat calcium loss was observed to decrease after one week of exercise in a hot environment (Conolazio et al., 1962). Another physiological adaptation observed is a decrease in mineral concentration over time. Serial sweat collections made during prolonged exercise have found that sweat zinc and iron concentrations decrease over time (DeRuisseau et al., 2002; Paulev et al, 1983; Tipton et al., 1993; Waller and Haymes, 1996). A similar decrease in sweat iron concentration over time was found when subjects sat in a sauna (Brune et al., 1986). Although sweat rates increase over time during exercise and sauna exposure, Brune et al. (1986) suggested the first sweat secreted by sweat glands may contain cellular debris and external contaminants. DeRuisseau et al. (2002) recently reported lower sweat iron and zinc concentrations during the second hour of exercise than the first hour. Sweat rates remained constant during the final 90 minutes of exercise.

All these research data point to apparent inconsistencies in sweat losses of minerals that may be due not only to differences in methods or laboratories but also to critical factors such as collection methods, environmental conditions, and acclimatization.

## SWEAT MINERAL CONCENTRATIONS DURING EXERCISE

### Calcium

Whole body sweat calcium concentrations were measured during exercise in two studies. Mean sweat calcium concentration was 52 ± 36 mg/L during exercise in a warm (34.5°C) humid environment (Shirreffs and Maughan, 1997). Costa et al. (1969) found exercise sweat calcium concentrations of 72 ± 10 mg/L and 74 ± 17 mg/L on two different diets that did not differ in calcium intake in a cooler (24.5°C) environment.

Several studies have used pads or sponges to collect sweat from various sites during exercise. Sweat calcium concentrations of 30 ± 5 mg/L and 44 ± 12 mg/L were found during exercise by runners and firefighters, respectively (Bullen et al., 1999; O'Toole et al., 2000). Verde et al. (1982) found lower sweat calcium concentrations during indoor (40 ± 20 mg/L) and outdoor (54 ± 46 mg/L) exercise than during a sauna (94 ± 46 mg/L). Klesges et al. (1996) collected sweat from the trunk of basketball players using t-shirts and found mean sweat calcium concentration was 65 ± 31 mg/L. Palacios et al. (2003) found patches placed on eight body sites for 24 hours overestimated total body dermal calcium loss by more than threefold. Whole body dermal calcium loss collected using cotton underwear, shirt, pants, and socks in these same subjects averaged 103 ± 22 mg/day (Palacios et al., 2003).

### Magnesium

Sweat magnesium concentrations during exercise measured using whole body techniques vary from 12 ± 12 mg/L (Shirreffs and Maughan, 1997) and 15 ± 3 mg/L (Costa et al., 1969) to 55 ± 2 mg/L (Costill et al., 1976). Regional sweat collections with sponges yielded mean magnesium concentrations of 7 ± 2 mg/L and 10 ± 2 mg/L during indoor and outdoor exercise, respectively (Verde et al., 1982). Verde and colleagues observed a decrease in sweat magnesium concentration as the sweat rate increased. Although dermal magnesium loss in young women was 35 ± 13 mg/day using a whole body technique, use of sweat patches to measure sweat magnesium also have been found to overestimate daily dermal magnesium loss (Palacios et al., 2003).

### Copper

Only one study was found that measured sweat copper concentrations during exercise. Aruoma et al. (1988) collected sweat samples from the back, chest, abdomen and arm by scraping the skin with plastic tube following heavy exercise. Sweat copper concentrations were 0.89 mg/L (abdomen), 0.73 mg/L (chest), 0.56 mg/L (back), and 0.52 mg/L (arm). Whole body dermal copper loss has been found to average 0.34 mg/day (Jacob et al., 1981). Mean sweat copper concentration collected in arm bags in the same study was 0.11 mg/L. Turnlund et al. (1990) also used arm bags to estimate dermal copper loss. Mean copper loss from the arm ranged from 0.5 to 5.7 μg/day, but this study was conducting with subjects at rest. Other studies that measure copper losses in the sweat have been conducted but they were using either questionable methods of copper quantification, sweat induction, or collection.

## Iron

Many studies have examined the concentration of iron in the sweat. Green et al. (1968) estimated dermal uptake and loss of iron using $^{59}Fe$. Mean dermal iron loss was 0.24 mg/day in sedentary men and women. Slightly higher dermal iron loss (0.33 ± 0.15 mg/day) was found using whole body dermal collection method by Jacob et al. (1983). Mean sweat iron concentration measured using an arm bag was 0.076 mg/L in the same subjects.

Wheeler et al. (1973) measured dermal iron loss using a whole body technique during habitual daily activity and with the addition of two hours of exercise with two different levels of dietary iron. Dietary iron intake and iron loss through the gastrointestinal and urinary tracts were simultaneously measured. Mean iron intake and losses are presented in Table B-11.

The subjects were in negative iron balance during the lower dietary iron intake phase of the study. Sweat iron concentrations were lower during the two exercise phases (0.13 mg/L and 0.15 mg/L) compared to the habitual physical activity phase (0.20 mg/L). However, subjects had higher sweat rates during the exercise phases.

Mean sweat iron concentrations during exercise also decrease over time. Paulev et al. (1983) observed sweat iron on the back decreased from 0.20 mg/L to 0.13 mg/L over 30 minutes of exercise. Waller and Haymes (1996) found arm bag sweat iron concentrations decreased from 30 to 60 minutes of exercise in

**TABLE B-11** Iron Intake and Losses During Habitual Activity With and Without 2 Hours of Exercise

| Trial | Iron Intake (mg/day) | Urinary Iron Loss (mg/day) | Dermal Iron Loss (mg/day) | Fecal Iron Loss (mg/day) |
|---|---|---|---|---|
| HA | 34.8 | 0.22 | 0.38 | 22.0 |
| HA/Ex1 | 36.8 | 0.23 | 0.32 | 26.0 |
| HA/Ex2 | 17.5 | 0.19 | 0.34 | 25.2 |

NOTE: HA = habitual daily exercise; HA/Ex = habitual daily exercise with additional hours of exercise.
SOURCE: Wheeler et al. (1973).

warm (0.21 mg/L to 0.08 mg/L) and neutral environments (0.31 mg/L to 0.14 mg/L). Significant decreases in sweat iron concentration were also found between 30 minutes (0.19 mg/L) and 120 minutes (0.11 mg/L) by DeRuisseau et al. (2002). Total sweat iron loss was significantly lower during the second hour of exercise. Regional sweat iron concentrations vary with higher concentrations found in sweat from the chest (0.50 mg/L) and abdomen (0.49 mg/L) than from the arm (0.28 mg/L) and back (0.20 mg/L) (Aruoma et al., 1988).

### Zinc

Dermal zinc loss measured using whole body techniques has been found to average 0.50 mg/day in men (Jacob et al., 1981) and 0.67 mg/day in women (Hess et al., 1977). Consumption of a low zinc diet by men reduced dermal zinc loss to 0.29 mg/day and zinc repletion increased dermal zinc loss to 0.62 mg/day (Milne et al., 1983).

Sweat zinc concentrations decrease over time during exercise. Tipton et al. (1993) found sweat zinc was lower after 60 minutes of exercise (0.41 mg/L) than at 30 minutes (0.97 mg/L). Similar findings were reported by DeRuisseau et al. (2002) with higher zinc concentrations during the first hour (0.90 mg/L) than the second hour (0.56 mg/L) of exercise. Lower sweat zinc concentrations were also observed during one hour of exercise in a warm environment (0.52 ± 0.41 mg/L) than in a neutral environment (0.87 ± 0.87 mg/L) (Tipton et al., 1993) but the total amount of zinc lost were not different in the two environments. Just like with the other minerals, Aruoma et al. (1988) found higher sweat concentrations on the abdomen (0.83 mg/L) than the back (0.48 mg/L), arm (0.44 mg/L) and chest (0.42 mg/L). Cordova and Navas (1998) observed significantly higher facial sweat zinc concentrations in athletes during the competitive season (0.83 mg/L) than during training (0.28 mg/L). Significantly higher serum cortisol levels were also found in the athletes during the competitive season.

## CONCLUSION

Mineral sweat concentrations measured during exercise are quite variable and it is obvious from the results presented in this paper that the methods of sweat collection need to be similar in order to compare results, preferably whole body collection methods. Sweat iron and zinc concentrations decrease over time during prolonged exercise and are lower in warm environments when the sweat rate is higher. Differences in sweat iron, zinc, and copper concentrations have been found from different regions of the body. Calcium and magnesium concentrations in exercise sweat samples also vary. Use of patches over small areas of skin surface leads to overestimation of dermal calcium and magnesium losses compared to whole body dermal loss techniques. There is not much data on sweat losses with exercise for selenium or other trace minerals.

For more accurate and comparable results, whole body collection as opposed to the use of patches or small skin areas should be the collection method of sweat and sweat should be collected over a period of time and under the specific environmental conditions of interest. For example, for military situations environmental conditions could be extreme and, therefore, temperature and humidity should mimic those extreme conditions while the study is being conducted. In addition, with acclimatization to the environment the amount of minerals in the sweat decreases. It would then be advisable to conduct studies that last for at least five days so that the effect of acclimatization on sweat mineral losses can be determined.

## REFERENCES


Aruoma OI, Reilly T, MacLane D, Halliwell B. 1988. Iron, copper and zinc concentrations in human sweat and plasma: The effect of exercise. *Clin Chim Acta* 177:81–88.

Brune MD, Magnusson B, Persson H, Hallberg L. 1986. Iron losses in sweat. *Am J Clin Nutr* 43:438–443.

Bullen DB, O'Toole ML, Johnson KC. 1999. Calcium losses resulting from an acute bout of moderate-intensity exercise. *Int J Sport Nutr* 9:275–284.

Consolazio, CF, Matoush, LO, Nelson, RA, Hackler, LR, Preston, EE. 1962. Relationship between calcium in sweat, calcium balance, and calcium requirements. J Nutr 78:78–88.

Consolazio, CF, Nelson, RA, Matoush, LO, Hughes, RC. 1964. The Trace Mineral Losses in Sweat. Denver, CO: U.S. Army Medical Research and Nutrition Laboratory, Report No. 284.

Cordova A, Navas FJ. 1998. Effect of training on zinc metabolism: Changes in serum and sweat zinc concentrations in sportsmen. *Ann Nutr Metab* 42:274–282.

Costa F, Calloway DH, Margen S. 1969. Regional and total body sweat composition of men fed controlled diets. *Am J Clin Nutr* 22:52–58.

Costill DL, Cote R, Fink W. 1976. Muscle water and electrolytes following varied levels of dehydration in man. *J Appl Physiol* 40:6–11.

DeRuisseau KC, Cheuvront SN, Haymes EM, Sharp RG. 2002. Sweat iron and zinc losses during prolonged exercise. *Int J Sport Nutr Exer Metab* 12:428–437.

Green R, Charlton R, Seftel H, Bothwell T, Mayet F, Finch C, Layrisse M. 1968. Body iron excretion in man. *Am J Med* 45:336–353.

Hess FM, King JC, Margen S. 1977. Zinc excretion in young women on low zinc intakes and oral contraceptive agents. *J Nutr* 107:1610–1620.

Jacob RA, Sandstead HH, Munoz JM, Klevay LM, Milne DB. 1981. Whole body surface loss of trace metals in normal males. *Am J Clin Nutr* 34:1379–1382.

Klesges RC, Ward KD, Shelton ML, Applegate WB, Cantler ED, Palmieri GMA, Harmon K, Davis JP. 1996. Changes in bone mineral content in male athletes: Mechanisms of action and intervention effects. *JAMA* 276:226–230.

Milne DB, Canfield WK, Mahalko JR, Sandstead HH. 1983. Effect of dietary zinc on whole body surface loss of zinc:impact on estimation of zinc retention by balance method. *Am J Clin Nutr* 38:181–186.

O'Toole ML, Johnson KL, Satterfield S, Bush AJ, Koo WW, Klesges RC, Applegate WB. 2000. Do sweat calcium losses affect bone mass during firefighter training? *J Occup Environ Med* 42:1054–1059.

Palacios C, Wigertz K, Weaver CM. 2003. Comparison of 24-hour whole body versus patch tests for estimating body surface electrolyte losses. *Int J Sport Nutr Exer* Metab 13:479–488.

Paulev PE, Jordal R, Pedersen NS. 1983. Dermal excretion of iron in intensely training athletes. *Clin Chim Acta* 127:19–27.

Shirreffs SM, Maughan RJ. 1997. Whole body sweat collection in humans:an improved method with preliminary data on electrolyte content. *J Appl Physiol* 82:336–341.

Tipton K, Green NR, Haymes EM, Waller M. 1993. Zinc loss in sweat of athletes exercising in hot and neutral temperatures. *Int J Sport Nutr* 3:261–271.

Turnlund JR, Keen CL, Smith RG. 1990. Copper status and urinary and salivary copper in young men and three levels of dietary copper. *Am J Clin Nutr* 51:658–664.

Verde T, Shephard RJ, Corey P, Moore R. 1982. Sweat composition in exercise and in heat. *J Appl Physiol* 53:1540–1545.

Waller MF, Haymes EM. 1996. The effects of heat and exercise on sweat iron loss. *Med Sci Exer Sport* 28:197–203.

Wheeler EF, El-Neil H, Willson JOC, Weiner JS. 1973. The effect of work level and dietary intake on water balance and the excretion of sodium, potassium and iron in a hot climate. *Br J Nutr* 30:127–137.

# Stress Factors Affecting Homeostasis: Weight Loss and Mineral Status

*Steven B. Heymsfield*
*Merck and Co. Inc., Rahway, New Jersey*

## INTRODUCTION

Weight loss in adults follows when energy losses as heat and solid matter exceed energy provided by foods. Negative energy balance is accompanied by corresponding losses of all major body compartments, including body cell mass (BCM), extracellular fluid, bone mineral, and fat. Minerals, with their respective multiple corresponding functions, are associated with each of these compartments and are hence lost from tissues with weight loss.

Minerals are ingested with foods, and are distributed to the tissue functional sites. Losses then follow through urine, stool, skin, and other portals of exit (Figure B-18). Under conditions of controlled weight loss on nutritionally adequate diets, the ensuing resorption of BCM and other lean compartments releases minerals into the available body pool.

Environmental, physical, and psychological demands during military training and operations may alter metabolism in ways that exacerbate the mineral losses already occurring during weight loss diets. Other stressful factors during military lifestyle that accompany negative energy balance may be heat or cold temperatures, increased physical activity, psychological stressors, and undesirable medical conditions such as diarrhea, vomiting, and fever. When subjects experience these conditions while ingesting diets that may be inadequate with respect to mineral and vitamins, disproportionate tissue mineral depletion with adverse functional consequences for health or performance might occur. Al-

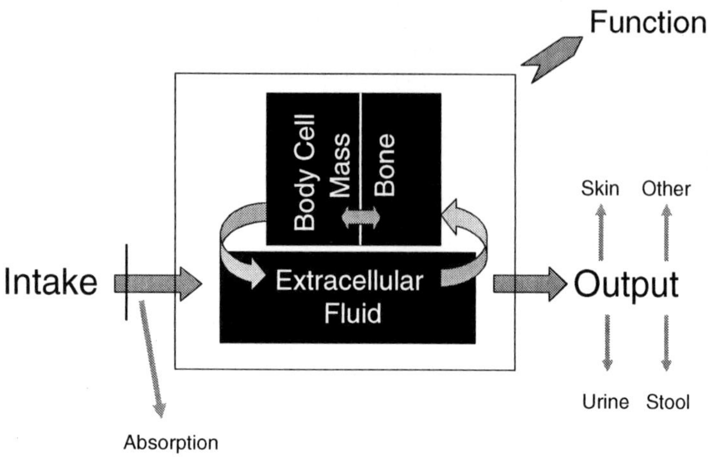


**FIGURE B-18** Intake, distribution, and losses of a representative mineral.

though an evaluation of all potential interventions would not be feasible, this paper reviews the potential adverse effects resulting from mineral inadequacies due to a number of different weight loss interventions, including surgeries or weight loss diets.

## REVIEW OF WEIGHT LOSS LITERATURE

Selective mineral depletion with related functional consequences develops with weight loss programs that provide poor quality diets or weight-loss procedures that interfere with normal absorptive processes. Moreover, selective mineral losses compounded on adverse environmental or medical conditions can facilitate depletion of mineral reserves, as for example that might follow with extreme heat and sodium loss.

### Intestinal Malabsorption

Depending on the intervention used to attain weight loss, intestinal malabsorption of nutrients may accompany weight loss; malabsorption can lead to a net disproportionate mineral loss. Two interventions can serve as models for the typical malabsorption response that may occur with weight loss.

The first intervention is that which is based on pharmaceutical that specifically decrease absorption of some nutrients. For example, a mild malabsorption that occurs with the use of the weight loss medication Xenical (orlistat) (Davidson et al., 1999). Orlistat is a gastrointestinal lipase inhibitor that limits absorption of dietary fat by about 30 percent. The result is a small, but clinically important, increase in fecal fat excretion. Chelation results in binding of divalent cations such as calcium and there are also increased losses of fat soluble vitamins. Long-term studies of up to four years (Davidson et al., 1999; Torgerson et al., 2004) show some reduction in selected fat soluble vitamins, with occasional values below the normal range. Minimal changes are observed in serum calcium levels and there are as of yet no reports of excessive osteoporosis risk, possibly because mineral and multivitamin supplementation is recommended with use of orlistat. Military personnel may use Xenical for weight loss along with popular diets, as discussed below, potentially compounding depletion of fat soluble vitamins and minerals such as calcium and magnesium.

A second more potent malabsorptive intervention involves surgical alterations of gastrointestinal anatomy to promote weight loss. The rate of bariatric surgery (surgery performed to reduce the size of the stomach or to bypass so that fewer calories are absorbed or both) use as a means of managing severe obesity is increasing rapidly. Bariatric surgical procedures provide a good model of malabsorptive weight loss effects on minerals.

Various alterations in gastrointestinal anatomy are accompanied by surgical procedures such as the jejunoileal bypass, roux-en-y gastric bypass, and biliopancreatic diversion (Bloomberg et al., 2005). Mineral and vitamin absorption can be compromised, depending on the specific procedure. The modern practice is to routinely provide oral multivitamin and mineral supplementation and parenteral vitamin $B_{12}$ as needed following the surgical procedure, although deficiencies are occasionally recognized. Iron, absorbed in the duodenum and proximal jejunum, is deficient in 6–36 percent of evaluated subjects (Alvarez-Leite, 2004; Bloomberg et al., 2005; Ortega et al., 2004). Calcium and vitamin D, with duodenal and proximal jejunal absorption, are reported deficient in 10–63 percent of patients evaluated following surgery, depending on the specific operation (Alvarez-Leite, 2004; Bloomberg et al., 2005; Ortega et al., 2004). Zinc deficiency is reported in 10–50 percent of patients and may be accompanied by alopecia (Alvarez-Leite, 2004; Bloomberg et al., 2005; Ortega et al., 2004). Data on magnesium and selenium is limited. Most of the available studies are based on non-randomly selected subject groups and the actual prevalence of mineral deficiency is unknown, although clearly a mechanistic basis and the accompanying population specific observations support disturbances in mineral pools with surgically-induced weight loss.

## Low-Quality Very Low Calorie Diets

Diets intended for weight loss vary in caloric content and can be generally divided into categories including: fasting; very low calorie diets (VLCDs) that provide less than 800 kcal/day; and low calorie diets that provide greater than 800 kcal/day but less than the caloric requirement for weight maintenance. Low calorie diets include a vast array of recommended intakes including balanced or even supplemented meals and popular diets such as Atkins, South Beach, The Zone, Weight Watchers, and SlimFast, or meal replacements.

Fasting as a means of weight control was first popularized by Bloom beginning in 1959 (Bloom, 1959). The treatment was usually carried out under medical supervision and water replacement prevented dehydration. Ketosis and metabolic acidosis were predictable components of the total fast, and popularity waned when reports emerged of total body potassium depletion, cardiac arrhythmias, and sudden death (Schucker and Gunn, 1978). Although the mechanism of disturbed cardiac function was never fully established, hypotheses included essential nutrient depletion and cardiac protein depletion with myofiber atrophy.

Fasting was replaced, in the late nineteen sixties, with the protein-sparing modified fast or VLCD. These diets usually provided ~300 kcal/day, mainly protein, along with some other essential nutrients including minerals and vitamins (Lockwood and Amatruda, 1984; Vertes et al., 1977). Weight loss on the early VLCDs was rapid and required medical supervision with frequent electrolyte and mineral evaluations. These VLCDs were often ketogenic and, as with total fasting, induced a metabolic acidosis.

In the mid nineteen seventies the closely monitored VLCD-type of program gave way to the widely used "liquid protein" diet popularized in diet books such as the "Last Chance Diet" (Linn and Stuart, 1976). These over-the-counter liquid diet formulas often included a poor-quality protein source and were lacking in minerals, vitamins, and other essential nutrients (Lantigua et al., 1980; Licata et al., 1981). Mineral and electrolyte deficiencies, accompanied by muscle weakness and cardiac arrhythmias, were reported in the medical literature (Isner et al., 1979; Michiel et al., 1978). Even after excluding patients with obvious deficiencies, there existed a sudden and near sudden-death group with a characteristic "torsade de pointes" form of ventricular fibrillation (Sours et al., 1981). The specific mechanism leading to sudden death was never fully elucidated, although Lantigua et al. reproduced cardiac rhythm disturbances in carefully monitored obese patients using a typical liquid protein formula (1980) along with negative balances of nitrogen, phosphorus, potassium, calcium, and magnesium (Figure B-19). Sodium balance remained near zero while early potassium loss was particularly rapid. The group later showed adequate diet mineral, vitamin, and trace element supplementation restored zero or near zero balances of nitrogen, phosphorus, potassium, calcium, and magnesium (Figure B-20) and also abolished the adverse cardiac effects (Amatruda et al., 1983, 1988). These and related observations led the modern "supplemented" VLCD that remains in use today.

Although the specific mechanism of fatal outcomes with VLCD dieting may never be known, there is uniform agreement that providing subjects with a low energy diet that lacks adequate minerals and vitamins can lead to serious adverse consequences. The specific required amount of minerals and electrolytes has not been rigorously established, but rather accomplished on an empirical basis using recommended daily allowance and other guideline values.

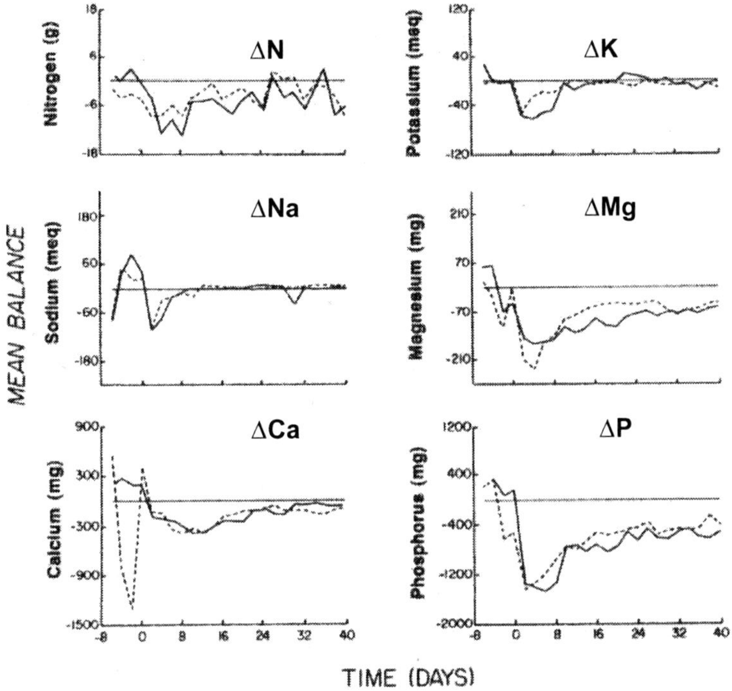


**FIGURE B-19** Mean nitrogen and mineral balances in obese subjects using a control days (–9 to 0) or a typical liquid protein formula (days 0 to 40). Subjects with arrhythmias are denoted by solid lines and subjects without them by dashed lines.
SOURCE: Lantigua et al. (1980).

### Refeeding as an Experimental Model

Adequacy of mineral and electrolyte requirements was engendered not only by events highlighted with nutritionally inadequate VLCDs, but also during the refeeding interventions of malnourished adults and children. Information regarding needs for minerals can also be gain from refeeding interventions. The classic study of Rudman et al. (1975) was carried out in the era following introduction of parenteral feeding solutions. The authors prepared various intravenous feeding solutions ranging from nutritionally complete to devoid of nitrogen, phosphorus, potassium, or sodium. These formulas were then fed to malnourished patients at a calorie level producing weight gain. The complete intravenous formula led to anabolism with corresponding positive balances of nitrogen, phosphorus, potassium, sodium, and calcium in proportions typical of "normal" protoplasm, extracellular fluid, adipose tissue, and bone. Elimination of formula nitrogen led to cessation of increments in protoplasm and extracellular fluid;

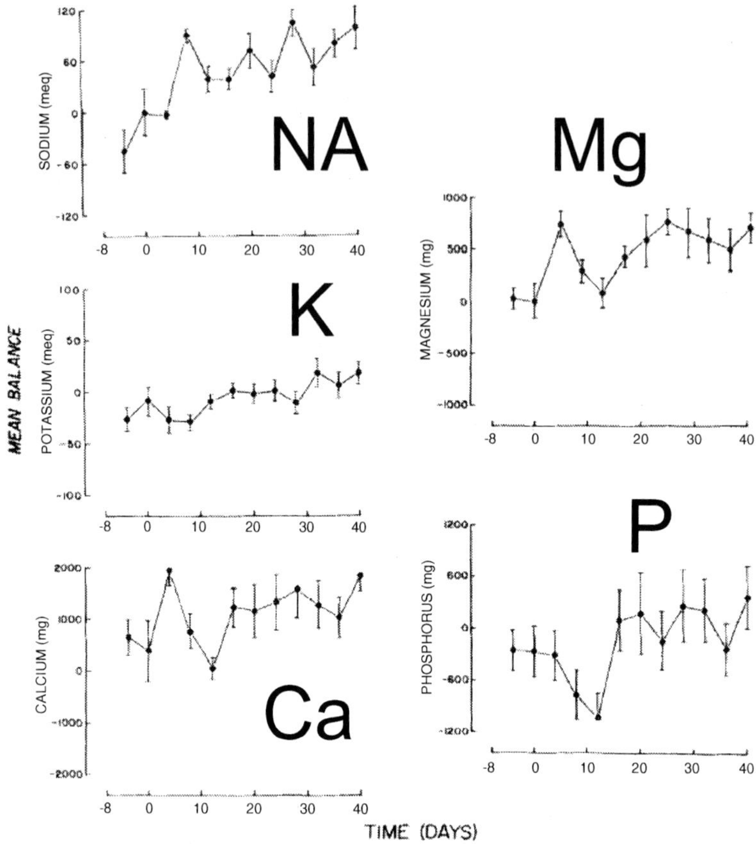


**FIGURE B-20** Mean mineral balances per four-day period in six obese subjects using a control (days –8 to 0) or typical liquid protein formula (days 0 to 40). The data represent the mean + / – SEM.
SOURCE: Amatruda et al. (1983).

bone mineral and adipose tissue growth continued. Likewise, feeding subjects with formulas lacking in phosphorus, potassium, or sodium led to corresponding failures to produce incremental gains in combinations of protoplasm, extracellular fluid, and bone. Withdrawal of phosphorus or sodium interrupted protoplasm, extracellular fluid, and bone repletion. Repletion of protoplasm was limited when the intravenous feeding solution was potassium-free. Refeeding from a malnourished state, whether from disease as in Rudman's patients or through a period of starvation-induced weight loss in a military setting, clearly benefits from an adequate intake of all essential minerals, electrolytes, and trace elements.

Malnutrition is common in children from developing nations and these experiences can also serve to inform about mineral needs. When these children are renourished, optimum growth may not be achieved if the administered diets are inadequate in zinc. Simmer et al. (1988) investigated whether zinc becomes deficient during malnutrition and, thus, limits the rate of weight recovery of malnourished children. The mean zinc intake was 3.7 mg/day and one group of children was supplemented with 50 mg for two weeks. The rate of early weight gain was similar in the un-supplemented and supplemented groups, but by the second refeeding week the supplemented group had a weight gain rate 73 percent greater than the un-supplemented group. The zinc content of polymorphonuclear cells increased in the zinc supplemented group ($p < 0.001$) but not in the un-supplemented group. Khanum et al. (1988) reported a similar observation in a larger group of malnourished children.

## Popular Diets

As with the general population, excess weight is a concern to military personnel and regulations regarding military weight standards may encourage those afflicted to attempt weight loss on a popular diet. Programs such as Weight Watchers are highly developed and the prescribed food intake is adequate in minerals and other essential nutrients. Similarly, other commercially available products, such as the liquid meal replacement SlimFast, are well studied and amply supplemented with minerals and vitamins. Of greater concern is the regular appearance of popular diets that are not rigorously developed with respect to the underlying weight loss nutritional theory or to the nutrient content of suggested foods. This section describes some potential health risks if military personnel would adhere to some of these diets.

The widely used Atkins diet promotes ketosis, early diuresis, and associated metabolic acidosis if rigorously adhered to. Some concern has been expressed for the potential renal effects of high protein intake and the potential for low vitamin D and calcium intake. Metabolic acidosis over the long term can lead to osteoporosis. Freedman et al. (2001) examined the three Atkin's Diet New Diet Revolution phases, induction, ongoing, and maintenance in relation to the Food Guide Pyramid and the dietary reference intakes. Calcium, magnesium, iron, and potassium intakes would be low across the three phases while phosphorus, sodium, and zinc intakes would be within an acceptable intake range.

Freedman et al. (2001) also provide an extensive tabulation of potential nutritional inadequacies, including low mineral content, for other popular plans including Carbohydrate Addict's diet, Sugar Busters!, and Ornish. As with Atkin's, these diet plans are low in calcium, magnesium, iron, and potassium.

Vasilaris and colleagues (2004) examined micronutrient intake in overweight subjects on an ad libitum fat-reduced, high simple-carbohydrate diet. The authors observed a lower zinc intake in men and lower vitamin $B_{12}$ intake in men and women ingesting a fat-reduced simple carbohydrate-rich diet compared to a habitual, normal-fat diet, but not below recommended levels.

More studies are needed of the mineral adequacy of popular diets potentially ingested by military personnel before recommending their use.

The intake of essential micronutrients by subjects in these diets has been reported in a few studies. As expected, a consequence of the diets being low in minerals is that most subjects embarking on a low calorie diet without professional guidance will often ingest inadequate minerals and vitamins (Cifuentes et al., 2004). Of particular note is the low calcium intake observed in overweight and obese women ingesting low calorie diets for weight loss. Riedt et al. (2005) examined the influence of energy restriction and calcium intake on bone mineral density in overweight post-menopausal women. Weight loss resulted in loss of bone at several anatomic sites (e.g., trochanter and spine) in women consuming 1 g Ca/day and was abolished at calcium intakes of ~1.7 g/day. A reduction in circulating estradiol or a rise in parathyroid hormone (PTH) and cortisol may explain bone mobilization, possibly because of Ca-PTH axis suppression.

## SUMMARY

These collective observations highlight the critical importance of mineral content of weight loss diets and the functional and pathological consequences that ensue when mineral supplementation is inadequate. Not only the weight loss diets, but surgical interventions that aim at decreasing absorption of energy sources, may have severe consequences in the mineral balance and therefore performance of soldiers. Of special concern is calcium, because studies have shown that even when meeting the adequate intake for calcium, weight loss diets can result in excessive bone loss, potentially increasing stress fractures.

Most of these studies have been carried out in otherwise healthy subjects living and working in stable developed environments. The additional burdens imposed by some military conditions, heat, intense physical activity, and other potential mineral pool stresses, may lead to serious deficiencies and related functional consequences when accompanying weight loss. Therefore, when adhering to interventions to attain a specific weight within the military, individuals should seek dietary guidance from appropriate experts so that micronutrient intake and, especially, mineral intake is adequate.

## REFERENCES

Alvarez-Leite JI. 2004. Nutrient deficiencies secondary to bariatric surgery. *Curr Opin Clin Nutr Metab Care* 7:569–575.

Amatruda JM, Biddle TL, Patton ML, Lockwood DH. 1983. Vigorous supplementation of a hypocaloric diet prevents cardiac arrhythmias and mineral depletion. *Amer J Med* 74:1016–1022.

Amatruda JM, Richeson JF, Welle SL, Brodows RG, Lockwood DH. 1988. The safety and efficacy of a controlled low-energy ("very-low-calorie") diet in the treatment of non-insulin-dependent diabetes and obesity. *Arch Inter Med* 148:873–877.

Bloom WL. 1959. Fasting as an introduction to the treatment of obesity. *Metabolism* 8:214–220.

Bloomberg RD, Fleishman A, Nalle JE, Herron DM, Kini S. 2005. Nutritional Deficiencies following Bariatric Surgery: What Have We Learned? *Obes Surg* 15:145–154.

Cifuentes M, Riedt CS, Brolin RE, Field MP, Sherrell RM, Shapses SA. 2004. Weight loss and calcium intake influence calcium absorption in overweight postmenopausal women. *Am J Clin Nutr* 80:123–130.

Davidson MH, Hauptman J, DiGirolamo M, Foreyt JP, Halsted CH, Heber D, Heimburger DC, Lucas CP, Robbins DC, Chung J, Heymsfield SB. 1999. Weight control and risk factor reduction in obese subjects treated for 2 years with Orlistat: A randomized controlled trial. *JAMA* 281:235–242.

Freedman M, King J, Kennedy E. 2001. Popular diets: A scientific review. *Obesity Research Suppl* 1:1S–40S.

Isner JM, Sours HE, Paris AL, Ferrans VJ, Roberts WC. 1979. Sudden, unexpected death in avid dieters using the liquid-protein-modified-fast diet. *Circulation* 60:1401–1412.

Khanum S, Alam AN, Anwar I, Akbar Ali M, Mujibur Rahaman M. 1988. Effect of zinc supplementation on the dietary intake and weight gain of Bangladeshi children recovering from protein-energy malnutrition. *Eur J Clin Nutr* 42:709–714.

Lantigua RA, Amatruda JM, Biddle TL, Forbes GB. 1980. Cardiac arrhythmias associated with a liquid protein diet for the treatment of obesity. *Med Intell* 303:735–738.

Licata AA, Lantigua R, Amatruda J, Lockwood D. 1981. Adverse effects of liquid protein fast on the handling of magnesium, calcium and phosphorus. *Amer J Med* 71:767–772.

Linn R., Stuart SL. 1976. *The Last Chance Diet*. Secaucus, NJ: Lyle Stuart.

Lockwood DH, Amatruda JM. 1984. Very low calorie diets in the management of obesity. *Ann Rev Med* 35:373–381.

Michael RR, Sneider JS, Dickstein RA, Hagman HH, Eich RH. 1978. Sudden death in a patient on a liquid protein diet. *N Engl J Med* 298:1005–1007.

Ortega J, Sala C, Flor B, Jimenez E, Escudero D, Martinez-Valls J, Lledo S. 2004. Vertical banded gastroplasty converted to Roux-en-Y gastric bypass: Little impact on nutritional status after 5-year follow-up. *Obes Surg* 638–643.

Riedt CS, Cifuentes M, Stahl T, Chowdhury HA, Schlussel Y, Shapses SA. 2005. Overweight postmenopausal women lose Bone with moderate weight reduction and 1g/day calcium intake. *J Bone Miner Res* 20:455–463.

Rudman D, Millikan WJ, Richardson TJ, Bixler TJ, Stackhouse J, McGarrity WC. 1975. Elemental balances during intravenous hyperalimentation of underweight adult subjects. *J Clin Invest* 55: 94–104.

Schucker RE, Gunn WJ. 1978. *A National Survey of the Use of Protein Products in Conjunction with Weight Reduction Diets Among American Women*. Atlanta, GA: Centers for Disease Control and Prevention.

Simmer K, Khanum S, Carlsson L, Thompson RP. 1988. Nutritional rehabilitation in Bangladesh—the importance of zinc. *Am J Clin Nutr* 47:1036–1040.

Sours HE, Frattali VP, Brand CD, Feldman RA, Forbes AL, Swanson RC, Paris AL. 1981. Sudden death associated with very low calorie weight reduction regimens. *Am J Clin Nutr* 34:453–461.

Torgerson JS, Hauptman J, Boldrin MN, Sjostrom L. 2004. XENical in the prevention of diabetes in obese subjects (XENDOS) study: A randomized study of orlistat as an adjunct to lifestyle changes for the prevention of type 2 diabetes in obese patients. *Diabetes Care* 27:155–161.

Vasilaras TH, Astrup A, Raben A. 2004. Micronutrient intake in overweight subjects is not deficient on an ad libitum fat-reduced, high-simple carbohydrate diet. *Euro J Clin Nutr* 58:326–336.

Vertes V, Genuth SM, Hazelton IM. 1977. Supplemented fasting as a large scale outpatient program. *JAMA* 238:2151–2153.

# Protein Turnover and Mineral Metabolism

*Henry C. Lukaski*
*USDA-ARS Grand Forks Human Nutrition Research Center, Grand Forks, North Dakota*

## INTRODUCTION

Military personnel are regularly exposed to multiple stressors during operational training and combat. Factors including food restriction, sleep deprivation, increased physical activity, psychological stressors, harsh environments, and infection promote weight loss and body composition changes, as well as impairments in some biological functions and altered nutritional status (Baker-Fulco, 1995; Shippee, 1993). Decreases in lean body mass (Friedl et al., 2000) that parallel increases in the circulating concentrations of minerals, specifically intracellular cations, such as magnesium, zinc, and copper (Shippee, 1993), suggest an important link between protein turnover and mineral excretion.

This review examines the effects of stressors on indirect measures of protein catabolism and biochemical indices of mineral nutritional status. It describes findings in injured patients and the limited observations in healthy adults participating in controlled exercise and dietary interventions. A summary of the findings of intensive, military training under diverse conditions is provided. This information is assembled into a model that integrates experimental findings that link protein catabolism and mineral excretion.

## PROTEIN AND MINERAL METABOLISM AFTER INJURY

Following moderate to severe injury, there is a period of excess protein breakdown as measured by increased urinary excretion of nitrogen, creatinine potassium, phosphorus, sulfur, magnesium, and zinc (Cuthbertson et al., 1972). Urinary nitrogen was significantly correlated with urinary zinc, potassium, and creatinine (r = 0.46–0.66) in patients with different types of trauma. These findings suggest a general association between a marker of protein breakdown, nitrogen, and intramuscular cations and metabolites.

Supportive information comes from data in which patients were labeled with radioactive zinc ($^{65}Zn$) that was incorporated into skeletal muscle, a major reservoir of zinc, before elective surgery (Fell et al., 1973). Urinary nitrogen and zinc excretions increased 80 and 100 percent, respectively, after surgery; these outputs were significantly correlated (r = 0.84–0.98). Compared to pre-surgical values, fractional $^{65}Zn$ excretion increased significantly from 10 percent to 20 percent after surgery. The authors concluded that the zincuria indicated loss of muscle.

Additional evidence of accelerated muscle breakdown and zinc losses is available. Significant increases in urinary excretion of 3-methylhistidine, an index of myofibrillar protein breakdown (Munro and Young, 1978), creatinine and zinc were observed in patients either undergoing orthopedic surgery or in response to trauma (Threlfall et al., 1981). The outputs were related to the severity of injury and reached peak values seven days after injury or surgery. Other investigators (Askari et al., 1982; Berger et al., 1996) have confirmed these findings and emphasized the need for adequate zinc intake to accommodate the increased zinc losses.

## OTHER STRESSORS AFFECTING PROTEIN AND MINERAL METABOLISM

Whereas the effects of severe injury on increased protein breakdown and mineral excretion is well established, there is a paucity of information describing metabolic perturbations with stressors that impose mild and moderate injury. An area of interest is the effect of increased physical activity on protein and mineral metabolism.

### Endurance Exercise

Studies have examined the effects of intense, endurance exercise on zinc homeostasis. Compared to pre-exercise values, plasma zinc concentrations increased (5–10 percent) in men immediately after a bout of prolonged, endurance running (Anderson et al., 1984; Cordova and Alvarez-Mon, 1995; Van Rij et al., 1986). However, 2 hours after completing the exercise, plasma zinc concentrations decreased significantly. Exercise, however, was associated with significant increases in urinary zinc ranging from 20 to 40 percent compared to values determined on days without exercise. While it is speculated that the decrease in plasma zinc concentration may be related to zinc sequestration in liver and other soft tissues (Oh et al., 1978; Shinogi et al., 1999), the increase in urinary zinc is the result of muscle breakdown and mobilization from other stores. The impact of differences in dietary zinc, however, should not be dismissed because zinc intake was not assessed.

Stressors such as prolonged endurance exercise increase amino acid oxidation and urinary nitrogen excretion (Lemon, 1998). Unfortunately, studies that have investigated metabolic responses to endurance exercise have not concurrently determined indices of muscle protein breakdown and mineral excretion.

### Effects of Energy Deficit and Exercise

An experimental model that may provide insight into the effects of multiple stressors on protein and mineral metabolism is reduced energy intake and increased physical activity. Briefly, obese women were studied on a metabolic unit for five months (Lukaski, unpublished results). During the first 28 day period, they received a nutritionally balanced diet with energy sufficient to maintain admission body weight. Energy intake was reduced by 25 percent during the next 28 days, and then further reduced to 50 percent of maintenance levels for the following two 28 day periods. Aerobic physical activity increased progressively with the start of the energy restriction. Body weight decreased modestly (3 percent) with a 25 percent reduction in energy intake; it decreased (8 percent and 14 percent) significantly with an energy restriction of 50 percent of weight maintenance levels. Urinary nitrogen excretion increased significantly at the end of each period of 50 percent energy reduction (1.5 to 1.7 g/day). Urinary zinc output increased significantly (0.1 mg/day) in parallel with the restricted energy intake. These findings indicate a concomitant loss of muscle protein and zinc with a 50 percent reduction of energy intake required to maintain body weight and increased physical activity.

## SEMISTARVATION IN A MULTISTRESSOR ENVIRONMENT

Training of candidates for Special Forces such as Rangers exposes military personnel to semi-starvation, heavy energy expenditures and other psychological and physical challenges (Moore et al., 1992). A number of metabolic perturbations have been observed (Friedl et al., 2000; Shippee, 1993). Hormonal responses include a significant decrease in testosterone, thyroid hormones and insulin-like growth factor 1 (IGF-1), and a significant increase in cortisol concentrations in blood. Metabolic parameters also were impacted. Blood urea nitrogen, β-hydroxybutyrate and lactate increased significantly during training. Magnesium, copper, zinc, and ferritin increased significantly (12, 30, 25, and 70 percent, respectively) whereas iron decreased significantly (30 percent). Taken together, these findings indicate that the conditions of Ranger training promoted catabolism of body protein and mobilization of minerals as a result of many factors including food deprivation, injury, and inflammatory processes.

## LINK BETWEEN PROTEIN CATABOLISM AND MINERAL OUTPUT

Situations and conditions that expose humans to multiple stressors elicit hormonal and immune responses that adversely impact protein and mineral metabolism (Figure B-21). Hypocaloric intake increases catabolic hormones (glucagon, catecholamines, and cortisol) and decreases anabolic hormone (insulin and IGF-1) concentrations in the circulation (Keys et al., 1950). The magnitude of the caloric deficit, by restriction and increased energy expenditure, directly influences these

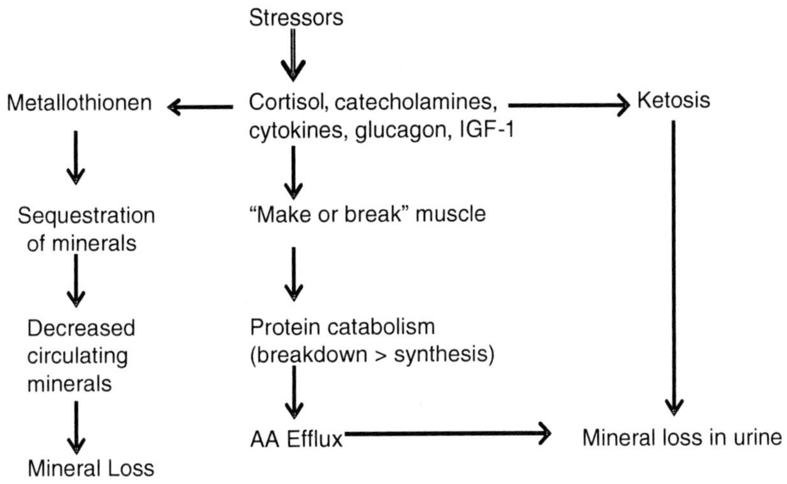


**FIGURE B-21** Effects of stress on protein turnover and mineral metabolism.
NOTE: AA = amino acids; IGF-1 = insulin-like growth factor-1.

hormonal responses. Similarly, inadequate energy intake and increased exercise, particularly in conjunction with injury, affect circulating cytokines. Tumor necrosis factor (TNF-α) and interleukin-1 (IL-1) and other immuno-regulatory proteins are involved in the acute phase response. Interestingly, IL-6 which is increased in response to exercise, is anti-inflammatory (Petersen and Pedersen, 2005). Because the circulating concentrations of these cytokines increase in response to energy stress, heavy exercise and injury, they, together with the catabolic hormones, up-regulate intracellular signal transduction pathways to increase protein catabolism and promote amino acid efflux (Glass, 2003; Tisdale, 2002). Caloric deprivation also increases fatty acid mobilization and promotes ketosis. Both amino acid efflux and ketosis increase mineral excretion in the urine.

Increases in circulating mineral concentrations stimulate metallothionein synthesis (Oh et al., 1978). Metallothionein removes minerals from the circulation and sequesters them in tissues such as the liver and kidney; it scavenges ionized minerals and reduces the potential for oxidative damage. The increase in synthesis of thionein requires about 2 hours. Thus, there is a period during which minerals are lost into the urine. However, with a half-life of 5–6 hours, metallothionein serves to attenuate loss of minerals acutely.

## SUMMARY AND CONCLUSIONS

Evidence from diverse sources indicates a clear link between muscle protein breakdown and losses of minerals. Studies in patients with acute phase response and healthy individuals participating in endurance exercise reveal increased losses of nitrogen and zinc in the urine. Obese adults participating in a program of energy restriction and increased aerobic physical activity also experience a similar pattern of increased urinary nitrogen and zinc loss. Studies of soldiers exposed to semi-starvation and other stressors show a hormonal pattern of increased catabolism and release of minerals into the circulation that suggests an increased loss of muscle and minerals, specifically zinc and magnesium, as part of an acute phase response.

There is a need to concurrently determine nutrient and mineral intakes, measures of mineral nutritional status, and losses together with hormonal and cytokine measurements in soldiers under conditions simulating strenuous training and operations. This information is needed to critically evaluate adequacy of minerals, particularly zinc and magnesium, in rations to compensate for losses during active training.

## DISCLAIMER

Mention of a trademark or proprietary product does not constitute a guarantee of the product by the United States Department of Agriculture and does not imply its approval to the exclusion of other products that may also be suitable. U.S. Department of Agriculture, Agricultural Research, Northern Plains Area is an equal opportunity/affirmative action employer and all agency services are available without discrimination.

## REFERENCES

Anderson RA, Polansky MM, Bryden NA. 1984. Strenuous running: Acute effects of chromium, copper, zinc, and selected clinical variables in urine and serum of male runners. *Biol Trace Elem Res* 6:327–336.

Askari A, Long CL, Blakemore WS. 1982. Net metabolic changes of zinc, copper, nitrogen, and potassium balances in skeletal trauma patients. *Metabolism* 31(12):1185–1193.

Baker-Fulco CJ. 1995. Overview of dietary intakes during military exercises. In: *Not Eating Enough*. Washington, DC: National Academy Press.

Berger MM, Cavadini C, Chiolero R, Dirren H. 1996. Copper, selenium and zinc status and balances after major trauma. *J Trauma* 40(1):103–109.

Cordova A, Alvarez-Mon M. 1995. Behavior of zinc in physical exercise: A special reference to immunity and fatigue. *Neurosci Biobehav Rev* 19(3):439–445.

Cuthbertson DP, Fell GS, Smith CM, Tilstone WJ. 1972. Metabolism after injury. I. Effects of severity, nutrition, and environmental temperature on protein, potassium, zinc, and creatine. *Br J Surg* 59(12):925–931

Fell GS, Fleck A, Cuthbertson DP, Queen K, Morrison C, Bessent RG, Husain SL. 1973. Urinary zinc levels as an indication of muscle catabolism. *Lancet* Feb. 10, 1(7798):280–282.

Friedl KE, Moore RJ, Hoyt RW, Marchitelli LJ, Martinez-Lopez LE, Askew EW. 2000. Endocrine markers of semistarvation in healthy lean men in a multistressor environment. *J Appl Physiol* 88:1820–1830.

Glass DJ. 2003. Molecular mechanisms modulating muscle mass. *Trends Mol Med* 9:344–350.

Keys A, Brozek J, Henschel A, Mickelsen O, Taylor HL.1950. *The Biology of Human Starvation*. Minneapolis, MN: University of Minnesota Press, vols. 1 and 2.
Lemon PWR. 1998. Effects of exercise on dietary protein requirements. *Int J Sport Nutr* 8(4): 426–447.
Moore RJ, Friedl KE, Tulley RT, Askew EW. 1993. Maintenance of iron status in healthy men during an extended period of stress and physical activity. *Am J Clin Nutr* 58:923–927.
Munro HN, Young VR. 1978. Urinary excretion of N gamma-methylhistidine (3-methylhistidine): a tool to study metabolic responses in relation to nutrient and hormonal status in health and disease of man. *Am J Clin Nutr* 31(9):1608–1614.
Oh SH, Deagen JT, Whanger PD, Weswig PH. 1978. Biological function of metallothionein. V. Its induction in rats by various stressors. *Am J Physiol* 234(3):E282–E285.
Petersen AMW, Pedersen BK. 2005. The anti-inflammatory effect of exercise. *J Appl Physiol* 98(4):1154–1162.
Shinogi M, Sakaridani M, Yokoyama I. 1999. Metallothionein induction in rat liver by dietary restriction or exercise and reduction of exercise-induced hepatic lipid peroxidation. *Biol Pharm Bull* 22(2):132–136.
Shippee RL. 1993. Nutritional status and immune function of Ranger trainees given increased caloric intake. Briefing for the National Academy of Sciences. In: Marriott BM, ed. Review of the Results of Nutritional Intervention, US Army Ranger Training Class 11/92 (Ranger II). Washington, DC: National Academy Press. Pp. 86–104.
Threlfall CJ, Stoner HB, Galasko CS. 1981. Patterns in the excretion of muscle markers after trauma and orthopedic surgery. *J Trauma* 21(2):140–147.
Tisdale MJ. 2002. Biochemical mechanisms of cellular catabolism. *Curr Opin Clin Nutr Metabol* 5(4):401–405.
Van Rij AM, Hall MT, Dohm GL, Bray JT, Pories WJ. 1986. Changes in zinc metabolism following exercise in human subjects. *Biol Trace Elem Res* 10:99–101.

# Physical Activity and Tyrosine Supplementation: Two Effective Interventions Against Stress-Induced Immunosuppression

*Monika Fleshner*
*University of Colorado, Boulder*

## INTRODUCTION

### Excessive Sympathetic Nervous System Output Is Detrimental to Health

Stimulation of the sympathetic nervous system (SNS) is a hallmark of the acute stress response (Goldstein, 1987). SNS activation has many physiological consequences such as increased heart rate, respiration and blood flow to muscles, that work in concert to promote the "fight or flight" response (Goldstein, 1996; Jansen et al., 1995). SNS activation is a powerful feature of the acute stress response that is adaptive when the response is acute and constrained. If, however, SNS activation is frequent or excessive, it can produce negative health consequences (Seals and Dinenno, 2004). For example, chronically elevated SNS responses are believed to mechanistically contribute to the etiology of "metabolic syndrome," a key antecedent to clinical atherosclerotic diseases that include visceral adiposity, glucose intolerance, insulin resistance, dyslipidemia and hypertension (Baron, 1990; Julius et al., 1992; Lind and Lithell, 1993). In addition, it has been reported in both the human and animal literatures that chronic or excessive SNS activation can lead to arterial wall thickening (Chen et al., 1995; Pauletto et al., 1991; Xin et al., 1997), hypertension (Lind and Lithell, 1993), α- and β- adrenergic receptor desensitization (Abrass, 1986; Dinenno et al., 2002; Xiao and Lakatta, 1992) and immunosuppression (Irwin, 1993; Kennedy et al., 2005a). The negative consequences of frequent or excessive SNS activity have been convincingly demonstrated in transgenic mice lacking functional $\alpha_{2A}$ adrenergic receptor (ADR) autoinhibition in the midbrain. Due to the lack of normal $\alpha_{2A}$ADR central nervous constraint on SNS drive, these mice have chronically activated peripheral SNS responses and rapidly develop cardiac dysfunction (Baum et al., 2002).

## Stress Modulates Immune Function

Exposure to physical or psychological stress modulates the immune response (Adell et al., 1988; Laudenslager, 1994; Maier et al., 1994; Plotnikoff, 1991). Stress is neither globally immunosuppressive nor immunopotentiating, but rather immunomodulatory. Factors that impact the effect of stress on the immune response include the following: the duration and intensity of stressor exposure (Monjan, 1976); the perceived controllability of the stressor (Laudenslager, 1983); the timing and measure of the immune response (e.g., days versus hours, acquired versus innate (Deak et al., 1999; Fleshner et al., 1998); and the physiological state of the organism (e.g., young versus old, anxious versus calm, healthy versus ill, and physically active versus sedentary (Ader et al., 1991; Bonneau 1997; Brown, 1988; Dishman, 1995; Fleshner et al., 2002; Moraska and Fleshner, 2001).

## Animal Model of Acute Stress

My laboratory has been studying the behavioral and physiological consequences of exposure to a well-characterized animal model of stress. This model of stress involves exposing rats to random, intermittent (average intertrial interval of 60 seconds), inescapable tailshocks (100 shocks of 1.6mA for a duration of 5 seconds), administered when the rats are lightly restrained in Plexiglas tubes. The use of this stressor is important for several reasons. First, a great deal is known about the behavioral, neural, endocrine, and immunological consequences of exposure to this acute stressor (Brennan, 1995, 1996; Campisi and Fleshner, 2003; Campisi et al., 2002, 2003; Day et al., 2004; Deak, 1997, 1999; Deak et al., 1997; Fleshner et al., 1993, 1995a,b,c,d, 1998, 2002; Gazda et al.,

2003; Greenwood et al., 2003a,b; Laudenslager, 1994; Maier, 1998; Maier et al., 1994; Milligan et al., 1998; Moraska and Fleshner, 2001; Moraska et al., 2002; Nguyen, 1998; Nguyen et al., 1998, 2000; O'Conner, 1999; Watkins, 1990). Second, the effects of acute stressor exposure on immune function are stressor dependent (Ader et al., 1991; Plotnikoff, 1991), therefore the use of a consistent stressor is necessary to advance our understanding of the mechanism responsible for stress-induced immunomodulation. Third, tail-shock stress allows the administration of a discrete, consistent, and quantifiable stressor that does not produce physical injury.

## SUPRESSION OF ACQUIRED IMMUNITY BY STRESS

### In Vivo Generation of Antibody Against Keyhole Limpet Hemocyanin as a Measure of Acquired Immunity

Acquired immunity is characterized by two primary features, exquisite antigen specificity and immunological memory. The effector cells of the acquired immune response include T cells and B cells. Our assessment of acquired immune function has been the generation of an immunoglobulin response to keyhole limpet hemocyanin (αKLH Ig). This measure of immune function has both experimental advantages, as well as clinical relevance that include the following: (1) the cells involved with the generation of this response remain in the hormonal milieu of the organism; (2) the kinetics of the developing response can be easily monitored; (3) use of a benign protein does not produce the behavioral confounds associated with the generation of sickness; (4) antibody reflects a functionally important end product of the immune system; (5) measurement of the antigen specific antibody response more accurately reflects the function of acquired immunity; (6) measurement of αKLH Ig is quantifiable making the results directly comparable across studies; (7) the cells involved with this response are T cells and B cells, two primary players in acquired immune responses; (8) the antibody response generated against KLH is similar to the immunological response generated after vaccination to tetanus toxoid; (9) a reduction in specific antibodies to bacteria, virus, or soluble toxin could render the organism more susceptible to disease caused by these pathogens; (10) KLH is clinically relevant because it is used as a immunotherapeutic in the treatment of cancer (Gilewski, 1996; Jurincic-Winkler, 1995, 1996; Lamm, 1993; Livingston, 1995), and stress-induced modulation of the antibody response to KLH could affect the efficacy of this type of vaccination and immunotherapy. Finally, results from measuring responses to KLH in animals can be easily tested in humans (Smith et al., 2004).

### Spleen Is Site for Stress-Induced KLH Antibody Suppression

Rats that are immunized with KLH and exposed to a single session of inescapable tailshock have a long-term (+ 21 days) reduction in serum levels of αKLH IgM, IgG and IgG2a (Fleshner et al., 1995d, 1998; Gazda et al., 2003; Laudenslager et al., 1988). We know that the final site of stress-induced immunomodulation is the spleen because if we remove the spleen from adult male rats prior to intraperitoneal immunization with KLH and stressor exposure, we eliminate the stress-induced reduction in αKLH Ig (Fleshner, 2005). Importantly, the stress-associated suppressive effect is specific to the generation of antibody to the antigen. Total serum IgM and IgG is not reduced (Fleshner et al., 1992; Smith et al., 2004).

### Cellular Mechanisms of Stress-Induced KLH Antibody Suppression

The generation of an antibody response to a T cell dependent soluble protein, such as KLH, involves the interaction of antigen presenting cells (APC; B cells or dendritic cells), T helper cells (Th) and B cells. Following intraperitoneal injection of KLH, antigen is transported to the draining lymph nodes and spleen. B cells expressing the B cell receptor that bind KLH must receive T cell help from the KLH-specific T helper cells in the form of co-stimulation and cytokines. The Th "help" facilitates B cell proliferation, B cell differentiation into antibody secreting cells (Clark and Ledbetter, 1994; Foy et al., 1996), and Ig isotype switching (IgM to IgG or IgG2a, [Stevens et al., 1988]). The proliferation of KLH-specific Th and B cells is greatest in the draining lymph nodes and spleen 4–7 days after KLH injection (Fleshner et al., 1995d, 1998; Gazda et al., 2003). Using flow cytometric analysis (Fleshner et al., 1995a; Fleshner et al., 1998), ELISPOT (Laudenslager, 1994), and antigen-specific proliferative assays (Gazda et al., 2003), we have determined that the suppression in αKLH Ig is likely due to a failure of the stressed rats to increase KLH-specific T helper cell numbers (Fleshner et al., 1995a, 1998). With fewer αKLH T helper cells, there is less T cell help, and fewer KLH-specific B in the spleen (Laudenslager, 1994). Fewer KLH-specific B cells lead to a reduction in serum αKLH Ig. Thus, tailshock-induced suppression of αKLH Ig is a well-characterized animal model of stress-induced immunosuppression.

### Excessive Sympathetic Nervous System Response Suppresses Acquired Immunity

Although the specific mechanism responsible for stress-induced suppression of αKLH Ig remains under investigation, excessive SNS output likely plays a role. Most primary and secondary lymphoid tissues (including the spleen) receive dense SNS innervation (Felten, 1987; Meltzer, 1997) and Th cells (Kohm and Sanders, 2000, 2001; Sanders, 1997; Swanson et al., 2001), B cells (Kasprowicz et al., 2000; Kohm et al., 2002; Podojil and Sanders, 2003; Podojil et al., 2004) and monocytes-macrophages-dendritic cells (Takahashi et al., 2004) express adrenergic receptors $\beta_2$ADR. If we focus on the role of the SNS in stress-induced immunomodulation, there is evidence that SNS contributes to stress-induced suppression of specifically the $\alpha$KLH Ig response (Irwin, 1993). Although earlier work suggested that high concentrations of norepinephrine (NE) could suppress various aspects of immunity, more recent data support the hypothesis that splenic NE depletion, not circulating or splenic NE elevation, may be responsible for stress-induced suppression of *in vivo* $\alpha$KLH Ig responses.

There are several lines of evidence to support this shift in dogma from "too much NE" to "too little NE." First, if one examines the past literature demonstrating that high levels of NE are immunosuppressive, many studies were done in vitro, examined mitogen-stimulated proliferative or cytokine responses, and tested pharmacological concentrations of NE (Malarkey et al., 2002; Ramer-Quinn, 1997). Under these circumstances, NE suppresses immune function and can be fatal to immune cells (Del Rey et al., 2003). Second, activation status of the immune cells was rarely considered in these earlier studies. For example, it was recently reported that modulation of dendritic cell function following NE exposure occurred only in the early phases of dendritic cell activation (Maestroni, 2002), and $\beta_2$ADR are differentially expressed on naïve versus stimulated B cells (Sanders et al., 2003). Thus, past research supporting a simple view that too much NE is responsible for stress-induced suppression of *in vivo* immune responses has limitations.

Recent evidence is consistent with the dogmatic shift that too little NE may be responsible for stress-induced suppression of *in vivo* antibody responses and that dynamic interactions between SNS and immune cells occur to produce optimal Ig responses. For example, during the generation of an *in vivo* antibody response to KLH, NE is released from peripheral nerves innervating the spleen (Kohm et al., 2000). NE binding to the B cell $\beta_2$ADR stimulates the expression of costimulatory molecules (Kohm et al., 2002), Ig production (Kasprowicz et al., 2000), and splenic germinal center formation (Kohm, 1999). In addition, splenic NE depletion produced by surgical denervation (Fleshner, 2006), pharmacological lesion [6-OHDA,] (Kohm and Sanders, 1999) or pharmacological competition ($\alpha$-methyl-p-tyrosine (Kennedy et al., 2005b) prior to immunization with KLH reduces the antibody response. Thus, splenic NE depletion in the absence of stress is sufficient to supress $\alpha$KLH Ig. Furthermore, central activation of the SNS in the absence of stressor exposure with an $\alpha_{2A}$ADR antagonist (Mirtazapine, Mirt) that acts in the brain to release the SNS from $\alpha_{2A}$ADR-mediated inhibition (Dazzi et al., 2002), elevates blood NE for longer duration and to a higher level than that produced by stress. Yet, in spite of high blood concentrations of NE at the time of immunization, Mirt produces neither splenic NE depletion nor $\alpha$KLH Ig suppression (Kennedy et al., 2005b). Blood NE is derived from spillover of NE released by nerve terminals in sympathetically innervated tissues. We speculate that the lack of splenic NE depletion in spite of equal or greater blood concentration on NE after Mirt injection may be due to a more global, whole body activation of the SNS; whereas tailshock stress may activate more selective central SNS circuits (Greenwood et al., 2003b) perhaps excessively driving SNS output to select tissues such as the spleen.

## BEHAVIORAL AND PHARMACOLOGICAL INTERVENTIONS TO PREVENT STRESS-RELATED ADVERSE EFFECTS ON IMMUNE SYSTEM

### Introduction

Based on our results it follows that to prevent the negative consequences of activation of the acute stress response one would need interventions that prevent splenic NE depletion by either (1) constraining excessive SNS output or (2) providing additional substrate to prevent splenic NE depletion in the face of intense SNS drive. Such approaches are optimal because they would not eliminate SNS responses. In that way, the stressed organism could reap the positive physiological effects of SNS activation but avoid the negative immunological consequences of excessive SNS activation and splenic NE depletion. We have evidence that exercise and tyrosine supplementation are both possible interventions that satisfy this goal.

### Physical Activity Constrains SNS Activation

We have conducted a series of studies investigating the impact of tailshock on various aspects of the stress response including SNS activation, splenic NE depletion and αKLH Ig suppression. Physical active status was varied in these studies by housing animals with either a mobile or locked running wheels. In these conditions, male F344 rats will run an average distance of 15 km/week (Campisi et al., 2003; Greenwood et al., 2003a,b). Nearly 100 percent of their running occurs during the dark part of their circadian cycle (Solberg, 1999). This level of activity produces physiological changes that are indicative of "metabolic fitness". In some rat strains, wheel running reduces body weight gain (Noble et al., 1999), body fatness (Podolin, 1999), triglycerides concentrations (Suzuki, 1995), and increases lipid metabolism (Podolin, 1999), HDL/LDL ratio (Kennedy et al., 2005a), muscular hypertrophy (triceps and plantaris (Ishihara et al., 1998), red blood cell hemoglobin content (Kennedy et al., 2005a), and endurance.

Animals that lived sedentary life styles with locked running wheels, and were exposed to tailshock stress, had excessive SNS responses leading to splenic NE depletion and αKLH Ig suppression (Kennedy et al., 2005b). In contrast, rats that were physically active for 6 weeks prior to exposure to tailshock stress,

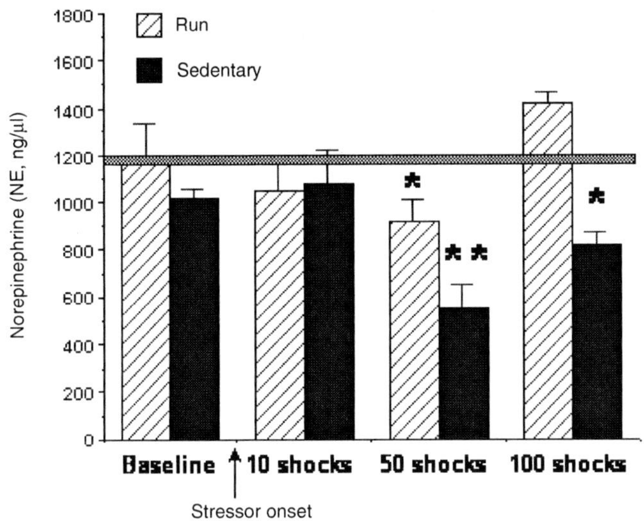


**FIGURE B-22** Effect of Physical Activity (freewheel running) on supression of stress-induced (10, 50, or 100 5-second, 1.6mA tailshocks) splenic NE depletion in adult male F344 rats. (*$P < 0.05$).
SOURCE: Greenwood et al. (2003b).

had constrained SNS responses such that tailshock elevated blood levels of NE but did not drive the response excessively, did not lead to splenic NE depletion (Figure B-22) and did not produce αKLH Ig suppression (Figure B-23) (Greenwood et al., 2003b; Moraska and Fleshner, 2001). Thus, physical activity prevented the negative effects of acute stress on acquired immunity by constraining SNS drive (Fleshner, 2005).

## Tyrosine Supplementation Prevents Stress-Induced Splenic NE Depletion

Tyrosine is a precursor for the synthesis of NE (and dopamine, DA), and during times of intense SNS drive can be rate limiting (Acworth et al., 1988; Gibson and Wurtman, 1977; Milner and Wurtman, 1987). It has been previously reported in rats that tyrosine administration can prevent stress-induced brain NE depletion (Lehnert et al., 1984) and stress-induced behavioral deficits (Brady et al., 1980; Reinstein et al., 1984). In addition, tyrosine supplementation has been used to reduce headaches, tension and fatigue in men exposed to cold stress (Banderet and Lieberman, 1989) and more recently tyrosine was used to reduce elevated blood pressure associated with combat training (Deijen and Orlebeke, 1994; Deijen et al., 1999). The possible effect that tyrosine could have in humans on stress-induced immunosupression has yet to be tested.

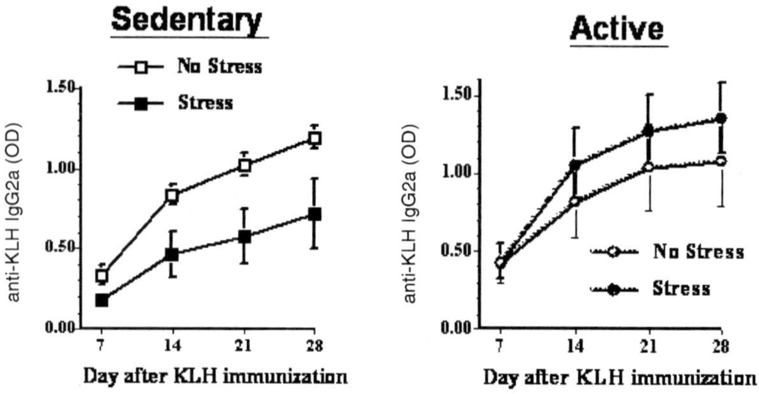


**FIGURE B-23** Prevention of stress-induced (tailshocks) supression of anti-keyhole limpet hemocyanin (KLH) IgG2a by physical exercise on running wheels in rats ($P < 0.01$). Physically active rats exposed to stress were protected against stress-induced immunosuppression.
SOURCE: Moraska and Fleshner (2001).

Using our animal model of stress-induced immunosuppression, we have recently reported (Kennedy et al., 2005b) that rats treated with tyrosine (400 mg/kg) 30 minutes prior to stressor exposure are protected from both stress-induced splenic NE depletion (Figure B-24) and αKLH Ig suppression (Figure B-25). In this study we also replicated the previous findings that tyrosine presents stress-induced brain NE depletion. Importantly, blood concentrations of NE in the tyrosine treated stressed rats were equal to saline treated stressed rats, yet tyrosine completely prevented the suppression in αKLH Ig. These data further support our hypothesis that stress-induced suppression of αKLH Ig requires splenic NE depletion and not circulating NE elevation (Kennedy et al., 2005b).

## CONCLUSION

The data presented here support the hypothesis that stress-induced immunosuppression is due to excessive activation of the sympathetic nervous system (SNS). Future work should strive to further develop interventions, such as exercise and tyrosine supplementation, that allow us to reap the positive physiological effects, while minimizing the maladaptive consequences, of activation of the acute SNS stress response.

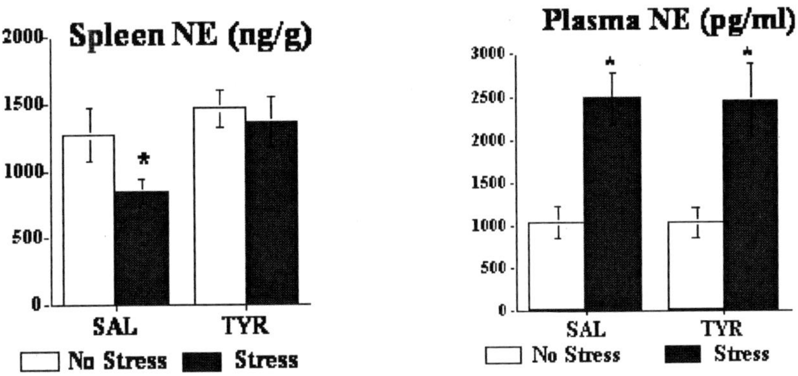


**FIGURE B-24** Prevention of stress-induced (tailshocks) splenic NE depletion by tyrosin (TYR) in rats. Prior injection of tyrosine before stressor exposure fully prevented splenic NE depletion. Stress also increased plasma concentrations of plasma NE and tyrosine treatment did not change this effect (*P < 0.01).
SOURCE: Kennedy et al. (2005b).

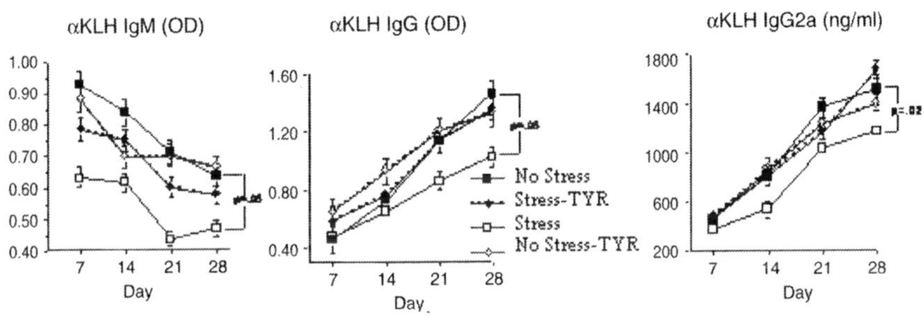


**FIGURE B-25** Prevention of stress-induced (tailshocks) KLH antibody (αKLH IgM, IgG and IgG2a) suppression by tyrosin (TYR) in rats. Prior injection of tyrosine before stressor exposure fully prevented the stress-induced immunosuppression (*P < 0.01).
SOURCE: Kennedy et al. (2005b).

## REFERENCES

Abrass IB. 1986. Catecholamine levels and adrenergic responsiveness in aging. In: Horan MJ, Steinberg GM, Dunbar JB, Hadley EC, eds. *NIH Blood Pressure Regulation and Aging*. New York: Biomedical Information Corporation.

Acworth IN, During MJ, Wurtman RJ. 1988. Tyrosine: Effects on catecholamine release. *Brain Res Bull* 21(3):473–477.

Adell A, Garcia-Marquez C, Armario A, Gelpi E. 1988. Chronic stress increases serotonin and noradrenaline in rat brain and sensitizes their responses to a further acute stress. *J Neurochem* 50(6):1678–1681.

Ader R, Felten DL, Cohen N. 1991. *Psychoneuroimmunology*. New York: Academic Press.

Banderet LE, Lieberman HR. 1989. Treatment with tyrosine, a neurotransmitter precursor, reduces environmental stress in humans. *Brain Res Bull* 22(4):759–762.

Baron A, Laakso M, Brechtel G, Hoit B, Watt C, Edelman S. 1990. Reduced postprandial skeltal muscle blood flow contributes to glucose intolerance in human obesity. *J Clin Endocrinol Metab* 70:1525–1533.

Baum PC, Kosek J, Patterson A, Bernstein D, Kobilka B. 2002. Abnormal cardiac function associated with sympathetic nervous system hyperactivity in mice. *Am J Physio* 283:H1838–H1845.

Bonneau RH, Brehm MA, Kern AM. 1997. The impact of psychological stress on the efficacy of anti-viral adoptive immunotherapy in an immunocomprimised host. *J Neurochem* 78:19–33.

Brady K, Brown JW, Thurmond JB. 1980. Behavioral and neurochemical effects of dietary tyrosine in young and aged mice following cold-swim stress. *Pharmacol Biochem Behav* 12(5):667–674.

Brennan FX, Fleshner M, Deak T, Watkins LR, Maier SF. 1995. Stress may suppress specific immunity by stimulating macrophages. *Society for Neuroscience Abstracts*.

Brennan FX, Fleshner M, Watkins LR, Maier SF. 1996. Macrophage stimulation reduces the cholesterol levels of stressed and unstressed rats. *Life Sci* 58:1771–1776.

Brown JD, Siegal JM. 1988. Exercise as a buffer of life stress: A prospective study of adolescent health. *Health Psychol* 7(4):341–353.

Campisi J, Fleshner M. 2003. Role of extracellular HSP72 in acute stress-induced potentiation of innate immunity in active rats. *J Appl Physiol* 94(1):43–52.

Campisi J, Leem TH, Fleshner M. 2002. Acute stress decreases inflammation at the site of infection. A role for nitric oxide. *Physiol Behav* 77(2–3):291–299.

Campisi J, Leem TH, Greenwood BN, Hansen MK, Moraska A, Higgins K, Smith TP, Fleshner M. 2003. Habitual physical activity facilitates stress-induced HSP72 induction in brain, peripheral, and immune tissues. *Am J Physiol Regul Integr Comp Physiol* 284(2):R520–R530.

Chen L, Xin X, Eckhart AD, Yang N, Faber JE. 1995. Regulation of vascular smooth muscle growth by alpha 1-adrenorecepotr subtypes in vitro and in vivo. *J. Biol. Chem* 270:30980–30988.

Clark EA, Ledbetter JA. 1994. How B and T cells talk to each other. *Nature* 367(6462):425–428.

Day HE, Greenwood BN, Hammack SE, Watkins LR, Fleshner M, Maier SF, Campeau S. 2004. Differential expression of 5HT-1A, alpha 1b adrenergic, CRF-R1, and CRF-R2 receptor mRNA in serotonergic, gamma-aminobutyric acidergic, and catecholaminergic cells of the rat dorsal raphe nucleus. *J Comp Neurol* 474(3):364–378.

Dazzi L, Ladu S, Spiga F, Vacca G, Rivano A, Pira L, Biggio G. 2002. Chronic treatment with imipramine or mirtazapine antagonizes stress- and FG7142-induced increase in cortical norepinephrine output in freely moving rats. *Synapse* 43(1):70–77.

Deak T, Meriwether JL, Fleshner M, Spencer RL, Abouhamze A, Moldawer LL, Grahn RE, Watkins LR, Maier SF. 1997. Evidence that brief stress may induce the acute phase response in rats. *Am J Physiol* 273(6 Pt 2):R1998–R2004.

Deak T, Nguyen KT, Fleshner M, Watkins LR, Maier SF. 1999. Acute stress may facilitate recovery from a subcutaneous bacterial challenge. *Neuroimmunomodulation* 6(5):344–354.

Deijen JB, Orlebeke JF. 1994. Effect of tyrosine on cognitive function and blood pressure under stress. *Brain Res Bull* 33(3):319–323.

Deijen JB, Wientjes CJ, Vullinghs HF, Cloin PA, Langefeld JJ. 1999. Tyrosine improves cognitive performance and reduces blood pressure in cadets after one week of a combat training course. *Brain Res Bull* 48(2):203–209.

Del Rey A, Kabiersch A, Petzoldt S, Besedovsky HO. 2003. Sympathetic abnormalities during autoimmune processes: Potential relevance of noradrenaline-induced apoptosis. *Ann N Y Acad Sci* 992:158–167.

Dinenno FA, Dietz NM, Joyner MJ. 2002. Aging and forearm postjunctional alpha-adrenergic vasoconstriction in healthy men. *Circulation* 106:1349–1354.

Dishman RK, Warren JM, Youngstedt SD, Yoo H, Bunnell BN, Mougey EH. 1995. Activity-wheel running attenuates suppression of natural killer cell activity after footshock. *J Appl Physiol* 78(4):1547–1554.

Felten DL, Ackerman KD, Wiegand SJ, Felten SY. 1987. Noradrenergic sympathetic innervation of the spleen I. Nerve fibers associate with lymphocytes and macrophages in specific compartments of the splenic white pulp. J *Neurosci Res* 18:28–36.

Felten SY, Olschowka J. 1987. Noradrenergic sympathetic innervation of the spleen II: Tyrosine hydroxylase (TH)- posititive nerve terminals from synaptic-like contacts on lymphocytes in splenic white pulp. *J Neurosci Res* 18:37–42.

Fleshner M. 2005. Physical activity & stress resistance: Sympathetic nervous system adaptations prevent stress-induced immunosuppression. *Exerc Sports Sci Rev* 33:120–126.

Fleshner M. 2006. Stress-induced sympathetic nervous activation contributes to both suppressed acquired and potentiated innate immunity: The role of splenic NE depletion and extracellular Hsp72. In: Welsh J, Meagher M, Sternberg E, eds. N*eural and Norendocrine Mechanisms in Host Defense and Autoimmunity*. New York: Kluwer Academic/Plenum Publishers: in press.

Fleshner M, Watkins LR, Lockwood LL, Bellgrau D, Laudenslager ML, Maier SF. 1992. Specific changes in lymphocyte subpopulations: A potential mechanism for stress-induced immunomodulation. *J Neuroimmunol* 41(2):131–142.

Fleshner M, Watkins LR, Lockwood LL, Brossard C, Laudenslager ML, Maier SF. 1993. Blockade of the hypothalamic-pituitary-adrenal response to stress by intraventricular injection of Dexamethasone: A method for studying the stress-induced peripheral effects of Glucocorticoids. *Psychoneuroendocrinology* 18(4):251–263.

Fleshner M, Bellgrau D, Watkins LR, Laudenslager ML, Maier SF. 1995a. Stress-induced reduction in the rat mixed lymphocyte reaction is due to macrophages and not to changes in T cell phenotypes. *J Neuroimmunol* 56(1):45–52.

Fleshner M, Deak T, Spencer RL, Laudenslauger ML, Watkins LR, Maier SF. 1995b. A long term increase in basal levels of corticosterone and a decrease in corticosteroid-binding globulin after acute stressor exposure. *Endocrinology* 136(12):5336–5342.

Fleshner M, Goehler LE, Hermann J, Relton JK, Maier SF, Watkins LR. 1995c. Subdiaphramatic vagotomy blocks hypothalamic NE depletion and attenuates serum corticosterone elevation produced by IL-1. *Brain Res Bul* 37:605–610.

Fleshner M, Hermann J, Lockwood LL, Laudenslager ML, Watkins LR, Maier SF. 1995d. Stressed rats fail to expand the CD45RC+CD4+ (Th1-like) T cell subset in response to KLH: Possible involvement of IFN-gamma. *Brain Behav Immun* 9(2):101–112.

Fleshner M, Nguyen KT, Cotter CS, Watkins LR, Maier SF. 1998. Acute stressor exposure both suppresses acquired immunity and potentiates innate immunity. *Am J Physiol* 275(3 Pt 2):R870–R878.

Fleshner M, Campisi J, Deak T, Greenwood BN, Kintzel JA, Leem TH, Smith TP, Sorensen B. 2002. Acute stressor exposure facilitates innate immunity more in physically active than in sedentary rats. *Am J Physiol Regul Integr Comp Physiol* 282(6):R1680–R1686.

Foy TM, Aruffo A, Bajorath J, Buhlmann JE, Noelle RJ. 1996. Immune regulation by CD40 and its ligand GP39. *Annu Rev Immunol* 14:591–617.

Gazda LS, Smith T, Watkins LR, Maier SF, Fleshner M. 2003. Stressor exposure produces long-term reductions in antigen specific T and B cell responses. *Stress* 6(4):259–267.

Gibson CJ, Wurtman RJ. 1977. Physiological control of brain catechol synthesis by brain tyrosine concentration. *Biochem Pharmacol* 26(12):1137–1142.

Gilewski T, Adluri R, Zhang S, Houghton A, Norton L, Livingston P. 1996. Preliminary results: Vaccination of breat cancer patients (pts) lacking identifiable disease (NED) with MUC-1-keyhole limpet hemocyanin (KLH) conjugate and QS21. *Proceedings of the Annual Meeting of the American Society of Clinical Oncology* 15:A1807.

Goldstein DS. 1987. Stress-induced activation of the sympathetic nervous system. *Baillieres Clin Endocrinol Metab* 1(2):253–278.

Goldstein DS. 1996. The sympathetic nervous system and the 'fight-or-flight' response: Outmoded ideas? *Mol Psychiatry* 1(2):95–97.

Greenwood BN, Foley TE, Day HE, Campisi J, Hammack SH, Campeau S, Maier SF, Fleshner M. 2003a. Freewheel running prevents learned helplessness/behavioral depression: Role of dorsal raphe serotonergic neurons. *J Neurosci* 23(7):2889–2898.

Greenwood BN, Kennedy S, Smith TP, Campeau S, Day HE, Fleshner M. 2003b. Voluntary freewheel running selectively modulates catecholamine content in peripheral tissue and c-Fos expression in the central sympathetic circuit following exposure to uncontrollable stress in rats. *Neuroscience* 120(1):269–281.

Irwin M. 1993. Brain corticotropin-releasing hormone and interleukin-1 beta-induced suppression of specific antibody production. *Endocrinology* 133:1352–1360.

Ishihara A, Roy RR, Ohira Y, Ibata Y, Edgerton VR. 1998. Hypertrophy of rat plantaris muscle fibers after voluntary running with increasing loads. *Journal of Applied Physiology* 84(6):2183–2189.

Jansen AS, Nguyen XV, Karpitskiy V, Mettenleiter TC, Loewy AD. 1995. Central command neurons of the sympathetic nervous system: basis of the fight-or-flight response. *Science* 270(5236): 644–646.

Julius S, Gudbrandsson T, Jamerson K, Andersson O. 1992. The interconnection between sympathetics, microcirculation, and insulin resistance in hypertension. *Blood Pressure* 1:9–19.

Jurincic-Winkler C, Metz KA, Beuth J, Sippel J, Klippel KF. 1995. Effect of keyhole limpet hemocyanin (KLH) and bacillus Calmette-Guerin (BCG) instillation on carcinoma in situ of the urinary bladder. *Anticancer Research* 15(6B):2771–2776.

Jurincic-Winkler C, von der Kammer H, Beuth J, Scheit KH, Klippel KF. 1996. Antibody response to keyhole limpet hemocyanin (KLH) treatment in patients with superficial bladder carcinoma. *Anticancer Research* 16(4A):2105–2110.

Kasprowicz DJ, Kohm AP, Berton MT, Chruscinski AJ, Sharpe A, Sanders VM. 2000. Stimulation of the B cell receptor, CD86 (B7-2), and the beta 2-adrenergic receptor intrinsically modulates the level of IgG1 and IgE produced per B cell. *J Immunol* 165(2):680–690.

Kennedy S, Smith TP, Fleshner M. 2005a. Resting cellular and physiological effects of wheel running. *Med Sci Sports Exerc* 63:79–83.

Kennedy SL, Nickerson M, Campisi J, Johnson JD, Smith TP, Sharkey C, Fleshner M. 2005b. Splenic norepinephrine depletion following acute stress suppresses in vivo antibody response. *Journal of Neuroimmunology* 165:150–160.

Kohm AP, Sanders VM. 2000. Norepinephrine: A messenger from the brain to the immune system. *Immunol Today* 21(11):539–542.

Kohm AP, Sanders VM. 2001. Norepinephrine and beta 2-adrenergic receptor stimulation regulate CD4+ T and B lymphocyte function in vitro and in vivo. *Pharmacol Rev* 53(4):487–525.

Kohm AP, Tang Y, Sanders VM, Jones SB. 2000. Activation of antigen-specific CD4+ Th2 cells and B cells in vivo increases norepinephrine release in the spleen and bone marrow. *J Immunol* 165(2):725–733.

Kohm AP, Mozaffarian A, Sanders VM. 2002. B cell receptor- and beta 2-adrenergic receptor-induced regulation of B7-2 (CD86) expression in B cells. *J Immunol* 168(12):6314–6322.

Lamm DL, DeHaven JI, Riggs DR, Ebert RF. 1993. Immunotherapy of murine bladder cancer with keyhole limpet hemocyanin. *Journal of Urology* 149(3):648–652.

Laudenslager ML, Fleshner M. 1994. Stress and Immunity: Of mice, monkeys, models, and mechanisms. In: Glaser R, Kiecolt-Glaser J, eds. *The Handbook of Human Stress and Immunity*. New York: Academic Press. Pp. 161–181.

Laudenslager ML, Ryan SM, Drugen RL, Hyson RL, Maier SF. 1983. Coping and immunosuppression: Inescapable but not escapable shock suppresses lymphocyte proliferation. *Science* 221: 568–570.

Laudenslager ML, Fleshner M, Hofstadter P, Held PE, Simons L, Maier SF. 1988. Suppression of specific antibody production by inescapable shock: Stability under varying conditions. *Brain Behav Immun* 2(2):92–101.

Lehnert H, Reinstein DK, Strowbridge BW, Wurtman RJ. 1984. Neurochemical and behavioral consequences of acute, uncontrollable stress: Effects of dietary tyrosine. *Brain Res* 303(2):215–223.

Lind L, Lithell H. 1993. Decreased peripheral blood flow in the pathogenisis of the metabolic syndrome comprising hypertension, hyperlimidemia and hyperinsulinemia. *Am Heart J* 125:1474–1497.

Livingston PO. 1995. Approaches to augmenting the immunogenicity of melanoma gangliosides: from whole melanoma cells to ganglioside-KLH conjugate vaccines. *Immunol Rev* 145:147–166.

Maestroni GJ. 2002. Short exposure of maturing, bone marrow-derived dendritic cells to norepinephrine: impact on kinetics of cytokine production and Th development. *J Neuroimmunol* 129 (1–2):106–114.

Maier SF, Watkins LR, Fleshner M. 1994. Psychoneuroimmunology: The interface between behavior, brain, and immunity. *Am Psychol* 49(12):1004–1017.

Maier SF, Fleshner M, Watkins LR. 1998. Neural, endocrine, and immune mechanisms of stress-induced immunomodulation. New Frontiers in Stress Research: Modulation of Brain Function. Harwood Academic Publishers. Pp. 117–126.

Malarkey WB, Wang J, Cheney C, Glaser R, Nagaraja H. 2002. Human lymphocyte growth hormone stimulates interferon gamma production and is inhibited by cortisol and norepinephrine. *J Neuroimmunol* 123(1–2):180–187.

Meltzer JCG, Greenberg AH, Nance DM. 1997. Enhanced immunohistochemical detection of autonomic nerve fibers, cytokines and inducible nitric oxide synthase by light and fluorescent microscopy in rat spleen. *J Histochem Cytochem* 45:599–610.

Milligan ED, Nguyen KT, Deak T, Hinde JL, Fleshner M, Watkins LR, Maier SF. 1998. The long term acute phase-like responses that follow acute stressor exposure are blocked by alpha-melanocyte stimulating hormone. *Brain Res* 810(1–2):48–58.

Milner JD, Wurtman RJ. 1987. Tyrosine availability: A presynaptic factor controlling catecholamine release. *Adv Exp Med Biol* 221:211–221.

Monjan A, Collector MI. 1976. Stress-induced modulation of the immune response. *Science* 196:307–308.

Moraska A, Fleshner M. 2001. Voluntary physical activity prevents stress-induced behavioral depression and anti-KLH antibody suppression. *Am J Physiol Regul Integr Comp Physiol* 281(2): R484–R489.

Moraska A, Campisi J, Nguyen KT, Maier SF, Watkins LR, Fleshner M. 2002. Elevated IL-1beta contributes to antibody suppression produced by stress. *J Appl Physiol* 93(1):207–215.

Nguyen KT, Deak T, Owens SM, Kohno T, Fleshner M, Watkins LR, Maier SF. 1998. Exposure to acute stress induces brain interleukin-1beta protein in the rat. *J Neurosci* 18(6):2239–2246.

Nguyen KT, Deak T, Will MJ, Hansen MK, Hunsaker BN, Fleshner M, Watkins LR, Maier SF. 2000. Timecourse and corticosterone sensitivity of the brain, pituitary, and serum interleukin-1beta protein response to acute stress. *Brain Res* 859(2):193–201.

Noble EG, Moraska A, Mazzeo RS, Roth DA, Olsson MC, Moore RL, Fleshner M. 1999. Differential expression of stress proteins in rat myocardium after free wheel or treadmill run training. *J Appl Physiol* 86(5):1696–1701.

O'Conner KA, Johnson JD, Nagel T, Fleshner M, Watkins LR, Maier SF. 1999. Role of hormones in stress-induced nitric oxide production. *Society for Neuroscience Abstract.*

Pauletto P, Scannapieco G, Pessina A. 1991. Sympathetic drive and vascular damage in hypertension and atherosclerosis. *Hypertension* 17 (Suppl):III75–III8.

Plotnikoff N, Murgo A, Faith R, Wybran J, eds. 1991. *Stress and Immunity.* Boca Raton, FL: CRC Press, Inc.

Podojil JR, Sanders VM. 2003. Selective regulation of mature IgG1 transcription by CD86 and beta 2-adrenergic receptor stimulation. *J Immunol* 170(10):5143–5151.

Podojil JR, Kin NW, Sanders VM. 2004. CD86 and beta2-adrenergic receptor signaling pathways, respectively, increase Oct-2 and OCA-B Expression and binding to the 3'-IgH enhancer in B cells. *J Biol Chem* 279(22):23394–23404.

Podolin DA, Wie Y, Paglizssotti J. 1999. Effects of a high-fat diet and voluntary wheel running on gluconeogenesis and lipolysis in rats. *J Appl Physiol* 86:1374–1380.

Ramer-Quinn DS, Baker RA, Sanders VM. 1997. Activated T helper 1 and T helper 2 cells differentially express the beta-2-adrenergic receptor. *J Immunol* 159:4857–4867.

Reinstein DK, Lehnert H, Scott NA, Wurtman RJ. 1984. Tyrosine prevents behavioral and neurochemical correlates of an acute stress in rats. *Life Sci* 34(23):2225–2231.

Sanders VM, Baker RA, Ramer-Quinn DS, Kasprowicz DJ, Fuchs BA, Street NE. 1997. Differential expression of the beta2-adrenergic receptor by Th1 and Th2 clones. *J Immunol* 158:4200–4210.

Sanders VM, Kasprowicz DJ, Swanson-Mungerson MA, Podojil JR, Kohm AP. 2003. Adaptive immunity in mice lacking the beta(2)-adrenergic receptor. *Brain Behav Immun* 17(1):55–67.

Seals D, Dinenno F. 2004. Collateral Damage: Cadiovascular consequences of chronic sympathetic activation with human aging. *Am J Physiol* 287:1895–1905.

Smith A, Vollmer-Conna U, Bennett B, Wakefield D, Hickie I, Lloyd A. 2004. The relationship between distress and the development of a primary immune response to a novel antigen. *Brain Behav Immun* 18(1):65–75.

Smith TP, Kennedy SL, Fleshner M. 2004. Influence of age and physical activity on the primary in vivo antibody and T cell-mediated responses in men. *J Appl Physiol* 97(2):491–498.

Solberg LC, Horton TH, Turek FW. 1999. Circadian rhythms and depression: Effect of exercise in an animal model. *American Journal of Physiology* 276:R152–R161.

Stevens TL, Bossie A, Sanders VM, Fernandez-Botran R, Coffman RL, Mosmann TR, Vitetta ES. 1988. Regulation of antibody isotype secretion by subsets of antigen-specific helper T cells. *Nature* 334(6179):255–258.

Suzuki K, Machida K. 1995. Effectivenss of lower-level voluntary exercise in disease prevention of mature rats: Cardiovascular risk factor modification. *Eur J Appl Physiol* 71:240–244.

Swanson MA, Lee WT, Sanders VM. 2001. IFN-gamma production by Th1 cells generated from naive CD4+ T cells exposed to norepinephrine. *J Immunol* 166(1):232–240.

Takahashi HK, Iwagaki H, Mori S, Yoshino T, Tanaka N, Nishibori M. 2004. Beta 2-adrenergic receptor agonist induces IL-18 production without IL-12 production. *J Neuroimmunol* 151 (1–2):137–147.

Watkins LR, Thurston CL, Fleshner M. 1990. Phenlyephrine-induced antinociception: Investigations of potential neural and endocrine bases. *Brain Res* 528:273–284.

Xiao RP, Lakatta EG. 1992. Deterioration of beta-adrenergic modulation of cardiovascular function with aging. *Ann N Y Acad Sci* 673:293–310.

Xin X, Yang N, Eckhart AD, Faber JE. 1997. Alpha1D-adrenergic receptors and mitogen-activated protein kinase mediate increased protein synthesis by arterial smooth muscle. *Mol Pharmacol* 51:764–775.

# Mineral Intake Needs and Infectious Diseases

*Davidson H. Hamer*
*Boston University and Tufts University, Boston, Massachusetts*

## INTRODUCTION

Several minerals play central roles in the immune response and thus may be integral to protective responses to pathogens causing human infections. The inflammatory response associated with acute infections, especially diarrheal disease, may result in enhanced excretion of certain essential minerals including copper, iron, and zinc, and thus contribute to deficiencies of these minerals. During the last decade, there has been extensive research in children in resource-poor areas of the world that has demonstrated the beneficial effects of zinc for the prevention and adjunctive treatment of common infectious diseases. In contrast, despite its important role in immune function, iron supplementation has been occasionally associated with a small increased risk of infection. Unfortunately, there is little data available regarding the role of mineral supplements in adults for prevention or treatment of infection with the exception of zinc for the common cold—these studies have shown variable results. Although military personnel are at increased risk for enhanced losses of minerals due to physical stress as well as exposure to infectious pathogens, there is a dearth of data regarding the potential role of mineral supplements in this population.

## IMPACT OF STRESS ON INFECTION

Numerous psychological and physical stressors exert immunomodulatory effects, which may increase the risk of infection acquisition or result in greater severity of infections (Peterson et al., 1991). Several stress-responsive neurotransmitters and neuropeptides have been shown to interact with cells of the immune system *in vitro*, resulting in either enhancement (e.g., β-endorphin) (Maestroni and Conti, 1989) or suppression (e.g., glucocorticoids) (Cupps and Fauci, 1982) of the immune response. Animal models of stress and viral infection have mostly shown increased mortality (reviewed in Peterson et al., 1991) or other complications such as paralysis in a poliomyelitis model in mice and monkeys. Similar results have been found in animal models of bacterial infection and stress (i.e., forced exercise), with the majority demonstrating increased mortality associated with stress (Peterson et al., 1991).

Relatively little pathogen-specific data exist on the association between stress and infections in humans. Most studies evaluated viral pathogens (e.g., poliomyelitis, hepatitis A, and herpes simplex virus) or upper respiratory infections, which are predominantly also due to viruses (see review by Peterson et al., 1991). With a few exceptions, the results of most studies suggested an association between physical or psychosocial stress and increased frequency, duration, or severity of symptoms. Two studies involved military trainees. A prospective study of marine recruits in North Carolina found, in addition to an association with winter, higher rates of colds in those who were white, well educated, and had slower promotion (Voors et al., 1968). A four-year prospective seroepidemiological study of infectious mononucleosis in West Point Military Academy cadets demonstrated an association between increased risk of clinical illness and three psychosocial factors: having fathers who were overachievers, being highly motivated, and struggling academically.

In summary, while animal models have consistently demonstrated an association between stress and increased mortality from infection, the limited human studies suggest an association between increased physical or psychological stress and enhanced morbidity from viral infections. Relatively little is known about the impact of stress on bacterial, fungal, or parasitic infections in humans. Although the evidence is limited, it is likely that the physical and severe psychological stressors to which the military are exposed increase the likelihood of acquisition while also potentially worsening the severity of infectious diseases.

## EFFECTS OF STRESS AND INFECTION ON MINERAL EXCRETION

Systemic infections produce an acute phase response that results in alterations of mineral status indicators including elevation of serum ferritin (Elin et al., 1977) and erythrocyte protophoryin (Stoltzfus et al., 2000), and reduction of plasma zinc concentrations (Duggan et al., 2005; Strand et al., 2004). In addition to their impact on measures of iron and zinc status, acute infections may also lead to accelerated losses of essential minerals.

### Fecal Mineral Losses

There are a number of different potential causes of mineral loss from the gastrointestinal tract (Box B-3). A consequence of mineral loss, whether due to infectious or malabsorptive processes, is a net negative balance. For example, acute and persistent diarrhea in children has been associated with low serum or plasma zinc concentrations (Castillo-Duran et al., 1988; Chaudhary et al., 1996; Naveh et al., 1982). Although the acute phase response during infectious diarrhea contributes to depression of plasma zinc, at least one study found low rectal mucosal zinc concentrations in children with chronic diarrhea (Sachdev et al., 1990), thus suggesting that the infectious process can lead to a net negative balance.

Two studies have rigorously evaluated the impact of acute diarrhea on trace mineral balance (Table B-12). Castillo-Duran and colleagues (1988) evaluated the magnitude of zinc and copper losses in young children with acute diarrhea requiring hospitalization. Fourteen infants, aged 3 to 14 months, with acute diar-

**BOX B-3**
**Causes of Fecal Mineral Loss**

1. Infectious Etiologies
   - Tropical sprue
   - Acute diarrhea
   - Persistent diarrhea

2. Non-Infectious Causes of Malabsorption
   - High phytate diets
   - High concentrations of competing divalent cations
   - Crohn's disease
   - Celiac disease
   - Short-bowel syndrome
   - Intestinal bypass
   - Pancreatic insufficiency

rhea were compared to a control group of 15 infants of similar age, birth weight, and nutritional status. Mean fecal losses of copper and zinc were higher in the diarrhea group during the initial 48 hours. When repeat metabolic balance studies were performed on days 6 and 7 of admission, fecal zinc losses were similar for the two groups whereas copper balance remained negative only for the diarrhea group. There was a strong correlation between fecal weight and fecal losses for both minerals, and a negative correlation between fecal and plasma zinc concentrations. A study of 24 male Guatemalan children, aged 7 to 23 months, with acute, dehydrating diarrhea found increased fecal excretion of copper, iron, and zinc during oral rehydration therapy (Ruz and Solomons, 1990). Although this study lacked a control group and did not carry out a follow-up evaluation after resolution of diarrhea, it nevertheless also demonstrated significant linear correlations between mineral excretion and fecal volume. These studies both demonstrate that fecal losses of copper, iron, and zinc during acute diarrhea are likely to induce a negative balance of these minerals.

Although limited data exist for adults, one study that evaluated zinc losses in patients with a variety of gastrointestinal disorders (primarily Crohn's disease and ischemic bowel) found substantial small intestinal zinc losses that persisted over time (Table B-12) (Wolman et al., 1979). Similar to the pediatric studies of acute diarrhea, this adult study found a significant correlation between intestinal zinc losses and the weight of contents lost or excreted. Positive zinc balance was nearly reached in patients receiving 6 mg of zinc per day intravenously and was easily achieved if 12 mg/day was administered. In contrast to the patients with diarrhea, positive zinc balance could be attained in those without diarrhea with only 3 mg of zinc per day. Although this study involved hospitalized patients

**TABLE B-12** Gastrointestinal Mineral Losses in Diarrhea

| Author | Study population | Fecal copper | Fecal iron | Fecal zinc |
|---|---|---|---|---|
| Castillo-Duran et al., 1988 | Infants with acute diarrhea | 55.7 ± 21.2 µg/kg body weight/day | Not evaluated | 159.4 ± 59.9 µg/kg body weight/day |
| | Healthy infants | 28.8 ± 6.7 µg/kg body weight/day | Not evaluated | 47.4 ± 6.4 µg/kg body weight/day |
| Ruz and Solomons, 1990 | Young children with acute diarrhea | 1.61 µg/kg/hour (38.6 µg/kg/day)[a] | 6.33 µg/kg/hour (151.9 µg/kg/day)[a] | 6.08 µg/kg/hour (145.9 µg/kg/day)[a] |
| Wolman et al., 1979 | Adults with gastrointestinal disease | Not evaluated | Not evaluated | 15.15 µg/g of intestinal content[b] |

[a]Estimated 24 hour output based on hourly measurement.
[b]Patients with intact small intestine.

with serious intestinal pathology, it nevertheless demonstrates the important contribution of diarrhea to fecal zinc losses and its negative impact on zinc balance.

## Urinary and Sweat Mineral Losses

There are a number of different factors that influence urinary mineral excretion including age, gender, physical exercise, urine pH, high protein food, high fiber food, coffee, tobacco, and alcohol. A study of healthy volunteers from the Canary Islands found urinary zinc levels that were 19-fold and nearly 8-fold greater than copper and iron, respectively (Rodriguez and Diaz, 1995). Men had significantly greater daily excretion of zinc than women although these differences were no longer significant when urinary excretion was controlled for creatinine, an indicator of glomerular filtration rate and overall renal function. In terms of copper and iron, women had greater daily urinary excretion of both these minerals than men. Routine exercise was associated with reduced urinary excretion of copper, iron, and zinc. Patients with increased urinary nitrogen excretion, due to probable hypercatabolism, had higher urinary zinc losses than those with lower urinary nitrogen excretion (Wilman et al., 1979).

Moderate amounts of iron and zinc can also be lost in sweat. Studies of young, physically fit adults have demonstrated that sweat losses of both iron and zinc are greatest in the first 30 minutes of exercise and thereafter diminish (DeRuisseau et al., 2002; Waller and Haymes, 1996). Estimated whole body iron loss is greater during exercise than at rest and is greater overall in men than women (Waller and Haymes, 1996). During two hours of exercise, sweat losses were 3 percent and 1 percent of the Recommended Daily Allowance (RDA) of iron RDA and 9 percent and 8 percent of the zinc RDA for men and women, respectively (DeRuisseau et al., 2002).

Of the different factors influencing the excretion of essential minerals, there are two that have implications for the mineral needs of the military. First, intensive sweating associated with physical exercise contributes to enhanced losses of iron and zinc; however, it appears that homeostatic mechanisms serve to reduce sweat losses of iron and zinc during prolonged exertion. Although data are limited regarding the impact of fever on sweat losses, it is likely that prolonged febrile illnesses will contribute to total body losses of iron and zinc. The second and potentially more significant factor is the enhanced fecal excretion of several minerals during acute and persistent diarrhea. Infectious diarrhea, especially if prolonged, is likely to result in a negative balance for copper, iron, magnesium, and zinc. Consequently, supplemental minerals, especially zinc, need to be considered for military personnel with diarrhea.

## ROLE OF ZINC IN THE PREVENTION OF INFECTION

### Subclinical Zinc Deficiency and Risk of Infection

Cross-sectional studies of children in Papua New Guinea and pregnant women in Malawi have shown associations between suboptimal zinc status, based on hair zinc levels, and falciparum malaria (Gibson and Huddle, 1998; Gibson et al., 1991). A prospective study of children aged 12 to 59 months who had recovered from a recent episode of acute non-dysenteric diarrhea was carried out in an urban slum in New Delhi (Bahl et al., 1998). Thirty two percent of children had low plasma zinc concentrations ($\leq$ 8.4 μmol/L). Children with low baseline plasma zinc levels had a 47 percent higher risk of diarrhea during the three month observation period than those with normal zinc. Although the overall risk of acute lower respiratory infection (ALRI) was not significantly higher in the low plasma zinc group, boys as opposed to girls with low plasma zinc had a four-fold higher risk of developing an episode of ALRI during the 90 day observation period. The prevalence of ALRI was about three-fold higher in zinc-deficient children, possibly as a result of longer duration episodes of ALRI in this group.

In summary, while the cross-sectional studies suggested an association between malaria and zinc deficiency, there were multiple other factors including poor zinc intake and high phytate intake that contributed to the poor zinc status. In contrast, the longitudinal design of the Indian study provides stronger evidence of an association between subclinical zinc deficiency and the subsequent risk of infection.

## Prevention of Childhood Diarrhea and Pneumonia with Zinc Supplements

Similarly to the studies on zinc deficiency above, there are, there are virtually no studies of the effect of zinc for the prevention of infections in adults. Therefore, this section will review the results of seminal studies in children, even though the results cannot be extrapolated to adults with any level of confidence. Several studies in recent years have shown that zinc supplementation in children normalizes immune function and dramatically reduce infectious disease morbidity and mortality (Sazawal et al., 1997, 1998; Sempertegui et al., 1996). A pooled analysis of studies of zinc supplementation for the prevention of diarrhea and pneumonia in children in developing countries found that, in trials that provided 1–2 times the RDA of elemental zinc 5 to 7 times per week, the pooled odds ratios (OR) for diarrheal incidence and prevalence were 0.82 (95 percent confidence interval, CI, ranging from 0.72 to 0.93) and 0.75 (95 percent CI ranging from 0.63 to 0.88), respectively (ZICG, 1999). The OR for pneumonia was 0.59 (95 percent CI ranging from 0.41 to 0.83) for zinc-supplemented children. This pooled analysis found a 33 percent reduction in the incidence of persistent diarrhea but this effect only trended towards significance (OR 0.67, 95 percent CI, ranging from 0.42 to 1.06). Similarly, zinc supplementation was associated with a non-significant reduction of dysentery of 13 percent. A more recent study of zinc supplementation given for a period of 14 days each time a child had an episode of diarrhea demonstrated reductions in the duration and incidence of diarrhea and a reduced incidence of ARI (acute respiratory infection) (Baqui et al., 2002). The non-injury death rate was also 51 percent lower in the zinc intervention clusters, suggesting that zinc supplementation reduced mortality.

## Prevention of Malaria with Zinc

In contrast to the extensive evidence base for the efficacy of zinc in the prevention of diarrheal disease and ALRI in children in resource-poor settings, there is relatively limited data regarding zinc and malaria prevention. A trial in The Gambia found that zinc supplementation was associated with a 32 percent reduction in health centre visits for slide-confirmed malaria, though this difference did not attain statistical significance (Bates et al., 1993). While this finding was provocative, the study was not optimally designed for this outcome, and had several important limitations including the lack of a precise definition of malarial illness and a small sample size. Subsequent work from Papua New Guinea provided more convincing evidence of a protective effect of zinc. In a community-based study, a 46-week period of zinc supplementation in preschool children significantly reduced *Plasmodium falciparum*-attributable health centre attendance by 38 percent ($p = 0.037$) (Shankar et al., 2000). Episodes accompanied by any level of parasitemia were also reduced by 38 percent ($p = 0.028$) and episodes with parasitemia ≥ 100,000 per µL were reduced by 69 percent (p = 0.009).

A community-based trial of zinc supplementation in Burkina Faso on the incidence of febrile episodes of falciparum malaria, the severity of malaria episodes, or anemia in children aged 6 to 31 months demonstrated that the cross-sectional prevalence of falciparum malaria and of *P. falciparum*, *P. malariae*, and *P. ovale* parasitemia were all significantly lower in children supplemented with zinc (p = 0.001) for all comparisons to placebo (Muller et al., 2001). In addition, the mean density of *P. falciparum* increased significantly (p = 0.001) during the study in the placebo group relative to the zinc group. Thus, zinc supplementation appeared to provide benefits in terms of several key malariometric measures. Other beneficial effects of zinc supplementation, such as a significant reduction of the number of days with diarrhea (p = 0.002) and a trend towards reduced mortality (relative risk, RR 0.41, 95 percent CI 0.15–1.19, p = 0.1) were also noted. However, this study failed to find any benefit of zinc on the incidence of clinical malaria episodes (defined as temperature ≥ 37.5°C and ≥ parasites/µL). There are several potential explanations for the lack of a protective effect of zinc for malaria in this study. First, the sample size was too small to measure this effect, since the proportion of febrile malaria episodes of all children with positive blood smears was quite small. Second, the prevalence of clinical zinc deficiency in the population under study was low. Using a cut-off point for zinc deficiency of 60 µg/dL (ZICG, 1999), only a small proportion of these children were zinc deficient at baseline, as the mean zinc concentration was 76.5 mg/dL. Theoretically, zinc might have a greater effect on clinical malaria if used in a population where zinc deficiency was widespread.

Thus, in summary there is ample evidence that zinc supplementation serves to protect children against diarrheal disease, ALRI, and possibly malaria. In addition, there is growing evidence that zinc supplementation may reduce mortality in young children (Baqui et al., 2002; Muller et al., 2001; Sazawal et al., 2001). At present there is no data available regarding the potential benefits of zinc supplementation for prevention of malaria in healthy adults.

## TREATMENT OF INFECTIONS WITH ZINC

### Treatment of Diarrheal Disease with Zinc

There are several potential mechanisms by which zinc might have a beneficial effect on the duration of diarrhea. These include improved absorption capacity (Golden and Golden, 1985), increased brush border disaccharidase activity (Gebhard et al., 1983), faster regeneration of intestinal epithelium (Bettger and O'Dell, 1981), a reduction of gut permeability, and an enhanced immune response (Shankar and Prasad, 1998), which may result in more rapid clearance of enteropathogens. Based on these potential mechanisms, a large number of studies have evaluated the role of zinc in the treatment of acute and persistent diarrhea in children.

Zinc supplementation, as an adjunct to oral rehydration therapy, reduced the duration and severity of acute and persistent diarrhea in several randomized controlled trials (Bhutta et al., 1999; Roy et al., 1997; Sachdev et al., 1988, 1990; Sazawal et al., 1995, 1997). A pooled analysis of randomized, controlled trials of zinc for acute diarrhea found that zinc reduced the mean duration of diarrhea by 16 percent (95 percent CI: 7 percent, 26 percent) (ZICG, 2000). Zinc-supplemented children also had a 15 percent lower probability of continuing diarrhea on a given day in the acute diarrhea studies and a 24 percent lower probability of continuing diarrhea in the persistent diarrhea trials. There was also a 42 percent lower rate of death or treatment failure in the persistent diarrhea studies. An analysis of the cost-effectiveness of zinc as adjunct therapy to standard management of acute childhood diarrhea, including dysentery, found that the use of zinc significantly improved the cost-effectiveness of standard treatment for both dysenteric and non-dysenteric diarrhea (Sommerfelt et al., 2004).

An alternative approach to the management of acute diarrhea that has been recently evaluated is the addition of zinc to oral rehydration solution (ORS). In a zinc-deficient rat model of diarrhea, treatment with ORS plus zinc resulted in a recovery of normal plasma zinc levels and improved histology of the intestinal villi relative to rats treated with ORS minus zinc, suggesting that the supplemental zinc helped to improve intestinal epithelial integrity (Altaf et al., 2002). Two studies in children have evaluated ORS-zinc in children. One of these, a small study of young children in Cuba, found no advantage of ORS-zinc over ORS alone (Bahl et al., 2001). In contrast, a study of young children with acute diarrhea in North India found that ORS-zinc was more efficacious than ORS alone for reducing the duration of an episode of diarrhea (Bahl et al., 2001). However, ORS-zinc was less efficacious than zinc supplements given separately from ORS. Although the addition of zinc to ORS was not associated with tolerability problems in these two studies, this approach does not appear to be as efficacious as oral zinc supplementation, perhaps because the total amount of zinc administered on a daily basis is greater when oral supplements are administered. To date there have been no evaluations of zinc for the management of diarrhea in adults.

### Treatment of Pneumonia, Measles, and Malaria with Zinc

Two studies evaluated the efficacy of zinc as an adjunct to antimicrobial therapy for children with severe ALRI (Brooks et al., 2004; Mahalanabis et al., 2004). In the first study, children aged 2–23 months with severe pneumonia received 20 mg of zinc per day plus standard antibiotics until hospital discharge (Brooks et al., 2004). Children who received zinc had a reduced duration of severe pneumonia including shorter duration of tachypnea, hypoxia, and chest in-drawing. The overall duration of pneumonia was 4 days in children treated with zinc versus 5 days in those who received placebo. The second study involved the administration of 10 mg of zinc twice daily for 5 days to children aged 2–24 months with severe ALRI (Mahalanabis et al., 2004). Zinc treatment significantly reduced the duration of fever and very ill clinical status as judged by the study pediatrician in boys but not girls. Since this finding arose from post hoc subgroup analysis, it needs to be validated in a gender-stratified, randomized controlled trial. These two studies provide early suggestions of a potential therapeutic effect of zinc for severe pneumonia in very young children. Whether zinc will prove to be a useful therapeutic adjunct for the treatment of pneumonia in older children or for selected respiratory pathogens remain open questions.

The utility of zinc supplementation for the treatment of measles has been evaluated in only one study (Mahalabis et al., 2002). Children, aged 9 months to 15 years, hospitalized in India for measles were randomized to zinc or placebo in addition to routine supportive care. Treatment with zinc had no impact on the time to recovery or the proportion of children who were judged to be cured by day six.

In order to evaluate the potential role of zinc as an adjunct in the treatment of acute, uncomplicated falciparum malaria, a randomized, placebo-controlled, multi-centre trial was undertaken (ZAP Study Group, 2002). Children (n = 1,087) between the ages of 6 months and 5 years with fever and ≥ 2,000/μL asexual forms of *P. falciparum* in a thick blood smear were enrolled at sites in Ecuador, Ghana, Tanzania, Uganda, and Zambia. Children were randomized to receive zinc (20 mg/day for infants, 40 mg/day for older children) or placebo for four days as well as chloroquine, the standard first line treatment for malaria in all sites at the time of study initiation. There was no effect of zinc on the median time to reduction of fever (zinc = 24.2 hr versus placebo = 24.0 hr, p = 0.37), reduction of parasitemia in the first 72 hr (zinc group = 73.4 percent; placebo group = 77.6 percent, p = 0.11), or hemoglobin concentration during the three day period of hospitalization or four week follow-up period. This carefully designed study thus failed to demonstrate any benefits of zinc as an adjunct to the treatment of malaria. As with prevention, there is no data available on the benefits of zinc supplementation for treatment of malaria in adults.

### Treatment of the Common Cold with Zinc

Viral upper respiratory tract infections are a major cause of physician visits and time lost from work or education in the United States. Because of its immunomodulatory activities (Shankar and Prasad, 1998) and in vitro inhibitory activity against rhinoviruses (Korant et al., 1974), zinc lozenges have been extensively evaluated as a therapeutic strategy for the common cold. Randomized controlled trials of zinc salt lozenges have yielded mixed results. A meta-analysis by Jackson and colleagues (1997), which included 6 trials, found a summary odds ratio of 0.5 (95 percent CI, 0.19–1.29) for the presence of any cold symptoms at 7 days. A subsequent study in adults with common cold symptoms for less than 24 hours found a significant reduction in the mean overall duration of cough, nasal discharge, and cold symptoms (4.5 versus 8.1 days) (Prasad et al., 2000). Although this carefully designed study showed a reduction of more than 3 days of cold symptoms in adults taking zinc acetate lozenges, a repeat meta-analysis failed to find evidence of the effectiveness of zinc for reducing the duration of the common cold (Jackson et al., 2000). Even though the revised meta-analysis did not include the study by Prasad and colleagues (2000), there nevertheless is little evidence to support the routine use of zinc for the treatment of the common cold. A recent IOM report also concluded that there is conflicting evidence arising from studies in the elderly population and that data on the effects of non-pharmacological levels of zinc on immunity in young healthy adults are not available (IOM 2005).

## IRON AND INFECTION

There are a number of harmful effects of iron deficiency on cellular immunity that are reversible with iron supplementation (reviewed in Oppenheimer, 2001). These include reduced neutrophil function, decreased numbers of T-lymphocytes associated with thymic atrophy, defective T-lymphocyte-induced proliferative responses, impaired natural killer cell activity, decreased production of macrophage migration inhibition factor, and impaired delayed-type hypersensitivity. On the other hand, there is little indication of major deficiencies of humoral immunity in iron-deficient humans. Despite the solid evidence of abnormalities of cellular immunity associate with iron deficiency, there has been a long standing controversy regarding the relationship between iron status and susceptibility to infection.

Iron is required for both the human host and pathogens for survival and replication. In the setting of acute infection, there is a rise in iron-binding proteins such as serum ferritin, which has been proposed as a defensive maneuver by the host that limits the amount of iron available to pathogens (Weinberg, 1978). Findings from studies in the 1970s suggested that iron treatment resulted in aggravation of pre-existing or latent bacterial or parasitic infections. Neonates with iron deficiency in New Zealand who were treated with parenteral iron dextran at birth had a 6-fold increase in gram-negative sepsis (Barry and Reeve, 1977). Similarly, adult Somali nomads with iron deficiency treated with oral iron supplementation had significantly increased clinical malaria attacks relative to a placebo control group (Murray et al., 1978). Subsequent studies also suggested that iron therapy increased a child's risk of developing malaria or aggravated the clinical severity of an episode (Oppenheimer et al., 1986; Smith et al., 1989). In contrast, other investigators did not find a negative effect of iron supplementation on malaria (Bates et al., 1987; Harvey et al., 1989).

During the last two decades, there have been a large number of randomized controlled trials of the effect of iron supplementation on the risk of infections in children. A systematic review of many of these studies found that the pooled estimate of the incidence rate ratio of infection episodes for iron versus placebo was 1.02 (95 percent CI 0.96–1.08) (Gera and Sachdev, 2002). Although there was a slight increased incidence of several infection types in iron supplemented children, the only forms of infection that was significantly increased was diarrheal disease (11 percent increased risk) and malaria parasitemia (43 percent increase). A meta-analysis that focused only on malaria found a 17 percent increased risk of *P. falciparum* parasitemia in randomized, controlled trials of iron supplementation (Shankar et al., 1998). There was also a non-significant 9 percent increase in the risk of clinical malaria. However, iron supplementation was associated with substantial benefits in terms of hemoglobin improvement and a reduced risk of severe anemia.

In summary there is limited evidence of a harmful effect of iron supplementation on risk of infection. Although there may be a small increased risk of malarial parasitemia, it appears that the risk of clinical malaria attacks is not significantly increased and that the benefits of iron in terms of improvement of hematological status far outweigh the risks of supplementation.

## IMPLICATIONS FOR MILITARY PERSONNEL MINERAL REQUIREMENTS

Physical and psychological stresses contribute to an enhanced risk of infection and accelerated mineral losses. Infections, especially diarrhea, may also contribute to increased losses of essential minerals. There has been a vast amount of research done in recent years on the importance of maintaining adequate zinc status for the prevention of infection. Although much of this work has been performed in young children in resource-poor countries, these results nevertheless have implications for military personnel. In circumstances where there is enhanced excretion of zinc, especially in the setting of acute or prolonged diarrhea, zinc supplementation plays an adjunctive role in the management of diarrhea. Based on the limited evidence available, zinc is most efficacious when provided as oral supplements rather than being mixed with ORS. Maintenance of adequate zinc status should be a priority as this should serve to reduce the risk of infection in military personnel.

In contrast to the ample evidence of the benefits of zinc supplementation or maintenance of zinc status for the treatment and prevention of infections at least in children, the role of iron in preventing or resisting infections is less clear. In the setting of anemia due to iron deficiency, there is a need for iron replacement.

However, in most other circumstances, there is insufficient evidence of a meaningful benefit of iron supplementation to decrease the incidence or severity of infections. In addition, there may be a slight risk of harm from this intervention since iron is also an essential element for many pathogens. Taking into consideration the potential risks and benefits that iron supplementation might impart to the immune system, it seems prudent to continue research efforts in this area before iron supplementation to improve immune responses is recommended.

## REFERENCES


Altaf W, Perveen S, Rehman KU. 2002. Zinc supplementation in oral rehydration solutions: Experimental assessment and mechanisms of action. *J Am Coll Nutr* 21:26–32.

Anonymous. 2001. Effect of zinc supplementation on clinical course of acute diarrhea. Report of a meeting, New Delhi, 7–8 May 2001. *J Health Popul Nutr* 19:338–346.

Bahl R, Bhandari N, Hambidge KM, Bhan MK. 1998. Plasma zinc as a predictor of diarrheal and respiratory morbidity in children in an urban slum setting. *Am J Clin Nutr* 68 (Suppl):414S–417S.

Baqui AH, Black RE, El Arifeen S. 2002. Effect of zinc supplementation started during diarrhoea on morbidity and mortality in Bangladeshi children: Community randomized trial. *Br Med J* 325:1–7.

Barry DMJ, Reeve AW. 1977. Increased incidence of gram-negative neonatal sepsis with intramuscular iron administration. *Pediatrics* 60:908–912.

Bates CJ, Powers HJ, Lamb WH, Gelman W, Webb E. 1987. Effect of supplementary vitamins and iron on malaria indices in rural Gambian children. *Trans R Soc Trop Med Hyg* 81:286–291.

Bates CJ, Evans PH, Dardenne M. 1993. A trial of zinc supplementation in young rural Gambian children. *Br J Nutr* 69:243–255.

Bettger WJ, O'Dell BL. 1981. A critical physiological role of zinc in the structure and function of biomembranes. *Life Sc* 28:1425–1438.

Bhutta ZA, Nizami SQ, Isani Z. 1999. Zinc supplementation in malnourished children with persistent diarrhea in Pakistan. *Pediatrics* 103:1–9.

Brooks WA, Yunus M, Santosham M. 2004. Zinc for severe pneumonia in very young children: Double-blind placebo-controlled trial. *Lancet* 363:1683–1688.

Castillo-Duran C, Vial P, Uauy R. 1988. Trace mineral balance during acute diarrhea in infants. *J Pediatr* 113:452–457.

Chaudhary S, Verma M, Dhawan V. 1996. Plasma vitamin A, zinc and selenium concentrations in children with acute and persistent diarrhoea. *J Diarrhoeal Dis Res* 14:190–193.

Cupps TR, Fauci AS. 1982. Corticosteroid-mediated immunoregulation in man. *Immunol Rev* 65: 133–155.

DeRuisseau KC, Cheuvront SN, Haymes EM, Sharp RG. 2002. Sweat iron and zinc losses during prolonged exercise. *International J Sport Nutr Exerc Met* 12:428–437.

Duggan C, MacLeod W, Krebs NF. 2005. Plasma zinc concentrations are depressed during the acute phase response in children with falciparum malaria. *J Nutr* 135:802–807.

Elin RJ, Wolf SM, Finch C. 1977. Effect of induced fever on serum iron and ferritin concentrations in man. *Blood* 49:147–153.

Gebhard RL, Karouani R, Prigge WF, McClain CJ. 1983. Effect of severe zinc deficiency on activity of intestinal disaccharidases and 3-hydroxy-3-methyl-glutaryl coenzyme A reductase in the rat. *J Nutr* 113:855–859.

Gera T, Sachdev HP. 2002. Effect of iron supplementation on incidence of infectious illness in children: systematic review. *Br Med J* 325:1142.

Gibson RS, Huddle JM. 1998. Suboptimal zinc status in pregnant Malawian women: Its association with low intakes of poorly available zinc, frequent reproductive cycling, and malaria. *Am J Clin Nutr* 67:702–709.

Gibson RS, Heywood A, Yaman C.1991. Growth in children from the Wosera subdistrict, Papua New Guinea, in relation to energy and protein intakes and zinc status. *Am J Clin Nutr* 53: 782–789.

Golden BE, Golden MHN. 1985. Zinc, sodium and potassium losses in the diarrhoeas of malnutrition and zinc deficiency. In: Mills CF, Bremner I, Chesters JK, eds. *Trace Elements in Man and Animals TEMA 5*. Aberdeen, UK: Rowett Research Institute.

Harvey PW, Heywood PF, Nesheim MC.1989. The effect of iron therapy on malarial infection in Papua New Guinean schoolchildren. *Am J Trop Med Hyg* 40:12–18.

Jackson JL, Peterson C, Lesho E. 1997. A meta-analysis of zinc salts lozenges and the common cold. *Arch Intern Med* 157:2373–2376.

Jackson JL, Lesho E, Peterson C. 2000. Zinc and the common cold: A meta-analysis revisited. *J Nutr* 130: S1512–S1515.

Korant BD, Kauer JE, Butterworth BE. 1974. Zinc ions inhibit replication of rhinoviruses. *Nature* 248:588–590.

Maestroni GJM, Conti A. 1989. Beta-endorphin and dynorphin mimic the circadian immunoenhancing and anti-stress effects of melatonin. *J Immunopharmacol* 11:333–340.

Mahalanabis D, Chowdhury A, Jana S, Bhattacharya MK, Chakrabarti MK. 2002. Zinc supplementation as adjunct therapy in children with measles accompanied by pneumonia: A double-blind, randomized controlled trial. *Am J Clin Nutr* 76:604–607.

Mahalanabis D, Lahiri M, Dilip P. 2004. Randomized, double-blind, placebo-controlled clinical trial of the efficacy of treatment with zinc or vitamin A in infants and young children with severe acute lower respiratory infection. *Am J Clin Nutr* 79:430–436.

Muller O, Becher H, van Zweeden AB. 2001. Effect of zinc supplementation on malaria and other causes of morbidity in West African children: Randomised double blind placebo controlled trial. *Brit Med J* 322:1–5.

Murray MJ, Murray AB, Murray MB, Murray CJ. 1978. The adverse effect of iron repletion on the course of certain infections. *Brit Med J* 2:1113–1115.

Naveh Y, Lightman A, Zinder O. 1982. Effect of diarrhea on serum zinc concentrations in infants and children. *J Pediatr* 101:730–732.

Oppenheimer SJ. 2001. Iron and its relation to immunity and infectious disease. *J Nutr* 131:16S–633S.

Oppenheimer SJ, Gibson FD, Macfarlane SB. 1986. Iron supplementation increases prevalence and effects of malaria: report on clinical studies in Papua New Guinea. *Trans R Soc Trop Med Hyg* 80:603–612.

Peterson PK, Chao CC, Molitor T. 1991. Stress and pathogenesis of infectious disease. *Rev Infect Dis* 13:710–720.

Prasad AS, Fitzgerald JT, Bao B, Beck FWJ, Chandrasekar PH. 2000. Duration of symptoms and plasma cytokine levels in patients with the common cold treated with zinc acetate. *Ann Intern Med* 133:245–252.

Rodriguez E, Diaz C. 1995. Iron, copper and zinc levels in urine: relationship to various individual factors. *J Trace Elem Med Biol* 9:200–209.

Roy S.K., Tomkins A. M., & Akramuzzaman SM (1997) Randomised controlled trial of zinc supplementation in malnourished Bangladeshi children with acute diarrhoea. *Arch Dis Child* 77: 196–200.

Ruz M, Solomons NW. 1990. Mineral excretion during acute, dehydrating diarrhea treated with oral rehydration therapy. *Pediatr Res* 27:170–175.

Sachdev HPS, Mittal NK, Mittal SK, Yadav HS. 1988. A controlled trial on utility of oral zinc supplementation in acute dehydrating diarrhea in infants. *J Pediatr Gastroenterol Nutr* 7:877–881.

Sachdev HPS, Mittal NK, Yadav HS. 1990. Oral zinc supplementation in persistent diarrhoea in infants. *Ann Trop Paediatr* 10:63–69.

Sazawal S, Black RE, Bhan MK. 1995. Zinc supplementation in young children with acute diarrhea in India. *N Engl J Med* 333:839–844.

Sazawal S, Black RE, Bhan MK.1997. Efficacy of zinc supplementation in reducing the incidence and prevalence of acute diarrhea—a community-based, double-blind, controlled trial. *Am J Clin Nutr* 66:413–418.

Sazawal S, Black RE, Jalla S. 1998. Zinc supplementation reduces the incidence of acute lower respiratory infections in infants and preschool children: A double-blind, controlled trial. *Pediatrics* 102:1–5.

Sazawal S, Black RE, Menon VP. 2001. Zinc supplementation in infants born small for gestational age reduces mortality: A prospective, randomized, controlled trial. *Pediatrics* 108:1280–1286.

Sempertegui F, Estrella B, Correa E. 1996. Effects of short-term zinc supplementation on cellular immunity, respiratory symptoms, and growth of malnourished Ecuadorian children. *Eur J Clin Nutr* 50:42–46.

Shankar AH, Prasad AS. 1998. Zinc and immune function: The biological basis of altered resistance to infection. *Am J Clin Nutr* 68:447S–463S.

Shankar AH, Fishman S, Goodman S, Stoltzfus RJ. 1998. Iron supplements and *Plasmodium falciparum* morbidity: A meta-analysis of controlled clinical trials of iron supplementation in malarious areas. Background paper for the ILSI-INACG.

Shankar AH, Genton B, Baisor M. 2000. The influence of zinc supplementation on morbidity due to Plasmodium falciparum: A randomized trial in preschool children in Papua New Guinea. *Am J Trop Med Hyg* 62:663–669.

Smith AW, Hendrickse RG, Harrison C, Hayes RJ, Greenwood BM. 1989. The effects on malaria of treatment of iron-deficiency anaemia with oral iron in Gambian children. *Ann Trop Paediatr* 9:17–23.

Sommerfelt H, Robberstad B, Stand T, Black RE. 2004. Cost-effectiveness of zinc as adjunct therapy for acute childhood diarrhoea in developing countries. *Bull World Health Organ* 82:523–531.

Stoltzfus RJ, Chwaya HM, Montresor A. 2000. Malaria, hookworms and recent fever are related to anemia and iron status indicators in 0- to 5-y old Zanzibari children and these relationships change with age. *J Nutr* 130:1724–1733.

Strand TA, Adhikari RK, Chandyo RK, Sharma PR, Sommerfelt H. 2004. Predictors of plasma zinc concentration in children with acute diarrhea. *Am J Clin Nutr* 79:451–456.

Voors AW, Stewart GT, Gutekunst RR, Moldow CF, Jenkins CD. 1968. Respiratory infection in Marine recruits. Influence of personal characteristics. *Am Rev Respir Dis* 98:801–809.

Waller MF, Haymes EM. 1996. The effects of heat and exercise on sweat iron loss. *Med Sci Sports Exerc* 28:197–203.

Weinberg ED. 1978. Iron and infection. *Microbiol Rev* 42:45–66.

Wolman SL, Anderson GH, Marliss EB, Jeejeebhoy KN. 1979. Zinc in total parenteral nutrition: Requirements and metabolic effects. *Gastroenterology* 76:458–467.

Zinc Against Plasmodium Study Group. 2002. Effect of zinc on the treatment of *Plasmodium falciparum* malaria in children: A randomized controlled trial. *Am J Clin Nutr* 76:805–812.

Zinc Investigators' Collaborative Group. 1999. Prevention of diarrhea and pneumonia by zinc supplementation in children in developing countries: Pooled analysis of randomized controlled trials. *J Pediatr* 135:689–697.

Zinc Investigators' Collaborative Group. 2000. Therapeutic effects of oral zinc in acute and persistent diarrhea in children in developing countries: Pooled analysis of randomized controlled trials. *Am J Clin Nutr* 72:1516–1522.

# Copper, Zinc, and Immunity

*Susan S. Percival*
*University of Florida, Gainesville*

## INTRODUCTION

When the body is invaded by a foreign agent, the immune response follows a sequential, methodological and functional process: recognition of that foreign agent, response of the immune cells and the eradication of the foreign agent (Box B-4). Each immune cell has a unique way of recognizing foreign agents, and must distinguish between self and non-self. Not much is known about nutritional influences on the recognition function. Immune cells must respond once the foreign invader is recognized. Such responses include traveling to the site of infection, proliferating and differentiating. Cytokine synthesis and secretion are also part of the cellular response and drive much of the subsequent reactions. More research has been performed regarding nutritional influences on these cellular processes compared to the amount of research on the recognition process.

**BOX B-4**
**Sequential, Methodological, and Functional Scheme of Immunity**

| | |
|---|---|
| Recognition of Foreign Agents | T-Cell Receptor<br>B-cell membrane bound receptor<br>Toll-like receptors<br>Major Histocompatibility Complex, class I and II<br>Co-stimulatory molecules<br>Co-inhibitory molecules |
| Cellular Responses | Chemotaxis<br>Proliferation<br>Differentiation<br>Cytokine signaling<br>Memory<br>Apoptosis |
| Eradication Functions | Phagocytosis<br>Oxidative burst<br>Antigen processing and presentation<br>Antibody production<br>Cell killing (cytolysis) |

MCH = Major Histocompatibility Complex

One of the cellular processes that has relatively more information relating nutrient status to immunity is proliferation of peripheral blood mononuclear cells (PBMC). Cells also develop memory and undergo apoptosis to down regulate the response. Finally, the third and last step is eradication of the foreign agent. Engulfing and digesting microorganisms, processing and presentation of antigen, antibody synthesis and cell perforation as some of the eradication mechanisms. Research has also been done in regards to nutrient deficiencies and eradication functions.

All nutrients are critical for an appropriate immune response. At rest, presumably the immune system can optimally function at Recommended Dietary Allowances (RDA) levels of nutrient intake. It is not known, however, if or how much nutrient requirements change to evoke an optimum response.

Immunity should be regarded as a continuum. We are always infected, but if immuno-surveillance is optimum, then we do not show symptoms. Only when a microorganism has found a way to overcome the system, do we get symptoms such as fevers or rashes. If immunity has been compromised due to inadequate nutrients or other factors, then it is easily overwhelmed and we constantly have symptoms associated with illness. However, on the other side of the continuum, if the immune system remains continually stimulated, chronic disease such as heart disease, autoimmunity, rheumatoid arthritis and some cancers may result.

While much of the research and discussion centers on peripheral blood cells, it should be remembered that the gut is an important immune organ, constantly sampling lumen contents, processing and presenting antigen, and having effector cell activity, cytotoxic activity and barrier function. More research is needed on the role of nutrients in the gut's immune function, particularly the barrier function.

## IMMUNE SYSTEM: INDICATORS OF FUNCTIONALITY

Historically, PBMC proliferation has been widely used as an indicator of immune status. But how much of a decline in PBMC proliferation is required to negatively impact the host? Murasko and colleagues studied PBMC proliferation as a predictor of mortality in the elderly. In a group of people who had a low response to mitogen, a greater percent of that group died in subsequent years than those that had a high or mid response (Table B-13; Murasko and Goonewardene, 1990; Murasko et al., 1987). The low responders were very low having lost 75–93 percent of the PBMC proliferative response compared to young controls. In another study, individuals who had post-surgical complications had a significantly lower PBMC proliferation value at baseline pre-surgery than those who did not have post-surgical complications (Takagi et al., 2001). Those that had post-surgical complications had 40 percent lower response to phytohaemagglutinin (PHA) and 35 percent lower response to ConA compare to the group without complications. The level of the reductions in PBMC proliferation suggests that overall host response is negatively impacted when PBMC proliferation

**TABLE B-13** Correlations Between Mortality and PBMC Proliferation

| Age | Mortality (4.5 year follow-up) % dead | PHA Response units | PHA Response % reduction | ConA Response units | ConA Response % reduction | PWM Response units | PWM Response % reduction |
|---|---|---|---|---|---|---|---|
| Young | NA | 184 | | 162 | | 56 | |
| Elderly | | | | | | | |
| Low | 33% | 23 | 87% | 12 | 93% | 14 | 75% |
| Mid | 16% | 70 | 62% | 43 | 73% | 43 | 23% |
| High | 11% | 135 | 27% | 103 | 37% | 60 | -7% |

NOTE: PHA = phytohaemagglutinin; ConA = concanavalin A; PWM = pokeweed mitogen
SOURCE: Adapted from Murasko et al. (1990).

is moderately reduced. In a study on energy intake deficit and high intensity exercise, PBMC proliferation was reduced 35 to 75 percent of the groups' baseline values (Kramer et al., 1997). This reduction was associated abscesses and other visual signs of impaired immunity (personal communication, K. Friedl and A. Young, U.S. Army Research Institute for Environmental Medicine, June 13, 2005).

## COPPER AND IMMUNITY: RESEARCH IN HUMANS

It is known that copper has an important role in immunity from multiple models, although the exact mechanism of copper's function is not known. Evidence from individuals with the genetic disorder, Menkes, or those who have been on extended total parenteral nutrition (TPN) solutions without copper demonstrate functional immune changes. These models, however, may have other nutritional, genetic, or immunological issues that were not measured in the research. Rodent models, not only weanling animals, but perinatal and marginal models have been used to study copper deficiency and immunity. Rodent models on marginal copper diets (Hopkins and Failla, 1995) and swine models (Bala et al., 1992) show impairment in immunity without changes in copper dependent enzymes or serum copper levels. This confirms that biomarkers of copper status are urgently needed (see Keen and Uriu-Adams 2005 in this Appendix).

A metabolic study of copper depletion was performed in healthy humans. Eleven humans were placed on a diet containing 0.66 mg of copper per day for 24 days and then further reduced to 0.38 mg/day until day 66 and then repleted with 2.5 mg per day until day 90 (Kelley et al., 1995). Peripheral blood mononuclear cell (PBMC) proliferation was impaired at the end of 0.38 mg/day but not at the end of 0.66 mg/day. The impairment was about two-third of the baseline values. These values did not return to baseline levels at the end of the repletion period.

The biological significance of a 33 percent reduction is not known. In the study where post-surgical complications were noted, reductions of 35–45 percent of control values were associated with host complications. It is possible that the reduction caused by copper deficiency impacts overall host resistance, but this is not known.

A reduction in serum interleukin (IL)-2 receptor concentrations by the end of the 0.38 mg/day period were observed (Kelley et al., 1995). Levels did not return to baseline after repletion. White blood cell numbers were not affected. Neutrophil copper concentrations were reduced by the end of 0.66 mg/day, further reduced at the end of 0.38 mg/day and did not return to baseline values after repletion (Table B-14) (Turnlund et al., 1997). Neutrophil copper concentration remained at about 66 percent of the baseline values at the end of the repletion phase. Phagocytic activity of the neutrophil was not affected by these copper changes, and no other neutrophil functional indices were measured.

High copper intake (7 mg) for 5 months resulted in some statistical changes in certain immune functional assays (Turnlund, et al., 2004) but the biological significance of these changes is not known (Table B-15). Antibody titer response to three flu viruses appeared lower, although only the response to one strain was

**TABLE B-14** Neutrophil Copper Concentrations

| Day | Concentration, means ± SD |
|---|---|
| 0 | 125 ± 61[a] |
| Mid MP2 | 91 ± 42[b] |
| End MP2 | 54 ± 27[c] |
| End MP3 | 79 ± 35[b,c] |

NOTE: MP = metabolic period.
[a, b, c]Values having different letters are significantly different at $p < 0.05$.
SOURCE: Turnlund et al. (1997).

**TABLE B-15** Immune Changes and High Copper Intake

| Indicator | Before | After |
|---|---|---|
| Neutrophils (× $10^9$/L) | 3.3 ± 0.2 | 3.2 ± 0.2* |
| Lymphocytes (× $10^9$/L) | 2.14 ± 0.06 | 2.48 ± 0.06* |
| IL-2R (pg/mL) | 33.1 ± 3.5 | 27.3 ± 2.2* |
| IL-6 (pg/mL) | 1.4 ± 0.5 | 2.3 ± 0.6 |

NOTE: pg = picogram.
*Significantly different from levels before copper supplementation, $P < 0.05$.
SOURCE: Turnlund et al. (2004).

**TABLE B-16** Changes in Vaccination Titers After High Copper Intake

| Vax titers (fold increase) | Controls | Experimental |
|---|---|---|
| Beijing | 47 ± 9 | 14 ± 4* |
| Sydney | 92 ± 55 | 14 ± 4 |
| Harben | 32 ± 14 | 12 ± 6 |

*Significantly different from control subjects, $P < 0.05$.
SOURCE: Turnlund et al. (2004).

statistically lower (Table B-16). However, individuals averaged a 14 fold titer increase and immunologists consider a 4-fold increase to be responsive to the vaccination.

## ZINC AND IMMUNITY: RESEARCH IN HUMANS

Like copper, many models of zinc and immunity have been reported. A genetic disorder of zinc metabolism, acrodermatitis enteropathica, showed changes in immunity. Likewise, the elderly, hemodialysis patients, and people in developing countries all show immune changes that respond to zinc supplementation. It is difficult to interpret these studies since multiple nutrients may be impacted and differences in genetics and diseases may confound the results. The models that have shown an impact on immunity in a human population by zinc deficiency are not germane to the military. Having said that, the indices of immunity that are reduced in zinc deficiency are drawn from those publications. As shown in Box B-5 almost all measured indices of immunity are impacted negatively by zinc deficiency.

In a controlled metabolic study of zinc depletion, eight men consumed 13.7 mg/day for 5 wk, were reduced to 4.6 mg/day for 10 weeks and then repleted for 5 weeks with 13.7 mg/day (Pinna et al., 2002). No changes were observed for plasma zinc, or two zinc-requiring enzymes, alkaline phosphatase or 5'nucleotidase throughout the course of the study. Leukocytes remained constant in number and in their percent distribution. Neutrophil superoxide generation did not change.

Proliferation of PBMC was significantly reduced by about 25–30 percent at the end of the depletion and did not return to baseline values after 5 wk of repletion. It is not clear whether this reduction will impact the host's overall immunity. Secretion of INF-$\gamma$ and tumor necrosis factor (TNF)-$\alpha$ were not altered. IL-2 receptor secretion was impaired at suboptimal levels of PHA stimulation, but not at maximal levels of stimulation.

**BOX B-5**
**Reductions in Immune Parameters in Zinc Deficient Models**

| | |
|---|---|
| Recognition of Foreign Agents | Major histocompatibility complex<br>Receptors with zinc-finger domains |
| Cellular Response | |
| NK | Chemotaxis |
| Neutrophils | Cytokine secretion |
| Macrophages | Proliferation |
| T cell | Cytokine secretion<br>Proliferation |
| B cell | Differentiation<br>Memory |
| Gut | Barrier function<br>Prolonged parasite survival (mice) |
| Eradication Functions | Phagocytosis<br>Cytotoxic function<br>Oxidative burst<br>Antibody production |

Although PBMC proliferation did not return to normal by the end of repletion, the authors believe that zinc deficiency may be prolonged due to the long lifespan of lymphocytes. They also suggested that it did not return to baseline values due to stresses associated with living in a metabolic ward. If additional stress in already compromised zinc status results in immune status changes, this would be relevant to the military. More research is needed. However, the subjects did not exhibit increased rates of infection and illness and all other immune parameters remained at baseline levels suggests that immunity is largely upheld during a marginal zinc intake for relatively short period of time.

During stress, zinc appears to be redistributed rather than lost from the body. Isotope tracer studies suggest that when plasma zinc goes down, it is taken up by the liver, thymus and bone marrow, important immune organs (Huber and Cousins, 1988). However, the plasma is not the only organ with reduced zinc levels, but concentrations of zinc in skin, bone and intestine are also reduced. Due to the gut's important role in immunity, more research is needed to understand zinc's role in gut immunity.

There is no evidence for increased susceptibility to specific diseases with low zinc status although many organisms have been studied and evidence shows an increase susceptibility to a broad range of infectious diseases with the following etiological agents:

- Virus (*Herpes simplex*)
- Bacteria (Listeria, Salmonella, *Mycobacterium tuberculosis*)
- Protozaoan parasites (trypanasoma, *Toxoplasma gondii*, Plasmodium)
- *Candida albicans*
- Helminthes (tricinella, schistosoma)

Similarly, there is no evidence that suggests zinc deficiency promotes one type of infection over another.

There is also no evidence that zinc is required by microorganisms and the acute phase response is to prevent organisms from using zinc. Levels of zinc in the plasma do not get low enough to prevent microorganisms from using it. Also, those levels return to normal rapidly—by about 24 hours.

## CONCLUSIONS

Human models of copper or zinc depletion indicate that PBMC proliferation may be impacted by low levels of consumption. Other indices of immune function do not seem to be affected under these metabolic conditions and the length of time studied. The PBMC proliferation rates in both cases did not return to prestudy levels. The extrapolation of these observations to infectious disease resistance is not straightforward, and depends upon the nature of the microbe, its own nutrient needs, and the relative importance of innate, as opposed to immunologic, defense mechanisms.

Research areas that need further investigation are (1) the impact of nutrients on the recognition function of immunity; (2) gut function, particularly barrier function and survival of foreign invaders; (3) immunity as impacted by stress and by heavy exercise, coupled with the potential for marginal nutrient deficiencies; (4) overall host resistance to infection needs to be correlated with PBMC proliferation; (5) the need for a great level of nutrients during a major immune response.

## REFERENCES

Bala S, Lunney JK, Failla ML. 1992. Effects of copper deficiency on T-cell mitogenic responsiveness and phenotypic profile of blood mononuclear cells from swine. *Am J Vet Res* 53(7):1231–1235.

Hopkins RG, Failla ML. 1995. Chronic intake of a marginally low copper diet impairs in vitro activities of lymphocytes and neutrophils from male rats despite minimal impact on conventional indicators of copper status. *J Nutr* 125(10):2658–2668.

Huber KL, Cousins RJ. 1988. Maternal zinc deprivation and interleukin-1 influence metallothionein gene expression and zinc metabolism of rats. *J Nutr* 118(12):1570–1576.

Kelley DS, Daudu PA, Taylor PC, Mackey BE, Turnlund JR. 1995. Effects of low-copper diets on human immune response. *Am J Clin Nutr* 62(2):412–416.

Kramer TR, Moore RJ, Shippee RL, Friedl KE, Martinez-Lopez L, Chan MM, Askew EW. 1997. Effects of food restriction in military training on T-lymphocyte responses. *Int J Sports Med* 18 (Suppl 1):S84–S90.

Murasko DM, Goonewardene IM. 1990. T-cell function in aging: Mechanisms of decline. *Annu Rev Gerontol Geriatr* 10:71–96.

Murasko DM, Weiner P, Kaye D. 1987. Decline in mitogen induced proliferation of lymphocytes with increasing age. *Clin Exp Immunol* 70(2):440–448.

Murasko, DM, Gold, M.J., Hessen, M.T. and Kaye, D. 1990. Immune reactivity, morbidity, and mortality of elderly humans. *Aging Immun and Infect Disease* 2:171–179.

Pinna K, Kelley DS, Taylor PC, King JC. 2002. Immune functions are maintained in healthy men with low zinc intake. *J Nutr* 132(7):2033–2036. Erratum in: *J Nutr* 2002 Nov;132(11):3431.

Takagi K, Yamamori H, Morishima Y, Toyoda Y, Nakajima N, Tashiro T. 2001. Preoperative immunosuppression: Its relationship with high morbidity and mortality in patients receiving thoracic esophagectomy. *Nutrition* 17(1):13–17.

Turnlund JR, Scott KC, Peiffer GL, Jang AM, Keyes WR, Keen CL, Sakanashi TM. 1997. Copper status of young men consuming a low-copper diet. *Am J Clin Nutr* 65(1):72–78.

Turnlund JR, Jacob RA, Keen CL, Strain JJ, Kelley DS, Domek JM, Keyes WR, Ensunsa JL, Lykkesfeldt J, Coulter J. 2004. Long-term high copper intake: Effects on indexes of copper status, antioxidant status, and immune function in young men. *Am J Clin Nutr* 79(6):1037–1044.

# Impact of Nutritional Deficiencies and Psychological Stress on the Innate Immune Response and Viral Pathogenesis

*John F. Sheridan, Patricia A. Sheridan, and Melinda A. Beck*
*Ohio State University, Columbus*

## INTRODUCTION

Many nutrients have been demonstrated to be essential to maintain an adequate immune system able to defend against infectious diseases. When in garrison training or combat operations, the stress, and often negative energy balance, may contribute to impairment of the immune system. The risk of contracting an infectious disease, foodborne or otherwise, needs to be managed in part by adequate nutrition. This paper provides scientific evidence that demonstrates the importance of an appropriate diet, especially selenium intake, in maintaining an optimal immune defense system, especially when faced with stressful situations.

Research presented from animal (mice) studies explores the potential relationship between selenium deficiency and infection by enteroviruses, in particular enteroviruses that can cause Keshan disease. Studies that explain the mechanisms by which the combination of selenium deficiency and enterovirus infection result in disease are described in detail. Further evidence that explains the onset of disease results from studies conducted to examine the host immune response of selenium deficiency versus selenium adequate mice in response to an experimental influenza viral infection.

## COXSACKIE VIRUS B3 AND SELENIUM DEFICIENCY

The discovery that the cardiomyopathy know as Keshan disease has a dual etiology that involves both a deficiency of the essential trace mineral selenium as well as an infection with an enterovirus provides the impetus for studies of the relationships between nutrition and viral infection. Enterovirus isolates from patients with Keshan disease in a selenium-deficient area of China were predominantly coxsackievirus group B. Thus, these viruses may contribute to the pathology of Keshan disease, as coxsackie B viruses are known etiologic agents of myocarditis (Peng et al., 2000).

The possible relationship between selenium deficiency and infection with coxsackievirus was explored further using an experimental animal model. Virulent strains of coxsackievirus B3 (CVB3) induce myocarditis in infected mice, although avirulent strains, such as CVB3/0, do not induce disease even though the avirulent strain replicates in heart muscle. To determine if a deficiency in selenium could influence the ability of an avirulent virus to cause disease, weanling mice were fed a diet that was either deficient or replete in selenium for 4 weeks prior to infection with the avirulent CVB3/0. Mice fed the selenium-sufficient diet did not develop cardiac inflammation, the hallmark of myocarditis. In contrast, the Se-deficient mice developed moderate to severe myocarditis (Beck et al., 1994a). To determine if the increase in virulence was due to host factors alone, or a result of genome changes, the virus was isolated from the hearts of selenium-deficient mice and passed back into selenium-adequate mice. If the induction of myocarditis in the selenium-deficient mice was due to host factors alone, then infecting the selenium-adequate mice with this viral isolate would not be expected to cause myocarditis. However, selenium-adequate mice infected with virus isolated from selenium-deficient mice developed myocarditis, while selenium-adequate mice infected with virus isolated from other selenium-adequate mice did not develop myocarditis (Beck et al., 1994a). These findings suggested that CVB3/0 virus that replicated in a selenium-deficient host underwent a genomic change. To confirm this finding, CVB3/0 viral isolates obtained from selenium-adequate and selenium-deficient hosts were sequenced.

Sequencing of the multiple viral isolates obtained from infected selenium-adequate and selenium-deficient mice confirmed that a viral genome change had occurred (Beck et al., 1995). Six nucleotide changes between the original CVB3/0 strain and the virus isolated from the selenium-deficient mice were found, whereas no changes were found in the genome of virus isolated from selenium-adequate mice. The mutations persisted, and myocarditis developed, when the newly virulent virus infected naïve selenium-adequate mice. Therefore, replication of an avirulent coxsackievirus in the selenium-deficient host led to specific viral mutations that resulted in altered viral virulence. Once these mutations occurred, normal selenium-adequate mice were susceptible to myocarditis following infection by the newly pathogenic virus.

## CVB3 MUTATIONS AND OXIDATIVE STRESS

Because selenium plays in important role in several antioxidant enzymes, a deficiency in selenium can lead to increased oxidative stress of the host. In order to determine if oxidative stress associated with selenium-deficiency can induce changes in a viral genome, glutathione peroxidase 1 (Gpx-1) knockout mice were used. Selenium is an essential component of the antioxidant enzyme Gpx-1. When selenium is limited in a diet Gpx-1 activity declines (Whanger and Butler, 1998). In order to determine if a decrease in Gpx-1 activity was a crucial step in selenium-associated changes in virulence, Gpx-1 knockout mice were infected with CVB3/0. Similar to selenium-deficient mice, the Gpx-1 knockout mice developed myocarditis, whereas infected wildtype mice did not (Beck et al., 1998). The virus isolated from knockout mice with myocarditis demonstrated mutation to the cardiovirulent genotype at seven nucleotide positions, of which six were identical to the mutations found in virus isolated from selenium-deficient mice (Beck et al., 1998). These results suggest that the change in viral genome in infected selenium-deficient mice is due to increased oxidative stress as a consequence of a deficiency in antioxidant protection. Further evidence that increased oxidative stress is the driving force for the viral mutations is provided by the finding that CVB3/0 infected mice deficient in vitamin E, a lipid soluble antioxidant that functions differently from Gpx-1, also develop myocarditis due to a change in the viral genome (Beck et al., 1994b).

## HOST NUTRITIONAL STATUS AND INFLUENZA VIRUS INFECTION

Influenza virus is a leading cause of morbidity and mortality in the U.S. According to the Centers for Disease Control, influenza kills more than 36,000 people annually and is responsible for more than 114,000 hospitalizations (CDC, 2004). Influenza is a single stranded-RNA virus with a segmented genome. It belongs to the Orthomyxoviridae family of viruses.

To determine whether selenium deficiency had an effect on a family of viruses other than enteroviruses, weanling mice were fed a diet either deficient or adequate in selenium. After 4 weeks, mice were infected with influenza A/Bangkok/1/79 (H3N2), a strain that causes mild pneumonitis in normal mice. At all time points examined, Se-deficient mice had greater lung pathology than selenium-adequate mice. Additionally, the lung pathology persisted longer in the selenium-deficient mice (Beck et al., 2001).

Three segments of the influenza viral genome were sequenced from selenium-adequate and selenium-deficient mice; hemagglutinin (HA), neuraminidase (NA) and the matrix gene (M). All three proteins have been associated with virulence. The HA and NA proteins are responsible for viral entry and exit from the infected cell, respectively. The M gene, which codes for both M1 and M2 proteins, is associated with viral replication. Mutations in the M gene were consistently found in virus recovered from the selenium-deficient mice. As with the coxsackievirus studies, when this virulent influenza viral isolate was passed back into selenium-adequate mice, enhanced lung pathology was observed (Nelson et al., 2001). Therefore, similar to what was found for coxsackievirus B3, host selenium deficiency leads to increased viral mutation in the influenza virus genome, resulting in a more virulent phenotype.

In order to understand the mechanisms by which host nutritional status promotes viral mutation, we also examined the host's innate immune response. The innate immune response plays an important role in controlling the replication of influenza, and in directing the magnitude of the subsequent adaptive immune response. As a critical part of the innate immune response, IFN-α and IFN-β are produced by infected cells. These anti-viral cytokines protect uninfected cells from becoming infected by acting in an autocrine or paracrine manner to inhibit viral replication and increase expression of the major histocompatibility complex (MHC) class I molecules and natural killer (NK) cell cytotoxicity (Bogdan, 2000; Sinigaglia et al., 1999).

Similar to interferon (IFN)-α and IFN-β, IFN-γ is a potent antiviral cytokine produced early after infection by NK cells. Additionally, IFN-γ activates macrophages, increases MHC expression, antigen processing and directs the subsequent cell-mediated immune response (Huang et al., 1993; Ruby and Ramshaw, 1991). In these studies, weanling male C57Bl/6 mice were fed either selenium-adequate or selenium-deficient diets for 4 weeks and subsequently infected with influenza A Bangkok/1/79 virus. In response to the influenza infection, selenium-adequate mice upregulated expression of IFN-α, IFN-β and IFN-γ 24h post infection (p.i). Although selenium-deficient mice increased IFN-α, IFN-β and IFN-γ expression after infection, expression of these genes was 2–4 fold lower than in the Se-adequate mice (Sheridan, et al., 2005). These data suggest that in response to an influenza viral infection, selenium deficiency impairs the early, anti-viral cytokine response. How these changes in gene expression may correlate with the emergence of the viral mutations is currently under investigation.

## STRESS AND INFLUENZA INFECTION

The response to stress, whether physical or psychological, involves a variety of adaptive neuroendocrine mechanisms designed to restore homeostasis (Selye, 1936). Although these neuroendocrine responses are designed to restore homeostasis, the mammalian response to stress involves the release of immunomodulatory hormones and peptides that influence the host's response to infection. Stress induced activation of the hypothalamic-pituitary-adrenal axis and sympathetic nervous system results in the release of glucocorticoids, catecholamines and opioids that modulate various aspects of innate immunity. Natural killer cell responses, a major element of human and animal natural resistance to infection, is affected by stress responses (Bonneau et al., 1991; Campbell et al., 2001; Coe et al., 2002; Dobbs et al., 1996; Hermann et al., 1995).

During an influenza viral infection, NK cells play an important role in the early, innate defense (Stein-Streilein and Guffee, 1986). They respond within 2–3 days of infection to kill virus-infected cells and to produce cytokines that begin to initiate and enhance the subsequent, specific anti-viral responses (Kos and Engelman, 1996). The study described here was designed to extend previous findings to a translational model where the consequences of stress-induced modulation of NK cell function could be examined in the context of an infectious disease. Mice were subjected to repeated, daily cycles of restraint (RST) and then infected intranasally with influenza A/PR8 virus. In this model, NK cells are an important component of the innate immune response involved in controlling viral replication and limiting the spread of virus (Kos and Engelman, 1996; Stein-Streilein and Guffee, 1986). Daily cycles of restraint significantly modulated NK cell trafficking and cytolytic activity and contributed to elevated virus replication. Daily cycles of restraint suppressed two key chemokines necessary for peak NK activity, monocyte chemoattractant protein (MCP)-1 and macrophage inflammatory protein (MIP)-1$\alpha$, in lungs of virus-infected mice. Suppression of these chemokines correlated with reduced NK cell number and activity in the lungs (Hunzecker et al., 2004). Reduced NK activity resulted in enhanced pathophysiology. This suggests that in stressed mice, NK cells are not appropriately called to the lungs to fight infection.

Interleukin-12, a cytokine critical during the innate response, is an antigen presenting cell-derived cytokine that stimulates NK cells to secrete interferon IFN-$\gamma$ and also augments the proliferation and cytolytic activity of NK cells (Fehniger et al., 1999). The stress due to RST also contributed to a decrease in IL-12 gene expression during the course of the influenza infection. These data suggest that not only does RST diminish the recruitment of NK cells to the sites of viral replication, but RST also inhibits the expression of several key genes involved in controlling NK cell effector function. Although influenza infections are resolved by the adaptive T cell response, the innate NK response is important for controlling influenza replication prior to activation of the antigen-specific response.

## CONCLUSIONS

These studies demonstrate that selenium-deficiency and other nutritional changes that lead to increased host oxidative stress result in changes in the viral genome of two different RNA viruses. The viruses that emerge are more virulent and induce significant pathology even in a nutritionally intact host. Together, these data demonstrate that host nutritional status can influence not only the host response to the pathogen, but can also influence the genetic make-up of the viral genome. This last point is extremely important as it represents a new paradigm for understand host-pathogen relationships. Developing countries are sites of widespread nutritional deficiencies; they are also areas of emergence of new viral diseases as well as old diseases with new properties.

Our data also demonstrate that mice fed selenium-deficient diets have lowered innate host defenses to influenza infection. Mice that are stressed and infected with an influenza virus also have lowered innate immune responses to influenza infection. As the innate immune response is critical to controlling viral infections and directing the subsequent cell-mediated immune response, alterations in the response may have profound consequences. New research indicates that oxidative stress may link psychological stress with alterations in immune response (Neigh et al., 2005). We propose that both nutritional deficiencies and psychological stress share a final common pathway of increased oxidative stress that impacts the host's innate defenses. The combination of nutritional deficiency with psychological stress may result in even greater oxidative stress and thus increased impact on host immune function and viral mutation rates. Therefore, adequate nutritional protection against oxidative stress is necessary to improve immune function and decrease the possibility of viral mutation.

## REFERENCES

Beck M, Kolbeck P, Rohr L, Shi Q, Morris V, Levander O. 1994a. Benign human enterovirus becomes virulent in selenium-deficient mice. *J Med Virol* 43:166–170.

Beck M, Kolbeck P, Rohr L, Shi Q, Morris V, Levander O. 1994b. Vitamin E deficiency intensifies the myocardial injury of coxsackievirus B3 infection of mice. *J Nutr* 124:345–358.

Beck M, Shi Q, Morris V, Levander O. 1995. Rapid genomic evolution of a non-virulent coxsackievirus B3 in selenium-deficient mice results in selection of identical virulent isolates. *Nat Med* 1:433–436.

Beck MA, Esworthy RS, Ho Y, Chu F. 1998. Glutathione peroxidase protects mice from viral-induced myocarditis. *FASEB J* 12:1143–1149.

Beck M, Nelson HK, Shi Q, Van Dael P, Schiffrin EJ, Blum S, Barclay D, Levander OA. 2001. Selenium deficiency increases the pathology of an influenza virus infection. *FASEB J* 15:1481–1483.

Bogdan C. 2000. The function of type I interferons in antimicrobial immunity. *Curr Opin Immunol* 12:419–424.

Bonneau RH, Sheridan JF, Feng NG, Glaser R. 1991. Stress-induced effects on cell-mediated innate and adaptive memory components of the murine immune response to herpes simplex virus infection. *Brain Behav Immun* 5:274–295.

Campbell T, Meagher MW, Sieve A, Scott B, Storts R, Welsh TH, Welsh CJR. 2001. The Effects of Restraint Stress on the Neuropathogenesis of Theiler's Virus Infection: I. Acute Disease. *Brain Behav Immun* 15:235–254.

Centers for Disease Control and Prevention. 2004. Prevalence of overweight and obesity among adults with diagnosed diabetes—United States, 1988–1994 and 1999–2002. MMWR *Morb Mortal Wkly Rep* 53:1066–1068.

Coe CL, Kramer M, Kirschbaum C, Netter P, Fuchs E. 2002. Prenatal stress diminishes the cytokine response of leukocytes to endotoxin stimulation in juvenile rhesus monkeys. *J Clin Endocrinol Metab* 87:675–681.

Dobbs CM, Feng N, Beck M, Sheridan JF. 1996. Neuroendocrine regulation of cytokine production during experimental influenza viral infection: Effects of restraint stress-induced elevation in endogenous Ecorticosterone. *J Immunol* 157:1870–1877.

Fehniger TA, Shah MH, Turner MJ, VanDeusen JB, Whitman SP, Cooper MA, Suzuki K, Wechser M, Goodsaid F, Caligiuri MA. 1999. Differential cytokine and chemokine gene expression by human NK cells following activation with IL-18 or IL-15 in combination with IL-12: Implications for the innate immune response. *J Immunol* 162:4511–4520.

Hermann G, Beck FM, Sheridan JF. 1995. Stress-induced glucocorticoid response modulates mononuclear cell trafficking during an experimental influenza viral infection. *J Neuroimmunol* 56: 179–186.

Huang S, Hendriks W, Althage A, Hemmi S, Bluethmann H, Kamijo R, Vilcek J, Zinkernagel RM, Aguet M. 1993. Immune response in mice that lack the interferon-gamma receptor. *Science* 259:1742–1745.

Hunzeker J, Padgett DA, Sheridan PA, Dhabhar FS, Sheridan JF. 2004. Modulation of natural killer cell activity by restraint stress during an influenza A/PR8 infection in mice. *Brain Behav Immun* 18:526–535.

Kos FJ, Engleman EG. 1996. Role of Natural Killer Cells in the Generation of Influenza Virus-Specific Cytotoxic T Cells. *Cell Immunol* 173:1–6.

Neigh GN, Samuelsson AR, Bowers SL, Nelson RJ. 2005. 3-Aminobenzamide prevents restraint-evoked immunocompromise. *Brain Behav Immun* 19:351–356.

Peng T, Li Y, Yang Y, Niu C, Morgan-Capner P, Archard LC, Zhang H. 2000. Characterization of Enterovirus Isolates from Patients with Heart Muscle Disease in a Selenium-Deficient Area of China. *J Clin Microbiol* 38:3538–3543.

Ruby J, Ramshaw I. 1991. The antiviral activity of immune CD8+ T cells is dependent on interferon-gamma. *Lymphokine Cytokine Res* 10:353–358.

Selye H. 1936. A syndrome produced by diverse nocous agents. *Nature* (Lond) 138:32.

Sheridan, P.A., Sheridan, J.F., Beck, M.A. 2005. Selenium deficiency alters the innate immune response during an influenza infection in mice. *FASEB J.* 19(4):A443.

Sinigaglia F, D'Ambrosio D, Rogge L. 1999. Type I interferons and the Thl/Th2 paradigm. *Dev Comp Immunol* 23:657–663.

Stein-Streilein J, Guffee J. 1986. In vivo treatment of mice and hamsters with antibodies to asialo GM1 increases morbidity and mortality to pulmonary influenza infection. *J Immunol* 136:1435–1441.

Whanger P, Butler J. 1998. Effects of various dietary levels of selenium as selenite or selenomethionine on tissue selenium levels and glutathione peroxidase activity in rats. *J Nutr* 118:846–852.

# The Influence of Minerals on Muscle Injury and Recovery

*Joseph G. Cannon*
*Medical College of Georgia, Augusta*

## MECHANISMS OF INJURY AND REPAIR

Muscle damage can be caused by overloading, atrophy, ischemia/reperfusion, toxins, blunt impact, freezing, or lacerations. The general response to injury is stereotyped, regardless of the mode of damage. However, the nature of the initial damaging event at the cellular level, and any foreign material (such as infectious microorganisms or toxins) within the tissue, can affect the types of cells recruited to the site of injury. For example, ischemia itself may cause little damage to muscle but activates the endothelium such that upon reperfusion, neutrophils contacting the endothelium release reactive oxygen species that can cause extensive damage. In contrast, mechanical overloading of muscle fibers causes direct damage to the structural proteins of the sarcomeres, but the magnitude of damage and time course of repair are unaffected in animals that have been depleted of neutrophils (Lowe et al., 1995). The presence of microbes in the wound draws in neutrophils and wound healing is usually delayed until the microbes are cleared by the phagocytic and cytotoxic activities of the neutrophils and macrophages.

The recruitment and activation of macrophages and fibroblasts are common responses to all modes of muscle injury, in fact common to all types of tissue injury. The sequence of events in muscle repair and regeneration illustrates the function of these cells (adapted from Bischoff, 1994).

## Cellular and Molecular Events Following Muscle Injury

An initial injury disrupts cell membranes and extracellular matrix. Liberated intracellular factors and matrix fragments bind to scavenger receptors on resident macrophages. Cytokines such as interleukin-1 beta (IL-1β) are secreted by the macrophages. These cytokines activate endothelial cells to express adhesion molecules (selectins) that facilitate leukocyte extravasation. The leukocytes secrete matrix metalloproteinases (MMPs) that break down endothelial basement membranes and extracellular matrix, allowing the cells to migrate out of the vasculature and into the damaged area.

Twenty-four human MMPs have been identified: all possess a modular structures, including a common catalytic domain containing a zinc binding site. They are pro-enzymes activated by proteolytic cleavage (Lee and Murphy, 2004). MMP-2 and MMP-9 cleave type IV collagen, which is a major constituent of basement membranes and extracellular matrix. MMP-9 is a major product of macrophages and neutrophils (Goetzl et al., 1996).

Monocytes recruited from the bloodstream differentiate into macrophages and phagocytize damaged tissue. Most damage is cleared within a few days, but macrophages remain in the area secreting chemoattractants and growth factors that recruit and activate fibroblasts and muscle precursor (satellite) cells. These satellite cells also secrete a matrix metalloproteinase to facilitate their migration, in this case MMP-2 is produced. Following myotoxin injury, MMP-9 was expressed early during inflammatory cell infiltration, while MMP-2 coincided with regeneration of fibers (Carmeli et al., 2004). Matrix metalloproteinases also activate latent forms of cytokines: MMP-2 and -9 activate transforming growth factor beta (TGFβ), IL-1β and tumor necrosis factor (TNFα), whereas MMP-1 and -3 release basic fibroblast growth factor (FGF-2) bound to extracellular matrix (McCawley and Matrisian, 2001).

After arriving at the site of injury, the satellite cells proliferate and then fuse together into myotubes that mature into new muscle fibers. Insulin-like growth factor-I (IGF-I) is an important stimulus for fusion and differentiation. In muscle, as in other tissues, much of the zinc is bound to metallothionein. While activated satellite cells are proliferating, the Zn/metallothionein complexes are localized in the nuclei. Upon fusion and differentiation, the complexes migrate to the cytosol (Apostolova et al., 2000). Meanwhile, fibroblasts produce collagen and other proteoglycans for reconstruction of basement membranes and extracellular matrix and the original tissue structure is restored.

Adhesion molecules, matrix metalloproteinases, macrophages, fibroblasts perform similar functions in the repair of skin, bone and other organs. However instead of satellite cells, new skin tissue is formed by epidermal cells and new bone is formed by osteoblasts. The function of these effector molecules and cells is under paracrine regulation by locally-produced cytokines and growth factors.

## INFLUENCE OF ZINC ON INDIVIDUAL EFFECTORS OF WOUND HEALING

In zinc deficiency, heart and skeletal muscle zinc concentrations are unchanged, but drop in plasma, liver, and bone. The normal plasma zinc concentration is about 15 μmole/L, with 84 percent bound to albumin, 15 percent bound to $\alpha_2$macroglobulin and 1 percent bound to amino acids. Zinc deficiency reduces osteoblast activity, collagen and proteoglycan synthesis, and platelet aggregation (Rude and Shils, 2006).

Zinc promotes antioxidant state by: (1) preserving metallothionein (as described below), (2) serving as a component of superoxide dismutase, and (3) interfering with iron-mediated free radical formation. Zinc also blocks caspase-6, a mediator of apoptosis (Tapiero and Tew, 2003).

### Metallothionein

Four isoforms of metallothionein are known: MT-1 and MT-2, which are ubiquitous, and MT-3 and MT-4, which are located in the brain and skin. Each metallothionein molecule binds 7 zinc atoms. Zinc induces the mRNA for apometallothionein (thionein), which is susceptible to proteolysis until zinc-binding confers resistance. Physical trauma, glucocorticoids, IL-1, IL-6, and reactive oxygen species induce metallothionein, which is thought to provide protection against oxidative damage and to serve as a reservoir of zinc that can be donated to "zinc finger" transcription factors and zinc-dependent enzymes (Davis and Cousins, 2000). Monocyte metallothionein mRNA correlates with zinc intake in adequate diets (Cao and Cousins, 2000). Topical application of zinc oxide increases metallothionein expression in rat skin wounds (Lansdown, 2002).

## Matrix Metalloproteinases

Matrix metalloproteinase gene expression does not appear to be affected by mild zinc deficiency or excess, based on dietary studies in mice (Moore et al., 2003). In these experiments, whole thymus was digested, mRNA was harvested and 48,000 transcripts were analyzed. Zinc metalloenzymes and zinc-finger transcription factors not affected. Nevertheless, matrix metalloproteinase activity does appear to be dependent upon zinc availability. For example, tetracycline analogs inhibited MMP activity in vitro in proportion to their ability to bind zinc and the inhibition could be partially antagonized by excess zinc (Ryan et al., 2001). In the same report, oral administration of analogs to streptozotocin-diabetic rats reduced MMP-9 activity in the skin. A zinc chelating protein released by activated neutrophils, calprotectin, may serve as an endogenous regulator of MMP activity (Isaksen and Fagerhol, 2001). Topical application of zinc oxide increases MMP activity in pig skin wounds (Agren, 1993).

## Cytokines and Growth Factors

There is no compelling evidence that zinc deficiency adversely affects cytokine production. In a study of five healthy subjects (23–38 years old), zinc deficiency was induced by a diet of soy-based protein and a phytic acid supplement to reduce zinc bioavailability. Total dietary zinc was 2–3.5 mg/day for 20–24 weeks. The subjects were then repleted with zinc acetate (25–50 mg/day) for 8–12 weeks. Peripheral blood mononuclear cells were isolated for analysis of cytokine secretion at baseline, end of the depletion phase, and end of the repletion phase. Zinc depletion resulted in significant reductions in interferon-gamma (IFN$\gamma$) and TNF$\alpha$ secretion, compared to baseline and repletion conditions, but had no significant influence on IL-1$\beta$, IL-4, IL-10 or IL-6 secretion (Beck et al., 1997). In a study of shorter duration, 8 healthy men (27–47 yrs) were placed on a zinc restricted diet (4.6 mg/day) for 10 weeks. No significant effect was observed on phytohemagglutinin-induced TNF$\alpha$ or IFN$\gamma$ secretion by peripheral blood mononuclear cells nor on phorbol myristic acetate-induced neutrophil superoxide production (Pinna et al., 2002).

On the other hand, IGF-I may be significantly affected by zinc availability. Serum IGF-I correlated with zinc intake in adequate diets (Devine et al., 1998) whereas zinc deficiency reduced serum IGF-I concentration (Cossack, 1991) and zinc supplementation increased it (Imamoglu et al., 2005). Topical application of zinc oxide increased IGF-I mRNA by 50 percent in pig skin wounds (Tarnow et al., 1994). In vitro, zinc decreased affinity of IGF binding protein-5 and increased the affinity of myoblast IGF receptor type 1 for both IGF-I and IGF-II (McCusker and Novakofski, 2003). This, in effect, increases the bioavailability of IGF-I to the muscle cell, one of the regulatory factors in cell growth and multiplication during muscle repair after injury.

### Phagocytic Activity

The limited evidence available suggests that zinc supplementation may have a negative effect on the function of phagocytic cells. In one study, 11 healthy adult men given 300 mg/day zinc sulfate orally for 6 weeks. Plasma zinc increased from 83 to 200 μg/dL by the 6th week. Neutrophil chemotactic migration and phagocytosis were reduced by ~50 percent, whereas bactericidal capacity (percent viable ingested bacteria at 2 hours) was unchanged. No data regarding incidence of infection were reported (Chandra, 1984). In another study, 39 marasmic infants (7–8 months old) were given formula with (1.9 mg/kg/day) or without (0.35 mg/kg/day) supplemental zinc for 105 days (Schlesinger et al., 1993). Monocyte phagocytosis and fungicidal activity were significantly less in the supplemented group. Furthermore, the supplemented group had more than 2 times as many days of impetigo episodes as the control group ($1.3 \pm 1.1$ versus $0.55 \pm 0.8$, $P < 0.02$).

## INFLUENCE OF ZINC ON INTEGRATED WOUND HEALING

Very little information exists regarding the influence of zinc on overall wound healing. In one study, groups of mice were placed on a normal or low-protein diet for 4 weeks prior to abdominal surgery (Nezu et al., 1999). After surgery, the mice were further subgrouped by placement on total parenteral nutrition with either normal zinc content or no zinc for 6 days. No differences were observed in bursting pressure of the anastomosed intestine. Low protein groups had ~33 percent, non-significant reduction in tensile strength of sutured abdominal wall muscle, but no influence of zinc was observed. Low protein caused a ~50 percent reduction in tensile strength of sutured skin. Zinc deficiency reduced skin tensile strength at the suture by 35 percent in normal protein condition and by 69 percent ($P < 0.05$) in low protein condition.

Perhaps the most extensively studied application of zinc to humans relates to the potential effectiveness of oral zinc in healing arterial or venous leg ulcers. The conclusions of two Cochrane Systematic reviews (Wilkinson and Hawke, 1998, 2005) are that oral zinc has little effect, except perhaps a small benefit for individuals with low serum zinc concentrations.

## CONCLUSIONS

The complete mechanism by which skeletal muscle initiates and completes a repair process is not well deciphered. The number of synchronized events is numerous and involved many cells and signaling factors whose functions remained unknown. During the process proteins that depend on zinc as a modulator of function or synthesis, such as methalothionin, metalloproteinases, are known to play a role but the relationship between zinc status or zinc intake and their function during muscle repair is unknown. Likewise, no response on cytokine production has been observed as a result of zinc deficiency in humans. Only IGF-1 levels in serum and bioavailability to muscle cells appears to be affected by zinc status, zinc deficiency being related to lower serum concentrations of IGF-1.

With so few suggestive data regarding the involvement of zinc or any other minerals in muscle repair processes, there currently appears to be little justification for increasing dietary intakes of minerals based on the potential for improved wound healing or muscle repair that may occur during the high intensity exercise or other traumatic injuries potentially occurring during military garrison training.

## REFERENCES

Agren MS. 1993. Zinc oxide increases degradation of collagen in necrotic wound tissue. *Br J Dermatol* 129:221–223.

Apostolova MD, Ivanova IA, Cherian MG. 2000. Signal transduction pathways and nuclear translocation of zinc and metallothionein during differentiation of myoblasts. *Biochem Cell Biol* 78:27–37.

Beck FW, Prasad AS, Kaplan J, Fitzgerald J, Brewer G. 1997. Changes in cytokine production and T cell subpopulations in experimentally induced zinc-deficient humans. *Am J Physiol* 272:E1002–E1007.

Bischoff R. 1994. The satellite cell and muscle regeneration. In: Engel AG, Franzini-Armstrong C., eds. *Myology*. New York: McGraw-Hill, Inc. 1:97–118.

Cao J, Cousins RJ. 2000. Metallothionein mRNA in monocytes and peripheral blood mononuclear cells and in cells from dried blood spots increases after zinc supplementation of men. *J Nutr* 130:2180–2187.

Carmeli E, Moas M, Reznick AZ, Coleman R. 2004. Matrix metalloproteinases and skeletal muscle: A brief review. *Muscle Nerve* 29:191–197.

Chandra RK. 1984. Excessive intake of zinc impairs immune responses. *JAMA* 252:1443–1446.

Cossack ZT. 1991. Decline in somatomedin-C (insulin-like growth factor-I) with experimentally induced zinc deficiency in human subjects. *Clin Nutr* 10:284–291.

Davis SR, Cousins RJ. 2000. Metallothionein expression in animals: A physiological perspective on function. *J Nutr 130*:1085–1088.

Devine A, Rosen C, Mohan S, Baylink D, Prince RL. 1998. Effects of zinc and other nutritional factors on insulin-like growth factor I and insulin-like growth factor binding proteins in postmenopausal women. *Am J Clin Nutr* 68:200–206.

Goetzl EJ, Banda MJ, Leppert D. 1996. Matrix metalloproteinases in immunity. *J Immunol* 156:1–4.

Imamoglu S, Bereket A, Turan S, Taga Y, Haklar G. 2005. Effect of zinc supplementation on growth hormone secretion, IGF-I, IGFBP-3, somatomedin generation, alkaline phosphatase, osteocalcin and growth in prepubertal children with idiopathic short stature. *J Pediatr Endocrinol Metab* 18:69–74.

Isaksen B, Fagerhol MK. 2001. Calprotectin inhibits matrix metalloproteinases by sequestration of zinc. *Clin Pathol Mo Pathol* 54:2289–2292.

Lansdown ABG. 2002. Metallothioneins: Potential therapeutic aids for wound healing in the skin. *Wound Rep Reg* 10:130–132.

Lee MH, Murphy G. 2004. Matrix metalloproteinases at a glance. *J Cell Sci* 117:4015–4016.

Lowe DA, Warren GL, Ingalls CP, Boorstein DB, Armstrong RB. 1995. Muscle function and protein metabolism after initiation of eccentric contraction-induced injury. *J Appl Physiol* 79:1260–1270.

McCawley LJ, Matrisian LM. 2001. Matrix metalloproteinases: They're not just for matrix anymore! *Curr Opin Cell Biol* 13:534–540.

McCusker RH, Novakofski J. 2003. Zinc partitions insulin-like growth factors (IGFs) from soluble IGF binding protein (IGFBP)-5 to the cell surface receptors of BC3H-1 muscle cells. *J Cell Physiol* 197:388–399.

Moore JB, Blanchard RK, Cousins RJ. 2003. Dietary zinc modulates gene expression in murine thymus: Results from a comprehensive differential display screening. *Proc Natl Acad Sci* 100:3883–3888.

Nezu R, Takagi Y, Ito T, Matsuda H, Okada A, 1999. The importance of total parenteral nutrition-associated tissue zinc distribution in wound healing. *Surg Today* 29:34–41.

Pinna K, Kelley DS, Taylor PC, King JC. 2002. Immune functions are maintained in healthy men with low zinc intake. *J Nutr* 132:2033–2036.

Rude RK, Shils ME. 2006. Magnesium. In: *Modern Nutrition in Health and Disease.* In: Shils ME, Shike M, Ross AC, Caballero B, Cousins RJ. Philadelphia, PA: Lippincott, Williams and Wilkins. Pp. 223–247.

Ryan ME, Usman A, Ramamurthy NS, Golub LM, Greenwald RA. 2001. Excessive matrix metalloproteinase activity in diabetes: Inhibition by tetracycline analogues with zinc reactivity. *Curr Med Chem* 8:305–316.

Schlesinger L, Arevalo M, Arredondo S, Lonnerdal B, Stekel A. 1993. Zinc supplementation impairs monocyte function. *Acta Paediatr* 82:734–738.

Tapiero H, Tew KD. 2003. Trace elements in human physiology and pathology: Zinc and metallothioneins. *Biomed Pharmacother* 57:399–411.

Tarnow P, Agren MS, Steenfos H, Jansson JO. 1994. Topical zinc oxide treatment increases endogenous gene expression of insulin-like growth factor-I in granulation tissue from porcine wounds. *Scand J Plast Reconstr Hand Surg* 28:255–259.

Wilkinson EAJ, Hawke CI. 1998. Does oral zinc aid the healing of chronic leg ulcers? A systematic literature review. *Arch Dermatol* 134:1556–1560.

Wilkinson EAJ, Hawke CI. 2005. Oral zinc for arterial and venous leg ulcers. *Cochrane Database*, Accession number: 00075320-100000000-00387.

# Physical Activity and Nutrition: Effects on Bone Turnover, Bone Mass, and Stress Fracture

*Jeri W. Nieves*
*Helen Hayes Hospital and Columbia University,*
*West Haverstraw, New York*

## INTRODUCTION

Bone mass accumulates throughout childhood and adolescence until peak bone mass is reached during the third decade of life (Heaney et al., 2000; Weaver, 2002), at a time when many individuals enter military service. When higher bone mineral density (BMD) is attained at a young age (peak bone mass) there is a subsequent reduction in the risk of childhood fractures, stress fractures, and possibly osteoporosis and osteoporotic fractures later in life (Goulding et al., 2001; Marx et al., 2001; Melton et al., 1998, 2003; Myburgh et al., 1990;

Torgerson et al., 1996). Studies indicate that a larger bone size is also related to a reduced risk of fracture. Genetic factors account for between 60–80 percent of the variance in peak bone mass and bone size (McGuigan et al., 2002; Mitchell et al., 2003; Nguyen et al., 2003; Orwoll et al., 2001). However, an individual may not achieve their genetically determined bone mass/size, if environmental and lifestyle conditions are not permissive. High levels of physical activity and adequate calcium intake have been shown to improve accrual of peak bone mass, although data in males are limited (HHS, 2004; Klesges et al., 1996; Moiso et al., 2004; Molgaard et al., 2001).

## BONE HEALTH IN THE MILITARY: A U.S. MILITARY ACADEMY STUDY

A recent study was conducted with military academy students, both men and women, to investigate the relationship between exercise and bone health and diet, particularly milk consumption and bone health. Results show that there is an association between eating disorders and bone health as well as between negative energy balance and bone health in women cadets. Those women with abnormal menstrual function had more bone loss compare with women with normal menstrual function, possibly due to the effects of excess exercise in menstrual function. In men cadets, milk consumption was associated with mineral content of bone and the benefits of exercise for bone health where only seen with higher intakes of milk. This study follows up previous studies with military personnel. Results from this recent study are presented in detail in the sections that follow. Other relevant studies are also described.

In this study, college aged subjects were recruited from the United States Military Academy (USMA) Class of 2002, West Point, NY. Exercise and milk intake were assessed by self-administered questionnaires. Eating disorders were determined using the Eating Disorders Inventory (EDI). Female cadets reported menstrual function for the prior year. The outcome measurements used as indicators of bone health were peripheral quantitative computed tomography (QTC) and tibial length, Peripheral QCT (Stratec XCT-2000; Germany) was used to image a single slice at the two-third distal tibia. The distal third of the tibia was determined by a manual measurement of tibial length between the base of the patella and the styloid process to the closest centimeter. Peripheral QCT provides bone density (volumetric or true density), as well as bone size and geometry including cortical thickness, periosteal circumference, and endosteal circumference.

## EXERCISE AND BONE MASS AND SIZE

In the recent Military Academy study, described above prior exercise in males was significantly correlated to tibial content ($r = 0.23$; $p < 0.001$) and there was a significant 5 percent difference in total tibial content between those in the highest exercise (> 11 hours per week) group versus all others ($p < 0.001$). Male cadets in the lowest exercise group when compared to those in the highest exercise groups had 7 percent lower cortical thickness ($p < 0.04$), and 3 percent smaller periosteal circumference ($p < 0.04$; Ruffing et al., in review).

Although exercise is beneficial to bone health, excessive exercise can lead to abnormal menstrual function, which may have a negative impact on bone health. In the Military academy study, female cadets who had regular menstrual cycles during the first year in the academy gained bone in the spine and total hip as compared to women who had fewer than 6 menstrual cycles per year who lost bone mass at the spine and hip (p-value < 0.05; Nieves et al., 2000).

## CALORIC INTAKE AND BONE MASS

Several studies show that athletes with energy expenditures in excess of caloric intake have low BMD; however, this is often confounded by abnormal menstrual function (Cobb et al., 2003). Even in male distance runners, without hormonal disturbances, bone mass is lower than in controls if energy balance is negative; it is hypothesized to result from an energy intake that is lower than required (Hetland et al., 1993). Clearly caloric restriction for weight loss is related to bone loss, this was demonstrated in a review by Shapses and Cifuentes (2004). In USMA female military cadets, BMD losses over 4 years occurred at both the spine and hip in cadets with sub-clinical eating disorders (EDI highest quartile) whereas there was no change in BMD or gains in those women in the lower quartiles of EDI ($p < 0.05$; Nieves et al., 2005).

## CALCIUM, MILK, AND BONE MASS

The most frequently studied mineral in relation to bone health is calcium. There have been 10 of 11 controlled trials of calcium supplementation (300–1,000 mg/day) that have shown a positive relationship, with BMD increases from 1–6 percent depending on the study duration and skeletal site measured (Bonjour et al., 2001; Chan et al., 1995; Chevalley et al., 2005; Dibba et al., 2000; Johnston et al., 1992; Lee et al., 1993; Matkovic et al., 2004; Merrilees et al., 2000; Nowson et al., 1997; Rosen, 2003). When calcium supplementation was discontinued some studies report gain in bone health was lost (Johnston et al., 1992; Lee et al., 1993) whereas in others the benefit remained (Bongour et al., 2001; Dibba et al., 2000; Matkovic et al., 2004). A review in premenopausal women (Welten et al., 1995) suggested that calcium supplementation to a total calcium intake from 1,500 to 2,500 mg/day produces an annual mean percentage difference in bone mass of 1.3 percent at multiple skeletal sites.

In some studies, milk supplementation has been evaluated rather than calcium alone. In an earlier study of milk supplementation in young adults there were significantly greater increases in total body bone mineral content and total body bone mineral density as compared to young adults given a placebo (Cadogan et al., 1997). In the recent study of male military cadets described above, milk consumption was related to tibial mineral content and there was a 6 percent higher tibial content between those consuming more than 3 glasses of milk per day as compared to those consuming 1 or fewer glasses ($p < 0.03$; Ruffing et al., in review). Daily milk consumption was positively associated with cortical thickness and periosteal circumference, such that cortical thickness was significantly greater in the highest milk intake categories compared to the lowest milk intake group ($p < 0.04$; $p < 0.01$). There was a significant interaction between milk intake and prior exercise in relation to cortical thickness (Ruffing et al., in review). Males who exercise more only showed a skeletal benefit of the exercise if milk intake was greater than one glass per day.

## OTHER MINERALS AND BONE MASS

The data relating trace minerals to bone health are very limited. There have been limited studies evaluating phosphorus intake and bone health in young adults. Individuals with a healthy diet who consume the RDA for phosphorus are unlikely to have any negative impact on bone health. It is likely that the relationships between calcium, protein, and phosphorus intakes are what are important for bone health (Lemke et al., 1998). Low intakes in the face of high calcium intake from supplements may create a relative phosphorus deficiency because availability of phosphorus decreases as calcium supplement intake increases (Heaney and Nordin, 2002). Magnesium deficiency, if severe, will disturb calcium homeostasis leading to impaired PTH (parathyroid hormone) secretion and a lack of skeletal and renal response to PTH leading to hypocalcemia. There are also some data that suggest that magnesium intakes are inversely related to bone resorption. However, in a cross-over study of 26 females aged 20–28 years, who were given 240 mg magnesium per day had no effect on bone turnover (Doyle et al., 1999). By contrast, magnesium administration (360 mg) in 12 males age 27–36, resulted in an initial significant suppression of bone formation and resorption, that was transient and lasted for 10 days out of 30 days (Dimai et al., 1998). Several cross-sectional studies have noted a positive association between magnesium intake and BMD in premenopausal women (Angus et al., 1988; Freudenheim et al., 1986; Houtkooper et al., 1995; New et al., 1997, 2000; Wang et al., 1997; Yano et al., 1985), although not all (Michaelsson et al., 1995). These inconsistent results may be related to the difficulty in trying to discriminate the effect of a diet deficient in magnesium versus other deficiencies that also may impact BMD. The concentration of zinc in bone is higher than in most other tissues and can be quickly depleted. Zinc has a structural role in the bone matrix where it complexes with fluoride into the hydroxyapetitie crystals of the bone. One study related low zinc levels to forearm bone mineral in premenopausal women (Angus et al., 1988). Zinc may diminish bone resorption and stimulate bone formation but these data is mostly the result of animal studies (Hosea et al., 1999). In rat studies zinc has been shown at the site of fracture healing, but there are no clinical studies on the role of zinc in fracture healing.

Copper deficiency has negative effects on bone but there is inconclusive evidence regarding any bone benefits of increasing copper intake (Roughead and Lukaski, 2003). There are limited data and no large trial data regarding the role of boron in bone health. Strontium has only been studied in very large doses (up to 1–2 g/day) and these high strontium intakes may be beneficial for bone and may prevent bone loss in older women (Reginster et al., 2002). Silicon deficiency has negative effects on bone and silicon intake was positively related to bone density of the hip in some (men and young women) but not postmenopausal women (Jugdaohsingh et al., 2004).

## BONE TURNOVER, STRESS FRACTURES, AND EXERCISE

The impact of exercise on PTH and bone turnover has been studied in several small studies and the results are not always in agreement and it appears that the type of exercise, duration, timing of samples all can influence the results (Eliakim et al., 1997; Karlsson et al., 2003). Probably one of the most relevant papers for this topic was an evaluation of changes in dioxypyridinoline (DPD) during Marine Recruit Training (n = 158 females and 58 males). Increases in bone resorption were found to correspond to an increase in miles of weight bearing exercise performed during training. The authors reported significant bone resorption at the end of Marine recruit training and attributed this to an accumulation of weight bearing exercise as well as an increase in marching miles (Sheehan et al., 2003). It is possible that basic training will lead to increased resorption followed by increased formation and that the window between increments in these two processes may be the period of greatest risk of stress fractures. In the study of marine recruits (Sheehan et al., 2003) weekly DPD levels for females with and without stress fractures were evaluated and, although the differences were not significant, there was a trend toward higher levels of urinary DPD in female recruits with stress fractures as compared to female recruits without stress fracture, which indicates bone resorption might be related to stress fractures.

If bone resorption was excessive as reported and if it were related to excess risk for stress fracture, then it would be expected that prophylactic treatment with risedronate would reduce the incidence of stress fracture during military training. When subjected to strains higher than usual bone will remodel to repair microdamage and to strengthen the bone. In a randomized controlled trial for 15 weeks, 324 new infantry recruits in Israel were given risedronate, a bisphosphonate that reduces bone resorption or a placebo. There was no significant difference between drug and placebo for tibial, femoral, metatarsal, or total stress fracture incidence (Milgrom et al., 2004).

It is possible that calcium and vitamin D supplementation may be capable of preventing stress fractures in female naval recruits; Dr. Joan Lappe, at Creighton University, is currently evaluating this hypothesis. In this trial the female naval recruits are provided supplementation with 2,000 mg calcium and 800 IU vitamin D (Oscal+D) given as 2 doses with meals for 8 weeks basic training (n = 5,200). There are no increases in adverse effects at this dose and by the end of 2005 the study should be completed (Personal communication, J. Lappe, Creighton University).

## SUMMARY

The studies presented here point to a need for a clearer understanding of the impact of exercise and other factors on bone turnover. Some of the conclusions from this discussion are that an adequate caloric intake must be maintained to meet energy expenditure or bone loss may occur. Higher bone losses might also occurred due to dermal losses during exercise. Bone loss will be exaggerated in females with loss of menstrual function or eating disorders. Micro-fracture repair is also dependent on calcium intake. To counteract any excess in bone turnover and meet the demands of the skeleton during intense activity calcium higher than the AI of 1,000 mg may be needed with intense exercise. Intakes of 1,500–2,500 mg/day may be needed to maintain or increase BMD in younger recruits since peak bone mass may not yet be achieved. Basic training appears to first lead to increased resorption (perhaps to compensate for calcium loss due to sweat or negative energy balance), but this is followed by increased formation (stimulated by intense training) and the window between increments in these two processes may be the period of greatest risk of stress fractures.

More data are clearly needed to understand the role of nutrition in stress fracture occurrence. Milk or similar products have the potential to provide calcium as well as other important nutrients but until now, data on calcium and stress fracture are limited with two negative and one positive studies. Ongoing research on the potential benefits of higher calcium intakes indicates that supplements of up to 2,000 mg of calcium are safe. Results from this study will be forthcoming soon and should shed more light on the prevention of stress fractures by calcium.

## REFERENCES

Angus RM, Sambrook PN, Pocock NA, Eisman JA. 1988. Dietary intake and bone mineral density. *Bone Miner* 4(3):265–277.

Angus RM, Pocock NA, Eisman JA. 1998. Nutritional intake of pre- and postmenopausal Australian women with special reference to calcium. *Eur J Clin Nutr* 42(7):617–625.

Bonjour JP, Chevalley T, Ammann P, Slosman D, Rizzoli R. 2001. Gain in bone mineral mass in prepubertal girls 3.5 years after discontinuation of calcium supplementation: A follow-up study. *Lancet* 358(9289):1208–1212.

Cadogan J, Eastell R, Jones N, Barker ME. 1997. Milk intake and bone mineral acquisition in adolescent girls: Randomised, controlled intervention trial. *BMJ* 15(7118):1255–1260.
Chan GM, Hoffman K, McMurry M. 1995. Effects of dairy products on bone and body composition in pubertal girls. *J Pediatr* 126(4):551–556.
Chevalley T, Bonjour JP, Ferrari S, Hans D, Rizzoli R. 2005. Skeletal site selectivity in the effects of calcium supplementation on areal bone mineral density gain: A randomized, double-blind, placebo-controlled trial in prepubertal boys. *J Clin Endocrinol Metab* 90(6):3342–3349.
Cobb KL, Bachrach, LK, Greendale G, Marcus R, Neer R, Nieves J, Sowers MF, Brown BW, Gopalakrishnan G, Luetters C, Tanner HK, Ward B, Kelsey JL. 2003. Disordered eating, menstrual irregularity, and bone mineral density in female distance runners. *Medicine and Science in Sports and Exercise* 35(5):711–719.
Dibba B, Prentice A, Ceesay M, Stirling DM, Cole TJ, Poskitt EM. 2000. Effect of calcium supplementation on bone mineral accretion in gambian children accustomed to a low-calcium diet. *Am J Clin Nutr* 71(2):544–549.
Dimai HP, Porta S, Wirnsberger G, Lindschinger M, Pamperl I, Dobnig H, Wilders-Truschnig M, Lau KH. 1998. Daily oral magnesium supplementation suppresses bone turnover in young adult males. *J Clin Endocrinol Metab* 83(8):2742–2748.
Doyle L, Flynn A, Cashman K. 1999. The effect of magnesium supplementation on biochemical markers of bone metabolism or blood pressure in healthy young adult females. *Eur J Clin Nutr* 53(4):255–261.
Eliakim A, Raisz LG, Brasel JA, Cooper DM. 1997. Evidence for increased bone formation following a brief endurance-type training intervention in adolescent males. *J Bone Miner Res* 12(10):1708–1713.
Freudenheim JL, Johnson NE, Smith EL. 1986. Relationships between usual nutrient intake and bone-mineral content of women 35–65 years of age: Longitudinal and cross-sectional analysis. *Am J Clin Nutr* 44(6):863–876.
Goulding A, Jones IE, Taylor RW, Williams SM, Manning PJ. 2001. Bone mineral density and body composition in boys with distal forearm fractures: A dual-energy x-ray absorptiometry study. *J Pediatr* 139(4):509–515.
Heaney RP, Nordin BE. 2002. Calcium effects on phosphorus absorption: Implications for the prevention and co-therapy of osteoporosis. *J Am Coll Nutr* 21(3):239–244.
Heaney RP, Abrams S, Dawson-Hughes B, Looker A, Marcus R, Matkovic V, Weaver C. 2000. Peak bone mass. *Osteoporos Int* 11(12):985–1009.
Hetland ML, Haarbo J, Christiansen C. 1993. Low bone mass and high bone turnover in male long distance runners. *J Clin Endocrinol Metab* 77(3):770–775.
Hosea HJ, Taylor CG, Wood T, Mollard R, Weiler HA. 2004. Zinc-deficient rats have more limited bone recovery during repletion than diet-restricted rats. *Exp Biol Med* (Maywood) 229(4):303–311.
Houtkooper LB, Ritenbaugh C, Aickin M, Lohman TG, Going SB, Weber JL, Greaves KA, Boyden TW, Pamenter RW, Hall MC. 1995. Nutrients, body composition and exercise are related to change in bone mineral density in premenopausal women. *J Nutr* 125(5):1229–1237.
Johnston CC Jr, Miller JZ, Slemenda CW, Reister TK, Hui S, Christian JC, Peacock M. 1992. Calcium supplementation and increases in bone mineral density in children. *N Engl J Med* 327(2):82–87.
Jugdaohsingh R, Tucker KL, Qiao N, Cupples LA, Kiel DP, Powell JJ. 2004. Dietary silicon intake is positively associated with bone mineral density in men and premenopausal women of the Framingham Offspring cohort. *J Bone Miner Res* 19(2):297–307.
Karlsson KM, Karlsson C, Ahlborg HG, Valdimarsson O, Ljunghall S, Obrant KJ. 2003. Bone turnover responses to changed physical activity. *Calcif Tissue Int* 72(6):675–680.
Klesges RC, Ward KD, Shelton ML, Applegate WB, Cantler ED, Palmieri GM, Harmon K, Davis J. 1996. Changes in bone mineral content in male athletes. Mechanisms of action and intervention effects. *JAMA* 276(3):226–230.

Lee WT, Leung SS, Ng MY, Wang SF, Xu YC, Zeng WP, Lau J. 1993. Bone mineral content of two populations of Chinese children with different calcium intakes. *Bone Miner* 23(3):195–206.

Lemke B, Whiting S, McKay H. 1998. Dietary Patterns of a Group of Children, Mothers and Grandmothers. *Can J Diet Pract Res* 59(2):62–66.

Lloyd T, Andon MB, Rollings N, Martel JK, Landis JR, Demers LM, Eggli DF, Kieselhorst K, Kulin HE. 1993. Calcium supplementation and bone mineral density in adolescent girls. *JAMA* 270(7):841–844.

Marx RG, Saint-Phard D, Callahan LR, Chu J, Hannafin JA. 2001. Stress fracture sites related to underlying bone health in athletic females. *Clin J Sport Med* 11(2):73–76.

Matkovic V, Landoll JD, Badenhop-Stevens NE, Ha EY, Crncevic-Orlic Z, Li B, Goel P. 2004. Nutrition influences skeletal development from childhood to adulthood: A study of hip, spine, and forearm in adolescent females. *J Nutr* 134(3):701S–705S.

McGuigan FE, Murray L, Gallagher A, Davey-Smith G, Neville CE, Van't Hof R, Boreham C, Ralston SH. 2002. Genetic and environmental determinants of peak bone mass in young men and women. J Bone Miner Res 17(7):1273–1279.

Melton LJ 3rd, Atkinson EJ, O'Connor MK, O'Fallon WM, Riggs BL. 1998. Bone density and fracture risk in men. *J Bone Miner Res* 13(12):1915–1923.

Melton LJ 3rd, Crowson CS, O'Fallon WM, Wahner HW, Riggs BL. 2003. Relative contributions of bone density, bone turnover, and clinical risk factors to long-term fracture prediction. *J Bone Miner Res* 18(2):312–318.

Merrilees MJ, Smart EJ, Gilchrist NL, Frampton C, Turner JG, Hooke E, March RL, Maguire P. 2000. Effects of diary food supplements on bone mineral density in teenage girls. *Eur J Nutr* 39(6):256–262.

Michaelsson K, Holmberg L, Mallmin H, Sorensen S, Wolk A, Bergstrom R, Ljunghall S. 1995. Diet and hip fracture risk: A case-control study. Study Group of the Multiple Risk Survey on Swedish Women for Eating Assessment. *Int J Epidemiol* (4):771–782.

Milgrom C, Finestone A, Novack V, Pereg D, Goldich Y, Kreiss Y, Zimlichman E, Kaufman S, Liebergall M, Burr D. 2004. The effect of prophylactic treatment with risedronate on stress fracture incidence among infantry recruits. *Bone* 35(2):418–424.

Mitchell BD, Kammerer CM, Schneider JL, Perez R, Bauer RL. 2003. Genetic and environmental determinants of bone mineral density in Mexican Americans: Results from the San Antonio Family Osteoporosis Study. *Bone* 33(5):839–846.

Moiso, KC, Hurwitz DE, Sumner DR. 2004. Dynamic loads are determinants of peak bone mass. *J Orthop Res* 22(2):339–345.

Molgaard C, Thomsen BL, Michaelsen KF. 2001. The influence of calcium intake and physical activity on bone mineral content and bone size in healthy children and adolescents. *Osteoporos Int* 12(10):887–894.

Myburgh, KH, J Hutckins, AM Fataar, SF Hough and TD Noakes. 1990. Low bone density is an etiologic factor for stress fractures in athletes. *Ann Intern Med* 113:754–759.

New SA, Bolton-Smith C, Grubb DA, Reid DM. 1997. Nutritional influences on bone mineral density: a cross-sectional study in premenopausal women. *Am J Clin Nutr* 65(6):1831–1839.

New SA, Robins SP, Campbell MK, Martin JC, Garton MJ, Bolton-Smith C, Grubb DA, Lee SJ, Reid DM. 2000. Dietary influences on bone mass and bone metabolism: Further evidence of a positive link between fruit and vegetable consumption and bone health? *Am J Clin Nutr* 71(1):142–151.

Nieves J, Ruffing J, Zion M, Lindsay R, Cosman F. 2000. Menstrual function predicts change in bone mass in elite female cadets. 22nd Annual Meeting of the American Society for Bone and Mineral Research (ASBMR) Toronto, Canada, September, 2000.

Nieves J, Zion M, Ruffing J, Garrett P, Lindsay R, Cosman F. 2005. *Eating Disorders and Amenorrhea are Strong Predictors of Change in Bone Mass in Physically Active Young Females*. 27th Annual Meeting of the American Society for Bone and Mineral Research (ASBMR) Nashville, TN.

Nguyen TV, Livshits G, Center JR, Yakovenko K, Eisman JA. 2003. Genetic determination of bone mineral density: Evidence for a major gene. *J Clin Endocrinol Metab* 88(8):3614–3620.

Nowson CA, Green RM, Hopper JL, Sherwin AJ, Young D, Kaymakci B, Guest CS, Smid M, Larkins RG, Wark JD. 1997. A co-twin study of the effect of calcium supplementation on bone density during adolescence. *Osteoporos Int* 7(3):219–225.

Orwoll ES, Belknap JK, Klein RF. 2001. Gender specificity in the genetic determinants of peak bone mass. *J Bone Miner Res* 16(11):1962–1971.

Reginster JY, Deroisy R, Dougados M, Jupsin I, Colette J, Roux C. 2002. Prevention of early postmenopausal bone loss by strontium ranelate: The randomized, two-year, double-masked, dose-ranging, placebo-controlled PREVOS trial. *Osteoporos Int* 13(12):925–931.

Rosen CJ. 2003. Insulin-like growth factor I and calcium balance: Evolving concepts of an evolutionary process. *Endocrinology* 144(11):4679–4681.

Roughead ZK, Lukaski HC. 2003. Inadequate copper intake reduces serum insulin-like growth factor-I and bone strength in growing rats fed graded amounts of copper and zinc. *Nutr* 133(2):442–448.

Ruffing JA, Cosman F, Zion M, Tendy S, Garrett P, Lindsay R, Nieves J. In Press. Exercise level and milk intake are positively related to bone mass and size at weight bearing sites.

Sheehan KM, Murphy MM, Reynolds K, Creedon JF, White J, Kazel M. 2003. The response of a bone resorption marker to marine recruit training. *Mil Med* 168(10):797–801.

Torgerson DJ, Campbell MK, Thomas RE, Reid DM. 1996. Prediction of perimenopausal fractures by bone mineral density and other risk factors. *J Bone Miner Res* 11(2):293–297.

U.S. Department of Health and Human Services. 2004. Bone Health and Osteoporosis: A Report of the Surgeon General.

U.S. Department of Health and Human Services, Office of the Surgeon General. Wang MC, Luz Villa M, Marcus R, Kelsey JL. 1997. Associations of vitamin C, calcium and protein with bone mass in postmenopausal Mexican American women. *Osteoporos Int* 7(6):533–538.

Weaver CM. 2002. Adolescence: The period of dramatic bone growth. *Endocrine* 17(1):43–48.

Yano K, Heilbrun LK, Wasnich RD, Hankin JH, Vogel JM. 1985. The relationship between diet and bone mineral content of multiple skeletal sites in elderly Japanese-American men and women living in Hawaii. *Am J Clin Nutr* 42(5):877–888.

Zelten DC, Kemper HC, Post GB, van Staveren WA. 1995. A meta-analysis of the effect of calcium intake on bone mass in young and middle aged females and males. *J Nutr* 125(11):2802–2813.

# Evaluating Nutritional Effects on Cognitive Function in Warfighters: Lessons Learned

*Harris R. Lieberman*
*U.S. Army Research Institute of Environmental Medicine, Natick, Massachusetts*

## INTRODUCTION

There is substantial information in the scientific literature regarding the effects of various nutritional interventions on cognitive performance. Some of this research was specifically conducted to address issues of military relevance. Most of the literature in the area addresses the acute effects of nutritional factors on cognitive function; only a few studies have examined the chronic effects of variations in diet or administration of dietary supplements for more than a day. To date, only a few nutritional interventions have been shown to alter cognitive performance in young, healthy, adequately nourished humans. From an evolutionary perspective, this is to be expected since it would not be desirable for short term variations in the diet to change behavioral functions, except those associated with seeking or consuming food. Consequently, perhaps the most important lesson to be learned from this literature is that subtle variations in the diet, or treatment with many of the dietary supplements purported to alter cognitive function, do not have observable effects on cognitive state.

This paper is intended to serve, in part, as the basis for recommendations to be made by the Committee on Mineral Requirements for Cognitive and Physical Performance of Military Personnel. This committee was charged with making recommendations on mineral requirements for military personnel engaged in military operations and in garrison. The committee was asked to consider maintenance and/or improvement of cognitive and physical performance when formulating military mineral requirements. Therefore, they provided several questions to scientists working in the area of military nutrition. This paper addresses the decrements in cognitive function and behavior that result from stressors faced by soldiers during training and combat operations. In particular, it addresses how cognitive function and mood are uniquely affected by military operations. It also addresses selection of appropriate methods to assess warfighter cognitive state and the use of such methods in military nutrition research studies. This paper is organized in a question and answer format to directly address the questions posed by the committee.

## GENERAL QUESTIONS

***Are there specific effects of high levels of physical and emotional stress on cognitive function or behavior?***

There are devastating effects of physical and psychological stress on cognitive function and behavior. These adverse effects have been documented in many studies conducted with various military populations and in some limited situations, with civilian volunteers (Haslam, 1984; Lieberman et al., 2005b; Ruby et al., 2002). There is no clear consensus regarding the contribution of each type of stressor to the overall degradation in cognitive performance seen following either acute or chronic operational (military) stress. Nevertheless, in operations or training conducted to simulate combat by U.S. infantry and special operations units, as well as studies conducted with soldiers from other nations, severe decrements in cognitive performance inevitably are observed after two days or less of sustained operational stress (Banderet and Stokes, 1980; Haslam, 1984;

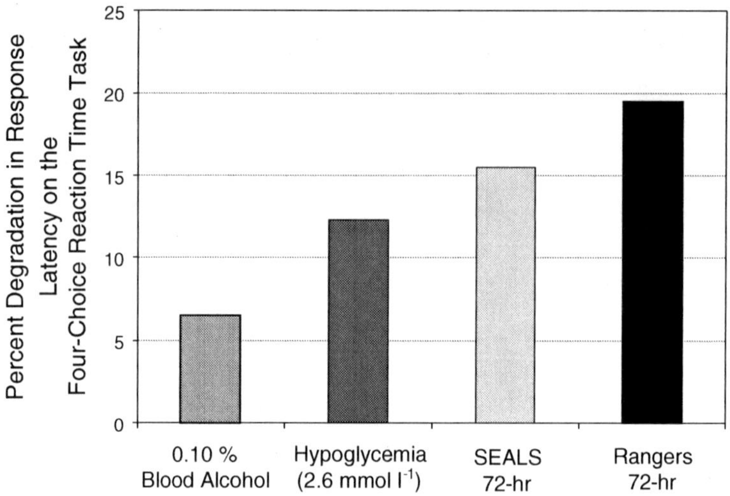


**FIGURE B-26** Percent degradation from baseline in mean response time on the Four-Choice Visual Reaction Time Test for the Ranger and SEAL studies (Lieberman et al., 2005; Lieberman et al., 2002b) compared with the effects of clinical hypoglycemia (2.6 mmol · $L^{-1}$) and a blood alcohol level of 0.10 percent, which is legally drunk in many localities (Strachan et al., 2001; Tiplady et al., 2001). In both studies with the SEALS and Rangers, volunteers were exposed to various stressors prior to cognitive testing including substantial sleep deprivation, environmental exposures, and psychological stress. The data from the SEAL trainees are only from those who received placebo treatment, not caffeine (Modified from Lieberman et al., 2005b).

McLellan et al., 2003). Typically, such short term operational stress includes sleep deprivation and, in many instances, exposure to environmental extremes and inadequate hydration and nutrition (Lieberman et al., 2005a; Opstad, 1994; Opstad et al., 1978). In several studies we have conducted in the field (Lieberman et al., 2002b, 2005a), in simulated combat-like scenarios, decrements in warfighter cognitive performance observed have exceeded those documented in studies of civilian volunteers who are legally drunk or suffering from clinical hypoglycemia (Figure B-26; Lieberman et al., 2005b; Strachan et al., 2001; Tiplady et al., 2001). Severe cognitive decrements are seen in most cognitive functions assessed in such studies, including simple and choice reaction time, logical reasoning, learning memory and vigilance. For a more detailed discussion see Lieberman et al. (2005b).

In studies where the principal "stressor" is inadequate nutrition there does not appear to be substantial adverse effects on cognitive performance, even after a month of substantial caloric deprivation (Lieberman, 1999; Lieberman et al.,

1997). This is consistent with the limited civilian literature in this area, in particular with the classic Minnesota Starvation studies (Keys et al., 1950).

***Is there any information regarding a "benefit" of altering nutritional status to improve cognitive behavior in individuals in the military?***

A number of studies have demonstrated that caffeine can enhance certain aspects of warfighter cognitive and physical performance in rested and sleep deprived volunteers (Amendola et al., 1998; Fine et al., 1994; Kamimori et al., 2003; LaJambe et al., 2005; Lieberman et al., 2002b; McLellan et al., 2004, 2005). In rested volunteers, the effects of caffeine in moderate doses are largely confined to tasks requiring sustained vigilance. They can also be observed on mood questionnaires that assess alertness, a mood state associated with changes in vigilance (for recent reviews see Institute of Medicine, 2001; Lieberman, 2003; Smith, 2005). These effects can also be observed in simulations of military activities such as sentry duty, where vigilance is a key factor (Johnson and Merullo, 2000). In sleep deprived volunteers, the effects of caffeine are observed not only on tests of vigilance and sentry duty, but on a wider variety of cognitive functions including learning, short term memory, and reasoning (Figure B-27; Kamimori et al., 2003; Lieberman et al., 2002b). It has been hypothesized that the more widespread cognitive effects of caffeine in sleep deprived individuals are not directly the result of caffeine's modulation of these higher order cognitive functions, but are secondary to the compound's ability to maintain alertness (Lieberman, 2003). An ad-hoc committee of the Committee on Military Nutrition Research has reviewed the literature in this area and concluded, ". . . caffeine in the range of 100 to 600 mg is effective in increasing speed of reaction time without affecting accuracy and in improving performance on visual and audio vigilance tasks" (Institute of Medicine, 2001).

A nutrient that has been extensively studied for its possible beneficial effects during acutely stressful environments is the amino acid tyrosine, a dietary precursor for the synthesis of dopamine and norepinephrine in the brain (for a recent review see Deijen, 2005). Studies conducted at a number of civilian and military laboratories suggest that high doses of tyrosine, greater than those present in single serving of foods, mitigate some of the adverse effects of acute stress on cognitive performance (Ahlers et al., 1994; Banderet and Lieberman, 1989; Magill et al., 2003). There are also some data suggesting that substantial doses of carbohydrate in beverage form can enhance cognitive performance of soldiers engaged in aerobic activities and who are not receiving fully adequate energy from rations (Figure B-28; Lieberman et al., 2002a). There is no question that carbohydrate supplementation enhances aerobic performance as demonstrated by numerous civilian and several military studies (for a recent review see Montain and Young, 2003). For a recent review of the cognitive literature in this area, particularly with regard to military nutrition issues, see Lieberman, 2003.

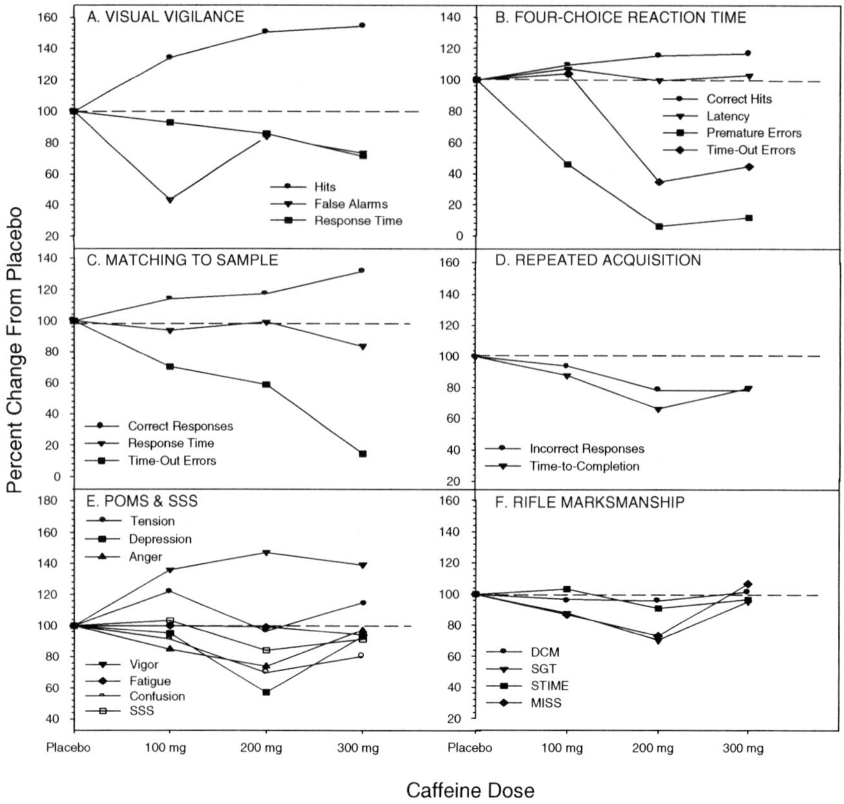


**FIGURE B-27** Percentage change in performance and mood following varying doses of caffeine compared to placebo treatment 1 hr after caffeine administration. Navy SEAL trainees undergoing Hell Week training were given 100, 200, or 300 mg of caffeine or placebo. The treatments were administered after 72 hours of sleep deprivation and exposure to stressors such as running, lifting, paddling inflatable boats, swimming, and calisthenics, as well as psychological stressors. At both 1 and 8 hours after caffeine administration, subjects were given several cognitive tests. Significant improvement was seen on many of the tests in a dose-dependent manner. (A) Percentage change from placebo on measures of visual vigilance. (B) Percentage change from placebo on the four-choice visual reaction time test. (C) Percentage change from placebo on the matching-to-sample test. (D) Percentage change on the repeated acquisition test. (E) Percentage change from placebo on the 6 sub-scales of the Profile of Mood States (POMS) and Stanford Sleepiness Scale (SSS). (F) Percentage change from placebo on measures of rifle marksmanship. Overall, caffeine appeared to be most effective at a dose of 200 mg, although on some tasks the optimal dose was 300 mg.

NOTE: DCM = Distance from Center of Mass; MISS = Percent of Targets Missed; SGT = Shot Group Tightness; STIME = Sighting Time

SOURCE: Lieberman et al. (2002a).

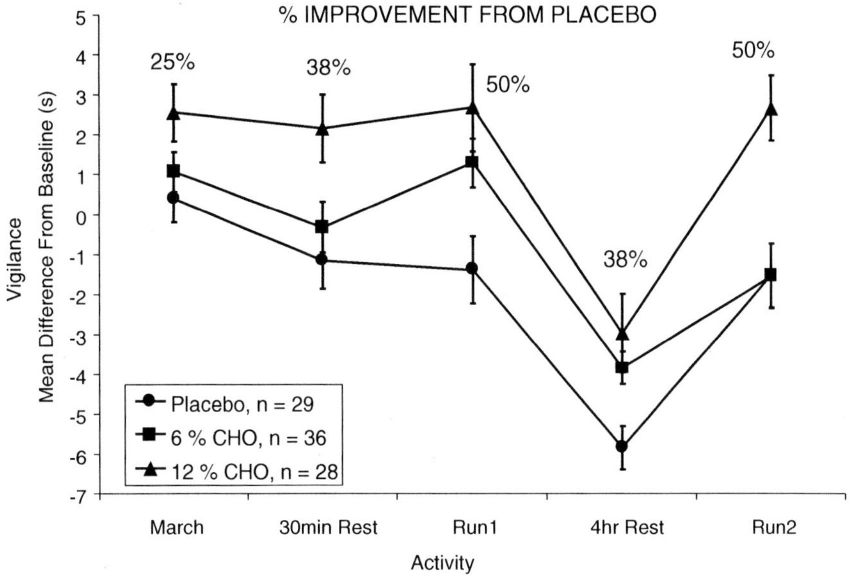


**FIGURE B-28** Mean (± SEM) differences from baseline in auditory vigilance reaction times over the 10 hour on study designed to evaluate the effects of carbohydrate on cognitive and physical performance (Lieberman et al., 2002a). This study examined the effects of carbohydrate supplementation on cognitive function during a day of sustained aerobic activity. Army Rangers received either 6 percent (by volume) carbohydrate, 12 percent (by volume) carbohydrate, or placebo beverage in 6 doses, in addition to two ration meals. During the day, volunteers completed a 19.3-km march, two 4.8-km runs, and live-fire marksmanship exercises. Each subject's vigilance was tested continuously by an ambulatory monitor worn on the nonpreferred wrist (Lieberman and Coffey, 2000; Lieberman et al., 2005c). Performance on the monitor was summed over 5 time periods that corresponded to the activity taking place. Because the values plotted are differences from baseline values, the higher the number on the *y* axis, the better the performance. Carbohydrate treatment had a positive, dose-dependent effect on mean reaction time vigilance difference scores. The interaction between treatment and time was also significant and reaction time was shorter with carbohydrate treatment that with placebo at every time period. Percent improvement on the 12 percent carbohydrate beverage relative to placebo treatment during the same activity is also provided above each activity.
SOURCE: Lieberman et al. (2002a).

## SPECIFIC QUESTIONS

***What cognitive functions are important when soldiers are engaged in military operations and in garrison?***

***What behaviors are important for performance when soldiers are engaged in military operations and in garrison?***

These two closely related questions are best addressed together. Cognitive functions are hypothetical constructs formulated to describe mental processes. When such processes are converted into an action, a behavior occurs. Therefore, from a practical perspective it is only the behavior that can be measured and is operationally relevant. Even the most concrete thought (cognitive process) cannot be observed unless some behavior occurs, except indirectly with technologies, such as brain scanning, that assess physiological correlates of mental activities. When behavioral psychologists study cognitive processes, they are in fact studying the behaviors which they hypothesize are the result of specific cognitive processes.

The relationship between cognitive processes and the behavior that results has to be inferred, and is always complex. Even simple tasks require multiple cognitive functions. For example, a seemingly simple cognitive test, such as visual choice reaction time, which produces a very simple behavior, pushing a button, requires a complex cascade of cognitive processes (Lieberman, 2003). Motivation to perform the task, allocation of attention, visual perception, visual processing, decision making, short and long term memory (recalling which stimulus is correct and recalling the instructions for the test), sensory-motor integration, and motor control are some of the cognitive processes required to perform the task. Given the behavioral complexity of such a simple task, attempting to objectively and quantitatively specify the critical cognitive parameters associated with the thousands of tasks associated with military operations in the field and garrison is, at present, impossible. There are hundreds of military specialties, each with hundreds of individual behaviors associated with performance of the job. Military performance is not unique in this regard, as few, if any of the behavioral processes required to adequately perform most civilian occupations have been specified.

In response to this complexity, psychologists have attempted to identify some key cognitive capabilities that appear to govern many aspects of human behavior and develop tests to assess them. Functions that can be assessed by cognitive tests include: sensation, perception, vigilance, attention, learning, memory, language, fine and gross motor performance, decision making, and complex mental processes, such as mathematical reasoning and face recognition. Cognitive psychologists who study military performance have attempted to choose functions from these categories that they believe are the most important for optimal military performance. In many instances, computerized cognitive test batteries can be administered to military populations to collect this information rapidly and with minimal hardware. The cognitive functions that seem to be frequently selected across various military laboratories, presumably because they are thought to be most important for warfighter operational performance, include: psychomotor tasks like simple and choice reaction time, vigilance, attention, short-term memory, and logical reasoning. More complex behaviors are also assessed such as marksmanship and performance in simulators of real world tasks. Performance on the more abstract and cognitive tests often predict performance on more realistic tasks (for examples see McLellan et al., 2003).

***Is there evidence from military studies that decrements in cognitive functions or behaviors occur in the field and may be related to mineral deficiencies?***

As discussed above in response to the first general question, cognitive performance rapidly degrades in operational scenarios designed to simulate combat. The loss of cognitive function associated with actual combat has been termed the 'fog of war' although the term has more general implications (Clausewitz, 1993; Kiesling, 2001; Lieberman et al., 2005b; Opstad et al., 1978). In developed countries, it seems unlikely that mineral deficiencies are associated with decrements in cognitive function on the battlefield or in garrison. An exception may be women, who are at greater risk of deficient mineral status than men. Of particular concern is iron status, due to the prevalence of iron deficiency and borderline iron deficiency seen in the young female population and in military population samples. Since iron status appears to be associated with physical and cognitive performance decrements there may be operational consequences in some women (Beard, 1995, 2003; Beard et al., 1995; Bruner et al., 1996; Cline et al., 1998; McClung et al., 2006).

***What makes military personnel unique regarding the use of tests for cognitive function and behavior?***

Military personnel are exposed to a great many physical and cognitive stressors that are unique to their profession. Some examples include: fear associated with severe injury or loss of life for the individual or his close associates in combat; long periods of time away from home; environmental stressors such as heat, cold and high altitude; acute and chronic sleep deprivation; exposure to environmental toxins unique to military operations such as depleted uranium, as well as more common pollutants; possible exposure to chemical and biological agents, and the simultaneous or consecutive combination of many of these stressors.

***What are the advantages and disadvantages of using self-report, such as the Profile of Mood States, to measure mood, fatigue, cognitive function, etc.?***

Mood questionnaires are frequently used to assess the effects of dietary constituents on behavioral state in civilian and military populations (this section has been adapted with minor modifications from Lieberman, 2005). When they are adequately standardized and have acceptable psychometric properties, mood questionnaires are accepted as valid measures of mental states and can be administered in a few minutes, unlike cognitive test batteries. This is an important advantage for military field studies since it is usually difficult for volunteers to spend a great deal of time taking comprehensive cognitive test batteries. One of the most widely employed mood questionnaires in nutrition-behavior research is the Profile of Mood States (POMS). This questionnaire provides six individual subscales: vigor, fatigue, tension, depression, anxiety, and anger, as well as an overall indication of mood state (McNair et al., 1971). Depending on the particular mood assessed, they can be highly correlated with tests of cognitive function (Bolmont et al., 2000; Glenville and Broughton, 1978; Nicholson and Stone, 1986). Although mood questionnaires do not have the cachet of tests of cognitive performance because they are mistakenly not considered to be objective, they are useful for documenting and explaining the effects of dietary constituents on human behavior. In fact, the distinction between an objective and a subjective test is more a matter of appearance than reality. Cognitive performance tests seem to be objective because they apparently bypass the emotional content of the behavior assessed, but in fact, when standardized, both cognitive performance and mood questionnaires are objective and reliable measures of particular aspects of human behavior. Each type of test requires the subject to make a response to a particular sequence of standardized stimuli.

Mood questionnaires are valuable in studies of dietary constituents as they explain and validate the results of cognitive performance tests. Furthermore, they can provide evidence that a dietary treatment or diet has effects not readily detected by cognitive tests. For example, caffeine alters a variety of mood states in a manner that would not be expected given its stimulant-like actions. Mood questionnaires have shown that in normal volunteers, given moderate doses of caffeine, depression and hostility are reduced and clarity of mind, imagination, and energy increase (Amendola et al., 1998; Leathwood and Pollet, 1982). This demonstrates the importance of administering mood questionnaires as complementary tests to explain certain cognition outcomes.

In general, if consistent effects are observed using different measurement techniques, such as performance tests and mood questionnaires, then the results of a study are more likely to be valid. As noted above, caffeine consistently affects tests of vigilance and closely related mood states such as vigor and fatigue (Lieberman, 2003; Smith, 2002). Drugs that are stimulants, like amphetamine, also have consistent effects on these outcomes (Magill et al., 2003). Use of mood questionnaires can also provide information regarding confounding factors, such as unanticipated changes in fatigue, anxiety, or depression of volunteers during testing.

Unfortunately, there is an unfounded, preconceived belief that standardized tests of mood state are less objective than tests of cognitive performance. In particular, military policy makers should consider results from such mood states questionnaires as valid data that provides pertinent information and together with cognitive tests results, can be used to develop strategies to improve military performance. In fact, cognitive tests can sometimes be worse predictors of actual military performance than mood questionnaires, as they are rarely standardized and appropriately validated in young, healthy populations.

***Can one extrapolate data on cognitive function or behavior from the civilian population to military personnel? What are study design characteristics or methods that need to be considered when making such extrapolations?***

Due to the unique nature of combat and the special requirements for many military occupations as discussed above, extrapolation from civilian to military populations is difficult. Under limited circumstances such generalization may be possible as a first approximation, but definitive data from appropriate military populations will usually be required. Moreover, such a determination can only be made on a case-by-case basis. Even key design characteristics and optimal methods for studies will vary from case-to-case. For a recent discussion of some of the critical methodological issues in the area of nutrition and behavior see Harris (2005) and Lieberman (2005). A conservative approach is necessary in relating nutrition to behavior across different populations since the effects in question are often modest.

## SUMMARY

There is abundant scientific evidence that the circumstances faced by soldiers during training and combat operations adversely affect their cognitive function and behavior. Some of these circumstances involve a variety of stressors, from physical to psychological, that impair normal brain function. Valid measures of cognitive performance and behavior are of critical importance to determine factors that alter cognitive domains and to implement strategies that may improve performance.

Measuring cognitive functions and behavior is a complex task that can only be conducted when the many domains that constitute cognition and behavior are examined. Therefore, many tests have been devised that explore these domains and have been used and standardized for both civilian and military populations. When developing strategies to improve military performance, policy makers should consider results from both mood states questionnaires and cognitive tests since, when standardized, both types provide pertinent information and compliment each other. That is, mood states questionnaires can help understand results from tests cognitive performance.

Although studies with the civilian population can initially be useful in exploring these issues, extrapolation to military personnel is in most cases challenging due to the differing situations and extreme demands often placed on military personnel. Therefore, it is advisable to duplicate the military environment to the extent possible (i.e., physical environment, physical activity, and other stressors) when conducting research intended to address military requirements.

## DISCLAIMERS

The opinions or assertions contained herein are the private views of the author and are not to be construed as official or as reflecting the views of the Army or the Department of Defense. Human subjects participated after giving their free and informed voluntary consent. The investigators adhered to the policies for protection of human subjects as prescribed in Army Regulation 70-25, and the research was conducted in adherence with the provisions of 45 CFR Part 46. Citations of commercial organizations and trade names in this report do not constitute an official Department of the Army endorsement or approval of the products or services of these organizations. Approved for public release; distribution is unlimited.

## REFERENCES


Ahlers ST, Thomas JR, Schrot J, Shurtleff D. 1994. Tyrosine and glucose modulation of cognitive deficits resulting from cold stress. In: B. Marriott, ed. *Food Components to Enhance Performance*. Institute of Medicine. Washington, DC: National Academy Press. Pp. 301–320.

Amendola CA, Gabrieli JDE, Lieberman HR. 1998. Caffeine's effects on performance and mood are independent of age and gender. *Nutr Neurosci* 1:269–280.

Banderet LE, Lieberman HR. 1989. Treatment with tyrosine, a neurotransmitter precursor, reduces environmental stress in humans. *Brain Res Bull* 24:147–150.

Banderet LE, Stokes JW. 1980. Simulated, sustained combat operations in the field artillery fire detection center (FOC): A model for evaluating biomedical indices. Technical Report No. T 9/80. Natick, MA: U.S. Army Research Institute of Environmental Medicine.

Beard J. 1995. One person's view of iron deficiency, development and cognitive function. *Am J Clin Nutr* 62:709–710.

Beard J. 2003. Iron deficiency alters brain development and functioning. *J Nutr* 133:1468S–1472S.

Beard JL, Feagans L, Frobose C. 1995. Cognitive dysfunction in iron deficient adolescents. *FASEB J* 9:A975.

Bolmont B, Thullier F, Abraini JH. 2000. Relationships between mood states and performances in reaction time, psychomotor ability, and mental efficiency during a 31-day gradual decompression in hypobaric chamber from sea level to 8848 m equivalent altitude. *Physiol Behav* 71:469.

Bruner AB, Joffe A, Duggan AK, Casella JF, Brandt J. 1996. Randomised study of cognitive effects of iron supplementation in non-anaemic iron-deficient adolescent girls. *Lancet* 348:992–996.

Clausewitz C von. 1993. *On War*. New York: Alfred A. Knopf.

Cline AD, Patton JF, Tharion WJ, Strowman SR, Champagne C, Arsenault J, Reynolds KL, Warber JP, Baker-Fulco C, Rood J, Tulley RT, Lieberman HR. 1998. Assessment of the relationship between iron status, dietary intake, performance, and mood state of female army officers in a basic training population. Technical Report No. T98-24. Natick, MA: U.S. Army Research Institute of Environmental Medicine.

Deijen JB. 2005. Tyrosine. In: Lieberman HR, Kanarek R, Prasad C, eds. *Nutritional Neuroscience*. Boca Raton, FL: CRC Press LLC. Pp. 363–381.

Fine BJ, Kobrick JL, Lieberman HR, Riley RH, Marlowe B, Tharion WJ. 1994. Effects of caffeine or diphenhydramine on visual vigilance. *Psychopharmacology* 114:233–238.

Glenville M, Broughton R. 1978. Reliability of the Stanford Sleepiness Scale compared to short duration performance tests and the Wilkinson Auditory Vigilance Task. *Adv Biosci* 21:235.

Harris RBS. 2005. Consideration of Experimental Design for Studies in Nutritional Neuroscience. In: Lieberman HR, Kanarek R, Prasad C, eds. *Nutritional Neuroscience*. Boca Raton, FL: CRC Press LLC. Pp. 11–23.

Haslam DR. 1984. The military performance of soldiers in sustained operations. *Aviat Space Environ Med* 55:216–221.

IOM (Institute of Medicine). 2001. *Caffeine for the Sustainment of Mental Task Performance: Formulations for Military Operations*. Washington, D.C.: National Academy Press.

Johnson RF, Merullo DJ. 2000. Caffeine, gender, and sentry duty: Effects of a mild stimulant on vigilance and marksmanship. In: Friedel K, Lieberman HR, Ryan DH, Bray GA, eds. *Pennington Center Nutrition Series Volume 10: Countermeasures for Battlefield Stressors.* Baton Rouge, LA: Louisiana State University Press. Pp. 272–289.

Kamimori GH, Johnson D, Thorne D. 2003. Efficacy of multiple caffeine doses for maintenance of vigilance during early morning operations. *Sleep* 26:A196.

Keys A, Brozek J, Henschel A, Mickelsen O, Taylor HL. 1950. The Biology of Human Starvation, Vol. 1. Minneapolis, MN: The University of Minnesota Press. Pp. 1255–1342.

Kiesling EC. 2001. *On war Without the Fog.* Fort Leavenworth, KS: Combined Arms Center.

LaJambe CM, Kamimori GH, Belenky G, Balkin TJ. 2005. Caffeine effects on recovery sleep following 27 h total sleep deprivation. *Aviat Space Environ Med* 76:108–113.

Leathwood PD, Pollet P. 1982. Diet-induced mood changes in normal populations. *J Psychiatric Res* 17:147.

Lieberman HR. 1999. Amino Acid and Protein Requirements: Cognitive performance, stress, and brain function. In: *The Role of Protein and Amino Acids in Sustaining and Enhancing Performance.* Washington, D.C.: National Academy Press. Pp. 289–307.

Lieberman HR. 2003. Nutrition, brain function, and cognitive performance. *Appetite* 40:245–254.

Lieberman HR. 2005. Human nutritional neuroscience: fundamental issues. In: Lieberman HR, Kanarek R, Prasad C, eds. *Nutritional Neuroscience.* Boca Raton, FL: CRC Press LLC. Pp. 3–10.

Lieberman HR, Coffey BP. 2000. Preliminary findings from a new device for monitoring performance and environmental factors in the field. In: Friedel K, Lieberman HR, Ryan DH, Bray GA, eds. *Pennington Center Nutrition Series Volume 10: Countermeasures for Battlefield Stressors.* Baton Rouge, LA: Louisiana State University Press. Pp. 126–159.

Lieberman HR, Askew EW, Hoyt RW, Shukitt-Hale B, Sharp MA. 1997. Effects of thirty days of undernutrition on plasma neurotransmitter precursors, other amino acids and behavior. *J of Nutr Biochem* 8:119–126.

Lieberman HR, Falco CM, Slade SS. 2002a. Carbohydrate administration during a day of sustained aerobic activity improves vigilance, assessed with a novel ambulatory monitoring device, and mood. *Am J Clin Nutr* 76:120–127.

Lieberman HR, Tharion WJ, Shukitt-Hale B, Speckman KL, Tulley R. 2002b. Effects of caffeine, sleep loss and stress on cognitive performance and mood during U.S. Navy SEAL training. *Psychopharmacology* 164:250–261.

Lieberman HR, Bathalon GP, Falco CM, Kramer FM, Morgan III CA, Niro P. 2005a. Severe decrements in cognition function and mood induced by sleep-loss, heat, dehydration and undernutrition during simulated combat. *Biol Psych* 57:422–429.

Lieberman HR, Bathalon GP, Falco CM, Morgan III CA, Niro P, Tharion WJ. 2005b. The fog of war: decrements in cognitive performance and mood associated with combat-like stress. *Aviat Space Environ Med* 76(7):C7–C14.

Lieberman HR, Kramer FM, Montain SJ, Niro P, Young AJ. 2005c. Automated ambulatory assessment of cognitive performance, environmental conditions and motor activities during military operations in obiomonitoring for physiological and cognitive performance during military operations. *Proceeding of SPIE* 5797:14–23.

Magill RA, Waters WF, Bray GA, Volaufova J, Smith SR, Lieberman HR, et al. 2003. Effects of tyrosine, phentermine, caffeine, d-amphetamine and placebo on cognitive and motor performance deficits during sleep deprivation. *Nutr Neurosci* 6:237–246.

McClung JP, Marchitelli LJ, Friedl KE, Young AJ. 2006. Prevalence of iron deficiency and iron deficiency anemia among three populations of female military personnel in the U.S. Army. *J Am Coll Nutr* 25:64–69.

McLellan TM, Bell DG, Lieberman HR, Kamimori GH. 2003. The impact of caffeine on cognitive and physical performance and marksmanship during sustained operations. *Canadian Mil J* 4:47–54.

McLellan TM, Bell DG, Kamimori GH. 2004. Caffeine improves physical performance during 24 h of active wakefulness. *Aviat Space Environ Med* 75:666–672.

McLellan TM, Kamimori GH, Bell DG, Smith IF, Johnson D, Belenky G. 2005. Caffeine maintains vigilance and marksmanship in simulated urban operations with sleep deprivation. *Aviat Space Environ Med* 76:39–45.

McNair DM, Lorr M, Droppleman LF. 1971. *Profile of Mood States Manual*. San Diego, CA: Educational and Industrial Testing Service.

Montain SJ, Young AJ. 2003. Diet and physical performance. *Appetite* 40:255–267.

Nicholson AN, Stone BM. 1986. Antihistamines: Impaired performance and the tendency to sleep. *Eur J Clin Pharmacol* 30:27.

Opstad K. 1994. Circadian rhythm of hormones is extinguished during prolonged physical stress, sleep and energy deficiency in young men. *Eur J Endocrinol* 134:56–66.

Opstad PK, Ekanger R, Nummestad M, Raabe N. 1978. Performance, mood, and clinical symptoms in men exposed to prolonged, severe physical work and sleep deprivation. *Aviat Space Environ Med* 49:1065–1073.

Ruby BC, Shriver TC, Zderic TW, Sharkey BJ, Burks C, Tysk S. 2002. Total energy expenditure during arduous wildfire suppression. *Med Sci Sports Exerc* 34:1048–1054.

Smith A. 2002. Effects of caffeine on human behavior. *Food Chem Toxicol* 40:1243.

Smith A. 2005. Caffeine. In: Lieberman HR, Kanarek R, Prasad C, eds. *Nutritional Neuroscience*. Boca Raton, FL: CRC Press LLC. Pp. 341–361.

Strachan MW, Deary IJ, Ewing FM, Fergusson SS, Young MJ, Frier BM. 2001. Acute hypoglycemia impairs the functioning of the central but not the peripheral nervous system. *Physiol Behav* 72:83–92.

Tiplady B, Drummond GB, Cameron E, Gray E, Hendry J, Sinclair W, Wright P. 2001. Ethanol, errors, and the speed-accuracy trade-off. *Pharmacol Biochem Behav* 69:635–641.

# Iron and Cognitive Performance

*John L. Beard and Laura E. Murray-Kolb*
*Pennsylvania State University, University Park*

## INTRODUCTION

Iron deficiency is the most common single nutrient deficiency in the world (WHO, 2002). Infants, children, and women of reproductive age are the most commonly affected though there is reason to believe there are functional consequences to iron deficiency in any individual, regardless of sex, age, and racial background (Beard, 1995). As many as 9–11 percent of women of reproductive age have iron deficiency (Looker et al., 1997); in military personnel > 50 percent of women in basic training were iron deficient (Westphal et al., 1995) suggesting a greater overall prevalence of iron deficiency in females in the military. The prevalence of iron deficiency specific to males and females in the military is not well documented nor is the stability of the prevalence estimates established

(Westphal et al., 1995). The special demands made upon military personnel in terms of physical and emotional stress may well lead to alterations in nutrient metabolism which in turn can be associated with cognitive and behavioral alterations (Cline et al., 1998). The purpose of this review is to present what is known regarding cognitive alterations that can be ascribed to iron deficiency with, or without anemia.

## MILITARY PERSONNEL

Several specific topics need to be addressed within this review: (1) Is there any direct evidence that iron deficiency and iron deficiency anemia alters cognitive functioning? (2) What is the evidence that the additional high physical and emotional stresses placed on military personnel will alter the relationship between iron nutritional status and cognitive performance? (3) What is known about the probable biological mechanisms for altered cognition in iron deficiency?

The existing scientific literature relating iron status to cognition and behavior is almost exclusively in the civilian population with the exception of several recent published reports (Booth, 2003) and one in-house report (Cline et al., 1998). This latter report was issued in 1998 from the U.S. Army Research Institute of Environmental Medicine regarding cognitive performance, and physical performance in a group of female officers going through basic training. One-third of the 57 subjects were low in serum ferritin while only seven percent were anemic at entry. After basic training, 64 percent of the women had low ferritin levels despite reported iron intakes > 16 mg/day. Intake of iron was < 80 percent of the military recommended dietary allowances in only 8 subjects suggesting dietary intakes of iron during training was close to adequate in most of the soldiers. The increase in prevalence of low ferritin however suggests the physical and emotional demands of basic training did increase iron losses; a finding consistent with the effect of physical training on iron balance (Murray-Kolb et al., 2001).

Importantly, there was no relationship between iron status and three negative emotions (tension, depression, anger) or the positive emotion scale (vigor) within the profile of mood states (POMS) battery that was administered. There was a positive correlation between "iron status" and confusion but the report is unclear regarding their definition of iron status in this regard so it is impossible to conclude if anemia or tissue iron deficiency were responsible for this statistically significant relationship. As a group, iron sufficient women did not differ from iron deficient women in any of these behavioral measures. The cognitive task, a four-choice reaction time paradigm, was also not different in iron deficient compared to iron sufficient subjects. Other reports on the relationship of iron status to cognition and behavior in military personnel are very sparse and not conclusive (Booth, 2003: Booth et al., 2003). In these two studies on Australian military personnel consuming either the fresh food diet or the combat ration pack, the soldiers had significant declines (approximately 15 percent) in serum ferritin and folate as well as a decline in antioxidant status while training during 12 or 23 days. Poor baseline antioxidant status improved in all the soldiers, especially those consuming the combat ration pack possibly due to the vitamin C fortified food items. Emotionally, there was increased fatigue and more negative affect but specific relationships to a micronutrient could not be established in either of these studies. The conclusions from the available studies in military personnel do not support a specific role for changes in iron status being related to mood, behavior, or cognitive performance but the extremely limited knowledge base makes this conclusion very tenuous.

## CIVILIAN PERSONNEL

There are a number of studies performed in adults and adolescents (Table B-17) that have had a focus on the relationship between iron status and cognitive or behavioral functioning. There are two cross sectional designs that looked at subscales of the General Health Questionnaire (GHQ) showing that both low ferritin and oral contraceptive use were required to observe a relationship between ferritin and depression (Fordy and Benton, 1994; Rangan et al., 1998). Other work using the Minnesota Multiphasic Personality Inventory (MMPI, the most widely used personality test in the U.S.) test and a set of French fatigue, depression, and anxiety scales showed no effect of iron status on these measures with the exception of a French study in which women with ferritin between 20–50 μg/L showed a 2.2 times greater benefit in terms of fatigue scores compared to women with ferritin > 50 μg/L (Hunt and Penland, 1999; Verdon et al., 2003). The former study was a blinded, placebo intervention trial but only for four weeks, which is unlikely to be sufficient time to replenish pools of essential iron (Youdim et al., 1989). One additional cross sectional study looked at depression in post-partum women and showed a doubling in amount of depression in anemic women but the study did not examine other iron status indicators so attribution of depression to iron deficiency anemia cannot be done (Corwin et al., 2003). Several blinded intervention and placebo controlled studies in adolescent girls (Bruner et al., 1996) and in women during the post partum period (Beard et al., 2005) provide more substantive data regarding the relationship of iron status to cognition and emotions. The iron deficient, but not anemic adolescent girls, that were provided iron supplements showed a significant and substantial improvement in verbal learning and memory but attention performance was unaffected. In contrast, iron deficient anemic mothers given iron for 28 weeks had much less depression and anxiety than anemic mothers given the placebo (Beard et al., 2005). This latter study was conducted in a complex environment of poverty, poor health care, and other confounding issues that comprise a situation of very high "stress," whereas the former study in inner city Baltimore was performed in individuals with much better opportunities for overall quality of life.

A research design that had a specific focus on iron status and cognition in women of reproductive age was recently completed in the U.S. (Murray Kolb et al., 2005, in revision). One hundred forty-nine women participated in the baseline testing while 113 completed the entire study. Blood samples were collected both before and after 16 weeks of treatment with either an iron supplement ($FeSO_4$) or a placebo (gelatin capsule). Cognitive testing was also conducted both at baseline and after 16 weeks of treatment.

The cognitive testing consisted of 8 self-administered and automated computerized tasks of basic cognition (Detterman et al., 1990) measuring three domains: attention (three tasks), memory (three tasks), and learning (two tasks). These tasks were developed to measure the "modal model" of information processing which offers the opportunity to test specific aspects of cognition. This model is composed of three memory stores (very short term memory, short term memory, and long term memory) which are served by a stimulus encoding mechanism for input, a retrieval mechanism for output, and an output mechanism which executes responses. It also contains an executive functioning mechanism which oversees movement of information through the system.

Analysis of data was conducted within each domain (memory, attention, and learning) as well as across all domains. Given the large number of variables for both the cognitive testing as well as the hematology measurements, factor analysis was used to reduce the number of variables and the probability of type 1 error. Factor analysis of the hematology variables resulted in four factors, storage, transport, pre-anemia, and anemia (Table B-18). Factor analysis of the cognitive variables resulted in two factors, performance and time (Table B-19). While iron researchers have traditionally categorized subjects as iron sufficient, iron deficient, or iron deficient anemic, the authors of this study recognize that iron status is a continuous measure and, therefore, should be assessed as such. Thus, to perform the baseline analyses, data were sorted according to each hematological factor (storage, transport, pre-anemia, anemia) and then divided into quintiles. The extremes of the distribution (upper versus lower quintile) were then compared.

When data were sorted by the storage factor and analyzed across all cognitive domains, a significant difference between the upper and lower quintiles was found with respect to performance but not with respect to time. The opposite was found when the data were sorted by the anemia factor. That is, a difference was found in time needed to complete the tasks while there were no differences with respect to performance.

Baseline data were then analyzed by cognitive domain (attention, memory, and learning) and quintiles of haematological factors. Sorting the data by the storage factor revealed a difference in performance for the attention, memory, and learning tasks. Although there was no difference on the time factor for the attention and learning domains, the amount of time needed to complete the memory tasks was significantly different between the upper and lower quintiles. In contrast, when the data were sorted by the anemia factor, those women in the

**TABLE B-17** Studies in Young Adults Focusing on the Relationship Between Iron Status and Cognitive or Behavioral Functioning

| Author | Design | Group Size | Length | Measures | Results (baseline) | Results (Follow-up) |
|---|---|---|---|---|---|---|
| Beard et al., 2005 | Double blinded placebo control (60 mg Fe/day) | 95 post partum women | 28 weeks | EPDS<br>RPMI<br>Perceived Stress | RPMI correlated with Hb | ↑depressive symptoms, ↑stress, and ↓ digit symbol in IDA<br>Iron treatment, normalized all variables |
| Bruner et al., 1996 | Double blind; placebo control (1,300 mg $FeSO_4$/d) | 81 adolescent girls | 8 weeks | Symbol digit<br>Visual acuity<br>Verbal learning<br>Attention<br>Memory | n/a | ↑verbal learning and memory with iron txt.<br>No effect on attention, visual acuity |
| Corwin et al., 2003 | Cross sectional | 37 post partum women | | CESD | Anemics had 2-fold ↑ in depressive symptoms | |
| Fordy and Benton, 1994 | Cross sectional | 297 males and females | | GHQ<br>Digit span<br>Reaction time<br>Attention | No overall effect<br>OCA and ↓ferritin → ↑depressive symptoms | |
| Hunt and Penland, 1999 | Cross sectional | 365 women | | MMPI | No effect | |

| | | | | | | |
|---|---|---|---|---|---|---|
| Murray Kolb et al., 2005 | Stratified blinded placebo intervention (60 mg iron/day) | 149 women | 16 weeks | CESD<br>Detterman Cognitive tasks<br>STAI<br>STAS | Attention, memory, learning in ID and IDA | ↑ iron status→, learning, memory, attention; errors and speed |
| Rangan et al., 1998 | Cross sectional | 255 women | | GHQ scale | Non-anemic>anemic<br>ID not different<br>OCA and ↓ferritin → ↑depression | |
| Verdon et al., 2003 | Double blind, placebo (80 mg $FeSO_4$) | 144 women | 4 weeks | Fatigue<br>Depression<br>Anxiety | n/a | 29% ↓ depression with iron treatment.<br>13% ↓ depression in placebo txt<br>Only if ferritin < 50 was there a relation. |

NOTE: CESD = Center for Epidemiological Studies Depression Scale; EPDS = Edinburgh Postnatal Depression Scale; GHQ = General Health Questionnaire; ID = iron deficiency; IDA = iron deficiency anemia; MMPI = Minnesota Multiphasic Personality Inventory; OCA = oral contraceptives; RPMI = Ravens Progressive Matrices Index; STAI = State-Trait Anxiety Inventory; STAS = State-Trait Anger Scale.

**TABLE B-18** Components of Hematological Factors

| Factor Name | Variables Loaded |
|---|---|
| Storage | sFt<br>-sTfR<br>-TfRIX*<br>Body Iron |
| Transport | Iron,<br>TfSat |
| Pre-anemia | MCV,<br>MCH,<br>MCHC,<br>-RDW |
| Anemia | Hb,<br>Hct,<br>RBC |

NOTE: Hb = hemoglobin; Hct = hematocrit; MCH = mean corpuscular hemoglobin; MCHC = mean corpuscular hemoglobin concentration; MCV = mean corpuscular volume; RBC = red blood cells; RDW = red cell distribution width; sFt = serum ferritin; sTfR = serum transferrin receptor; TfRIX = transferrin receptor index; TfSat = transferrin saturation.
*Calculated as log(sTfR/sFt).

**TABLE B-19** Components of Cognitive Factors

| Domain | Performance Factor* | Time Factor |
|---|---|---|
| Attention | RT, SD, TT # incorrect<br>TT # attempted trials | RT, SD, TT trial time<br>RT, SD, TT decision time<br>RT, SD, TT movement time |
| Memory | PR, RC % correct<br>ST # incorrect | PR, RC, ST trial time<br>RC, ST decision time<br>RC, ST movement time<br>PR, RC reaction time |
| Learning | LR # attempted trials<br>LR # blocks achieved<br>LR % correct<br>PM # correct | LR trial time<br>LR, PM reaction time |
| All Domains | all of the variables listed above | all of the variables listed above |

NOTE: LR = learning task; PM = progressive matrices task; PR = probed recall task; RC = recognition memory task; RT = reaction time task; SD = stimulus discrimination task; ST = Sternberg memory search task; TT = tachistoscopic threshold task.
*For those tasks measuring "negative" performance, the absolute values of the scores were used; therefore, a higher score on the performance factor is always indicative of better performance.

highest quintile completed the tasks in the attention domain significantly faster than those women in the lowest quintile and approached a significantly faster time for the memory as well as learning domains. On the other hand, performance on the attention, memory, and learning domains was not affected when data were sorted by the anemia factor.

After the 16 weeks of supplementation, an improvement in overall performance on the cognitive tasks was found for those women who significantly improved their ferritin status. In women whose iron status improved, whether due to iron supplementation or other unknown reasons, attention and learning improved more than five fold compared to those whose iron status remained low. This improvement was seven times greater for the memory domain for those whose iron status improved. No differences were observed with respect to time necessary to complete the tasks in those women who improved their ferritin levels versus those who did not.

Women who significantly improved their hemoglobin concentration over the 16 weeks of the study also had a significant improvement in processing speed in attention and memory tasks; this was not the case for those women who had no change in hemoglobin concentration. Importantly, no relationship was found with respect to "correctness" on the cognitive tasks and hemoglobin concentration. The careful screening of subjects for the study identified the anemia as being due to iron deficiency and not other causes.

## OTHER STUDIES

Several other pertinent observations exist that may explain possible biological mechanisms whereby iron deficiency in adults can alter cognitive and behavioral functioning. Variations in iron status, as reflected by variations in serum ferritin, are related to EEG asymmetry (Tucker et al., 1981, 1982, 1984). The authors demonstrated a strong relationship of activity recorded in occipital electrodes to variations in plasma ferritin, the studies were not conducted to establish specific relationships between brain regional activity and cognition and iron. The biochemical explanation for these alterations in electrical activity may lie in fundamental alterations in brain energy metabolism with brain iron deficiency (DeUngria et al., 2000) as well as in neurotransmission efficacy and degree of myelination alterations (Beard and Connor, 2003).

There are a few examples that have used humans to study the relation ship of brain functioning and iron deficiency. For example, individuals with Restless Legs Syndrome (RLS) have alterations in brain iron content and also have clinical manifestions such as aphasic contractions of peripheral limb muscles. Known treatments are L-DOPA or iron relieve the symptoms and in the case of iron supplementation, may actually "cure" the disease in some patients (Earley et al., 2000). Another example of the association between iron status in adults and neural functioning is the treatment of renal dialysis patients with recombinant human eytthropoietin and aggressive oral iron therapy; the standard clinical practice in place now for more than a decade and a half. Studies that have examined cognitive performance after treatment often see 8–10 point improvements in the Wechsler global intelligence scores (Temple et al., 1992) and, significant improvement in cerebral oxygen tension and brain oxygen extraction. This occurs when the hematocrit is moved from around 30 percent up to the normal 45 percent packed red cells and occurs with an associated change in EEG signals and improved attention (Metry et al., 1999; Pickett et al., 1999). However, many other biological factors are changing with the dialysis treatment and comparisons with healthy age matched controls may provide some strong clues as to specific mechanisms whereby iron treatment of iron deficiency anemia results in improved cognitive performance and emotionality.

## CONCLUSION

Although the few studies with military subjects do not show a clear association between iron status and cognitive function, the experiments with civilian women reviewed in this report strongly suggest that military personnel with poor iron nutritional status, usually women, may suffer from impaired performance, specifically in domains representing learning, memory, and attention tasks and that they may benefit from higher iron intakes. They may also have more depression and anxiety in situations in which there is "high stress." The evidence data relative to the association between iron status and cognitive performance and mood states need to be collected from appropriate study designs, performed with military personnel under circumstances that paralled the physical, psychological and environmental stressors during military operations and training.

## REFERENCES

Beard JL. 1995. One persons' view of iron deficiency, development, and cognitive function. *Am J Clin Nutr* 62:709–710.

Beard JL, Connor JR. 2003. Iron status and neural functioning. *Annual Rev Nutr* 23:41–58.

Beard JL, Hendricks MK, Perez EM, Murray-Kolb L, Berg A, Vernon-Feagans L, Irlam J, Isaacs W, Sive A, Tomlinson M. 2005. Effects of maternal iron deficiency anemia. Part 1: Maternal emotions and cognition in postpartum iron deficiency. *J Nutr* 135:267–272.

Booth CK. 2003. Combat rations and military performance-do soldiers on active service eat enough? *Asia Pac J Clin Nutr* 12:S2.

Booth CK, Coad RA, Forbes-Ewan CH, Thomson GF, Niro PJ. 2003. The physiological and psychological effects of combat ration feeding during a 12-day training exercise in the tropics. *Mil Medicine* 168:63–70.

Bruner AB, Joffe A, Duggan AK, Casella JF, Brandt J. 1996. Randomized study of cognitive effects of iron supplementation in non-anemic iron-deficient adolescent girls. *Lancet* 348:992–996.

Cline A, Patton JF, Tharion WJ. 1998. Assessment of the relationship between iron status, dietary intake, performance, and mood state of female army officers in a basic training population. USARIEM Technical Report T98-24.

Corwin EJ, Murray-Kolb L, Beard JL. 2003. Low hemoglobin level is a risk factor for postpartum depression. *J Nutr* 133(12): 4139–4142.

Detterman DK. 1990. CAT: Computerized Cognitive Abilities Tests for research and teaching. *MicroPsychol Network* 4:51–62.

DeUngria M, Rao R, Wobken JD, Luciana M, Nelson CA, Georgieff MK. 2000. Perinatal iron deficiency decreases cytochrome c oxidase (CytOx) activity in selected regions of neonatal rat brain. *Pediatr Res* 48(2):169–176.

Earley CJ, Allen RP, Beard JL, Connor JR. 2000. Insight into the pathophysiology of Restless Legs Syndrome. *J Neuroscience Res* 62(5):623–628.

Fordy J, Benton D. 1994. Does low iron status influence psychological functioning? *J Human Nutr Dietetics* 7:127–133.

Hunt JR, Penland JG. 1999. Iron status and depression in premenopausal women: An MMPI study. *Behav Med.* 25:61–68.

Looker AC, Harris TB, Wahner HW. 1991. Comparing serum ferritin values from different population surveys. *Vital Health Stat* 2(111):1–19.

Metry G, Wiksotrom B, Valind S, Sandhagen B, Linde T, Beshara B, Langstrom B, Danielson BG. 1999. Effect of normalization of hematocrit on brain circulation and metabolism in hemodialysis patients. *J Am Soc Nephrol* 10:854–863.

Murray-Kolb LE, Beard JL, Joseph LJ, Davey SL, Evans WJ, Campbell WW. 2001. Resistance training affects iron status in older men and women. *IJSN* 11:287–298.

Murray-Kolb L, Whitefield K, Beard JL. 2005. Iron status is related to cognitive functioning in young adult women. *AmJ Clin Nutrition* (in revision).

Pickett JL, Theberge DC, Brown WS, Schweitzer SU, Nissenson AR. 1999. Normalizing hematocrit in dialysis patients improves brain function. *Am J Kidney Dis* 33:1122–1130.

Rangan AM, Blight GD, Binns CW. 1998. Iron status and non-specific symptoms of female students. *Am College Nutr* 17: 351–355.

Temple RM, Langan SJ, Deary IJ, Winney RJ. 1992. Recombinant EPO improves cognitive function in chronic haemodialysis patients. *Mephrol Dial Transplant* 7:240–245.

Tucker DM, Sandstead HH. 1981. Spectral electroencephalographic correlates of iron status: Tired blood revisited. *Physiol Behav* 26:439–449.

Tucker DM, Sandstead HH, Swenson RA, Sawler BG, Penland JG. 1982. Longitudinal study of brain function and depletion of iron stores in individual subjects. *Physiol Behav* 29:737–740.

Tucker DM, Sandstead HH, Penland JG, Dawson SL, Milne DB. 1984. Iron status and brain function: Serum ferritin levels associated with asymmetries of cortical electrophysiology and cognitive performance. *Am J Clin Nutr* 39:105–113.

Verdon F, Furnand B, Fallab-Stubi CL, Bonaard C, Graff M, Michaud A. 2003. Iron supplementation for unexplained fatigue in non-anemic women: Double blind randomized placebo controlled trial. *Br Med J* 326:1124–1128.

Westphal KA, Friedl KE, Sharp MA. 1995. Health, performance, and nutritional status of U.S. Army women during basic combat training. USARIEM Technical Report T96-2.

World Health Organization (WHO). 2002. The World Health Report, 2002. Reducing Risks, Promoting Healthy Life. [Online]. Available: http://www.who.int/whr/2002/en/whr02_en.pdf [accessed March, 2, 2006].

Youdim MBH, Ben-Schachar D, Yehuda S. 1989. Putative biological mechanisms on the effects of iron deficiency on brain metabolism. *Am J Clin Nutr* 50:607–617.

# Zinc and Other Mineral Nutrients Required for Cognitive Function and Behavior in Military Personnel

*James G. Penland*
*USDA-ARS Grand Forks Human Nutrition Research Center, Grand Forks, North Dakota*

## INTRODUCTION

A recent review of energy requirements of military personnel (Tharion et al., 2005) indicates that energy requirements are higher on average for soldiers than civilians, but vary dramatically depending on factors such as the type of task (e.g., support, training, or combat), the physical environment (e.g., temperature and altitude), and the presence of additional stressors (e.g., extreme physical activity, restricted sleep, or psychological stress). Energy requirements are also higher on average for male than female soldiers, although that difference largely disappears when adjusted for body size and physical activity.

During field operations, soldiers may decrease food consumption up to 50 percent resulting in suboptimal intake of energy and micronutrients (Baker-Fulco, 1995; Shippee, 1993), including minerals such as zinc, magnesium, selenium, copper, and phosphorus. In addition to negative affects on immune function and physical performance, failure to meet energy requirements is known to impair psychological function and behavior in both military personnel and civilians (see below for a brief review of those findings). However, little is known about requirements for micronutrients, including minerals such as zinc, iron, and magnesium, and the impact of inadequate intakes on military performance. Data from civilians suggest that these nutrients are essential to optimal psychological function and behavior relevant to performance of military duties. Moreover, specific groups of military personnel (e.g., male soldiers involved in first-strike assault operations) may have mineral requirements that exceed those of the majority of military personnel. Repeated assault operations may result in mineral depletion because inadequate intake and increased turnover and losses of minerals may promote marginal deficiencies under stressful conditions. Also, entry into operations with marginal mineral status may put these soldiers at risk for reduced mineral nutritional status and result in impaired physiological and psychological function and performance, particularly when assaults occur repetitively without replenishment of depleted mineral reserves.

This paper describes the research studies conducted on animals, the civilian population, and military personnel that shed light on questions regarding mineral requirements for military personnel. In particular, the following specific questions have been addressed:

- What is the evidence that zinc intake and status is related to cognitive function and behavior of soldiers? Does varying zinc intake and status affect the ability of soldiers to perform mental tasks?
- What is the evidence that zinc intake and status is related to cognitive function and behavior of civilians? What are the effects of zinc deficiency in cognitive function and behavior?
- What are the likely mechanisms of action for zinc effects on cognitive function and behavior? What brain regions are excited or depressed in association with changes in zinc intake and status?
- What other minerals interact with zinc and what is the effect of the interaction on their homeostasis and roles in neural function?
- Does supplementation with zinc affect cognitive function or behavior? Will supplementation with zinc restore or improve mental performance of soldiers with impairments in cognitive function due to sleep deprivation, energy deficits, physical activity, or other stressors? If so, at what level and for how long is supplementation needed?
- What is the evidence that magnesium, selenium, copper, and phosphorus intake or status are related to behavior and cognitive function?

Unfortunately, studies with military personnel that would answer to these questions are scarce. Therefore, this paper responds to these questions with available relevant data from studies with civilian adults with supporting evidence from animal studies or studies in children. This paper focuses on zinc, magnesium, selenium, copper, and phosphorus. The important role of iron nutrition in cognitive function and behavior is discussed elsewhere in this Appendix (Beard, 2005). Although there has been no direct examination of the possible role of specific mineral nutrients in cognitive performance and mood states of soldiers during training and field operations, the effects of caloric restriction, alone and in combination with other stressors, has been studied and a summary of the conclusions is also presented here.

The studies presented make evident some of the current limitations of the data collected. For instance, blood biochemical markers of nutritional status do not reveal overt mineral deficiencies among military personnel but this may be explained by a lack of sensitive biochemical markers of mineral status, brief durations of restricted intakes, and mineral mobilization from stores into the blood with increased metabolic demands and loss of body weight.

Another major limitation is the need to extrapolate results of mineral nutrition studies with civilians to military personnel; that soldiers are subject to multiple and often severe stressors in many different domains (e.g., physical fatigue, extreme environmental conditions, sleep deprivation, food restriction, depression, anxiety, fear). Data from civilian studies that evaluate mineral effects on cognitive function and behavior under conditions of multiple demands (e.g., dual-tasks) and stressors would be most relevant to the military.

## THE EFFECT OF STRESSORS ON COGNITIVE FUNCTION AND BEHAVIOR OF MILITARY PERSONNEL

As noted in previous reports from the *Committee for Military Nutrition Research* (e.g., Mays, 1995), underconsumption of military rations for short periods (10–45 days) in the absence of significant environmental, physical, and mental stress reliably reduces weight (up to 6 percent) but produces no meaningful degradation of cognitive performance as measured by multiple methods. Moderate levels of underconsumption may actually enhance performance. Underconsumption by 50 percent or more may result in subjective reports of impaired concentration and memory, along with non-cognitive behavioral (i.e., mood) changes. When severe caloric restriction is combined with additional stressors, including increased physical exercise, sleep deprivation, and mental stress, cognitive performance may fall by as much as 35 percent within a few days (Shippee et al., 1994).

A controlled study (Booth et al., 2003) of the biochemical, physiological and psychological effects of caloric restriction during a 12-day field training exercise in Australian soldiers found weight loss, suppressed immune function (IgA and IL-2R), a decline in iron status (ferritin), dehydration, impaired sleep, increased fatigue, reduced vigor, and increased feelings of confusion in soldiers, regardless of the diet (i.e., diets provided either negative or zero energy balance). However, there was no meaningful impact on physical fitness or cognitive performance (reaction time, vigilance, perception, and memory). In contrast, Lieberman et al. (2005) recently showed that the combined stressors of sleep deprivation, physical activity, psychological stress, noise, hot and humid temperatures, dehydration, and general undernutrition during a 53-hour Army simulated combat exercise led to severe declines in cognitive performance on tasks measuring attention, memory and reasoning, and to deterioration in mood states, including increased confusion, anxiety, depression, and fatigue.

Longer periods of exposure to multiple stressors, nutritional, environmental, physical and mental, such as the 60+ days involved in Ranger training, clearly result in impaired cognitive performance, including attention (decoding), perception, memory, and reasoning (Mays, 1993). Shippee et al. (1994) found decreased iron status and increased zinc and copper status in Ranger II; however, dietary intakes were not measured so it is unclear whether the changes were due to decreased intake, inflammation, or some other factor. Pre-existing marginal nutritional status, rest, psychological state, etc., also likely exacerbate the impact of underconsumption, alone or in combination with other stressors typical of field training and combat operations.

At least one study (Crowdy et al., 1982) found no significant decrements in cognitive performance (vigilance, math, and coding) when soldiers consumed 47 percent energy expenditure during 12 days of rigorous training exercises in the Tropics. It is possible that relatively brief periods of caloric restriction, similar to sleep restriction and deprivation, do not degrade performance because soldiers may sacrifice speed to maintain performance accuracy (i.e., speed-accuracy trade-off) (Belenky et al., 1994; Mays, 1993).

## EFFECTS OF MINERAL NUTRITION ON COGNITIVE FUNCTION AND BEHAVIOR OF CIVILIANS

Controlled studies with civilian adult men and women are not extensive but provide important clues about how specific mineral nutrients may affect cognitive performance and mood states of military personnel.

### Zinc

Zinc is required for the structure and activity of more than 300 enzymes (Vallee and Falchuk, 1993). Frederickson et al. (2005) provide a comprehensive discussion of the broad role of zinc in central nervous system function indicating several potential mechanisms linking zinc and cognitive function and behavior. Zinc is concentrated in the cortex and limbic system (especially the hippocampus and amygdala). Zinc is contained in glutamatergic neurons, active in the vesicle, synaptic cleft, and post-synaptic neuron. Zinc modulates brain excitability primarily through its effects on both excitatory and inhibitory receptors (e.g., N-methyl-D-aspartate [NMDA] or, γ-aminobutyric acid [GABA] receptors). Zinc may also affect cognition and behavior through non-CNS (central nervous system) actions (Golub et al., 1995). These include involvement in neurotransmitter precursor production in the liver, hormone and growth factor transport and receptor binding, hormone and toxicant metabolism in the liver and testes, and pancreatic insulin production and glucose metabolism. Dreosti (1993) has suggested that zinc-deficiency effects on behavior and brain function may result from impaired activity of several zinc-dependent enzymes in the brain. Because zinc functions in all physiological systems, adequate zinc status is essential for optimal physiological and psychological performance.

The majority of studies relating zinc intake or status to cognitive function and behavior have been conducted in infants and children. In these groups, improved zinc nutrition has consistently benefited psychomotor skills, but has inconsistently affected attention, memory, reasoning, and psychosocial adjustment.

In civilian adults, low zinc intakes and status have been related to deficits in memory, perception, attention, and motor skills while zinc supplementation has improved memory (Table B-20). Clinical evaluation of mental status revealed impaired short-term memory, increased emotional lability, and perceptual deficits in adults with progressive systemic sclerosis whose zinc status was altered by histidine administration (Henkin et al., 1975). Goldstein and Pfeiffer (1978) administered zinc or a placebo to schizophrenics and assessed brain function by electroencephalogram (EEG) 4 hours after supplementation. There was a greater reduction in EEG amplitude (toward normal) in zinc-supplemented schizo-

**TABLE B-20** Effects of Zinc and Other Mineral Nutrients on Cognitive Function and Behavior in Civilian Adults

| Mineral | Subjects | Study Design | Outcome[a] | Reference |
|---|---|---|---|---|
| Zinc | Men | 5 vs. 15 mg/day | ↓ Memory, ↓ Perception | Tucker and Sandstead, 1984 |
| | Men | 1–4 vs. 10 mg/day | ↓ Psychomotor, ↓ Attention<br>↓ Perception, ↓ Memory | Penland, 1991 |
| | Men | 5 vs. 14 mg/day | ↓ Memory | Kretsch et al., 2000 |
| | Women | 3 vs. 53 mg/day | ↓ Memory | Penland et al., 2000 |
| | Women | 30 mg/day[b] | ↑ Perception ↑ Memory | Darnell and Sandstead, 1991 |
| | Women | 30 mg/day[b] | ↑ Psychomotor ↑ Reasoning | Penland et al., 2002 |
| Magnesium | Men and Women | Hypomagnesmia | ↓ EEG Alpha Activity | Delorme et al., 1992 |
| | Women | 113 vs. 315 mg/day | ↑ EEG Total Activity,<br>↑ % Theta Activity | Penland, 1995 |
| Selenium | Women | 100 μg/day[b] | ↓ Anxiety, ↓ Depression<br>↑ Energy | Benton and Cook, 1991 |
| | Men | 13 vs. 356 μg/day | ↓ RBC Se, ↓ Depression<br>↓ Hostility | Hawkes and Hornbostel, 1996 |
| | Men | 28 vs. 239 μg/day | ↑ Confusion, ↑ Depression<br>↓ GSH-Px, ↓ Positive Mood | Penland and Finley, 1995 |
| | Women | 0 vs. 10–40 μg/day | ↑ Hostility, ↑ Total Disturbance<br>↓ Confidence, ↓ Energy | Penland et al., 2005 |
| Copper | Women | 1 vs. 3 mg/day | ↓ Sleep Time, ↑ Sleep Latency<br>↑ Feeling Restless<br>↑ Depression, ↑ Confusion | Penland, 1988 |
| | Women | 1 vs. 3 mg/day | ↓ Short-term Memory<br>↑ Distraction | Penland et al., 2000 |

NOTE: See text for additional details. Refer to the workshop paper by Beard in this volume for a discussion of iron nutrition and cognitive performance.

[a]Effect of lower compared to higher dietary intake or supplement compared to placebo in supplementation studies.

[b]Supplementation study, included placebo condition.

phrenics compared to controls, but both groups showed a decrease in EEG activity. Henrotte et al. (1977) found a relationship between low red blood cell (RBC) zinc and photic responsivity, and determined that people with a Type A personality are characterized by a higher RBC and urinary zinc than those with Type B personality (Henrotte et al., 1985; Henrotte et al., 1986). Humphries et al. (1989) reported biochemical indices of zinc deficiency in 54 percent of a group of anorexic patients and 40 percent of a group of bulimic patients. Unfortunately, neither of these last two studies reported dietary zinc intakes so it is impossible to draw useful conclusions about associations between zinc intake level and cognitive function from those studies. In healthy men participating in a controlled feeding study, Sandstead et al. (1983) found a correlation between plasma zinc and brain electrical activity in three of five subjects; the principal finding was increased left and decreased right hemisphere amplitudes in the occipital lobes in the lower frequencies of the EEG. The meaning of these changes in brain electrophysiology for cognitive function remains unknown.

In a zinc depletion experiment with healthy young males, Tucker and Sandstead (1984) found that low serum zinc in these otherwise well-nourished men was correlated with faster but less accurate performance on memory for digits and several perceptual tasks. Darnell and Sandstead (1991) found that 30 mg/day zinc added to a vitamin-mineral supplement improved visual memory, but not verbal memory, in sideropenic women, whereas a vitamin-mineral supplement alone did not. Penland (1991) administered a battery of tasks assessing cognitive processes and psychomotor skills to 14 healthy men, aged 21–38 years, participating in a 6-month, live-in metabolic study of zinc nutrition. The men were fed 1, 2, 3, or 4 mg/day zinc during each of four consecutive 35-day deprivation periods administered in a random, double blind manner. Contrasted to a control period when the men were fed 10 mg/day zinc, low zinc intakes were associated with poorer performance on at least one task from each of five functional categories; those categories were, psychomotor function (tracking and connect-the-dots tasks), attention (orienting and misdirection tasks), perception (search-count task), memory (letter, shape and cube recognition tasks), and spatial function (maze task). However, a dose-response effect of dietary zinc on performance was not observed. Penland et al. (2002) also found improved performance on memory and reasoning tasks in adult women supplemented with 30 mg/d zinc for 8 weeks. In a double-blind metabolic study of 8 healthy young men (Kretsch et al., 2000), reaction times during word recall were significantly slower when men were fed 4.6 compared to 13.7 mg/day zinc for 70 days. In a double-blind metabolic study of 23 healthy postmenopausal women (Penland et al., 2000), immediate recall of word lists was improved when women were fed a total of 53 compared to 3 mg/day zinc for 90 days, when the diet was also low (< 1 mg/day) in copper. In the only intervention study of elderly with dementia, Potocnik et al. (1997) found "modest" improvements on the Mini Mental State Examination in 4 Alzheimer's patients following supplementation with 30 mg/day zinc for 12 months.

Zinc may play a role in the regulation of mood states, particularly depression. Henkin et al. (1975) reported irritability, anger, paranoia and depression in adults made severely zinc deficient by histidine administration (histidine binds zinc normally bound to albumine and depletes tissue zinc levels). Aggett (1989) reported that loss of affect and emotional lability were pronounced in children with acrodermatitis enteropathica and in early zinc deficiency of TPN (total parenteral nutrition) patients. See also Levenson 2005 in this appendix for a detailed review of zinc and depression. Nowak and Szewczyk (2002) provide a recent discussion of possible mechanisms linking zinc and depression.

There have been no studies in soldiers or civilians that address whether the effects of stressors on cognition and behavior can be mitigated by varying zinc intakes. There is only one study with rats that points to increased stress responses (corticosterone and anxiety) with zinc deficiency (Chu et al., 2003).

There are animal studies that suggest that zinc plays a role in regulating appetite and food consumption; however, studies looking at the possible role of zinc in regulating human food behavior find highly complex food behavior patterns, and the role of zinc is still unclear (Shay and Mangian, 2000).

Rats begin to reduce their food intake within 3–5 days of severe (< 1 ppm/day) zinc deprivation and continued deprivation may result in intakes 50 percent that of zinc-adequate controls (Rains and Shay, 1995). Zinc repletion increases intake almost immediately. Most of the reduced intake is in carbohydrates and the pattern of feeding (timing and number of meals) is disrupted (Rains et al., 1998). Both neuropeptide Y release (Levenson, 2003) and leptin (Mantzoros et al., 1998) are reduced during zinc deficiency and are associated with decreased intake and anorexia nervosa. As noted earlier, Humphries et al. (1989) reported biochemical indices of zinc deficiency in 54 percent of a group of anorexic patients and 40 percent of a group of bulimic patients.

In summary, data from the few available studies with civilian adults suggesting that zinc nutrition may have roles in cognitive function (particularly memory) and mood (particularly depression) is supported also by studies with animals, infants and children, and the existing putative mechanisms. At this time however, data are insufficient to identify specific zinc intakes needed to support and maximize cognitive function and behavior in either civilians or military personnel.

## Magnesium

Magnesium is a cofactor in more than 300 enzymes and influences DNA and protein synthesis, intracellular signal transduction, and cell growth and differentiation (Shils, 1997). Magnesium, thus, is a potentially limiting nutrient for cognitive function and behavior. In the central nervous system, magnesium plays an important role in glutamatergic neurotransmission, inhibiting excitatory NMDA (Cooper et al., 1996), and affects monoaminergic and serotonergic systems (Singewald et al., 2004). Magnesium is also involved in regulation of the hypothalmus-pituitary-adrenocortical (HPA) system and corticotropin releasing factor (Murck, 2002). The role of magnesium as an NMDA antagonist and GABA agonist is a likely mechanism responsible for the effects of magnesium on sleep (Held et al., 2002). The relationships between magnesium and mood are linked to increased HPA activity, which is frequently observed in depression and anxiety (Holsboer, 2000).

There are no previous studies that have directly correlated the intake or status of magnesium to cognitive function or behavior in soldiers, and few data exist from studies of civilians.

Severe magnesium deficiency has been associated with numerous neurological and psychological problems, including convulsions, dizziness, neuromuscular hyperexcitability (Chvostek and Trousseau signs), hyperemotionality (irritability and marked agitation), anxiety, confusion, depression, apathy, loss of appetite, and insomnia (Dubray and Rayssiguier, 1997; Durlach, 1980). Brain function assessed with the EEG has shown increased cortical excitability, characterized as diffuse, slow wave activity of the type commonly found in metabolic disorders, and "diffuse irritative tracings" in the absence of focal effects, marked by spiked alpha and increased theta activity (Durlach, 1985). Popoviciu et al. (1987) reported a disruption of normal sleep architecture in magnesium-deficient subjects, including greatly reduced deep, slow wave sleep, and decreased rapid eye movement sleep.

However, there are few data on neuropsychological effects of marginal magnesium restriction (Table B-20). In an early study that successfully induced magnesium deficiency by dietary restriction, Shils (1969) did not observe any changes in the EEG of subjects fed less than 10 mg/day magnesium for as long as 105 days. However, Shils' study was limited to 7 subjects and EEG analysis was visual rather than quantitative. Contrasting quantitative EEG of athletes (44 male and female kayakists) with low versus normal erythrocyte magnesium, Delorme et al. (1992) found significantly less relative alpha (7.25–12.5 Hz) activity, particularly in the right occipital region, in the low magnesium group. However, magnesium intakes were not experimentally controlled in that study. Penland (1995) fed either 115 or 315 mg/day magnesium for 42 days each to 13 healthy postmenopausal women living on a metabolic research unit; EEG activity (i.e., hyperexcitability) increased, suggesting that relatively short periods of marginal magnesium deprivation can affect brain function. Compared to high dietary magnesium, the low magnesium intake increased total EEG activity in the frontal regions and right temporal and parietal regions, and resulted in frequency-specific increases in left occipital delta (1–3 Hz) activity, theta (4–7 Hz) activity in all but the left temporal region, alpha (8–12 Hz) activity in the right frontal and right temporal regions, and beta (13–18 Hz) activity in the frontal regions. The proportion of theta to total activity in the parietal regions also increased with the low magnesium intake. Increased electrical activity across frequencies and increased theta activity have been associated with neurological disorders, behavioral hyperactivity, increasing sleep loss, and impaired cognition, especially memory.

Magnesium deficiency leads to reduced offensive and increased defensive behavior in rats (Kantak, 1988) and impaired learning and memory in mice (Bardgett et al., 2005), but there have been no studies showing these effects in humans. Magnesium deficiency in rats also leads to increased pain sensitivity (Begon et al., 2001). Again, this effect has not been investigated in humans.

Magnesium may play an important role in regulating sleep. Animal studies have shown that magnesium deficiency increases wakefulness and decreases slow wave sleep (Depoortere et al., 1993) and total sleep time (Poenaru et al., 1984). Intravenous magnesium administration in healthy young men increased EEG activity power in sigma frequencies (11–29 Hz) during non-REM sleep (Murck and Steiger, 1998). Magnesium supplementation (10–30 mmol/day [240 mg/day]) of elderly (60–80 years old) increased EEG power in the delta (1–3 Hz) and sigma frequencies (Held et al., 2002). A recent study found that sleep restriction over a 4 week period resulted in decreased intracellular magnesium in college males (Takase et al., 2004).

Magnesium may also be involved in regulating mood states. Many correlational studies have shown a positive association between blood magnesium concentrations and mood disorders, although a few have found either no association or a negative relationship (Imada et al., 2002). However, supplemental and intravenous magnesium have been effective in treating depression (Murck, 2002).

In summary, the importance of magnesium for cognitive function and behavior has received little attention and is largely unknown. Available data suggest that magnesium is involved in regulating brain electrical activity and that increasing intake may benefit sleep modulation and mood states.

## Selenium

Selenium acts through its association with proteins as an antioxidant and a regulator of thyroid hormone metabolism. Selenium-dependent enzymes in the brain are involved in antioxidant defense and redox regulation which may be relevant for neurodegenerative diseases caused by oxidative stress (Schweizer et al., 2004), but a role for selenium in cognitive function and behavior of younger adults has not been investigated. In individuals with low selenium intakes and status who have impaired deiodinase synthesis and activity, reduced conversion of thyroxine ($T_4$) to triiodothyronine ($T_3$) may result in sub-clinical thyroid hormone deficiency that impairs mood states (Beckett et al., 1993; Sait-Gonen et al., 2004). In individuals with adequate selenium intake and status, selenium may affect brain function and impair mood states by increasing dopamine turnover (Castano et al., 1997) or increasing the ratio of n-6/n-3 fatty acids (Yao and Reddy, 2005). Low glutathione peroxidase (GSH-Px) activity in women has been associated with elevated fasting glucose and glucose intolerance (Hawkes et al., 2004); elevated glucose and glucose intolerance have been associated with depression.

There are no previous studies that have directly correlated the intake or status of selenium to cognitive function or behavior in soldiers. However, several studies have shown an effect of selenium intakes and status on mood states in civilian men and women (Table B-20). Benton and Cook (1991) supplemented 33 women and 17 men with 100 μg/day selenium or a placebo for 5 weeks, in a double-blind crossover design with a 6-month washout period between treatments. Higher selenium intakes were related to less anxiety, less depression and more energy as reported on the Profile of Mood States—BiPolar Form (POMS-BI). Penland and Finley (1995) and Finley and Penland (1998) fed 30 healthy men, aged 21–44 years, typical Western diets containing 30 or 230 μg/day selenium for 15 week. Men fed high selenium reported less confusion and depression on the POMS-BI over the course of the study. Anxiety, hostility, uncertainty and tiredness also appeared to be less with higher selenium intakes, but subject variability was large and the effects were not statistically significant. Within the group fed low selenium, the activity of the selenium enxyme GSH-Px in platelets was significantly correlated with all six mood states measured by the POMS-BI; higher activity was associated with less anxiety, hostility, depression, uncertainty, tiredness, and confusion. Hawkes and Hornbostel (1996) fed 11 healthy men living on a metabolic research unit either 13 or 356 μg/day of selenium for 99 days. Although selenium intakes were not significantly related to mood states by the POMS-BI, a significant positive relationship was found between erythrocyte selenium concentrations and elated (versus depressed) and agreeable (versus hostile) mood states in the group fed low selenium; this finding suggests a greater range in mood and selenium status in the low selenium group.

Several recent studies show conflicting results. New Zealand adults, 33 females and 18 males, with typically low selenium intakes were supplemented with 0, 10, 20, 30 or 40 μg/day selenium for approximately 6 months (Penland et al., 2005). Monthly POMS-BI tests showed the female group increased agreeableness, confidence and energy, and less total mood disturbance as the study progressed (slope analysis). Males showed no dietary effects on mood states, which may be due to the low statistical power of the small sample size for males. In another study, 60 Chinese men (aged 18–49 years) with low selenium status, baseline plasma selenium concentration was negatively associated with anxiety, depression, tiredness, confusion, and with total mood disturbance (Penland et al., 2006). Plasma selenium concentration was also positively associated with performance on two perceptual tasks, search and matching. However, subsequent food fortification providing 200 μg/day selenium for 15 weeks markedly improved selenium status but did not improve mood or cognitive performance. In another study (Rayman et al., 2005), supplementation with 100–300 μg/day selenium for 6 months resulted in no significant improvement in mood states; however, subjects in that study were between 60–74 years of age, much older than participants in the studies showing a benefit of increased selenium intake for mood.

In summary, the importance of selenium for cognitive function and behavior has received little attention and is largely unknown. The limited available data suggest that selenium status is associated with mood states and that increasing selenium intake may benefit mood (Rayman, 2002), but such interventions have not always been effective (Raymon et al., 2005; Shor-Posner et al., 2003).

## Copper

Copper impacts biological function as a catalyst of enzyme activity. It regulates iron absorption, neurotransmitter metabolism, antioxidant defense and oxygen utilization. Thus, copper status may affect diverse biological functions, including cognitive function and behavior. The activıties of two copper-dependent enzymes may at least partially explain the diverse putative effects of copper intake on memory, mood, and sleep. Dopamine-β-monooxygenase is required for the synthesis of norepinephrine from dopamine, and Cu/Zn superoxide dismutase protects catecholamines from oxidation by reactive oxygen species (Johnson, 2005). Long-term alterations of the synaptic strength, gene transcription modulation and other processes are modulated by norepinephrine which supports a role for this neurotransmitter in alterations of neural function and behavior (Berridge and Waterhouse, 2003). Through its role in several enzymatic functions, adequate intake of copper appears to be important for fully functional cognition and behavior.

There are no previous studies that have directly correlated the intake or status of copper to cognitive function or behavior in soldiers, and only two studies from one laboratory have been conducted with civilians.

Restricted dietary copper has been associated with impaired verbal memory and disrupted sleep and mood states of women (Table B-20). In a double-blind, metabolic study of 23 healthy postmenopausal women (Penland et al., 2000), short-term memory and immediate recall of a list of words presented verbally worsened when women were fed low compared to high copper (1 versus 3 mg/day), when the diet was also high (53 mg/day) in zinc. Low copper intakes were also associated with increased difficulty in discriminating between relevant and irrelevant responses. Plasma copper and ceruloplasmin were positively associated with improved verbal memory and long-term memory, and increased clustering of verbal material (which indicates improved strategy), but fewer intrusions (reduced distractions) during recall (Penland et al., 2000).

In a depletion-repletion experiment (Penland, 1988; 1989), increased sleep times, longer latency to sleep, and feeling less rested upon awakening as well as increased confusion, depression, and total mood disturbances were reported when dietary copper was low (0.8 versus 2 mg/day). Review of the medical charts of participants in these long-term, live-in metabolic studies for the incidence of requests for medication to relieve pain unrelated to injury or illness found increased requests for pain medication during periods of low copper intake (unpublished data).

In summary, the importance of copper for cognitive function and behavior has received little attention and is largely unknown. Two studies in one laboratory suggest that copper nutrition may affect sleep and memory performance.

### Phosphorus

Inadequate phosphorus intake results in abnormally low serum phosphate levels (hypophosphatemia), resulting in loss of appetite, anemia, muscle weakness, bone pain, osteomalacia, increased susceptibility to infection, numbness and tingling of the extremities, and difficulty walking. There are no controlled studies that have directly correlated the intake or status of phosphorus to cognitive function or behavior in soldiers or civilians.

## SUMMARY

There are no previous studies relating zinc intake or status to cognitive function or behavior in soldiers. Data from the few available studies with civilian adults suggest that zinc nutrition may have roles in cognitive function (particularly memory) and mood (particularly depression). This conclusion is supported by data from studies with animals, infants and children, and reasonable putative mechanisms can be identified. At this time however, data are insufficient to identify specific zinc intakes needed to support and maximize cognitive function and behavior in either civilians or military personnel.

The importance of magnesium, selenium, copper, and phosphorus for cognitive function and behavior has received little attention and is largely unknown. Available data suggest that magnesium is involved in regulating brain electrical activity and possibly sleep and mood. Increasing selenium intake may benefit mood. Two studies in one laboratory suggest that copper nutrition may affect sleep and memory performance. There are no data to suggest any putative role for phosphorus in cognitive function or behavior.

Evidence shows that military personnel fail to consume adequate amounts of zinc and magnesium. These minerals, as well as selenium, copper, and phosphorus may play important roles in promoting optimal cognitive function and behavior. Limited data on mineral intakes and status of soldiers in various types of training do not provide evidence of overt nutritional deficiencies, but this may be due to a lack of sensitive biochemical markers of nutritional status. It is difficult to discriminate the independent effect of severely restricted energy intake on potential micronutrient impairments. Nevertheless, cognitive and psychological impairments found in civilians with marginal mineral deficits are consistent with problems in these areas reported in soldiers during active training and operations.

## RESEARCH RECOMMENDATIONS

There is a need to conduct studies of zinc nutrition and cognitive function and behavior with military personnel in there garrison and in the field, and while engaged in support, training and combat, in the context of moderating variables. These variables include gender, body composition and fitness, task, physical demand, extreme environmental conditions, sleep deprivation, food restriction, and psychological stressors (e.g., depression, anxiety, fear). A direct examination of the role of zinc nutrition in moderating biochemical and physiological responses to stressors of varying types is needed. Further there is a need to determine the possible role of zinc nutrition in regulating the food intake of soldiers.

There is also a need to determine the benefits of increasing magnesium, selenium, copper, and phosphorus intakes for cognitive function and behavior in the context of moderating variables affecting military personnel. In particular, there is a need to determine whether increasing magnesium intake will improve sleep, protect against the effects of sleep deprivation, and regulate mood, and whether increasing selenium intake will benefit mood. Exploratory studies on the possible benefits of copper and phosphorus for cognitive function and behavior may be undertaken with a lower priority.

This information is needed to critically evaluate the adequacy of current rations provided to and consumed by soldiers, and if indicated will provide a foundation for developing new rations that supply specific mineral nutrients required to support optimal cognitive function and behavior of military personnel operating in the presence of multiple demands and stressors with diverse needs. Such information may also be useful to better understanding the determinants of food intake by soldiers (Hirsch and Kramer, 1993).

## REFERENCES

Aggett PJ. 1989. Severe zinc deficiency. In: Mills CF, ed. *Zinc in Human Biology*. New York: Springer-Verlag. Pp. 259–279.

Baker-Fulco CJ. 1995. Overview of dietary intakes during military exercises. In: Marriott BM, ed. *Not Eating Enough: Overcoming Underconsumption of Military Operational Rations*. Washington, DC: National Academy Press. Pp. 121–149.

Bardgett ME, Schultheis PJ, McGill DL, Richmond RE, Wagge JR. 2005. Magnesium deficiency impairs fear conditioning in mice. *Brain Res* 1038(1):100–106.

Beckett GJ, Nicol F, Rae PW, Beech S, Guo Y, Arthur JR. 1993. Effects of combined iodine and selenium deficiency on thyroid hormone metabolism in rats. *Am J Clin Nutr* 57(2 Suppl):240S–243S.

Begon S, Pickering G, Eschalier A, Mazur A, Rayssiguier Y, Dubray C. 2001. Role of spinal NMDA receptors, protein kinase C and nitric oxide synthase in the hyperalgesia induced by magnesium deficiency in rats. *Br J Pharmacol* 134(6):1227–1236.

Belenky G, Penetar DM, Thorne D, Popp K, Leu J, Thomas M, Sing H, Balkin T, Wesenten N, Redmond D. 1994. The effects of sleep deprivation on performance during continuous combat operations. In: Marriott BM, ed. *Food Components to Enhance Performance: An Evaluation of Potential Performance-Enhancing Food Components for Operational Rations.* Washington, DC: National Academy Press. Pp.127–136.

Benton D, Cook R. 1991. The impact of selenium supplementation on mood. *Biol Psychiatry* 29(11): 1092–1098.

Berridge CW, Waterhouse BD. 2003. The locus coeruleus-noradrenergic system: modulation of behavioral state and state-dependent cognitive processes. *Brain Res Rev* 42(1):33–84.

Booth CK, Coad RA, Forbes-Ewan CH, Thomson GF, Niro PJ. 2003. The physiological and psychological effects of combat ration feeding during a 12-day training exercise in the tropics. *Mil Med* 168(1):63–70.

Castano A, Ayala A, Rodriguez-Gomez JA, Herrera AJ, Cano J, Machado A. 1997. Low selenium diet increases the dopamine turnover in prefrontal cortex of the rat. *Neurochem Int* 30(6):549–555.

Chu Y, Mouat MF, Harris RBS, Coffield JA, Grider A. 2003. Water maze performance and changes in serum corticosterone levels in zinc-deprived and pair-fed rats. *Physiol Behav* 78(4–5):5 69–578.

Cooper JR, Bloom FE, Roth RH. 1996. *The Biochemical Basis of Neuropharmacology.* New York: Oxford.

Crowdy JP, Consolazio CF, Forbes AL, Halsman MF, Worsley DE. 1982. Nutrition in adverse environments, 3. The metabolic effects of a restricted food intake on men working in a tropical environment. *Hum Nutr Appl Nutr* 36(5):325–344.

Darnell LS, Sandstead HH. 1991. Iron, zinc and cognition. *Am J Clin Nutr* 53(3):P16.

Delorme O, Bourdin H, Viel JF, Simon-Rigaud MLS, Kantelip JP. 1992. Spectral analysis of electroencephalography data in athletes with low electrolyte magnesium. *Magnesium Res* 5(4): 261–264.

Depoortere H, Francon D, Llopis J. 1993. Effects of a magnesium-deficient diet on sleep organization in rats. *Neuropsychobiology* 27(4):237–245.

Dreosti IE. 1993. Zinc in brain development and function. In: Prasad AS, ed. *Essential and Toxic Trace Elements in Human Health and Disease: An Update.* New York: Wiley-Liss. Pp. 81–90.

Dubray C, Rayssiguier Y. 1997. Magnesium, inflammation and pain. In: Theophanides TM, Anastassopoulou J, eds. *Magnesium: Current Status and New Developments: Theoretical, Biological, and Medical Aspects.* Dordrecht Netherlands: Kluwer Academic. Pp. 303–311.

Durlach J. 1980. Clinical aspects of chronic magnesium deficiency. In: Cantin M, Seelig MS, eds. *Magnesium in Health and Disease.* New York: Spectrum Publications. Pp.883–909.

Durlach J. 1985. Neurological disturbances due to magnesium imbalance. In: Gabay S, Harris J, Ho BT, eds. *Metal Ions in Neurology and Psychiatry.* New York: Alan R. Liss. Pp. 121–128.

Finley JW, Penland JG. 1998. Adequacy or deprivation of dietary selenium in healthy men: Clinical and psychological findings. *Biol Trace Elem Res* 11(1):11–27.

Frederickson CJ, Koh JY, Bush AI. 2005. The neurobiology of zinc in health and disease. *Nat Rev Neurosci* 6(6):449–462.

Goldstein L, Pfeiffer CC. 1978. Effects of single oral doses of trace elements on the quantitated EEG of normal subjects and chronic schizophrenics. *Psychopharm Bull* 14(3):55–57.

Golub MS, Keen CL, Gershwin ME, Hendrickx AG. 1995. Developmental zinc deficiency and behavior. *J Nutr* 125(8 Suppl):2263S–2271S.

Hawkes WC, Hornbostel L. 1996. Effects of dietary selenium on mood in healthy men living in a metabolic research unit. *Biol Psychiatry* 39(2):121–128.

Hawkes WC, Alkan Z, Lang K, King JC. 2004. Plasma selenium decrease during pregnancy is associated with glucose intolerance. *Biol Trace Elem Res* 100(1):19–29.

Held K, Antonijevic IA, Kunzel H, Uhr M, Wetter TC, Golly IC, Steiger A, Murck H. 2002. Oral Mg(2+) supplementation reverses age-related neuroendocrine and sleep EEG changes in humans. *Pharmacopsychiatry* 35(4):135–143.

Henkin RI, Patten BM, Re PK, Bronzert DA. 1975. A syndrome of acute zinc loss: cerebellar dysfunction, mental changes, anorexia, and taste and smell dysfunction. *Arch Neurol* 32(11): 745–751.

Henrotte JG. 1986. Type A behavior and magnesium metabolism. *Magnesium* 5(3–4):201–210.

Henrotte JG, Veadreaux G, Manod H. 1977. Relations entre re taux du zinc and guin et les modifications de le EEG sous le influence de le nyerpnee chez le homme narmole. [Relationship between blood zinc level and EEG changes under the influence of hyperpnea in normal subjects]. *L-Encephale* 3(2):159–164.

Henrotte JG, Plouin PF, Levy-Leboyer C, Moser G, Sidoroff-Girault N, Franck G, Santarromana M, Pineau M.1985. Blood and urinary magnesium, zinc, calcium, free fatty acids and catecholamines in type A and type B subjects. *J Am Coll Nutr* 4(2):165–172.

Hirsch ES, Kramer FM. 1993. Situational influences on food intake. In: Marriott BM, ed. *Nutritional Needs in Hot Environments: Applications for Military Personnel in Field Operations.* Washington, DC: National Academy Press. Pp. 215–243.

Holsboer F. 2000. The corticosteroid receptor hypothesis of depression. *Neuropsychopharmacology* 23(5):477–501.

Humphries L, Vivian B, Stuart M, McClain CJ. 1989. Zinc deficiency and eating disorders. *J Clin Psychiatry* 50(12):456–459.

Imada Y, Yoshioka S, Ueda T, Katayama S, Kuno Y, Kawahara R. 2002. Relationships between serum magnesium levels and clinical background factors in patients with mood disorders. *Psychiatry Clin Neurosci* 56(5):509–514.

Johnson WT. 2005. Copper and brain function. In: Lieberman HR, Kanarek RB, Prasad C, eds. *Nutritional Neuroscience.* Boca Raton, FL: Taylor & Francis. Pp. 289–305.

Kantak KM. 1988. Magnesium deficiency alters aggressive behavior and catecholamine function. *Behav Neurosci* 102(2):304–311.

Kretsch MJ, Fong, AKH, Penland JG, Sutherland B, King JC. 2000. Cognitive effects of adaptation to a low zinc diet in healthy men. In: Roussel AM, Favier AE, Anderson RA, eds. *Trace elements in man and animals—10: Proceedings of the Tenth International Symposium on Trace Elements in Man and Animals.* New York: Kluwer Academic/Plenum Publishers. Pp. 999–1001.

Levenson CW. 2003. Zinc regulation of food intake: New insights on the role of neuropeptide Y. *Nutr Rev* 61(7):247–249.

Lieberman HR, Bathalon GP, Falco CM, Kramer FM, Morgan CA, Niro P. 2005. Severe decrements in cognitive function and mood induced by sleep loss, heat, dehydration, and undernutrition during simulated combat. *Biol Psychiatry* 57(4):422–429.

Mantzoros CS, Prasad AS, Beck FW, Grabowski S, Kaplan J, Adair C, Brewer GJ. 1998. Zinc may regulate serum leptin concentrations in humans. *J Am Coll Nutr* 17(3):270–275.

Mays MZ. 1993. Cognitive function in a sustained multi-stressor environment. In: Marriott BM, ed. *Review of the Results of Nutritional Intervention, U.S. Army Ranger Training Class 11/92 (Ranger II).* Washington, DC: National Academy Press. Pp. 199–214.

Mays MZ. 1995. Impact of underconsumption on cognitive performance. In: Marriott BM, ed. *Not Eating Enough: Overcoming Underconsumption of Military Operational Rations.* Washington, DC: National Academy Press. Pp. 285–302.

Murck H. 2002. Magnesium and affective disorders. *Nutr Neursci* 5(6):375–389.

Murck H, Steiger A. 1998. Mg2+ reduces ACTH secretion and enhances spindle power without changing delta power during sleep in men—possible therapeutic implications. *Psychopharmacology* [Berlin] 137(3):247–252.

Nowak G, Szewczyk B. 2002. Mechanisms contributing to antidepressant zinc actions. *Pol J Pharmacol* 54(6):587–592.

Penland JG. 1988. Effects of trace element nutrition on sleep patterns in adult women. *FASEB J* 2(4):A434.

Penland JG. 1989. Relationship between essential trace element nutrition and self-reported mood states. *N Dak Acad Sci Proc* 43:68.

Penland JG. 1991. Cognitive performance effects of low zinc (Zn) intakes in healthy adult men. *FASEB J* 5(5):A938.

Penland JG. 1995. Quantitative analysis of EEG effects following experimental marginal magnesium and boron deprivation. *Magnes Res* 8(4):341–358.

Penland JG, Finley JW. 1995. Dietary selenium and mood states in healthy young men. *N Dak Acad Sci Proc* 49:26.

Penland JG, Milne DB, Davis CD. 2000. Moderately high zinc intake impairs verbal memory of healthy postmenopausal women on a low copper diet. In: Roussel AM, Favier AE, Anderson RA, eds. *Trace Elements in Man and Animals—10: Proceedings of the Tenth International Symposium on Trace Elements in Man and Animals*. New York: Kluwer Academic/Plenum Publishers. Pp.1025–1030.

Penland JG, Egger NG, Ramanujam VMS, Dayal HH, Sandstead HH. 2002. Zinc (Zn) and iron (Fe) repletion improves cognitive function of mildly deficient women. *FASEB J* 16(5):A974.

Penland JG, Duffield-Lillico AJ, Tompson CD. Submitted. Selenium supplementation and mood states of adults with low-selenium status.

Penland JG, Finley JW, Gao J. 2006. Selenium status is associated with mood states and cognitive function in Chinese men with low selenium status. *FASEB J* 20:A1070.

Poenaru S, Rouhani S, Durlach J, Aymard N, Belkahla F, Rayssiguier Y, Iovino M. 1984. Vigilance states and cerebral monoamine metabolism in experimental magnesium deficiency. *Magnesium* 3(3):145–151.

Popoviciu L, Corfariu O, Fagaraseanu M, Kollo K, Bagathai I. 1987. Polysomnographic research in sleep disorders associated with magnesium deficiency. *Rev Roum Méd Neurol Psychiat* [Neurol Psychiatr] 25(2):83–90.

Potocnik FC, van Rensburg SJ, Park C, Taljaard JJ, Emsley RA. 1997. Zinc and platelet membrane microviscosity in Alzheimer's disease. The in vivo effect of zinc on platelet membranes and cognition. *S Afr Med J* 87(9):1116–1119.

Rains TM, Shay NF. 1995. Zinc status specifically changes preferences for carbohydrate and protein in rats selecting from separate carbohydrate-, protein-, and fat-containing diets. *J Nutr* 125(11): 2874–2879.

Rains TM, Hedrick S, Randall AC, Lee RG, Kennedy KJ, Shay NF. 1998. Food intake patterns are altered during long-term zinc deficiency in rats. *Physiol Behav* 65(3):473–478.

Rayman MP. 2002. The argument for increasing selenium intake. *Proc Nutr Soc* 61(2):203–215.

Rayman M, Thompson A, Warren-Perry M, Galassini R, Catterick J, Hall E, Lawrence D, Bliss J. 2005. Impact of selenium on mood and quality of life: A randomized, controlled trial. *Biol Psychiatry* 51:147–154.

Sait Gonen M, Kisakol G, Savas Cilli A, Dikbas O, Gungor K, Inal A, Kaya A. 2004. Assessment of anxiety in subclinical thyroid disorders. *Endocr J* 51(3):311–315.

Sandstead HH, Wallwork JC, Halas ES, Tucker DM, Dvergsten CL, Strobel DA. 1983. Zinc and central nervous function. In: Sarkar B, ed. *Biological Aspects of Metals and Metal-Related Diseases*. New York: Raven Press. Pp. 225–241.

Schweizer U, Brauer AU, Kohrle J, Nitsch R, Savaskan NE. 2004. Selenium and brain function: A poorly recognized liaison. *Brain Res Rev* 45(3):164–178.

Shay NF, Mangian HF. 2000. Neurobiology of zinc-influenced eating behavior. *J Nutr* 130(5 Suppl): 1493S–1499S.

Shils ME. 1969. Experimental human magnesium depletion. *Medicine* 48(1):61–85.

Shils ME. 1997. Magnesium. In: O'Dell BL, Sunde RA, eds. *Handbook of Nutritionally Essential Mineral Elements.* New York: Marcel Dekker. Pp. 117–152.
Shippee RL. 1993. Nutritional status and immune function of Ranger trainees given increased caloric intake. In: Marriott BM, ed. *Review of the Results of Nutritional Intervention, U.S. Army Ranger Training Class 11/92 (Ranger II).* Washington, DC: National Academy Press. Pp. 86–104.
Shippee R, Friedl K, Kramer T, Mays M, Popp K, Askew EW, Fairbrother B, Hoyt R, Vogel J, Marchitelli L, Frykman P, Martinez-Lopez L, Bernton E, Kramer M, Tulley R, Rood J, Delaney J, Jezior D, Arsenault J, Nindl B, Galloway R, Hoover D. 1994. *Nutritional and Immunological Assessment of Ranger Students with Increased Caloric Intake.* Technical Report T95-5. Natick, MA: U.S. Army Research Institute of Environmental Medicine.
Shor-Posner G, Lecusay R, Miguez MJ, MorenoBlack G, Zhang G, Rodriguez N. 2003. Psychological burden in the era of HAART: Impact of selenium therapy. *Intl J Psychiatry Med* 33:55–69.
Singewald N, Sinner C, Hetzenauer A, Sartori SB, Murck H. 2004. Magnesium-deficient diet alters depression- and anxiety-related behavior in mice–influence of desipramine and Hypericum perforatum extract. *Neuropharmacology* 47(8):1189–97.
Takase B, Akima T, Satomura K, Ohsuzu F, Mastui T, Ishihara M, Kurita A. 2004. Effects of chronic sleep deprivation on autonomic activity by examining heart rate variability, plasma catecholamine, and intracellular magnesium levels. *Biomed Pharmacother* 58(1 Suppl):S35–S39.
Tharion WJ, Lieberman HR, Montain SJ, Young AJ, Baker-Fulco CJ, Delany JP, Hoyt RW. 2005. Energy requirements of military personnel. *Appetite* 44(1):47–65.
Tucker DM, Sandstead HH. 1984. Neuropsychological function in experimental zinc deficiency in humans. In: Frederickson CJ, Howell GA, Kasarskis EJ, eds. *The Neurobiology of Zinc. Part B: Deficiency, Toxicity, and Pathology.* New York: Alan R. Liss. Pp. 139–152.
Vallee BL, Falchuk KH. 1993. The biochemical basis of zinc physiology. *Physiol Rev* 73(1):79–118.
Yao JK, Reddy RD. 2005. Metabolic investigation in psychiatric disorders. *Mol Neurobiol* 31(1–3): 193–204.

# Zinc, Magnesium, and Copper Requirements and Exercise

*Henry C. Lukaski*
*USDA-ARS Grand Forks Human Nutrition Research Center, Grand Forks, North Dakota*

## INTRODUCTION

Soldiers are expected to perform physically and mentally at high levels despite concurrent exposure to environmental and operational stressors. During deployment, military personnel may reduce food intake up to 50 percent resulting in suboptimal intakes of energy and micronutrients (Baker-Fulco, 1995). Short duration (< 1 week) decreases in energy and macronutrient intakes are suggested to have minor effects on components of physical performance in young men (Taylor et al., 1957) unless body weight, and hence muscle, loss is significant (5–10 percent) and then strength is reduced (Friedl, 1995). Montain and Young (2003) recently concluded that decrements in maximal oxygen consumption occur with short-term energy restriction and that these decrements have implications for performance impairments during non-weight bearing tasks. The impact of reduced intake of micronutrients, specifically minerals, and of increased mineral losses on the physical performance of soldiers remains to be determined.

Surveys of mineral intakes by soldiers are scarce but data from a few studies suggest that their intakes of some minerals are inadequate. The limited surveys report that zinc and magnesium intakes of male soldiers during training and in garrison are less than those recommended by the Institute of Medicine (IOM, 2001) (for review see Lukaski and Penland, 2006). Although these findings suggest the potential for sub-clinical zinc and magnesium deficits, corresponding biochemical assessments of nutritional status did not reveal evidence of depletion possibly because of mineral mobilization in association with increased protein catabolism (Lukaski, 2005 in this Appendix) or the lack of sensitive biomarkers of marginal deficiencies. Thus, the impact of these short-term decreased intakes of minerals per se on physical performance is unknown. There are no data available on copper intakes by military personnel.

This review examines the current knowledge about zinc and magnesium and copper needs of soldiers in training and operations. It summarizes civilian studies conducted to assess the effects of exercise on circulating zinc and magnesium concentrations and describes redistribution of minerals in the body and their excretion in the urine. It also reviews the effects of restricted intakes of zinc and magnesium on components of physical performance and describes the time-course of depletion and repletion with supplemental zinc and magnesium. Information on copper intakes and losses of military personnel is not available. However, new information describing the effects of dietary copper on energy use during exercise is provided. The adequacy of the current Meal, Ready-to-Eat (MRE) and the First Strike Ration (FSR) to meet zinc and magnesium requirements of soldiers in training is evaluated.

## EXERCISE AND MINERAL METABOLISM

Zinc, magnesium, and copper play key roles in supporting physiological functions during physical activity. These minerals express their biological activities as metalloproteins and co-factors for enzymes. Via their role as enzyme cofactors, they regulate energy metabolism, integrate physiological systems, facilitate cellular energy production, coordinate the balance between aerobic and anaerobic energy metabolism, and provide defense against free radicals produced during periods of increased energy production (Lukaski, 2004).

### Exercise Effects on Mineral Metabolism

Exercise is a provocative stressor that causes redistribution of certain minerals (Oh et al., 1978). This finding stimulated the investigation of the effects of exercise and diet on circulating zinc and magnesium.

## Zinc

Maximal exercise induces hemoconcentration or reduction of plasma volume that increases plasma zinc concentrations. Young men fed zinc in amounts of 4 (low), 9 (adequate), and 34 (luxuriant) mg/day underwent progressive, maximal exercise tests on cycle ergometers after an overnight fast (Lukaski et al., 1984). Regardless of zinc intake, plasma zinc concentrations increased significantly immediately after exercise. However, pre- and post-exercise plasma zinc concentrations were significantly less when dietary zinc was low (4 mg/day) compared to the adequate and luxuriant intakes. To control for plasma volume reduction during intense exercise, plasma zinc concentrations were corrected with a previously validated method (Van Beaumont et al., 1973). Low, compared to adequate or supplemental, dietary zinc was associated with a significant decrease in total plasma zinc content. A significant relationship was found between total plasma zinc content and change in body zinc retention. Plasma zinc content paralleled changes in zinc balance during periods of low, adequate, and supplemental zinc intake. This finding suggested that zinc mobilization, assessed indirectly by using the total plasma zinc content, was impaired when dietary zinc was restricted.

Other studies have extended these observations. Plasma zinc concentrations of men who completed a 6-mile run increased immediately after exercise (Anderson et al., 1984) which is consistent with other reports (Cordova and Alvarez-Man, 1995). Other investigators reported, however, no change in plasma zinc concentration in men who completed a 10-mile run (van Rij et al., 1986). Differences in the timing of phlebotomies and uncontrolled fluid intakes explain the divergent observations (Keen, 1993). Two hours after completion of the runs, however, plasma zinc concentrations decreased significantly to pre-exercise values in all runners (Anderson et al., 1984; Cordova and Alvarez-Mon, 1995; van Rij et al., 1986). Similar findings were reported by Singh et al. (1994) who studied changes in plasma zinc concentrations after a standardized, prolonged endurance run of trained male runners supplemented with 50 mg/day of zinc or placebo for 6 days each in a double-blind cross-over study. These findings indicate that high-intensity exercise promotes mobilization of zinc from body stores. Also, recovery after exercise (2 hours) is associated with a sequestration of minerals, particularly zinc, probably as a result of metallothionein induction in liver and kidney (Oh et al., 1978).

There is some evidence that physically active adults have disrupted tissue pools of zinc. Trained female runners had intakes of zinc (10 mg/day), consistent with the current recommendation (IOM, 2001), but significantly reduced plasma zinc concentrations and significantly increased urinary zinc losses compared to age-matched untrained women with a similar intake of zinc (Deuster et al., 1989). In response to a $^{65}Zn$ infusion, the area under the plasma $^{65}Zn$ curve was significantly reduced in the trained women (35 versus 44 μmol in 4 hours). This finding suggests that zinc in muscle, the largest body pool of zinc, might also be depleted in the trained runners.

The interaction of dietary zinc and exercise on urinary losses of zinc has been examined. Fourteen physically active men were fed diets high (~19 mg/day) and low (~4 mg/day) in zinc for 9 weeks in a double-blind, randomized cross-over trial (Lukaski, 2005). Plasma zinc concentrations in both groups increased significantly compared to pre-exercise values after 45 minutes of high-intensity exercise. However, the magnitude of the increase was significantly greater when the high-zinc diet was consumed. Urinary zinc losses were significantly greater on the day of exercise (0.2 versus 0.1 mg/day) when the higher zinc was fed. Parallel changes in urinary nitrogen were observed. These findings indicate that the increased zinc mobilization and excretion night be related to muscle protein catabolism.

Intense exercise affects zinc metabolism (Figure B-29); based on the studies described here a hypothesis for the mechanisms of redistribution of zinc with metabolism can be proposed. The initial response is a decrease in plasma volume (hemoconcentration) that appears to increase the concentration of zinc in plasma and serum. Concomitantly, surface losses (sweat and cell sloughing) of water and minerals could also contribute to changes in circulating zinc. During exercise, zinc is likely mobilized from soft tissues into the circulation. This response, which is also influenced by the degree of protein breakdown and gluconeogen-

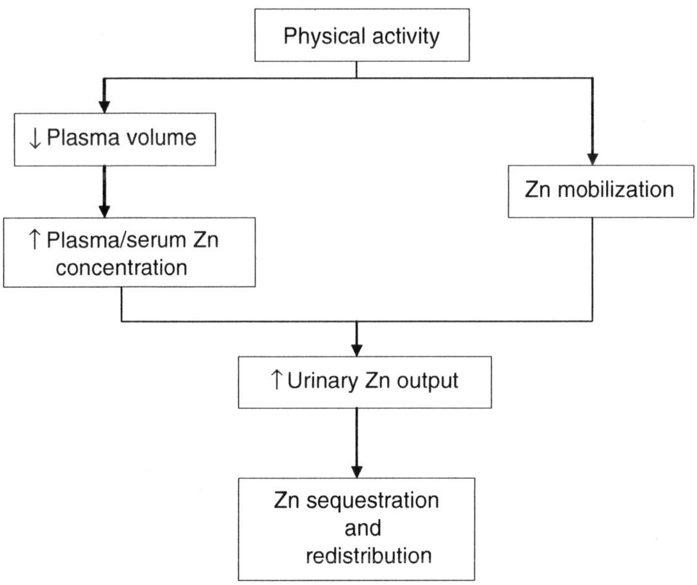


**FIGURE B-29** Schematic representation of the effect of physical activity on zinc metabolism.

esis, may contribute to the increased circulating zinc concentration. At least two hours after the cessation of exercise, it appears that zinc redistribution and sequestration into soft tissues begins with the up-regulation of metallothionein synthesis; the half-life of hepatic metallothionein is about six hours (Oh et al., 1978). Urinary output of zinc increases on days of exercise compared to non-exercise periods. Under conditions of adequate zinc intake, homeostatic adaptations of increased zinc absorption and decreased excretion in sweat and urine could accommodate for losses associated with physical activity. The extent of the homeostatic adaptation and, therefore, the additional needs for zinc intake during intense exercise is unknown.

### *Military Training and Zinc Metabolism*

One study, in which soldiers participated in field operations, reported altered zinc status (Miyamura et al., 1987). During a 4 week training period, energy intake was unchanged and body weight decreased (~2 kg). Dietary zinc intake (16–19 mg/day) was constant and exceeded military recommendations (U.S. Departments of Army, Navy and Air Force, 2001). However, plasma zinc decreased significantly and urinary zinc losses increased significantly. Although these findings suggest that zinc intake was inadequate to maintain zinc status (see below Adequacy of Zinc in Military Rations), more research is needed to decipher alterations of zinc metabolism during military training before firmly concluding that levels of dietary zinc should be higher than currently established (MDRI = 15 or 12 mg for men and women, respectively).

## Magnesium

Acute bouts of exercise affect magnesium metabolism. Serum magnesium concentration significantly increased immediately after short-duration, high-intensity exercise (Deuster et al., 1987) or prolonged endurance exercise (Deuster and Singh, 1994; Lijnen et al., 1988). Buchman et al. (1998) reported significant decreases (~15 percent) in serum magnesium in men and women following a marathon compared to measurements made on non-exercise days. Urinary magnesium outputs decreased during and immediately following strenuous exercise (Buchman et al., 1998) but increased during the next 24 hours (Deuster et al., 1987; Lijnen et al., 1988). Thus, exercise intensity and duration alter magnesium homeostasis.

Surface losses of magnesium during exercise can be appreciable. Men performing controlled work for 8 hours on cycle ergometers in the heat (37.8°C) lost 15–18 mg of magnesium daily in sweat and cellular exfoliation collected from a lower arm site (Consolazio et al., 1963). Surface losses of magnesium accounted for 4–5 percent of daily magnesium intake and 10–15 percent of total magnesium excretion.

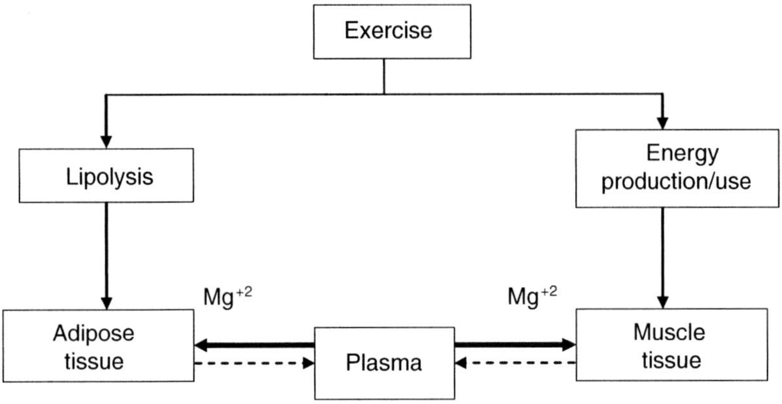


**FIGURE B-30** Magnesium (Mg) fluxes during aerobic exercise. Solid arrows indicate magnesium movement from plasma into specific tissues during aerobic exercise. Abbreviated arrows show redistribution of magnesium from soft tissues into the circulation. SOURCE: Adapted from Resina et al. (1995).

Changes in circulating and urinary magnesium suggest redistribution among body pools (Figure B-30). Resina et al. (1995) proposed that aerobic exercise promotes a relocation of magnesium from plasma into adipose tissue to enhance lipolysis and into working muscle to maintain activity of magnesium-containing enzymes. Thus, magnesium concentrations in serum may decline because of redistribution and sweat losses. After the cessation of exercise, magnesium re distributes from soft tissues into the plasma with concomitant increases in urinary magnesium output.

## MINERAL DEPLETION AND PHYSICAL PERFORMANCE

Evidence is accumulating that intakes of zinc and magnesium in amounts less than recommended are associated with impaired physical performance. Limited findings suggest that supplementation of these minerals can enhance responses to physical training. Differences in experimental designs pose difficulties in the interpretation of some findings.

### Zinc

Observational studies report decreased physical performance in people with low zinc status (Table B-21). Muscular strength and power were significantly less in adolescents (Brun et al., 1995) and men (Khaled et al., 1997), respec-

**TABLE B-21** Zinc (Zn) Intake or Status and Performance Measures

| Sample | Zn intake or status indicator | Design | Low Zn effects | Reference |
|---|---|---|---|---|
| Women | 135 mg/day | Cross-over | ↑ strength | Krotkiewski et al., 1988 |
| Adolescents | ↓ serum Zn | Observational | ↓ strength | Brun et al., 1995 |
| Male athletes | ↓ serum Zn | Observational | ↓ power | Khaled et al., 1997 |
| Men | 1 vs. 12 mg/day<br>↓ serum Zn | Controlled feeding | ↓ strength<br>↓ work capacity | Van Loan et al., 1999 |
| Men | 4 vs. 19 mg/day<br>↓ plasma Zn<br>↓ Zn retention | Controlled feeding | ↓ peak $O_2$ and $CO_2$<br>↑ $O_2$, HR & $V_E$ and<br>↓ $CO_2$ during submaximal exercise | Lukaski, 2005 |

NOTE: $CO_2$ = carbon dioxide output; HR = heart rate; $O_2$ = oxygen uptake; $V_e$ = ventilatory volume.

tively, with low serum zinc compared to age- and sex-matched controls with serum zinc concentrations in the range of normal values.

Controlled studies with different amounts of dietary zinc demonstrate physiological impairments with inadequate zinc intake. Men fed 1 compared to 12 mg of zinc daily had significantly decreased serum zinc concentrations and marked reductions in upper and lower body strength and work capacity (Van Loan et al., 1999). Similarly, cardiorespiratory function (heart and ventilation rates) as well as oxygen consumption and carbon dioxide production were significantly altered in physically active men consuming diets containing 3.7 compared to 18.7 mg zinc daily (Lukaski, 2005). Measures of zinc status (plasma zinc concentration, erythrocyte carbonic anhydrase activity and zinc retention) decreased when the low-zinc diet was fed.

Zinc supplementation during physical training resulted in significant gains in muscular strength. Older women supplemented with zinc (135 mg/day) compared to placebo in a double-blind, cross-over trial experienced greater gains in strength after 4 weeks of strength training (Krotkiewski et al., 1982). These findings are questionable because neither total dietary zinc intake nor zinc status was assessed. To add to the lack of clear evidence of benefits of supplementation, other studies suggest that supplementation with zinc does not improve performance (Sing et al., 1992, 1994, 1999; Telford et al., 1992; Weight et al., 1988).

## Magnesium

Magnesium status has been related to physical performance in a few groups of athletes. Observational studies of male, collegiate athletes (Lukaski et al., 1983) and adolescent swimmers (Conn et al., 1988) found significant correlations between peak oxygen uptake and plasma or serum magnesium concentrations. Dietary magnesium also was a significant predictor of swim performance in male and female collegiate swimmers (Lukaski, 1995).

Magnesium supplementation of physically active adults improved metabolic responses to training and during controlled exercise (Table B-22). Young men supplemented with magnesium (250 mg/day) in a blinded-randomized trial and enrolled in resistance training increased power significantly more than placebo-treated controls (Brilla and Haley, 1992). Physically active men (Ripari et al., 1989) and collegians (Brilla and Gunther, 1995) had significantly reduced heart rate, decreased oxygen consumption or increased endurance time, and decreased oxygen uptake during submaximal exercise, with magnesium supplementation (250 mg/day). Although these findings suggest a benefit of magnesium supplementation, they fail to indicate if functional improvements are limited to individuals with reduced magnesium intake or status.

Studies of individuals with low magnesium status demonstrate the benefit of increased magnesium intake on performance measures. Elite rowers with serum magnesium concentrations at the low end of the range of normal values and

**TABLE B-22** Magnesium (Mg) Intake and Responses to Exercise

| Sample | Mg intake, mg/d | Design | Low Mg effects | Reference |
|---|---|---|---|---|
| Men | 250 vs. 450 | Supplement[a] | ↑ HR, ↑$V_E$ | Ripari et al., 1989 |
| Men | 250 vs. 507 | Supplement[a] | ↓ strength gain | Brilla & Haley, 1992 |
| Women | Placebo vs. 360 | Supplement[a] | ↑ $O_2$ | Golf et al., 1993 |
| Men & Women | 290 vs. 540 | Supplement[a] | ↑ $O_2$ and HR, ↓ endurance | Brilla & Gunther, 1995 |
| Women | 153 vs. 322 vs. 360 | Controlled feeding | ↑ $O_2$, HR, and $V_E$ during submax exercise | Lukaski & Nielsen, 2003 |

NOTE: $O_2$ = oxygen uptake; $CO_2$ = carbon dioxide output; HR = heart rate; $V_E$ = ventilatory volume.
[a]Double-blind supplementation trial.

supplemented with 250 mg of magnesium daily used significantly less oxygen during submaximal rowing ergometer tests compared to placebo (Golf et al., 1994). Also, postmenopausal women fed diets containing 330–360 compared to 150 mg of magnesium responded with increased muscle and erythrocyte magnesium concentrations, and magnesium retention; they had reduced heart rate, ventilation rate, and oxygen use during exercise (Lukaski and Nielsen, 2003). Thus, magnesium supplementation of people with sub-optimal magnesium status, regardless of physical activity level (e.g., trained or untrained), improves physiological function during exercise and magnesium nutritional status. Conversely, magnesium supplementation (365 mg/day for 10 weeks) of marathon runners with normal magnesium status had no beneficial effects on performance or biochemical indicators of magnesium nutritional status (Terblanche et al., 1992).

### Copper

Only recently has there been interest in determining the effect of copper intake on energy metabolism and performance. The mechanisms of action apparently is reduced activity of a copper-containing enzyme, cytochrome c oxidase (CCO). Dietary copper restriction results in metabolic and functional impairments. In rodents, copper deprivation consistently resulted in decreased activity of CCO in brain, liver, heart, skeletal muscle (Prohaska, 1990) with the greatest reductions in muscle (Reeves et al., 2005). Davidson et al. (1993) found significantly decreased CCO activity in the soleus muscle and a blunted response to submaximal, aerobic training of adult, male Long-Evans rats fed a diet low compared to adequate in copper (< 1 versus 6 mg/kg diet). Exercise training was associated with a significantly reduced increase in muscle CCO in the copper-restricted compared to copper-adequate animals. The copper-deprived rats were unable to complete the exercise training regimen. Physically active young men fed copper at the recommended level of intake (0.9 mg/day; IOM, 2001) had adverse responses to submaximal exercise (Lukaski, submitted). Compared to a higher intake (1.6 mg/day), muscle cytochrome c oxidase activity decreased significantly when dietary copper was 0.9 mg/day. Plasma lactate concentration increased significantly with the low compared to the higher dietary copper. These findings suggest that copper needs of active men may exceed the recommended dietary copper intake for the general public.

## FACTORS CONTRIBUTING TO ZINC, MAGNESIUM AND COPPER DEPLETION

Many factors contribute to the depletion of body minerals and can lead to sub-clinical deficiency states. Intakes of minerals at the Recommended Dietary Allowance (RDA) minimize the probability of nutritional inadequacy. Thus, the RDA is a target intake for an individual (IOM, 2001).

Increased losses of minerals can affect mineral nutritional status. Exposure to conditions that increase urinary, fecal or surface losses, including cell sloughing and sweat, can reduce body stores of minerals. Conditions that decrease gastrointestinal transit time, such as diarrhea, increase fecal losses of minerals. Similarly, factors that increase urinary output of minerals, including catabolism of muscle and use of diuretics, promote excretion of minerals. Restricted intake of minerals, however, generally decreases mineral losses in urine.

Environmental conditions that increase surface losses may adversely impact mineral balance or retention. Under thermoneutral conditions, whole-body surface losses of zinc, copper, and iron were 0.5, 0.34, and 0.33 mg/day or 4, 26, and 2 percent, respectively, of dietary intake (Jacob et al., 1981). Exposure to a hot climate increased losses of minerals in arm sweat. Consolazio et al. (1964) reported zinc and copper losses of 2.2 and 1.5 mg/day or 19 and 48 percent of daily intake, respectively, during approximately 8 hours of exposure to 38°C daily during a 16-day heat exposure study and limited exercise (30 min/day). Similarly, iron and magnesium arm surface losses were 1 and 17 mg/day or 5 and 6 percent, respectively (Consolazio et al., 1963). Although data on whole-body surface losses of minerals during periods of heavy physical activity are lacking, one study (DeRuisseau et al., 2002) reported that arm sweat losses of zinc were 9 and 8 percent of the RDA for men and women, respectively, during a 2 hour period of controlled exercise. For a more detailed discussion on mineral sweat losses with exercise, see Haymes (2005) in this appendix.

The principal factor in precipitating copper depletion is intake less than needed to accomodate losses in urine, feces and sweat. Urinary copper losses tend to be small and negligible. Adaptation in absorption is the principal homeostatic regulation of copper status (Klevay et al., 1984). Although whole-body losses of copper in sweat appear to be small (~0.35 mg/day), they represent more than 25 percent of daily copper intake in healthy men (Jacob et al., 1981). This value is less than that previously reported by Consolazio et al. (1963) for copper losses in arm sweat. Regardless of collection site, surface loss of copper is appreciable.

## ADEQUACY OF ZINC IN MILITARY RATIONS

An evaluation of the adequacy of zinc intake for military personnel is limited by the lack of comprehensive data on mineral intake and losses. Thus, an assessment requires compilation of information from different sources. The principal source of data is a report from Miyamura et al. (1987) who studied male soldiers participating in a 34 day intensive training exercise. The soldiers experienced a significant decrease in plasma zinc concentration and a significant increase in urinary zinc loss despite a daily zinc intake of 17 mg.

Zinc losses could include about 1 mg/day in urine (Miyamura et al., 1987), 2.3 mg/day in sweat (Consolazio et al., 1964) and 12 mg in feces, assuming a

30 percent absorption of dietary zinc (Lukaski, 2005). Thus, estimated zinc losses could total as much as 15.3 mg/day. Assuming an average zinc intake of 17 mg/day (Miyamura et al., 1987) and a loss of 15.3 mg/day, the balance is calculated to be + 1.7 mg/day (17–15.3).

According to military regulation, operational rations, including the MRE and FSR, should be planned to provide either 15 or 8 mg of zinc daily, respectively (U.S. Departments of Army, Navy and Air Force, 2001). Assuming that the estimated daily losses of zinc could exceed 15 mg/day, the recommended contents of the MRE (15 mg) and FSR (8 mg) would not meet the needs to overcome daily losses.

The paucity of information describing intakes and losses of magnesium and copper limit the discussion of the adequacy of levels of these minerals in military rations. As summarized previously (Lukaski and Penland, 2006), intakes of zinc and magnesium by military personnel participating in a variety of operational activities are less than recommended levels. Moreover, estimates of daily copper intakes are not available. Evidence that recomended intakes of magnesium and copper are need for optimal physiological and psychological performance reinforces the need to ascertain intakes of these minerals among active duty military personnel.

## EFFECTS OF MULTI-MINERAL AND VITAMIN SUPPLEMENTS PHYSICAL PERFORMANCE

Limited studies have examined the effects of multiple vitamin and mineral supplements in exercising adults and measures of physical performance. Thirty male long distance runners participated in a blinded, cross-over supplementation trial with a washout (3 months) between treatment periods (3 months) to evaluate the effects of supplements containing the RDA or recommended intake of vitamins and minerals on nutritional status and physical performance (Weight et al., 1988a,b). Blood biochemical measures of nutritional status were within the ranges of normal values before and after supplementation with no adverse effects identified. Active supplementation failed to elicit any improvement in peak oxygen uptake, peak running speed, and peak post-exercise lactate accumulation. Similarly, 86 Australian male and female elite athletes (basketball, gymnastics, swimming, and rowing) participated in a 7–8 month placebo-controlled trial of a multiple vitamin and mineral supplement that contained recommended intakes of the nutrients (Telford et al., 1992a,b). Supplementation improved blood concentrations of vitamin $B_1$, $B_6$, $B_{12}$, and folate in athletes with lower levels at entry with no effects on mineral nutritional status indicators. Supplementation did not improve performance measures. Twenty two physically active men received no benefit in peak aerobic capacity, endurance capacity or muscle strength from a high potency (e.g., exceeding recommended intake levels) multivitamin-mineral supplement compared to placebo

(Singh et al., 1992). In each study, dietary intake of vitamins and minerals was consistent with population recommendations. Thus, consumption of a multiple vitamin and mineral supplement that meets recommended intakes neither adversely affects nutritional status nor enhances various physical performance assessed by a variety of measures.

## SUMMARY AND CONCLUSIONS

Evidence from controlled feeding studies and supplementation trials demonstrate that measures of physical performance including muscle strength, cardiorespiratory function and energy metabolism are adversely affected when intakes of zinc and magnesium are less than recommended. If military personnel fail to consume adequate amounts of zinc and magnesium, they also may experience impaired performance, although there are inconsistent results regarding the magnesium effects.

Acute bouts of exercise and heavy physical training increase losses of minerals in urine and sweat. These losses are appreciable and may exceed 10–20 percent of daily intakes. It is estimated that the contents of the MRE and FSR, as currently composed, are inadequate to meet the potential daily losses of zinc by soldiers during physical training.

There is a paucity of data on mineral intakes and losses by soldiers under the stressful conditions of training and adverse environmental conditions. This information is required to develop appropriate recommendations for mineral intakes, specifically zinc, magnesium, and copper.

## DISCLAIMERS

Mention of a trademark or proprietary product does not constitute a guarantee of the product by the United States Department of Agriculture and does not imply its approval to the exclusion of other products that may also be suitable.

U.S. Department of Agriculture, Agricultural Research Service, Northern Plains Area is an equal opportunity/affirmative action employer and all agency services are available without discrimination.

## REFERENCES

Anderson RA, Polansky MM, Bryden NA. 1984. Strenuous running: Acute effects of chromium, copper, zinc, and selected clinical variables in urine and serum of male runners. *Biol Trace Elem Res* 6:327–336.

Baker-Fulco CJ. 1995. Overview of dietary intakes during military exercises. In: *Not Eating Enough: Overcoming Underconsumption of Military Operational Rations.* Washington, DC: National Academy Press.

Brilla LR, Gunther KB. 1995. Effect of magnesium supplementation on exercise time to exhaustion. *Med Exerc Nutr Health* 4:230–233.

Brilla LR, Haley TF. 1992. Effect of magnesium supplementation on strength training in humans. *J Am Coll Nutr* 11:326–329.

Brun JF, Dieu-Cambrezy C, Charpiat A, Fons C. Fedou C, Micallef JP, Fussellier M, Bardet L, Orsetti A. 1995. Serum zinc in highly trained adolescent gymnasts. *Biol Trace Elem Res* 47:273–278.

Buchman AL, Keen CL, Commisso J, Killip D, Ou C-N, Rognerud CL, Dennis K, Dunn JK. 1998. The effect of a marathon run on plasma and urine mineral and metal concentrations. *J Am Coll Nutr* 17(2):124–127.

Conn CA, Schemmel RA, Smith BW, Ryder E, Heusner WW, Ku P-K. 1988. Plasma and erythrocyte magnesium concentrations and correlations with maximal oxygen consumption in nine-to-twelve-year-old competitive swimmers. *Magnesium* 7:27–36.

Consolazio CF. 1983. Nutrition and performance. In: Johnson RE, ed. *Progess in Food and Nutrition Science,* vol 7. Oxford, UK: Pergamon Press.

Consolazio CF, Matoush LO, Nelson RA, Harding RS, Canham JE. 1963. Excretion of sodium, potassium, magnesium, and iron in human sweat and the relation of each to balance and requirements. *J Nutr* 79:407–415.

Consolazio CF, Nelson RA, Matoush LO, Hughes RC, Urone P. 1964. *Trace Mineral Losses in Sweat.* Report 284. U.S. Army Medical Research & Nutrition Laboratory. Fitzsimmons General Hospital, August 18. Denver, CO.

Cordova A, Alvarez-Mon M. 1995. Behavior of zinc in physical exercise: A special reference to immunity and fatigue. *Neurosci Biobehav Rev* 19(3):439–445.

Davidson J, Medeiros DM, Hamlin RL, Jenkins JE. 1993. Submaximal, aerobic exercise training exacerbates the cardiomyopathy of postweanling Cu-depleted rats. *Biol Trace Elem Res* 38:251–272.

DeRuisseau KC, Cheuvront SN, Haymes EM, Sharp RG. 2002. Sweat iron and zinc losses during prolonged exercise. *Int J Sport Nutr Exerc Metab* 12:428–437.

Deuster PA, Singh A. 1993. Responses of plasma magnesium and other cations to fluid replacement. *J Am Coll Nutr* 12:286–293.

Deuster PA, Dolev E, Kyle SB, Anderson RA, Schoomaker EB. 1987. Magnesium homeostasis during high-intensity aerobic exercise in men. *J Appl Physiol* 62:545–550.

Deuster PA, Day BA, Singh A, Douglass L, Moser-Veillon PB. 1989. Zinc status of highly trained women runners and untrained women. *Am J Clin Nutr* 49:1295–1301.

Friedl KE. 1995. When does energy deficit affect soldier physical performance? In: *Not Eating Enough: Overcoming Underconsumption of Military Operational Rations.* Washington, DC: National Academy Press.

Golf SW, Bohmer D, Nowacki PE. 1994. Is magnesium a limiting factor in competitive sport? A summary of relevant literature. In: Golf S, Dralle D, Vecchiet L, eds. *Magnesium* 1993. London: John Libbey.

IOM (Institute of Medicine). 2001. *Dietary Reference Intakes for Vitamin A, Vitamin K, Arsenic, Boron, Chromium, Copper, Iodine, Iron, Manganese, Molybdenum, Nickel, Silicon, Vanadium, and Zinc.* Washington, DC: National Academy Press.

Jacob RA, Sandstead HH, Munoz JM, Klevay LM, Milne DB. 1981. Whole body surface loss of trace metals in normal males. *Am J Clin Nutr* 34:1379–1383.

Keen CL. 1993. The effect of exercise and heat on mineral metabolism and requirements. In: *Nutritional Needs in Hot Environments.* Washington, DC: National Academy Press.

Khaled S, Brun JF, Micallef JP, Bardet L, Cassanas G, Monnier JF, Orsetti A. 1997. Serum zinc and blood rheology in sportsmen (football players). *Clin Hemorheol Microcirc* 17:47–58.

Klevay LM, Inman L, Johnson LK, Lawler M, Mahalko JR, Milne DB, Lukaski HC, Bolonchuk W, Sandstead HH. 1984. Increased cholesterol in plasma in a young man during experimental copper depletion. *Metabolism* 33:1112–1118.

Krotkiewski M, Gudmundsson M, Backstrom P, Mandroukas K. 1982. Zinc and muscle strength and endurance. *Acta Physiol Scand* 116:309–311.

Lijnen P, Hespel P, Fagard R, Lysens R, Vanden Eynde E, Amery A. 1988. Erythrocyte, plasma, and urinary magnesium in men before and after a marathon. *Eur J Appl Physiol* 58:252–256.

Lukaski HC. 1995. Interactions among indices of mineral element nutriture and physical performance of swimmers. In: Kies CV, Driskell JA, eds. *Sports Nutrition: Minerals and Electrolytes.* Boca Raton, FL: CRC Press.

Lukaski HC. 2004. Vitamins and minerals: Effects on physical performance. *Nutrition* 20:632–644.

Lukaski HC. 2005. Low dietary zinc decreases erythrocyte carbonic anhydrase activities and impairs cardiorespiratory function in men during exercise. *Am J Clin Nutr* 81:1045–1051.

Lukaski HC. 2006. Protein turnover and mineral metabolism. In: *Mineral Requirements for Military Personnel.* Washington, DC: The National Academies Press.

Lukaski HC, Johnson PE. Submitted. Copper depletion and altered energy metabolism during exercise in men fed copper at the recommended intake. *Eur J Appl Physiol.*

Lukaski HC, Nielsen FH. 2002. Dietary magnesium depletion affects metabolic responses during submaximal exercise in postmenopausal women. *J Nutr* 132:930–935.

Lukaski HC, Penland JG. 2006. Zinc, magnesium, copper, iron, selenium, and calcium in assault rations: Roles in promotion of physical and mental performance. In: *Nutrient Composition of Rations for Short-Term, High-Intensity Combat Operations.* Washington, DC: The National Academies Press

Lukaski HC, Bolonchuk WW, Klevay LM, Milne DB, Sandstead HH. 1983. Maximal oxygen consumption as related to magnesium, copper and zinc nutriture. *Am J Clin Nutr* 37:407–415.

Lukaski HC, Bolonchuk WW, Klevay LM, Milne DB, Sandstead HH. 1984. Changes in plasma zinc content after exercise in men fed a low-zinc diet. *Am J Physiol* 247:E88–E93.

Miyamura JB, McNutt SW, Lichton IJ, Wenkam NS. 1987. Altered zinc status of soldiers under field conditions. *J Am Diet Assoc* 87(5):595–597.

Montain SJ, Young AJ. 2003. Diet and physical performance. *Appetite* 40:255–267.

Oh SH, Deagen JT, Whanger PD, Weswig PH. 1978. Biological function of metallothionein. V. Its induction in rats by various stressors. *Am J Physiol* 234:E282–E285.

Prohaska JR. 1990. Biochemical changes in copper deficiency. *J Nutr Biochem* 1:452–461.

Reeves PG, DeMars LCS, Johnson WT, Lukaski HC. 2005. Dietary copper deficiency reduces iron absorption and duodenal enterocyte hephaestin protein in male and female rats. *J Nutr* 135:92–98.

Resina A, Gatteschi L, Rubenni MG, Galvan P, Parise G, Tjouroudis N, Viroli L. 1995. Changes in serum and erythrocyte magnesium after training and physical exercise. In: Vecchiet L, ed. *Magnesium and Physical Activity.* London: Parthenon Publishing.

Ripari P, Pieralisi G, Giamberardino MA, Resina A, Vecchiet L. 1989. Effects of magnesium pidolinate on cardiorespiratory submaximal effort parameters. *Magnesium Res* 2:71–75.

Singh A, Moses FM, Deuster PA. 1992. Chronic multivitamin–mineral supplementation does not enhance physical performance. *Med Sci Sports Exerc* 24(6):726–732.

Singh A, Failla ML, Deuster PA. 1994. Exercise-induced changes in immune function: Effects of zinc supplementation. *J Appl Physiol* 76(6):2298–2303.

Taylor HL, Buskirk ER, Brozek J, Anderson JT, Grande F. 1957. Performance capacity and effects of caloric restriction with hard physical work on young men. *J Appl Physiol* 10:421–429.

Telford RD, Catchpole EA, Deakin V, McLeay AC, Plank AW. 1992a. The effect of 7 to 8 months of vitamin/mineral supplementation on the vitamin and mineral status of athletes. *Int J Sports Nutr* 2(2):123–134.

Telford RD, Catchpole EA, Deakin V, McLeay AC, Plank AW. 1992b. The effect of 7 to 8 months of vitamin/mineral supplementation on the athletic performance. *Int J Sports Nutr* 2(2):135–154.

Terblanche S, Noakes TD, Dennis SC, Marais DW, Eckert M. 1992. *Int J Sports Nutr* 2(2):154–164.

U.S. Departments of Army, Navy, and Air Force. 2001. *Nutrition Standards and Education*. AR 40-25/BUMEDINST 10110.6/AFI 44-141. Washington, DC: U.S. Department of Defense Headquarters.
Van Beaumont W, Strand JC, Petrofsky JS, Hipskind SG, Greenleaf JE. 1973. Changes in total plasma content of electrolytes and proteins with maximal exercise. *J Appl Physiol* 34:102–106.
Van Loan MD, Sutherland B, Lowe NM, Turnlund JR, King JC. 1999. The effects of zinc depletion on peak force and total work of knee and shoulder extensor and flexor muscles. *Int J Sport Nutr* 9(2):125–135.
Van Rij AM, Hall MT, Dohm GL, Bray JT, Pories WJ. 1986. Changes in zinc metabolism following exercise in human subjects. *Biol Trace Elem Res* 10:99–105.
Weight LM, Myburgh KH, Noakes TD. 1988a. Vitamin and mineral supplementation: Effect on the running performance of trained athletes. *Am J Clin Nutr* 47:192–195.
Weight LM, Noakes TD, Labadarios D, Graves J, Jacobs P, Berman PA. 1988b. Vitamin and mineral status of trained athletes including the effects OF SUPPLEMENTation. *Am J Clin Nutr* 47:186–191.

# The Effects of Iron Deficiency on Physical Performance

*Jere D. Haas*
*Cornell University, Ithaca, New York*

## INTRODUCTION

Iron deficiency is the most prevalent micronutrient deficiency in both the industrialized and non-industrialized world. In the United States iron deficiency affects approximately 3–4 percent of men and 12–14 percent of women between 18 and 45 years, the age of the majority of military personnel in the U.S. (Looker et al., 1997). While the most common consequence of iron deficiency is anemia, or blood hemoglobin concentration below a specified level, the prevalence of anemia underestimates the amount of iron deficiency in the population. WHO (2001) estimates that the prevalence of iron deficiency is more than twice the prevalence of anemia in any given population. Also, while iron deficiency accounts for the majority of anemia in the U.S. population, there are numerous additional causes of anemia, including other micronutrient deficiencies.

Numerous studies of the effect of iron deficiency on physical performance have been conducted over the past 35 years with conclusive evidence for a causal relationship (Haas and Brownlie, 2001). Most of the evidence from these studies indicates that low hemoglobin concentration and consequent reduced oxygen transport to working muscles is the primary mechanism for reduced performance due to iron deficiency. However, evidence from animal studies and more recently in human studies of non-anemic human subjects suggest that iron deficiency may affect physical performance through other mechanisms. This review addresses the evidence for the effects of iron depletion in non-anemic individuals.

## ASSESSING MODERATE IRON DEFICIENCY

There are a number of indicators of iron nutritional status that when used together can reveal a fairly comprehensive picture of the various body iron pools that are significant for understanding the functional consequences of iron deficiency. Figure B-31 shows the progress of iron status from normal to deficient states and the course taken by the major indicators of iron status in common use. The body iron stores reflect the functional iron status of an individual. With increased iron loss or decreased iron intake to compensate for losses, the body iron stores decline to a point indicated as "deficient." The best single indicator of the depletion of iron stores is serum ferritin. Hemoglobin concentration does not start to fall until after iron stores are depleted, and anemia is defined as a hemoglobin level that is achieved during the decline in hemopoiesis. There is a stage of body iron depletion when the iron stores are completely depleted but hemoglobin has not yet reached a level that indicates anemia; this is the iron deficient, non-anemic state (IDNA). Another indicator of iron status that is not represented in Figure B-31 is the blood plasma concentration of the soluble transferrin receptor (sTfR). It follows a course similar to that for free erythrocyte protoporphyrin (FEP), and increasing levels indicate a increased demand for iron at the muscle

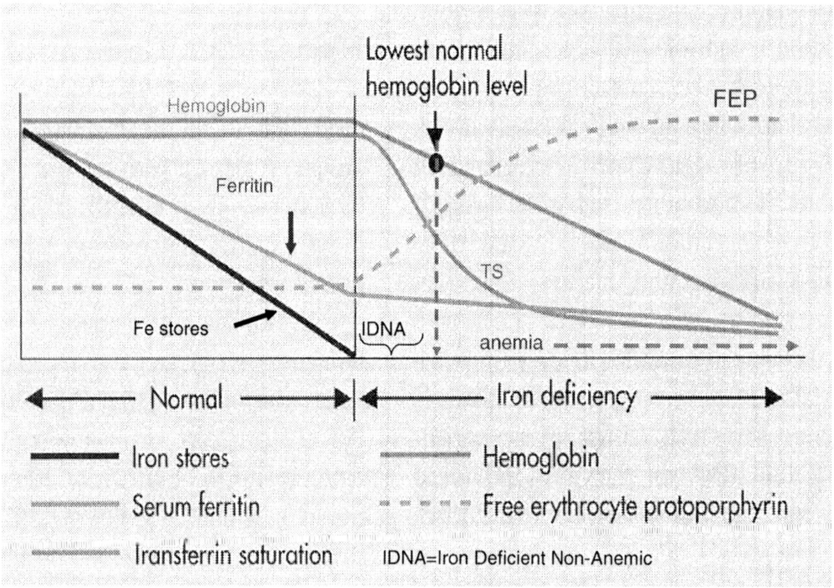


**FIGURE B-31** Relationship between various indicators of iron status and the body's level of iron stores.
SOURCE: Modified from Guthrie and Picciano (1995).

tissue level which is not being met by circulating iron in the iron depleted individual. This indicator appears to identify non-anemic individuals who will benefit from iron supplementation as it affects physical performance (Brownlie et al., 2004). Cook and colleagues (Cook et al., 2003) have developed an algorithm to estimate total body iron from the log of the ratio of soluble transferrin receptor and serum ferritin.

## EVIDENCE FOR THE EFFECT OF IRON DEFICIENCY ON PHYSICAL PERFORMANCE IN ANEMIC SUBJECTS

Most of the research on iron deficiency effects on physical performance has focused on anemic subjects. This literature has been reviewed extensively by Haas and Brownlie (2001) who conclude that there is considerable evidence to support a direct causal relationship. One of the more recent studies that used an experimental design that included randomization of subjects to consume either an iron supplement or a placebo was conducted by Li and colleagues (Li, 1993; Li et al., 1995), who studied the effects of iron deficiency on work capacity in female Chinese factory workers. They assessed changes in physical performance with the $VO_2$max test, an assessment of aerobic power, after 12 weeks of consuming either an iron supplement or a placebo. The results are summarized in Figure B-32. Li (1993) reported a 5 percent improvement in $VO_2$max in the iron supplemented group which corresponded to a 13g/L increase in hemoglobin concentration. There was a range of hemoglobin values in this sample and the great-

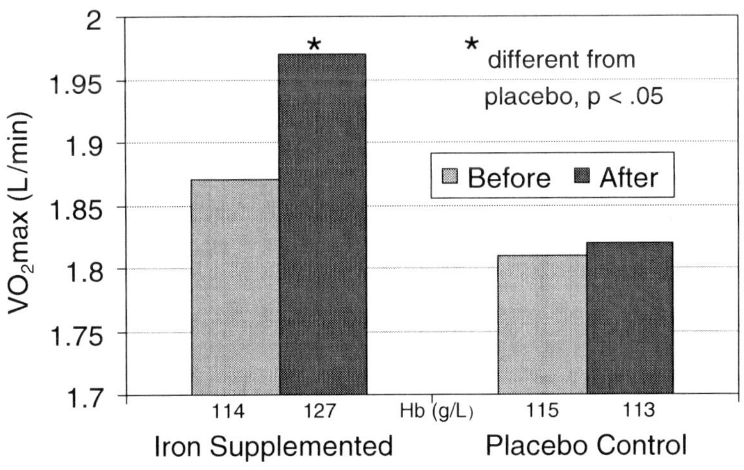


**FIGURE B-32** $VO_2$max in Chinese female cotton mill workers before and after 12 weeks of iron supplementation.
SOURCE: Li (1993, unpublished thesis).

est effects of iron supplementation on $VO_2$max were seen in the anemic women. The authors also reported an increase in productivity in the workplace after 12 weeks of iron supplementation (Li et al., 1995).

There have been a large number of studies of the effects of iron deficiency on physical performance using experimental animals. One of the most interesting was conducted by Davies et al. (1982) with post-weaning rats that developed iron deficiency after consuming a low-iron diet and then repleted rapidly by iron therapy. The results are summarized in Figure B-33. This study confirmed previous studies in animals and humans of an improvement in $VO_2$max, which paralleled an increase in hemoglobin concentration following iron therapy. This study is significant because it also followed changes in another measure of physical performance, endurance capacity, and a measure of tissue oxidative capacity, muscle pyruvate oxidase, throughout the 7-day period following iron repletion. The course of change in endurance lagged behind that of $VO_2$max and paralleled the increase in pyruvate oxidase. These findings indicate that physical performance may be only partially mediated by the effect of iron deficiency on oxygen transport in the blood, and that tissue iron depletion may also limit performance.

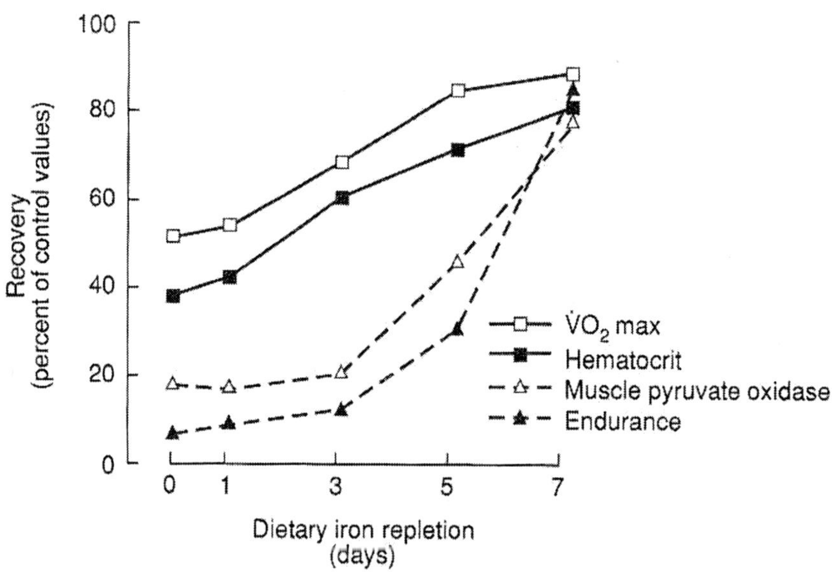


**FIGURE B-33** The relationship of iron repletion to hemoglobin response, maximal aerobic capacity ($VO_2$max), muscle pyruvate oxidase activity and endurance capacity in rats made iron deficient post-weaning.
SOURCE: Davies et al. (1982). Used with permission.

They also indicate that different types of physical performance tests need to be considered when studying severe compared to moderate iron deficiency.

## PHYSICAL PERFORMANCE IN IRON DEPLETED NON-ANEMIC SUBJECTS

This section reviews evidence for the effects of iron deficiency on physical performance, focused primarily on non-anemic individuals. Before the evidence is described, a brief review is presented of the rationale for why these affects should be observable and important.

### Rationale

The animal experiments represented by Davies et al. (1982) provide partial rationale for exploring relationships between iron depletion and performance in non-anemic human subjects. Further justification exists when one considers that iron plays an import role in muscle metabolism beyond the transport of oxygen by hemoglobin to the tissue sites for energy conversion to muscular work. Figure B-34 presents a list of iron-containing compounds that are affected by body iron depletion. Approximately 5 percent of the body iron is found in iron-containing enzymes and 10 percent is found in myoglobin. Many of these compounds are involved in transformation of chemical to mechanical energy. A second rationale

| | |
|---|---|
| **Heme Compounds** | Myoglobin<br>Cytochromes<br>Catalase<br>Peroxidases |
| **Non-Heme Compounds** | NADH dehydrogenase<br>Succinic dehydrogenase<br>Xanthine oxidase<br>Aldehyde oxidase<br>Alphaglycerophosphate oxidase<br>Phenylalanine hydroxylase<br>Ribonucleotide reductase? |
| **Iron-Dependent Enzymes** | Lipid peroxidase<br>Proline hydroxylase<br>Lysine hydroxylase<br>Monoamine Oxidase?<br>Tryosine hydroxylase?<br>Tryptophan hydroxylase? |

**FIGURE B-34** Iron containing compounds that are affected by iron deficiency.

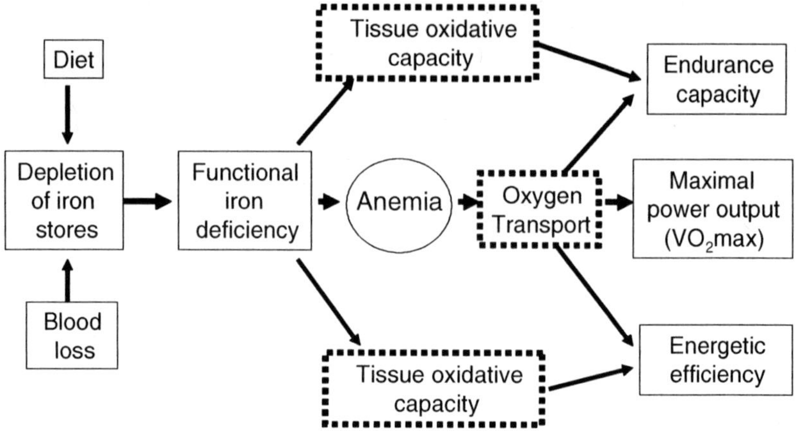


**FIGURE B-35** Conceptual model of iron deficiency effects on physical performance.

is the relatively large number of individuals in a population that may be affected by iron deficiency. This is a number that exceeds the prevalence of anemia in the population (WHO, 2001). While the effects of iron depletion without anemia may be less severe than the effects of iron deficiency, there is growing evidence that the impact on physical performance is not trivial.

The proposed mechanisms for the action of iron deficiency on physical performance are summarized in Figure B-35. Body iron stores become depleted due to an imbalance of iron loss and dietary gain. When levels of body iron become too low there is the beginning of a functional iron deficiency which affects compounds associated with muscle metabolism but probably does not affect hemoglobin synthesis and oxygen transport in the blood. Under conditions of more severe depletion, hemoglobin synthesis is compromised along with skeletal muscle compounds resulting iron deficiency anemia (IDA). Under IDA a broad range of physical performance measures are affected. The anemia results in reduced oxygen transport that limits aerobic power, endurance, and muscular energetic efficiency. The reduced levels and activity of iron-dependant, muscular tissue compounds seen in non-anemic, iron deficiency (IDNA) contribute to reduced endurance and energetic efficiency, but do not limit aerobic power, since blood oxygen transport is not compromised.

### Evidence for Effects of Iron Depletion in Non-Anemic Women

While the functional effects of iron deficiency have been well documented in those individuals who are anemic, the effects of IDNA have only recently been examined in some detail (Haas and Brownlie, 2001). Three recent iron supplementation trials with iron deficient non-anemic women provided evidence that supports the general conceptual model presented in Figure B-35 (Brutsaert et al., 2003; Hinton et al., 2000; Zhu and Haas, 1998). All of the studies used a similar research design. Female subjects between 18 and 45 years were identified through population screening to be non-anemic (hemoglobin > 120 g/L), but iron depleted (serum ferritin < 20 μg/L). Subjects were randomly assigned to consume either supplemental iron (100 to 135 mg $FeSO_4$/day) or a placebo daily for 6 or 8 weeks, following a double blind protocol. A battery of measures of iron status and various measures of physical performance were assessed at baseline and at the end of the supplementation period. The results of these studies are summarized as follows.

### *Metabolic Response to Exercise*

Zhu and Haas (1998) studied thirty-seven non-anemic, iron-deficient (ferritin < 16 μg/L) university women who consumed 135 mg/day of $FeSO_4$ (50 mg Fe/day) or a placebo for 8 weeks. Physical performance was assessed by $VO_2$max and time to complete a simulated 15-km time trial with a cycle ergometer, an indicator of endurance. Serum ferritin values increased in the supplemented group but hemoglobin did not change, and there was no group difference in $VO_2$max at the end of the trial. While the iron supplemented group did not complete the time trial in less time than the placebo group, they completed the task at a lower percentage of their $VO_2$max (82 versus 88 percent) and with 5.1 percent less energy expended than the placebo group. While one can conclude that iron deficient women are less efficient at doing heavy work, it is not known whether these effects of iron deficiency on performance can be observed under less rigorous levels of exertion. The next study addresses this question.

### *Energetic Efficiency in Mexican Women*

The studies described here (Brutsaert et al., 2003; Haas et al., 2002; Seymour, 2002) investigated the effects of iron supplementation for women on outcomes of physical performance while cycling at different intensities. Forty-three non-anemic, iron deficient (ferritin < 20 mg/L), female Mexican office workers and students consumed 18 mg/day of elemental iron as $FeSO_4$ or a placebo for 6 weeks (Haas et al., 2002). Serum ferritin increased while hemoglobin did not change in the iron supplemented group when compare to the placebo group, and estimated $VO_2$max did not differ between the groups after supplementation. Energy cost of performing 30 and 60 watts of work on a cycle ergometer was assessed at baseline and after 6 weeks. At 60 watts the iron supplemented women showed a 5.2 percent lower energy cost to perform the work after 6 weeks of supplementation (Seymour, 2002). As shown in Figure B-36 this resulted in a

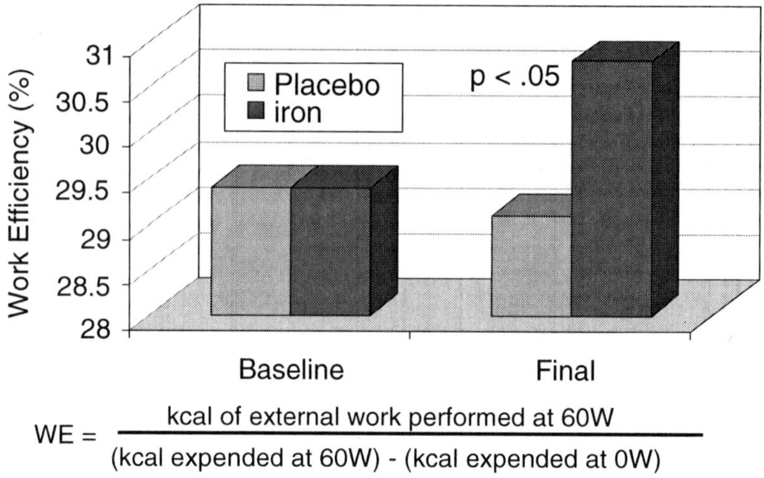


**FIGURE B-36** Work efficiency (WE) at 60 watts in Mexican women before and after 6 weeks of iron supplementation.
SOURCE: Seymour (2002, unpublished thesis).

significantly higher net work efficiency which was related to increased iron intake and decreases in tissue iron status, based on the soluble transferrin receptor concentration (sTfR). In a sub-sample of 20 women from this study, an additional test of a maximal voluntary static contraction (MVC) on a dynamic knee extension exercise was administered to assess local muscle fatigue (Brutsaert et al., 2003). The iron supplemented women performed the task with significantly less muscle fatigue than the placebo group after 6 weeks of supplementation.

*Adaptation to Physical Training*

Several papers have reported on a study of the effects of iron status and supplementation on improvements on performance outcomes due to adaptation to physical training (Brownlie et al., 2002, 2004; Hinton et al., 2000). In this study, 42 non-anemic, iron-deficient university women were randomly assigned to consume either 100mg/day of $FeSO_4$ or a placebo for 6 weeks. In addition, an additional exercise intervention for all subjects consisted on 20 days of aerobic training during the final 4 weeks of the supplementation trial. It was reported that both groups benefited from the training by increasing their $VO_2$max and reducing their times on a simulated 15-km time trial with a cycle ergometer. As shown in Figure B-37, the iron supplemented group improved its time in the time trial by 3.4 minutes compared to a 1.6 minute improvement in the placebo group (Hinton et al., 2000). The effect of iron treatment was mediated by changes in serum ferritin but not by changes in hemoglobin. $VO_2$max also improved

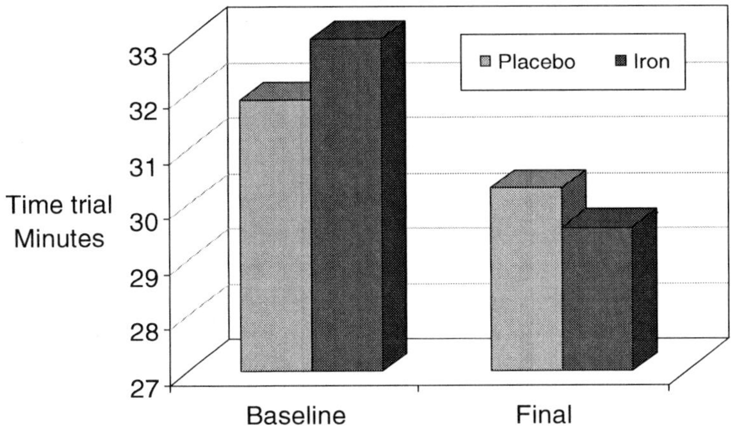


**FIGURE B-37** Improvements in times for women to complete a 15 km bicycle time trial after 4 weeks training while consuming supplemental iron or placebo. Iron group completed final trial 1.6 min faster than placebo group, after adjusting for differences in initial times and work rate, $p < 0.05$.
SOURCE: Hinton et al. (2000).

more in the iron supplemented group and the greatest improvement in time-trial time and work efficiency was seen in the iron supplemented women who were most depleted in tissue iron (sTfR) at baseline (Brownlie et al., 2004). From this study one can conclude that iron deficiency reduces the potential benefits of aerobic training in both endurance and $VO_2$max. It remains to be tested whether the effects of iron deficiency on adaptation to aerobic training can be observed in individuals who are already physically fit.

## CONCLUSIONS

We can draw several conclusions from the research literature on physical performance in iron deficiency anemia and from the recent experiments described in this paper on iron depleted non-anemic women:

- Iron deficiency anemia (IDA) has clear functional consequences across a wide range of tests of physical work capacity and productivity
- The mechanisms for IDA effects on performance include compromise to both oxygen transport and tissue level oxidative capacity
- Iron deficiency without anemia (IDNA) is more prevalent than IDA in the general population and carries measurable but less severe consequences to human performance

• The impact of IDNA is observed for physical endurance rather than aerobic power, and on reducing the ability to adapt to aerobic training.

For relevance to physical performance of military personnel, one can conclude:

• The results on the effects of iron deficiency anemia on physical performance should apply to all individuals
• The results on moderate iron deficiency without anemia in females should be extrapolated to males who experience a similar degree of iron deficiency and level of fitness
• Military personnel should be screened for anemia and body iron status
• Iron deficiency should be corrected in the long term by dietary adjustments and by mineral and vitamin supplementation in the short term, as conditions warrant.

Future research should consider assessing the effects of moderate iron deficiency on energetic efficiency and adaptation to training in more physically fit subjects and under conditions such as basic training. Additional research should consider assessing dietary iron requirements for military personnel which are based on potential iron loss from heavy exertion as well as additional demands to support physical training and maintenance of high levels of endurance.

## REFERENCES

Brownlie T, Utermohlen V, Hinton PS, Giordano C, Haas JD. 2002. Marginal iron depletion without anemia reduces adaptation to physical training in previously untrained women. *Am J Clin Nutr* 75:734–742.

Brownlie T, Utermohlen V, Hinton PS, Haas JD. 2004. Tissue-iron deficiency without anemia impairs endurance adaptation among previously untrained women. *Am J Clin Nutr* 79:437–443.

Brutsaert T, Hernandez-Cordero S, Rivera J, Viola T, Hughes G, Haas JD. 2003. Progressive muscle fatigue during dynamic work in iron deficient Mexican women. *Am J Clin Nutr* 77:441–448.

Cook JD, Flowers H, Skikne BS. 2003. The quantitative assessment of body iron. *Blood* 101:3359–3364.

Davies KJA, Maguire JJ, Brooks GA, Dallman PR, Packer L. 1982. Muscle mitochondrial bioenergetics, oxygen supply, and work capacity during dietary iron deficiency and repletion. *Am J Physiol* 242:E418–E427.

Guthrie H, Picciano MF. 1995. *Human Nutrition*. St. Louis, MO: Mosby-Year Book.

Haas JD, Brownlie T. 2001. Iron deficiency and reduced work capacity: A critical review of the research to determine a causal relationship. *J Nutr* (suppl) 131:676S–688S.

Haas JD, Seymour J, Hernandez-Cordero S, deHaene J, Villalpando S, Rivera J. 2002. Iron depletion increases the energy cost of work in non-anemic Mexican women. *Am J Phys Anthropol* (Suppl) 34:80.

Hinton PS, Giordano C, Brownlie T, Haas JD. 2000. Iron supplementation improves endurance after training in iron-deficient, non-anemic women. *J Appl Physiol* 88:1103–1111.

Li R. 1993. *Functional Consequences of Iron Supplementation in Iron-Deficient, Chinese Female Workers*. Unpublished doctoral dissertation. Wageningen, The Netherlands: Wageningen Agricultural University.

Li R, Chen X, Yan H, Durenberg P, Garby L, Hautvast JGAJ. 1995. Functional consequences of iron supplementation in iron-deficient, female cotton workers in Beijing, China. *Am J Clin Nutr* 59:908–913.

Looker AC, Dallman PR, Carroll MD, Gunter EW, Johnson CL. 1997. Prevalence of iron deficiency in the United States. *J Am Med Assoc* 277:973–976.

Seymour JM. 2002. Iron deficiency decreases efficiency of intermittent exercise in marginally iron deficient non-anemic Mexican women. Unpublished masters thesis. Ithaca NY: Cornell University.

WHO (World Health Organization). 2001. *Iron deficiency Anemia: Assessment, Prevention, and Control. A Guide for Program Managers*. Geneva, Switzerland: *World Health Organization*.

*Zhu YI, Haas JD. 1998. Altered metabolic response in iron-depleted non-anemic women during a 15-km time trial. J Appl Physiol 84:1768–1775.*

# C

# Tables

## NUTRIENT COMPOSITION OF RATIONS FOR SHORT-TERM, HIGH-INTENSITY COMBAT OPERATIONS SUMMARY TABLES

**TABLE C-1** Ration Nutrient Composition Recommended by the Committee on Optimization of Nutrient Composition of Military Rations for Short-Term, High-Stress Situations

| Nutrient or Energy Intake | Recommended Amount | Comments |
|---|---|---|
| *Energy Intake* | 2,400 kcal in basic ration | Additional 400 kcal should be supplemented as carbohydrate in form of candy, gels, or powder to add to fluids, or all three. |
| *Macronutrients* | | |
| Protein | 100–120 g | Protein should be of high biological value<br>Preferable to add sources of protein with low sulfur amino acids and low oxalate levels to minimize risk of kidney stone formation. |
| Carbohydrate | 350 g<br>100 g as a supplement | Additional 100 g should be supplemented as carbohydrate in form of candy, gels, or powder to add to fluids, or all three.<br>Amount of fructose as a monosaccharide should be limited to $< 25$ g. |
| Fiber | 15–17 g | Naturally occurring or added.<br>A mix of viscous, nonfermentable and nonviscous fermentable fiber should be in the ration for gastrointestinal tract function. |

**TABLE C-1** continued

| Nutrient or Energy Intake | Recommended Amount | Comments |
|---|---|---|
| Fat | 22–25% kcal<br>58–67 g | Fat added to the ration should have a balanced mix of saturated, polyunsaturated, and mono-unsaturated fatty acids with palatability and stability the prime determinants of the specific mixture. Fat should contain 5–10% linoleic acid and 0.6–1.2% α-linolenic acid. |
| *Vitamins* | | |
| Vitamin A | 300–900 µg RAE[a] | Could be added as preformed vitamin A or provitamin A carotenoids. |
| Vitamin C | 180–400 mg | Highly labile in processed food.<br>If added to foods, encapsulation should be considered to prevent degradation through interaction with pro-oxidants. |
| Vitamin D | 12.5–15 µg | Estimates of dietary intake are not available. Range based on ensuring serum levels of 25 hydroxy vitamin D. |
| Vitamin E (α-tocopherol) | 15–20 mg | Should be added to foods since natural foods are mainly sources of γ- rather than α-tocopherol. |
| Vitamin K | No recommended level | Amount in foods would be adequate provided ration is at least 50% whole foods.[b] |
| Thiamin | 1.6–3.4 mg | Dependent on energy use and intake.<br>Amount in foods would be adequate provided ration is at least 50% whole foods. |
| Riboflavin | 2.8–6.5 mg | Dependent on energy use. |
| Niacin | 28–35 mg | Dependent on energy use. The amount added to the ration should not be over 35 mg. |
| Vitamin $B_6$ | 2.7–3.9 mg | Dependent on negative energy balance and loss of lean tissue. If a higher protein level is provided, the amount of vitamin $B_6$ should be increased proportionally. |
| Folate | 400–560 µg | Fortification may be needed. |
| Vitamin $B_{12}$ | No recommended level | Amount in foods would be adequate provided ration is at least 50% whole foods. |
| Biotin | No recommended level | Amount in foods would be adequate provided ration is at least 50% whole foods. |
| Pantothenic Acid | No recommended level | Amount in foods would be adequate provided ration is at least 50% whole foods. |
| Choline | No recommended level | Amount in foods would be adequate provided ration is at least 50% whole foods. |

**TABLE C-1** continued

| Nutrient or Energy Intake | Recommended Amount | Comments |
|---|---|---|
| *Minerals* | | |
| Calcium | 750–850 mg | Major concern for higher levels is the potential formation of kidney stones. |
| Chromium | No recommended level | Amount in foods would be adequate provided ration is at least 50% whole foods. |
| Copper | 900–1,600 μg | If added to foods, encapsulation should be considered due to its pro-oxidant activity. |
| Iodine | 150–770 μg | Could be added as iodized salt. |
| Iron | 8–18 mg | If added to foods, encapsulation should be considered due to its pro-oxidant activity. Palatability should determine the amount in ration foods. |
| Magnesium | 400–550 mg | No more than 350 mg of magnesium salts should be present to meet the minimum daily amount of magnesium recommended. The rest should come from food sources. Also, if it needs to be added and taste problems result, encapsulation should be considered. |
| Manganese | No recommended level | Amount in foods would be adequate provided ration is at least 50% whole foods. |
| Molybdenum | No recommended level | Amount in foods would be adequate provided ration is at least 50% whole foods. |
| Phosphorus | 700–2,500 mg | Because inorganic phosphates may cause diarrhea, it is recommended that they are added only up to 700 mg. Intakes above this amount should come from food sources only. |
| Potassium | Aim to 3.3–4.7 g | Foods naturally high in potassium should be included in ration; if added to foods to achieve recommended levels, taste problems might be encountered. |
| Selenium | 55–230 μg | No clear evidence of effects as an enhancer of immune function or performance |
| Sodium | 3 or more g up to 12 g as supplement | For individuals who lose salt in excess or when in extremely hot or strenuous situations, sodium could be supplemented up to 12 g total. Part of this amount should be included in the form of candy, gels, or powder to add to fluids. Palatability will limit addition of sodium to these products; therefore, salt tablets should also be provided under medical guidance. |
| Zinc | 11–25 mg | If it needs to be added and taste problems result, encapsulation should be considered. |

**TABLE C-1** continued

| Nutrient or Energy Intake | Recommended Amount | Comments |
|---|---|---|
| *Ergogenics* | | |
| Caffeine | 100–600 mg | Not more than 600 mg in a single dose<br>There is no evidence of dehydration at this level. |

[a]RAE: retinol activity equivalents.
[b]Whole foods = food items prepared to preserve natural nutritive value.
SOURCE: IOM (2006).

**BOX C-1**
**General Design of the Recommended Ration: Approximate Energy and Macronutrient Content of the Assault Ration**

| | |
|---|---|
| Protein | 100–120 g (400–480 kcal; 17–20% kcal) |
| Carbohydrate | 350 g (1,400 kcal; 58% kcal) |
| Fat | 58–67 g (520–600 kcal; 22–25% kcal) |
| Water | 105 g (assuming an average of 17% moisture) |
| Total weight (kcal) | 613–642 g (2,400 kcal) |
| **Carbohydrate (and Electrolyte) Supplement:** | |
| Carbohydrate | 100 g (400 kcal) |
| Water | 17 g (assuming an average of 17% moisture) |
| Sodium | up to 12 g (based on palatability) |
| Potassium | up to 3.3–4.7 g (based on palatability) |
| Total Weight (kcal) | 117 g (400 kcal) |
| **Salt Tablets (available through medical personnel):** | |
| Sodium | up to 12 g |
| Potassium | up to 4.7 g |
| Total Weight | 8.7–16.7 g |
| **Packaging:** | 181 g |
| **Total Weight** | **0.95 kg** |
| **Total Energy Content** | **2,800 kcal** |

NOTE: This ration is intended for use over 3- to 7-day missions for up to a month. Prolonged and continuous use of these rations as a sole source of sustenance may lead to substantial weight loss. Constraints: weight of 1.36 kg and volume of 0.12 cubic feet.
SOURCE: IOM (2006).

**TABLE C-2** Average Mineral and Macronutrient Composition of Meal, Ready-to-Eat XXII Menus*

| | Weight (g) | Calories | Protein (g) | CHO (g) | Fat (g) | Calcium (mg) | Iron (mg) | Magnesium (mg) | Selenium (μg) | Sodium (mg) | Zinc (mg) |
|---|---|---|---|---|---|---|---|---|---|---|---|
| MRE XXII average | 513.53 | 1279.70 | 44.95 | 165.47 | 49.88 | 511.13 | 7.92 | 114.16 | 10.10 | 2045.90 | 4.20 |
| 1/3 NSOR | NA | 1200.00 | 33.30 | 147.00 | 53.30 | 267.00 | 6.00 | 133.00 | 18.33 | 2334.00 | 5.00 |
| % 1/3 NSOR | NA | 107% | 135% | 113% | 94% | 191% | 132% | 86% | 55% | 88% | 84% |

NOTE: NA = not applicable.
*Personal communication, C.Baker-Fulco, U.S. Army Research Institute of Environmental Medicine, October, 2005.

**TABLE C-3** Average Mineral and Macronutrient Composition of Meal, Ready-to-Eat XXIII Menus*

| | Weight (g) | Calories | Protein (g) | CHO (g) | Fat (g) | Calcium (mg) | Iron (mg) | Magnesium (mg) | Selenium (μg) | Sodium (mg) | Zinc (mg) |
|---|---|---|---|---|---|---|---|---|---|---|---|
| MRE XXIII average | 515.74 | 1284.54 | 43.88 | 170.09 | 49.70 | 526.62 | 8.62 | 177.15 | 11.89 | 2050.80 | 4.17 |
| MDRI | NA | 1200.00 | 30.30 | 165.00 | 50.00 | 333.00 | 5.00 | 140.00 | 18.30 | 2334.00 | 5.00 |
| % MDRI | NA | 107% | 145% | 103% | 99% | 158% | 172% | 127% | 65% | 88% | 83% |

NOTE: NA = not applicable.
*Personal communication, C.Baker-Fulco, U.S. Army Research Institute of Environmental Medicine, October, 2005.

**TABLE C-4** Average Mineral and Macronutrient Composition of Meal, Ready-to-Eat XXIV Menus*

| | Weight (g) | Calories | Protein (g) | CHO (g) | Fat (g) | Calcium (mg) | Iron (mg) | Magnesium (mg) | Selenium (µg) | Sodium (mg) | Zinc (mg) |
|---|---|---|---|---|---|---|---|---|---|---|---|
| MRE XXIV Average | 522.51 | 1311.16 | 44.26 | 174.01 | 50.94 | 557.45 | 9.02 | 140.55 | 12.50 | 2181.06 | 4.71 |
| MDRI | NA | 1200.00 | 30.30 | 165.00 | 50.00 | 333.00 | 5.00 | 140.00 | 18.30 | 2334.00 | 5.00 |
| % MDRI | NA | 109% | 146% | 105% | 102% | 167% | 180% | 100% | 68% | 93% | 94% |

NOTE: NA = not applicable.
*Personal communication, C.Baker-Fulco, U.S. Army Research Institute of Environmental Medicine, October, 2005.

**TABLE C-5** Summary and Comparison to Military Standards of the Average Meal, Ready-to-Eat Mineral and Macronutrient Menu Composition

| | MRE XXII[a] | MRE XXIII[a] | MREXXIV[a] | 1/3 NSOR[b] (operational rations) | MDRI[b] |
|---|---|---|---|---|---|
| Weight (g) | 513.53 | 515.74 | 522.51 | NA | NA |
| Calories | 1,279.70 | 1,284.54 | 1,311.16 | 1,200 | 1,200 |
| Protein (g) | 44.95 | 43.88 | 44.26 | 33.3 | 30.30 |
| Carbohydrate (g) | 165.47 | 170.09 | 174.01 | 147.00 | 165.00 |
| Fat (g) | 49.88 | 49.70 | 50.94 | 53.3 | 50.00 |
| Calcium (mg) | 511.13 | 526.62 | 557.45 | 267.00 | 333.00 |
| Iron (mg) | 7.92 | 8.62 | 9.02 | 6.00 | 5.00 |
| Magnesium (mg) | 114.16 | 177.15 | 140.55 | 133.00 | 140.00 |
| Selenium (μg) | 10.10 | 11.89 | 12.50 | 18.33 | 18.30 |
| Sodium (mg) | 2,045.90 | 2,050.80 | 2,181.06 | 2,334.00 | 2,334.00 |
| Zinc (mg) | 4.20 | 4.17 | 4.71 | 5.00 | 5.00 |

NOTE: Average meal should meet one-third of the Nutrition Standards for Operational Rations (NSOR). MDRI = military dietary reference intakes; NA = not applicable.

[a]Personal communication, C.Baker-Fulco, U.S. Army Research Institute of Environmental Medicine, October, 2005.

[b]U.S. Departments of the Army, Navy, and Air Force (2001).

## FIRST STRIKE RATION AVERAGE MENU MACRONUTRIENT AND MINERAL COMPOSITION

**TABLE C-6** Average Mineral and Macronutrient Composition in First Strike Ration Menus

| | Menu Average[a] | 1/3 NSOR (restricted rations)[b] |
|---|---|---|
| Weight (g) | 915 | NA |
| Calories | 2961 | 500 |
| Protein (g) | 105.1 | 16.67 |
| Carbohydrate (g) | 375.8 | 66.67 |
| Fat (g) | 112.2 | Should not exceed 35% of total calories |
| Calcium (mg) | 673 | 166.67 |
| Iron (mg) | 16.97 | 2.67 |
| Magnesium (mg) | 386 | 70 |
| Selenium (μg) | 100.2 | 9.33 |
| Zinc (mg) | 11.86 | 2.67 |

NOTE: Average meal should meet one-third of the Nutrition Standards for Operational Rations (NSOR). NA = not applicable.

[a]Personal communication, C.Baker-Fulco, U.S. Army Research Institute of Environmental Medicine, October, 2005.

[b]U.S. Departments of the Army, Navy, and Air Force (2001).

# UNITIZED GROUP RATIONS AVERAGE MENU MACRONUTRIENT AND MINERAL COMPOSITION

**TABLE C-7** Average Mineral and Macronutrient Composition in Unitized Group Rations Heat and Serve Menus

| | Breakfast Menu Average[a] | Lunch and Dinner Menu Average[a] | 1/3 NSOR[b] (operational rations) | MDRI[b] |
|---|---|---|---|---|
| Weight (g) | 1,203.70 | 1,358.65 | NA | NA |
| Calories | 1,391.33 | 1,325.72 | 1,200 | 1,200 |
| Protein (g) | 49.46 | 50.18 | 33.3 | 30.30 |
| Carbohydrate (g) | 178.48 | 181.18 | 147.00 | 165.00 |
| Fat (g) | 56.75 | 47.70 | 53.3 | 50.00 |
| Calcium (mg) | 466.91 | 472.39 | 267.00 | 333.00 |
| Iron (mg) | 7.21 | 9.68 | 6.00 | 5.00 |
| Magnesium (mg) | 110.63 | 189.81 | 133.00 | 140.00 |
| Selenium (μg) | 9.19 | 16.14 | 18.33 | 18.30 |
| Sodium (mg) | 2,579.62 | 2,464.98 | 2,334.00 | 2,334.00 |
| Zinc (mg) | 6.91 | 7.63 | 5.00 | 5.00 |

NOTE: Average meal should meet one-third of the Nutrition Standards for Operational Rations (NSOR). MDRI = military dietary reference intakes; NA = not applicable.

[a]Personal communication, C.Baker-Fulco, U.S. Army Research Institute of Environmental Medicine, October, 2005.

[b]U.S. Departments of the Army, Navy, and Air Force (2001).

# REFERENCES

IOM (Institute of Medicine). 2006. Nutrient Composition of Rations for Short-Term, High-Intensity Combat Operations. Washington, DC: The National Academies Press.

U.S. Departments of Army NaAF. 2001. *Nutrition Standards and Education*. AR 40-25/BUMEDINST 10110.6/AFI 44-141. Washington, DC: U.S. Department of Defense Headquarters.

# D

# Biographical Sketches of Workshop Speakers

**Carol (Cory) J. Baker-Fulco,** M.S., R.D., is a research dietitian in the Military Nutrition Division of the U.S. Army Research Institute of Environmental Medicine. She received a Master of Science degree in nutrition from the University of Bridgeport, Connecticut. She serves as a principal investigator responsible for applied research in support of studies on nutrition and operational medicine. Her research area includes assessment of the dietary and nutritional status of military personnel and evaluation of feeding systems and operational rations. Her areas of concentration include and dietary assessment, sports nutrition, nutrient requirements in environmental extremes, and nutrition education. Ms. Baker-Fulco developed *Performance Power: The Nutrition Connection* program, a video-based sports nutrition education program for military personnel distributed Army wide. Ms. Baker-Fulco is a member of the American Dietetic Association, the Research Dietitian Practice Group, and the Practice Group on Sports, Cardiovascular, and Wellness Nutrition.

**John L. Beard,** Ph.D., is a professor of nutrition in the Department of Nutrition at Pennsylvania State University. He earned degrees in organic chemistry in 1970 (B.S.), and 1972 (M.S.) from the Stevens Institute of Technology and the University of California–Santa Cruz, respectively; and his Ph.D. degree from Cornell University (1979) in human nutrition. His research interests include: role of iron in dopamine metabolism and action; effect of early life iron deficiency on brain development and functioning; relationship of brain iron metabolism to monoamine metabolism in Restless Legs Syndrome and; food based approaches to the eradication of iron deficiency. Dr. Beard serves as an associate editor of the Journal of Nutrition.

**Joseph G. Cannon,** Ph.D., is a professor in the Departments of Physiology and Biomedical Technologies at the Medical College of Georgia (MCG), and Associate Dean for Research in the School of Allied Health Sciences at MCG. Formerly, he was a professor of applied physiology at the Pennsylvania State University. He earned his Ph.D. in physiology from the University of Michigan, his M.S. in engineering from the University of California at Los Angeles, and his B.S. in engineering from Michigan State University. Dr. Cannon's primary research interests include (a) immunological mechanisms involved in skeletal muscle repair following injury, and (b) nutritional and hormonal influences on leukocyte function. He holds the Kellett Chair in Allied Health Sciences at MCG. Dr. Cannon has served on the editorial boards of the American Journal of Physiology and Journal of Applied Physiology, and is the author or co-author of over 100 articles in scientific publications.

**Gerald F. Combs, Jr.,** Ph.D., is center director of the U.S. Department of Agriculture's Grand Forks Human Nutrition Research Center. He also is Professor Emeritus at the Division of Nutritional Sciences, Cornell University, and an adjunct professor in the School of Medicine at the University of North Dakota. Previously, he was a professor of nutrition in the Division of Nutritional Sciences at Cornell University, having been on that faculty since 1975. Dr. Combs earned his B.S. degree in zoology in 1969, his M.S. degree in entomology in 1971, and his Ph.D. degree in nutrition in 1973. Dr. Combs is internationally recognized for his research in the nutritional biochemistry of trace elements and vitamins. His special interests have concerned the metabolism and physiological actions of the antioxidant nutrients selenium, vitamin E, vitamin C, and factors that can affect their metabolic functions and dietary needs (e.g., vitamin A, carotenoids, iron, copper, zinc), particularly as they relate to health maintenance in and reduction of chronic disease (e.g., cancer) risks in humans and animals.

**J. Mark Davis,** Ph.D., is a professor and director of Graduate Programs and Research in the Department of Exercise Science, which is part of the University of South Carolina's Arnold School of Public Health. He's been there almost 22 years since completing a Ph.D. degree at Purdue University in exercise physiology/neuroscience followed by a post-doctoral fellowship in neuroendocrinology at Mt. Sinai Medical School in New York. He is a Fellow of the American College of Sports Medicine where he is currently a member of the Board of Trustees. He also serves on the Sports Medicine Review Board of the Gatorade Sports Science Institute. Davis is an international authority (> 95 publications) on the effects of exercise and nutrition on (1) mental and physical fatigue and (2) immune function as related to defense against infection and cancer. His current research funding includes, among others, a large grant from the U.S. Army to develop novel herbal supplements to delay mental and physical fatigue, enhance recovery from intense exercise, and optimize immune function in soldiers.

**Monika Fleshner,** Ph.D., is an associate professor in the Department of Integrative Physiology, a member of the Center for Neuroscience, and director of the Neuroimmunophysiology laboratory at the University of Colorado at Boulder. Dr. Fleshner received her Ph.D. in behavioral neuroscience from the University of Colorado in 1990, and completed postdoctoral work in Immunology at the University of Colorado Health Sciences Center 1992. Dr. Fleshner is interested in understanding the impact of acute and chronic stress (mental, physical, or aging) on many aspects of integrative physiology. Specifically, her research examines the impact of stress on behavior, neural, hormonal and immunological function and how these systems interact to affect the whole organism She has published over 100 peer-reviewed articles, serves as a reviewer for over a dozen scientific journals, and is an assistant editor for the *Journal of Applied Physiology*.

**Karl E. Friedl,** Ph.D., is the commander of the U.S. Army Research Institute of Environmental Medicine in Natick, Massachusetts, a laboratory specialized in human performance and metabolic responses in harsh environments. Prior to this assignment, Colonel Friedl directed the Military Operational Medicine Research Program at the U.S. Army Medical Research and Materiel Command in Frederick, Maryland, including management of the DoD Gulf War Illnesses research portfolio and Congressional special interest programs such as bone health research, neurotoxin exposure treatment (Parkinson's) research, nutrition research, and the Defense Womens' Health Research Program. In earlier assignments he specialized in physiological limits of prolonged, intensive military training and endocrine physiology. He received his Ph.D. in physiology in 1984 from the Institute of Environmental Stress at the University of California, Santa Barbara. He has published original articles on diverse physiological investigations such as: functional consequences of semi starvation in high intensity field training; body composition methods and standards for DoD fitness regulations; nerve agent antidote delivery systems; steroid regulation of spermatogenesis for potential male contraception; and noninvasive physiological measurement systems to monitor hemorrhage and resuscitation.

**Jere D. Haas,** Ph.D., is the Nancy Schlegel Meinig Professor of Maternal and Child Nutrition in the Division of Nutritional Sciences at Cornell University. He received his Ph.D. in biological anthropology from the Pennsylvania State University and has been on the Cornell faculty for 30 years. He is currently conducting research on the functional consequences of iron deficiency on physical and reproductive performance. The emphasis is on the effects of moderate iron deficiency on various aspects of physical performance and behavior in young women and how measures of performance relate to everyday productivity and social and economic well-being. He conducts research on this and related topics in maternal and child nutrition in the United States, Mexico, the Philippines, Guatemala, Bolivia, and Bangladesh. Dr. Haas served as vice-president and president of the American Association of Physical Anthropologists and serves on the Expert Advisory Panel for Nutrition of the World Health Organization and the Technical Advisory Group on Food and Nutrition of the Pan American Health Organization. He served as director of the Division of Nutritional Science at Cornell from 1998 to 2003.

**Davidson H. Hamer,** M.D., is an associate professor of international health at the Boston University School of Public Health, an adjunct associate professor of nutrition at the Gerald J. and Dorothy R. Friedman School of Nutrition Science and Policy, and a visiting scientist in the Department of Nutritional Immunology at the Jean Mayer USDA Human Nutrition Research Center. Dr. Hamer is based at the Center for International Health and Development where he provides the lead technical support for applied research on micronutrients, malaria, and neonatal diseases as well as technical support for the diarrheal disease, respiratory disease, and antimicrobial resistance programs. During the last decade, Dr. Hamer has worked closely with local scientists on policy-relevant research involving evaluations of interventions for the treatment and prevention of malaria, micronutrient deficiencies, diarrheal disease, and acute respiratory infections in young children in resource-poor countries.

**Emily M. Haymes,** Ph.D., is a professor in the Department of Nutrition, Food and Exercise Sciences at Florida State University. She received her B.A. from Drury College in 1961, her M.S. from Florida State University in 1962, and her Ph.D. from Pennsylvania State University in 1973. Prior to joining the faculty at Florida State in 1979, she taught at the University of Colorado–Boulder for five years. An exercise physiologist, her primary research interests are iron depletion in athletes, field measurements of physical activity and energy expenditure, and the response of males and females to exercise in warm and cold environments. She co-authored the book *The Environment and Human Performance* with Christine Wells. Dr. Haymes has published papers in several journals including the *Journal of Applied Physiology, Medicine and Science in Sports and Exercise, International Journal of Sports Medicine, International Journal of Sport Nutrition, Exercise Metabolism, and the Physician and Sportsmedicine.* Dr. Haymes served a three-year term as president of the Research Consortium and a two-year term as vice president of the American College of Sports Medicine. She is a Fellow of the American Academy of Kinesiology and Physical Education, American College of Sports Medicine, and the Research Consortium of the American Alliance for Health, Physical Education, Recreation, and Dance.

**Steven B. Heymsfield,** M.D., is the executive director of clinical sciences at Merck pharmaceutical company. In this capacity he leads clinical obesity drug development in Company's metabolism division. Dr. Heymsfield was the former director of the Human Body Composition Laboratory and Weight Control Unit and the deputy director of the NIH-supported New York Obesity Research Center at St. Luke's-Roosevelt Hospital. In addition, he was a professor of medicine at Columbia University College of Physicians and Surgeons and a visiting scientist at Rockefeller University and the Brookhaven National Laboratory. Dr. Heymsfield maintains an appointment at the medical center and his research there continues. Dr. Heymsfield received his bachelor's degree from Hunter College in New York, and his degree in medicine from Mount Sinai School of Medicine in New York. He completed his medical internship and residency at Emory University in Atlanta, continuing on to become a fellow in medicine prior to his Columbia appointments in 1986. He moved to Merck in November of 2004. Dr. Heymsfield has published more than 300 articles covering topics such as obesity, anorexia nervosa, bulimia nervosa, malnutrition, pregnancy, body composition, and caloric expenditure. He developed a mathematical expression, the lithogenic index, for characterizing bile proclivity for cholesterol gallstone formation that has been used worldwide for over two decades.

**Janet R. Hunt,** Ph.D., R.D., is the research leader of the Micronutrient Absorption and Metabolism Unit at the U.S. Department of Agriculture/Agricultural Research Service (USDA/ARS) Human Nutrition Research Center in Grand Forks, North Dakota, and is an adjunct professor of nutrition and dietetics at the University of North Dakota. Dr. Hunt received her Ph.D. in nutrition from the University of Minnesota. An active member of the American Society for Clinical Nutrition, the American Society for Nutritional Sciences, the International BioIron Society and the American Dietetic Association (ADA), she has served on the ADA board of directors and the ADA journal's editorial board, and has co-authored ADA's Position Statements on Vitamin and Mineral Supplements. Dr. Hunt investigates human iron and zinc requirements as influenced by dietary bioavailability, and has published extensively on these topics.

**Carl Keen,** Ph.D., is a professor in nutrition and internal medicine and chair of the Department of Nutrition, University of California–Davis. He has served on numerous government boards. He has been a member of California's Scientific Advisory Board for the Office of Environmental Health Hazard Assessment since 1993. He has been a member of EPA Environmental Health Grant Review Panels (1990–1999), USDA Human Nutrient Requirements Study (1987–1992), and several NIH panels (Nutrition Study Section 1997–1999; ALTOX Study Section 2002–2004; XNDA Study Section 2004–present). He is past president of the California Nutrition Council (1998). He is a member of the American Society for Nutritional Sciences, the American Society of Clinical Nutrition, the Teratology Society, the Society for Experimental Biology and Medicine, and the American Association for the Advancement of Science. Dr. Keen has served on numerous editorial boards and has chaired and organized national and international scientific conferences.

**Cathy W. Levenson,** Ph.D., is currently an associate professor in the Department of Nutrition, Food and Exercise Sciences, and in the Program in Neuroscience at Florida State University. She holds a B.A. in neurobiology from the University of Virginia, an M.S. from the Department of Nutrition at Florida State University, and a Ph.D. from the Department of Medicine at the University of Chicago. Her research is focused on the role of the trace metals zinc, copper, and iron in the central nervous system with a particular interest in the role these nutrients play in gene expression that directs neuronal death and survival.

**Harris R. Lieberman,** Ph.D., is a research psychologist in the Military Nutrition Division of the U.S. Army Research Institute of Environmental Medicine (USARIEM) in Natick, Massachusetts. Dr. Lieberman is an internationally recognized expert in the area of nutrition and behavior and has published over 125 original, full-length papers in scientific journals and edited books. He has been an invited lecturer at numerous national and international conferences, government research laboratories and universities. Dr. Lieberman received his Ph.D. in physiological psychology in 1977 from the University of Florida and then conducted postdoctoral research at the Department of Psychology and Brain Science at the Massachusetts Institute of Technology (MIT). From 1980–1990, he was on the research staff at MIT where he examined the effects of food constituents and drugs on human behavior and brain function. In 1990, Dr. Lieberman joined the civilian research staff of USARIEM where he has continued his work in nutrition, behavior and stress. From 1994 to 2000, he was chief or deputy chief of the Military Nutrition program at USARIEM. His recent research has addressed the effects of various nutritional factors, diets and environmental stress on animal and human performance, brain function and behavior. His work has focused on developing and applying a variety of emerging technologies in nutrition, neuroscience and microelectronics to sustaining and enhancing human performance in stressful environments. He holds two patents for novel technologies to assess and enhance cognitive performance. Dr. Lieberman currently chairs an International Defense Panel on Protection and Sustainment of Human Physical and Cognitive Performance.

**Henry C. Lukaski,** Ph.D., is assistant center director and research physiologist at the U.S. Department of Agriculture, Agricultural Research Service, Grand Forks Human Nutrition Research Center and adjunct professor of medicine, and physical education and exercise science at the University of North Dakota. Since receiving his Ph.D. in physiology with a minor in nutrition from the Pennsylvania State University, Dr. Lukaski has developed a productive research program in determining functional roles of bioactive components of food, including mineral elements, and developing methods for human body composition assessment. He has published numerous articles and reviews in peer reviewed journals, book chapters, and position papers for professional organizations. He has provided consultation and advice to the World Health Organization, Medical Subcommittee of the International Olympic Committee and U.S. Olympic Committee, federal organizations including National Institutes of Health, Department of Defense and National Aeronautics and Space Agency, and research and development organizations such as Gatorade and GlaxoSmithKline. He has served or is a member of the editorial boards of *British Journal of Nutrition, Journal of Nutrition, Medicine and Science in Sports and Exercise, International Journal of Sports Nutrition and Metabolism, Nutrition, International Journal of Applied Sports Science, Current Nutrition and Food Science,* and *CRC Press Series on Nutrition and Sport*. Dr. Lukaski is a fellow of the American College of Sports Medicine, Human Biology Council and the Mexican Institute of Nutrition.

**Jeri W. Nieves,** Ph.D., is from the Helen Hayes Hospital in New York, where she is director of bone density testing. Dr. Nieves is also an assistant professor of clinical epidemiology at Columbia University. Dr. Nieves has co-authored over 60 journal articles, reviews, and book chapters on nutrition, epidemiology, and osteoporosis. She is a graduate of Columbia University where she received her Ph.D. in epidemiology, following a Masters degree in nutrition from Cornell University. Her current main interest is in calcium and vitamin D and the prevention and treatment of osteoporosis. She is a recipient of a grant from the National Institute of Health to study the effect of vitamin D supplementation for osteoporosis treatment in black postmenopausal women. She is currently working on two studies of young adults to determine the role of nutrition, exercise and menstrual function on peak bone mass and stress fractures. She serves on the Editorial Board of Osteoporosis International.

**James G. Penland**, Ph.D., is a research psychologist with the USDA, Agricultural Research Service, Grand Forks Human Nutrition Research Center, and adjunct professor of psychology at the University of North Dakota, where he received his doctoral degree in experimental cognitive psychology in 1984. Dr. Penland directs a comprehensive research program to study the effects of mineral nutrition (including copper, iron, magnesium, selenium, and zinc) on a broad range of human and animal neuropsychological function and behavior throughout the life span. During the past 20 years, Dr. Penland has conducted metabolic unit and community based feeding and supplementation studies, and designed and implemented a mobile nutrition laboratory for studies in schools, nursing homes, and rural communities. In addition to many research collaborations in the United States, Dr. Penland has participated in nutrition studies in Guatemala, New Zealand and the Peoples Republic of China. Dr. Penland has authored or co-authored nearly 100 scientific publications and served on many expert panels and scientific advisory groups. Dr. Penland has been honored as a Distinguished Alumni at the University of North Dakota and received the USDA Honor Award for Excellence.

**Susan S. Percival,** Ph.D., is a professor of nutritional sciences in the Department of Food Science and Human Nutrition at the University of Florida. Her educational background includes an M.S. degree from the University of California–Davis, and a Ph.D. from the University of Texas–Austin. She did postdoctoral research in the Department of Biochemistry and Biophysics at Texas A&M University. From 1978 to 1981 she was tenure track faculty at the University of Rhode Island prior to an educational leave to pursue her doctorate. At the University of Florida, she was an undergraduate coordinator for over 700 undergraduate students from 1994 to 2002. Dr. Percival is a member of several professional organizations including the American Society for Nutritional Sciences and the Institute of Food Technologists. She has been a member of the editorial board of the *Journal of Nutrition* since 2000 and previously served as an IFT Scientific Lecturer. She is completing a leave of absence from the University of Florida at the National Institutes of Health, National Cancer Institute, Division of Cancer Prevention, Nutritional Sciences Research Group. Her current research deals with how dietary components influence immunity.

**Michael N. Sawka,** Ph.D., is chief of the Thermal and Mountain Medicine Division at the U.S. Army Research Institute of Environmental Medicine. Dr. Sawka's research interests are environmental (heat, cold, altitude) and exercise physiology, fluid/electrolyte balance, and rehabilitation medicine. He has published over 285 full-length scientific papers as well as edited graduate textbooks on environmental physiology and on exercise physiology. He has presented over 65 invited Symposia and Keynote Lectures at scientific meetings. Dr. Sawka is a member of several editorial boards including *American Journal of Physiology, Journal of Applied Physiology, Medicine and Science in Sports and Exercise, International Journal of Sports Medicine.* He served on many scientific panels and professional committees such as those for the Institute of Medicine; National Institutes of Health; U.S. Anti-Doping Agency; Olympic Scientific Committees. He is active within the American Physiological Society and the American College of Sports Medicine. He is frequently cited and interviewed by the press.

**John F. Sheridan,** Ph.D., is a professor of immunology and director of a T32 training grant titled *Comprehensive Training in Oral and Craniofacial Biology.* He currently holds the George C. Paffenbarger Alumni Endowed Research Chair, and is the associate director of the Institute for Behavioral Medicine Research at the Ohio State University. He received a B.S. degree in biology from Fordham University, and his M.S. and Ph.D. degrees in microbiology from the Waksman Institute of Microbiology at Rutgers University. He did postdoctoral training in microbiology/immunology at the Duke University Medical Center and the Johns Hopkins School of Medicine. He is a founding member and past president of the Psychoneuroimmunology Research Society. His major research interests include neuroendocrine regulation of gene expression in inflammatory and immune responses, stress-induced susceptibility to infectious disease, viral pathogenesis, and host immunity.

**Connie M. Weaver,** Ph.D., is a distinguished professor and head of the Department of Foods & Nutrition at Purdue University–West Lafayette, Indiana. In 2000, she also became director of a National Institutes of Health funded Botanical Center to study dietary supplements containing polyphenolics for age-related diseases. Her research interests include mineral bioavailability, calcium metabolism, and bone health. Dr. Weaver is past-president of American Society for Nutritional Sciences and is on the board of trustees of the International Life Sciences Institute. For her contributions in teaching, Dr. Weaver was awarded Purdue University's Outstanding Teaching Award. In 1993, she was honored with the Purdue University Health Promotion Award for Women, and in 1997, she received the Institute of Food Technologists Babcock Hart Award. In April 2003, she received the USDA A.O. Atwater Lecturership Award at the annual Experimental Biology meeting. Dr. Weaver was appointed to the 2005 U.S. Dietary Guidelines Advisory Committee. She has published over 100 research articles. Dr. Weaver received a Bachelor of Science and Master of Science in food science and human nutrition from Oregon State University. She received a Ph.D. in food science and human nutrition from Florida State University and holds minors in chemistry and plant physiology.

**Andrew J. Young,** Ph.D., is a research physiologist and chief of the Military Nutrition Division at the U.S. Army Research Institute of Environmental Medicine (USARIEM) in Natick, Massachusetts. He obtained a B.S. in biology at Virginia Military Institute, and a Ph.D. in physiology at North Carolina State University, and then served in the U.S. Army with assignments at USARIEM (1977–1981) and at the Walter Reed Army Institute of Research (1981–1983). After leaving the Army, Dr. Young continued as a civilian scientist at USARIEM. His research has concerned the biological basis for, and strategies to mitigate performance degradations in people experiencing intense physical exertion, sleep restriction, nutritional deprivation and exposure to extremes of heat, cold, and high altitude, all of which are characteristics of sustained combat operations. Dr. Young is a member of the American Physiological Society, a fellow of the American College of Sports Medicine. He is also associate editor-in-chief of the American College of Sports Medicine's flagship scientific journal, *Medicine and Science in Sports and Exercise*, and was recently named to become editor-in-chief for that journal beginning in July of 2005.

# E

# Biographical Sketches of Committee Members and Staff

**Robert M. Russell,** M.D., (Chair) is a professor of medicine and nutrition at Tufts University and director of the Jean Mayer USDA Human Nutrition Research Center on Aging at Tufts University in Boston, Massachusetts. As a senior scientist at the Jean Mayer USDA Human Nutrition Research Center on Aging, Dr. Russell's primary work involves studying the effects of aging on gastrointestinal absorptive function. He is a noted expert in the area of human metabolism of retinoids and carotenoids. Dr. Russell is a member of numerous professional societies and has served as a councilor and president to the American Society for Clinical Nutrition and a member of the Board of Directors of the American College of Nutrition. Dr. Russell co-authored the standards for parenteral and enteral nutrition to be used in U.S. long-term care facilities. He has served on the editorial boards of five professional journals and is a staff gastroenterologist at the New England Medical Center Hospitals. He has served on national and international advisory boards including the F.D.A., National Digestive Diseases Advisory Board, USDA Human Investigation Committee (chairman), U.S. Pharmacopoeia Convention, National Dairy Council Scientific Advisory Board, and the American Board of Internal Medicine. He received his B.S. degree from Harvard University and his M.D. degree from Columbia University.

**John L. Beard,** Ph.D., is a professor of nutrition in the Department of Nutrition at Pennsylvania State University. He earned degrees in organic chemistry in 1970 (B.S.) and 1972 (M.S.) from the Stevens Institute of Technology and the University of California–Santa Cruz, respectively; and his Ph.D. degree from Cornell University (1979) in human nutrition. His research interests include: role of iron in dopamine metabolism and action; effect of early life iron deficiency on brain development and functioning; relationship of brain iron metabolism to monoamine metabolism in Restless Legs Syndrome and; food-based approaches to the eradication of iron deficiency.

**Melinda Beck,** Ph.D., is a professor in the Departments of Nutrition and Pediatrics at the University of North Carolina–Chapel Hill. Dr. Beck's research focuses on the exploration of the relationship between antioxidant nutrition and infectious disease. She received her Ph.D. degree in immunology from Ohio State University in 1987. Dr. Beck's research focuses on the exploration of the relationship between antioxidant nutrition and infectious disease. She is particularly interested in determining the mechanism of viral genetic mutation that is driven by replication in an oxidatively stressed host. In addition, she conducts collaborative research involving the use of technology of homologous recombination to knockout specific genes of interest. These studies will assist in defining the role inflammation plays in specific viral infections, and by using both knockout mice and dietary manipulations; further understanding of the effect of oxidative stress on both the host and pathogen can be explored.

**Bruce R. Bistrian,** M.D., Ph.D., is a professor of medicine at Harvard Medical School and chief of clinical nutrition at the Beth Israel Deaconess Medical Center. Formerly he was co-director of hyperalimentation services at the New England Deaconess Hospital, and a lecturer in the Department of Nutrition and Food Science, Massachusetts Institute of Technology (MIT). He earned his M.D. degree from Cornell University, his M.P.H. degree from Johns Hopkins University, and his Ph.D. degree in nutritional biochemistry and metabolism from MIT. Dr. Bistrian is board certified in Internal Medicine and Critical Care Medicine. Dr. Bistrian's primary research interests include nutritional assessment, metabolic effects of acute infections, nutritional support of hospitalized patients, and the pathophysiology of protein-calorie malnutrition. He is a fellow of the American College of Physicians, and has received an honorary M.A. degree from Harvard University. Dr. Bistrian is the 2004 recipient of the Goldberger Award of the American Medical Association. Dr. Bistrian has been president of the American Society for Parenteral and Enteral Nutrition, President of the American Society of Clinical Nutrition, and is President-Elect of the Federation of American Societies of Experimental Biology. Dr. Bistrian has served on the editorial boards of numerous nutrition and medical journals, and is the author or co-author of over 400 articles in scientific publications.

**Joseph G. Cannon,** Ph.D., is a professor in the Departments of Physiology and Biomedical Technologies at the Medical College of Georgia (MCG), and associate dean for research in the School of Allied Health Sciences at MCG. Formerly, he was a professor of applied physiology at the Pennsylvania State University.

He earned his Ph.D. degree in physiology from the University of Michigan, his M.S. degree in engineering from the University of California–Los Angeles, and his B.S. degree in engineering from Michigan State University. Dr. Cannon's primary research interests include the immunological mechanisms involved in skeletal muscle repair following injury, and nutritional and hormonal influences on leukocyte function. He holds the Kellett Chair in Allied Health Sciences at MCG. Dr. Cannon has served on the editorial boards of the American Journal of Physiology and Journal of Applied Physiology, and is the author or co-author of over 100 articles in scientific publications.

**Gerald F. Combs, Jr.,** Ph.D., is center director of the U.S. Department of Agriculture's Grand Forks Human Nutrition Research Center. He also is Professor Emeritus at the Division of Nutritional Sciences, Cornell University, and an adjunct professor in the School of Medicine at the University of North Dakota. Previously, he was a professor of nutrition in the Division of Nutritional Sciences at Cornell University, having been on that faculty since 1975. Dr. Combs earned his B.S. degree in zoology in 1969, his M.S. degree in entomology in 1971, and his Ph.D. degree in nutrition in 1973. Dr. Combs is internationally recognized for his research on the nutritional biochemistry of trace elements and vitamins. His special interests have concerned the metabolism and physiological actions of the antioxidant nutrients selenium, vitamin E, vitamin C, and factors that can affect their metabolic functions and dietary needs (e.g., vitamin A, carotenoids, iron, copper, zinc), particularly as they relate to health maintenance in and reduction of chronic disease (e.g., cancer) risks in humans and animals.

**Johanna T. Dwyer,** D.Sc., R.D., is director of the Frances Stern Nutrition Center at New England Medical Center and is a professor in the Departments of Medicine and of Community Health at the Tufts Medical School and the School of Nutrition Science and Policy in Boston. She is also a senior scientist at the Jean Mayer USDA Human Nutrition Research Center on Aging at Tufts University. She is currently on part-time assignment to the National Institutes of Health Office of Dietary Supplements. Dr. Dwyer's work centers on life-cycle related concerns such as the prevention of diet-related disease in children and adolescents and maximization of quality of life and health in the elderly. Dr. Dwyer is currently the editor of *Nutrition Today* and on the editorial boards of *Family Economics* and *Nutrition Reviews*. She received her D.Sc. and M.Sc. degrees from the Harvard School of Public Health, her M.S. degree from the University of Wisconsin, and completed her undergraduate degree with distinction from Cornell University. She is a member of the Institute of Medicine, the Technical Advisory Committee of the Nutrition Screening Initiative, past president of the American Society for Nutritional Sciences, past secretary of the American Society for Clinical Nutrition, and past president of the Society for Nutrition Education.

**John W. Erdman, Jr.,** Ph.D., is a professor of nutrition and food science in the Department of Food Science and Human Nutrition and a professor in the Department of Internal Medicine at the University of Illinois at Urbana–Champaign. His research interests include the effects of food processing on nutrient retention, the metabolic roles of lycopene and beta-carotene, and the bioavailability of minerals from foods. Dr. Erdman has published over 140 peer-reviewed research papers. He chaired the 1988 Gordon Conference on Carotenoids, and has served as a Burroughs Wellcome Visiting Professor in Basic Medical Sciences at the University of Georgia, and the G. Malcolm Trout Visiting Scholar at Michigan State University. His awards include the Borden Award from the American Society for Nutritional Sciences and the Babcock-Hart Award from the Institute of Food Technologists. Dr. Erdman has served on many editorial boards, and he has served as president of the American Society for Nutritional Sciences and on various committees of the Institute of Food Technologists and the National Academy of Sciences. He was elected a fellow of the Institute of Food Technologists and the American Heart Association. Dr Erdman was elected to the Institute of Medicine in 2003. Dr. Erdman received his M.S. and Ph.D. degrees in food science from Rutgers University.

**Emily M. Haymes,** Ph.D., is a professor in the Department of Nutrition, Food and Exercise Sciences at Florida State University. She received her B.A. degree from Drury College in 1961, her M.S. degree from Florida State University in 1962, and her Ph.D. degree from Pennsylvania State University in 1973. Prior to joining the faculty at Florida State in 1979, she taught at the University of Colorado at Boulder for five years. An exercise physiologist, her primary research interests are iron depletion in athletes, field measurements of physical activity and energy expenditure, and the response of males and females to exercise in warm and cold environments. She co-authored the book *The Environment and Human Performance* with Christine Wells. Dr. Haymes has published papers in several journals including the *Journal of Applied Physiology, Medicine and Science in Sports and Exercise, International Journal of Sports Medicine, International Journal of Sport Nutrition,* and *the Physician and Sportsmedicine.* Dr. Haymes served a three-year term as president of the Research Consortium and a two-year term as vice president of the American College of Sports Medicine. She is a Fellow of the American Academy of Kinesiology and Physical Education, American College of Sports Medicine, and the Research Consortium of the American Alliance for Health, Physical Education, Recreation, and Dance.

**Janet R. Hunt,** Ph.D., R.D., is the research leader of the Micronutrient Absorption and Metabolism Unit at the U.S. Department of Agriculture/Agricultural Research Service (USDA/ARS) Human Nutrition Research Center in Grand Forks, North Dakota, and is an adjunct professor of nutrition and dietetics at the University of North Dakota. Dr. Hunt received her Ph.D. degree in nutrition from the University of Minnesota. An active member of the American Society for Clinical Nutrition, the American Society for Nutritional Sciences, the International BioIron Society and the American Dietetic Association (ADA), she has served on the ADA board of directors and the ADA journal's editorial board, and has co-authored ADA's Position Statements on Vitamin and Mineral Supplements. Dr. Hunt investigates human iron and zinc requirements as influenced by dietary bioavailability, and has published extensively on these topics.

**Helen W. Lane,** Ph.D., R.D., is the Chief Nutritionist for the National Aeronautics and Space Administration, and Chief Scientist for the Johnson Space Center's Habitability, Environmental Factors, and Bioastronautics Office. She has served as the assistant to the director for Advanced Program Coordination and Research and branch chief for Biomedical Operations and Countermeasures. Dr. Lane was an associate professor of nutrition at the University of Texas Medical Center from 1977 to 1984, and a professor of nutrition at Auburn University from 1984 to 1989. At present, she serves as an adjunct professor, Department of Preventive Medicine and Community Health, at the University of Texas Medical Branch in Galveston. She has led efforts to define nutritional requirements for healthy crew members during spaceflight. Dr. Lane has completed research on body composition and on nutritional requirements for energy, water, electrolytes, protein, calcium, and iron, as well as clinical and basic research on selenium and breast cancer. As a registered dietitian, she is active in the American Dietetic Association (ADA). She is also a member of the American Society for Nutritional Sciences and the American Society for Clinical Nutrition.

**James G. Penland,** Ph.D., is a research psychologist and acting research leader of the Micronutrient Determinants of Health Unit at the USDA Grand Forks Human Nutrition Research Center, and adjunct professor of psychology at the University of North Dakota, where he received his doctoral degree in experimental cognitive psychology in 1984. Dr. Penland directs a comprehensive research program to study the effects of mineral nutrition (including copper, iron, magnesium, selenium, and zinc) on a broad range of human and animal neuropsychological function and behavior throughout the life span. During the past 20 years, Dr. Penland has conducted metabolic unit and community based feeding and supplementation studies, and designed and implemented a mobile nutrition laboratory for studies in schools, nursing homes, and rural communities. In addition to many research collaborations in the United States, Dr. Penland has participated in nutrition studies in Guatemala, New Zealand and the Peoples Republic of China. Dr. Penland has authored or co-authored nearly 100 scientific publications. Dr. Penland is a recipient of the USDA Honor Award for Excellence.

**Susan S. Percival,** Ph.D., is a professor in the Food Science and Human Nutrition Department at the University of Florida. Her research interests include: nutrition and immunity; effects of botanicals, phytochemicals, and trace elements on immune function; antioxidant bioavailability and impact on immunity; efficacy of dietary supplements in humans; and mechanistic studies in animal and cell culture models. Dr. Percival earned her B.S. degree in foods and nutrition from the University of Rhode Island in 1976, her M.S. degree in nutritional sciences in 1978 from the University of California–Davis, and her Ph.D. degree in biological sciences from the University of Texas–Austin in 1985.

**Connie M. Weaver,** Ph.D., is a distinguished professor and head of the Department of Foods & Nutrition at Purdue University. In 2000, she became the director of a National Institutes of Health funded Botanical Center to study dietary supplements containing polyphenolics for age-related diseases. Her research interests include mineral bioavailability, calcium metabolism, and bone health. She has published over 100 research articles. She was a member of the Institute of Medicine panel to develop new recommendations for requirements for calcium and related minerals. Dr. Weaver is past-president of American Society for Nutritional Sciences and is on the Board of Trustees of the International Life Sciences Institute. Dr. Weaver earned her B.S. (1972) and M.S. (1974) degrees in nutrition from Oregon State University, and her Ph.D. degree in nutrition (1978) from Florida State University. Dr. Weaver was a member of the 2005 U.S. Dietary Guidelines Advisory Committee.

## Institute of Medicine Staff

**Maria P. Oria,** Ph.D., is the study director for the Committee on Military Nutrition Research and its related committees. She is also the director of the Food Forum, an Institute of Medicine activity by which expert members from the various sectors dialogue about issues of concern in food and nutrition areas. She joined the Food and Nutrition Board (FNB) of the Institute of Medicine (IOM) in February 2002. Her work with the FNB has included serving as program officer for *Scientific Criteria to Ensure Safe Food* and as study director for *Infant Formula: Evaluating the Safety of New Ingredients*, and for *Monitoring Metabolic Status: Predicting Decrements in Physiological and Cognitive Performance.* Prior to joining the National Academies she was a staff scientist for the Institute of Food Technologists, coordinating projects on food safety and human nutrition under a contract with the Food and Drug Administration. She received her B.S. degree in biology from the University of Navarra (Spain), her M.S. degree in animal science from the University of Wyoming, and her Ph.D. degree in food science and nutrition from Purdue University. Her research interests include the cross-cutting areas between food production and food safety/quality and the impact of food production systems in the environment.

**Jon Q. Sanders,** B.A., is a senior program assistant with the Food and Nutrition Board of the Institute of Medicine. Since joining the National Academies in

2001, Mr. Sanders has worked on a variety of studies ranging from Everglades restoration to review of the WIC food packages. He is currently working on two FNB studies—the first is assessing the progress in childhood obesity prevention efforts at local, state, and national levels based on the recommendations of the IOM report *Preventing Childhood Obesity: Health in the Balance* (2005), and the second is a military nutrition study to asses the mineral requirements for cognitive and physical performance of military personnel. Mr. Sanders received his B.A. degree in anthropology from Trinity University, and is currently doing graduate work at Johns Hopkins University. He is a member of the Society for Applied Anthropology and the American Indian Science and Engineering Society. He is coauthor of *Sitting Down at the Table: Mediation and Resolution of Water Conflicts* (2001). Mr. Sanders' research interests include political ecology and environmental decision making.

**Leslie J. Sim,** B.S., is a research associate in the FNB at the IOM and also provides web support for all of the FNB activities. In 2003, she received recognition within the FNB as a recipient of an IOM inspirational staff award. Leslie has previously worked both as a teaching assistant and laboratory assistant for an undergraduate Food Science Laboratory class. She is currently working on two IOM studies—the first is directing a workshop on the impact of pregnancy weight on maternal and child health, and the second is a military nutrition study on mineral requirements for cognitive and physical performance of military personnel. Previously, she has worked on other military nutrition reports including: *Caffeine for the Sustainment of Mental Task Performance; High-Energy, Nutrient–Dense Emergency Relief Food Product; Weight Management: State of the Science and Opportunities for Military Programs; Monitoring Metabolic Status: Predicting Decrements in Physiological and Cognitive Performance; and Nutrient Composition of Rations for Short-Term, High-Intensity Combat Operations.* Leslie also provided research support for the IOM reports, *Infant Formula: Evaluating the Safety of New Ingredients; Dietary Reference Intakes: Applications in Dietary Planning; and Food Marketing to Children and Youth: Threat or Opportunity?* She received her B.S. degree in biology with an emphasis on food science from Virginia Tech University and took classes in food science at North Carolina State University.

# F

# Acronyms and Abbreviations

| | |
|---|---|
| ACE | Angiotensin converting enzyme |
| ADR | Adrenergic receptor |
| AI | Adequate Intake |
| $AI_{MGT}$ | Adequate Intake for military garrison training |
| Al | Aluminum |
| ALRI | Acute lower respiratory infection |
| AMDR | Acceptable macronutrient distribution range |
| APC | Antigen presenting cells |
| APP | Amyloid precursor protein |
| AR | Army regulation |
| ATP | Adenosine triphosphate |
| | |
| B | Boron |
| BCM | Body cell mass |
| BHMMR | Bone Health and Military Medical Readiness |
| BMC | Bone mineral content |
| BMD | Bone mass density |
| BMD | Bone mineral density |
| | |
| C | Celsius |
| Ca | Calcium |
| $CaCO_3$ | Calcium carbonate |
| cal | Calorie |
| CBC | Complete blood count |

| | |
|---|---|
| CCK | Cholecystokinin |
| CCS | Copper chaperone for Cu/Zn superoxide dismutase |
| CDC | U.S. Centers for Disease Control and Prevention |
| CESD | Center for Epidemiological Studies Depression |
| $(CH_3)_3Se+$ | Trimethylslenonium |
| $CH_3SeCH_3$ | Dimethylselenide |
| $CH_3SeH$ | Methylselenol |
| CI | Confidence interval |
| CID | Cold-induced diuresis |
| CK | Creatine kinase |
| Cl | Chlorine |
| CMNR | Committee on Military Nutrition Research |
| ConA | Concanavalin A |
| Cp | Ceruloplasmin |
| Cr | Chromium |
| CRP | Combat ration pack |
| Cu | Copper |
| CuZnSOD | Copper/Zinc superoxide dismutase |
| CVB3 | Coxsackievirus B3 |
| DA | Dopamine |
| DASH diet | Dietary Approaches to Stop Hypertension diet |
| DCT | Divalent cation transporter |
| DFE | Dietary folate equivalent |
| DHHS | U.S. Department of Health and Human Services |
| DI | Deiodinase |
| dL | Deciliter |
| DMT | Divalent metal transporters |
| DoD | Department of Defense |
| DPD | Dioxypyridinoline |
| DRI | Dietary Reference Intake |
| DSM IV | Diagnosis and Statistical Manual IV |
| DV | Daily value |
| DWHRP | Defense Women's Health Research Program |
| DXA | Dual energy x-ray absorptiometers |
| EAR | Estimated Average Requirement |
| $EAR_{MGT}$ | Estimated Average Requirement for military garrison training |
| EDI | Eating Disorders Inventory |
| EEG | Electroencephalogram |
| ELISA | Enzyme-linked immunosorbent assay |

| | |
|---|---|
| EPA | U.S. Environmental Protection Agency |
| EPDS | Edinburgh Postnatal Depression Scale |
| | |
| F | Fahrenheit |
| F | Fluorine |
| FAO | Food and Agriculture Organization |
| FDA | Food and Drug Administration |
| Fe | Iron |
| FEP | Free erythrocyte protoporphyrin |
| FEV | Forced expiratory volume |
| FGF | Fibroblast growth factor |
| fL | Femtoliters |
| FNB | Food and Nutrition Board |
| FOS | Food Operations Sergeants |
| FSR | First Strike Ration |
| ft | Foot |
| | |
| g | Gram |
| GABA | $\gamma$-aminobutyric acid |
| GHQ | General Health Questionnaire |
| Gpx | Glutathione peroxidase |
| GHS-Px | Glutathione peroxidase |
| GSSeH | Glutathioneselenol |
| GSSeSG | Selenodiglutathione |
| | |
| h | Hour |
| Hb | Hemoglobin |
| HCl | Hydrochloric acid |
| Hct | Hematocrit |
| hCtr1 | Hepatocyte copper transport protein one |
| HDL | High-density lipoprotein |
| HFE | Hemochromatosis gene product |
| HIV/AIDS | Human Immunodeficiency Virus/Acquired Immunodeficiency Syndrome |
| HOX1 | Heme oxygenase |
| HP2000 | Healthy People 2000 program |
| HPA | Hypothalmus-pituitary-adrenocortical |
| HR | Heart rate |
| $H_2Se$ | Hydrogen selenide |
| Hz | Hertz |

| | |
|---|---|
| I | Iodine |
| ID | Iron deficiency |
| IDA | Iron deficiency anemia |
| IDNA | Iron deficient, non-anemic state |
| IFN | Interferon |
| Ig | Immunoglobulin |
| IGF | Insulin-like growth factor |
| IL | Interleukin |
| IOM | Institute of Medicine |
| IRE | Iron responsive molecule |
| IU | International units |
| IUNS | International Union of Nutrition Scientists |
| IZiNCG | International Zinc Nutrition Consultative Group |
| | |
| K | Potassium |
| kcal | Kilocalorie |
| kg | Kilogram |
| kJ | Kilojoules |
| KLH | Keyhole limpet hemocyanin |
| km | Kilometer |
| | |
| lb | Pound |
| LDL | Low-density lipoprotein |
| L-DOPA | L-3,4-dihydroxyphenylalanine |
| LH | Luteinized hormone |
| LR | Learning task |
| | |
| mA | Milliamps |
| MCH | Mean corpuscular hemoglobin |
| MCHC | Mean corpuscular hemoglobin concentration |
| MCP | Monocyte chemoattractant protein |
| MCV | Mean corpuscular volume |
| MDQ | Menstrual Distress Questionnaire |
| MDRI | Military dietary reference intake |
| Mg | Magnesium |
| mg | Milligram |
| MGT | Military garrison training |
| MHC | Major Histocompatibility Complex |
| MIP | Macrophage inflammatory protein |
| MJ | Megajoule |
| mM | Millimolar |
| mmol | Millimole |
| MMP | Matrix metalloproteinases |

| | |
|---|---|
| MMPI | Minnesota Multiphasic Personality Inventory Test |
| Mn | Manganese |
| Mo | Molybdenum |
| MP | Metabolic period |
| mph | Mile per hour |
| MRDA | Military recommended dietary allowances |
| MRE | Meal, Ready-to-Eat |
| mRNA | Messenger ribonucleic acid |
| MT | Metallothionein |
| MVC | Maximal voluntary static contraction |
| | |
| Na | Sodium |
| NaCl | Sodium chloride |
| NAS | National Academy of Sciences |
| NE | Norepinephrine |
| NF | Nuclear factor |
| NHANES | National Health and Nutrition Examination Survey |
| Ni | Nickel |
| NMDA | N-methyl-D-aspartate |
| nmol | Nanomol |
| NOAEL | No adverse effect level |
| NPY | Neuropeptide Y |
| NRC | National Research Council |
| NSC | Natick Soldier Center |
| NSOR | Nutritional Standards for Operational Rations |
| | |
| O | Oxygen |
| OC | Oral contraceptive |
| OR | Odds ratio |
| ORS | Oral rehydration solution |
| OTC | Officer Training Corps |
| | |
| P | Phosphorus |
| PAM | Peptidylglycine alpha-amidating monooxygenase |
| PBMC | Peripheral blood mononuclear cells |
| pH | Potential of hydrogen |
| PHA | Phytohaemagglutinin |
| PM | Progressive Matrices Task |
| PMS | Premenstrual syndrome |
| POMS | Profile of Mood States |
| POMS-BI | Profile of Mood States–BiPolar Form |
| ppm | Parts per million |
| pQCT | Peripheral quantitative computed tomography |

| | |
|---|---|
| PR | Probed recall task |
| PTH | Parathyroid hormone |
| PWM | Pokeweed mitogen |
| | |
| QCT | Quantitative computed tomography |
| | |
| RBC | Red blood cell |
| RC | Recognition memory task |
| RDA | Recommended Dietary Allowance |
| $RDA_{MGT}$ | Recommended Dietary Allowance for military garrison training |
| RDW | Red cell distribution width |
| RLS | Restless Legs Syndrome |
| RNA | Ribonucleic acid |
| RNS | Reactive nitrogen species |
| ROS | Reactive oxygen species |
| RPMI | Ravens Progressive Matrices Index |
| RR | Relative risk |
| RT | Reaction time task |
| | |
| S | Sulphur |
| SD | Standard deviation |
| SD | Stimulus discrimination task |
| Se | Selenium |
| SEAL | U.S. Navy's Sea, Air and Land Special Forces |
| SeCys | Selenocysteine |
| SEM | Standard error of the mean |
| SeMet | Selenomethionine |
| $SeO_2$ | Selenium dioxide |
| SeP | Selenium protein |
| sFt | Serum ferritin |
| Si | Silicon |
| SNS | Sympathetic nervous system |
| SOD | Superoxide dismutase |
| SSS | Stanford Sleepiness Scale |
| ST | Sternberg Memory Search Task |
| STAI | State-Trait Anxiety Inventory |
| STAS | State-Trait Anger Scale |
| sTfR | Serum transferrin receptor |
| | |
| TfR | Transferrin Receptor |
| TfRIX | Transferrin receptor index |
| TfSat | Transferrin saturation |

| | |
|---|---|
| Tgf | Transforming growth factor |
| Th | T helper type cell |
| TIBC | Total iron binding capacity |
| TNF | Tumor necrosis factor |
| TPN | Total parenteral nutrition |
| TR | Thioredoxine reductase |
| tRNA | Transfer ribonucleic acid |
| TT | Tachistoscopic Threshold Task |
| | |
| μg | Microgram |
| μM | MicroMolar |
| UL | Tolerable Upper Intake Level |
| UHT | Ultra high temperature |
| USUHS | Uniformed Services University of Health Sciences |
| U.S. | United States |
| USARIEM | U.S. Army Research Institute of Environmental Medicine |
| USARMRMC | U.S. Army Medical Research and Materiel Command |
| USDA | U.S. Department of Agriculture |
| USDA-ARS | U.S. Department of Agriculture Agricultural Research Service |
| USMA | United States Military Academy |
| USP | United States Pharmacopoeia |
| | |
| VCLD | Very low calorie diet |
| Ve | Ventilatory volume |
| $VO_2$max or peak | Maximum oxygen consumption |
| VOC | Volatile organic compounds |
| | |
| WE | Work efficiency |
| WHO | World Health Organization |
| wk | Week |
| | |
| ZIP proteins | Zrt/IRT-like proteins |
| Zn | Zinc |
| ZnT | Zn transporter |

# G

# Glossary

| | |
|---|---|
| Acceptable Macronutrient Distribution Range | A range of intakes (represented as percent of energy intake) for a particular energy source that is associated with reduced risk of chronic disease while providing adequate intakes of essential nutrients. |
| Adequate Intake, AI | The recommended average daily intake level based on observed or experimentally determined approximations or estimates of nutrient intake by a group (or groups) of apparently healthy people that are assumed to be adequate—used when an RDA cannot be determined (IOM, 2004). |
| basal metabolic rate | The rate at which energy is used by the body to maintain basal metabolism when a person is awake but inactive and has fasted for 14 to 18 hours. The BMR typically accounts for 60 to 70 percent of daily energy use, but its value depends on body weight and other factors. |
| body mass index | A key index for relating a person's body weight to their height. The body mass index is a person's weight in kilograms (kg) divided by their height in meters (m) squared and is associated with body fat and health risk. |

| | |
|---|---|
| Chvostek sign | Tap over the facial nerve about 2 cm anterior to the tragus of the ear. Depending on the calcium level, a graded response will occur: twitching first at the angle of the mouth, then by the nose, the eye, and the facial muscles. |
| delayed type skin hypersensitivity | Test used as an indicator of the immune system function and that shows skin tissue injury due to phagocytic cell activation and inflammation induced by cell-mediated immunity. In experimental animal models, the injury is characterized by a granulomatous response consisting of macrophages, monocytes, and T lymphocytes. |
| Dietary Reference Intake | Quantitative estimates of nutrient intakes that can be used for planning and assessing diets for apparently healthy people. |
| Estimated Average Requirement | The average daily nutrient intake level estimated to meet the requirement of half the healthy individuals in a particular life stage and gender group (IOM, 2004). |
| garrison feeding | Food consumption by military personnel who are under a variety of scenarios that range from administrative duties to support tasks performed by personnel to soldiers training for or performing missions while living on a military base. |
| generally recognized as safe | Status of a food ingredient based on common knowledge about the safety of the ingredient through the scientific community that is knowledgeable in food toxicology and related disciplines specific to the safety and intended use of the ingredient under consideration. |
| military dietary reference intake | Nutritional standards, based on the Food and Nutrition Board's Dietary Reference Intakes, and intended for use by professional personnel involved in menu development, menu evaluation, nutrition education, nutrition research, and food research and development. |

| | |
|---|---|
| niacin equivalent | Because, 60 mg of the amino acid tryptophan is equivalent to 1 mg of preformed dietary niacin, niacin equivalents are estimated by adding preformed niacin intake plus 1/60th of tryptophan intake. |
| operational feeding | Consumption of either full- or restricted-calorie rations while engaged in military operations or training. |
| Profile of Mood States | A 65-item, adjective rating subjective scale that measures moods and was used in the National Hospice Study and The Study to Understand Prognoses and Preferences for Outcomes, and Risks of Treatments. |
| Recommended Dietary Allowance | The average daily dietary nutrient intake level sufficient to meet the nutrient requirement of nearly all (97 to 98 percent) healthy individuals in a particular life stage and gender group (IOM, 2004). |
| retinol equivalent | The specific biological activity of 1.0 microgram of all-trans retinol, 6.0 micrograms of b-carotene, or 12.0 micrograms of other provitamin A carotenoids; it is equivalent to 3.3 international units of vitamin A activity from retinol (10 from b-carotene). |
| Tolerable Upper Intake Level | The highest average daily nutrient intake level that is likely to pose no risk of adverse health effects to almost all individuals in the general population. As intake increases above the UL, the potential risk of adverse effects may increase (IOM, 2004). |
| Trousseau sign | Inflation of a blood pressure cuff above the systolic pressure causes local ulnar and median nerve ischemia, resulting in carpal spasm. |
| $VO_2max$ | The maximum amount (usually expressed as a volume, liter) of oxygen that an individual can consume in a defined period of time (usually 1 |

minute). It may be expressed per kilogram of body weight (ml/kg/min). It reflects the upper limit of aerobic metabolism and limited by the amount of oxygen that can be delivered into the working muscle cells. Basically a product of the maximal cardiac output and maximal arterial-venous oxygen difference at the capillary-cell interface.

## REFERENCE

IOM (Institute of Medicine). 2004. *Dietary Reference Intakes: Water, Potassium, Sodium, Chloride, and Sulfate*. Washington, DC: The National Academies Press.